Bacteria and Intracellularity

Bacteria and Intracellularity

EDITED BY

Pascale Cossart
Institut Pasteur, Paris, France

Craig R. Roy
Yale University School of Medicine, New Haven, Connecticut

Philippe Sansonetti
Institut Pasteur, Paris, France

ASM PRESS
Washington, DC

WILEY

Editorial Correspondence:
ASM Press, 1752 N Street, NW, Washington, DC 20036-2904, USA

Registered Offices:
John Wiley & Sons, Inc., 111 River Street, Hoboken, NJ 07030, USA

For details of our global editorial offices, customer services, and more information about Wiley products, visit us at www.wiley.com.

Wiley also publishes its books in a variety of electronic formats and by print-on-demand. Some content that appears in standard print versions of this book may not be available in other formats.

Library of Congress Cataloging-in-Publication Data

Names: Cossart, Pascale, editor. | Roy, Craig R., editor. | Sansonetti, P. J., editor.
Title: Bacteria and intracellularity / editors, Pascale Cossart, Institut Pasteur, Paris, France, Craig R. Roy, Yale University School of Medicine, New Haven, Connecticut, Philippe Sansonetti, Institut Pasteur, Paris, France.
Description: Hoboken : Wiley; Washington DC: American Society for Microbiology [2020] | Includes bibliographical references and index. | Description based on print version record and CIP data provided by publisher; resource not viewed.
Identifiers: LCCN 2019040621 (print) | LCCN 2019040622 (ebook) | ISBN 9781683670261 (adobe pdf) | ISBN 9781683670254 (hardback) | ISBN 9781683670254 (hardback) | ISBN 9781683670261 (adobe pdf)
Subjects: LCSH: Bacteria–Physiology. | Cell interaction.
Classification: LCC QR96.5 (ebook) | LCC QR96.5 .B325 2020 (print) | DDC 571.6/38293–dc23
LC record available at https://lccn.loc.gov/2019040621

Cover: Recapitulating the developing peripheral nervous system in a dish for studying *Mycobacterium leprae* interaction with Schwann cells in an *in vivo*-like microenvironment. Outgrowth of axons and migrating Schwann cells from embryonic mouse dorsal root ganglion. E14 mouse DRG neurites were labeled with neurofilament antibody (green) and Schwann cell nuclei were labeled with Hoechst dye (blue). Image taken on a Zeiss LSM 710 confocal microscope with 20× objective. Courtesy of Samuel Hess and Anura Rambukkana.

Cover design by Debra Naylor, Naylor Design, Inc.

Printed in the United States of America

V10015678_112019

Contents

I. CELLULAR MICROBIOLOGY IN THE STUDY OF TISSUE AND ORGAN INFECTIONS

v

II. SUBCELLULAR MICROBIOLOGY

III. AUTONOMOUS DEFENSE PATHWAYS IN THE CELL

IV. NEW TECHNOLOGIES TO MOVE CELLULAR MICROBIOLOGY TO ORGANS AND TISSUES

Contributors

CARMEN AGUILAR
Host RNA Metabolism Group, Institute for Molecular Infection Biology (IMIB),
University of Würzburg, Würzburg, Germany

LAURENCE ARBIBE
INSERM U1151, CNRS UMR 8253, Institut Necker Enfants Malades,
INEM Institute Department of Immunology, Infectiology and Hematology,
Paris, France

STEPHEN BAKER
Department of Medicine, University of Cambridge, Cambridge,
United Kingdom, and Oxford University Clinical Research Unit (OUCRU),
The Hospital for Tropical Diseases, Ho Chi Minh City, Vietnam

JOSEFIN BARTHOLDSON SCOTT
Department of Medicine, University of Cambridge, Addenbrooke's Hospital,
Hills Road, Cambridge, United Kingdom

PETR BROZ
Department of Biochemistry, University of Lausanne, Switzerland

DIRK BUMANN
Focal Area Infection Biology, Biozentrum, University of Basel, Basel, Switzerland

ROSALYN CASEY
Department of Microbial Sciences, School of Biosciences and Medicine,
University of Surrey, Guilford, Surrey, United Kingdom

JEAN CELLI
Paul G. Allen School for Global Animal Health, Washington State University,
Pullman, Washington

SIMON CLARE
Wellcome Sanger Institute, Wellcome Genome Campus, Hinxton, Cambridge,
United Kingdom

MICHAEL CONNOR
Institut Pasteur, G5 Chromatine et Infection, Paris, France

PASCALE COSSART
Institut Pasteur, Unité des Interactions Bactéries-Cellules (UIBC);
Institut National de la Santé et de la Recherche Médicale (INSERM), U604; and
Institut National de la Recherche Agronomique (INRA), USC2020, Paris, France

JAMES P. DI SANTO
Innate Immunity Unit, Immunology Department, Institut Pasteur,
and INSERM U1223, Paris, France

GORDON DOUGAN
Department of Medicine, University of Cambridge, Addenbrooke's Hospital,
Cambridge, United Kingdom

GUILLAUME DUMÉNIL
Pathogenesis of Vascular Infections, Institut Pasteur, INSERM, Paris, France

JOST ENNINGA
Institut Pasteur, Dynamics of Host-Pathogen Interactions Unit, Cell Biology
and Infection Department, Paris, France

ANA EULALIO
Host RNA Metabolism Group, Institute for Molecular Infection Biology (IMIB),
University of Würzburg, Würzburg, Germany, and RNA & Infection Group,
Center for Neuroscience and Cell Biology (CNC), University of Coimbra,
Coimbra, Portugal

ALYSSA C. FASCIANO
Department of Molecular Biology and Microbiology and Program in
Immunology, Sackler School of Biomedical Sciences, Tufts University School
of Medicine, Boston, Massachusetts

CELIA W. GOULDING
Department of Molecular Biology & Biochemistry and Department of
Pharmaceutical Sciences, University of California Irvine, Irvine, California

CHRISTINE HALE
Wellcome Sanger Institute, Wellcome Genome Campus, Hinxton, Cambridge,
United Kingdom

MELANIE HAMON
Institut Pasteur, G5 Chromatine et Infection, Paris, France

WOLF-DIETRICH HARDT
Institute of Microbiology, D-BIOL ETH Zurich, Zurich, Switzerland

ANNIKA HAUSMANN
Institute of Microbiology, D-BIOL ETH Zurich, Zurich, Switzerland

SAMUEL HESS
MRC Centre for Regenerative Medicine, University of Edinburgh, Edinburgh,
United Kingdom

SUZIE HINGLEY-WILSON
Department of Microbial Sciences, School of Biosciences and Medicine,
University of Surrey, Guilford, Surrey, United Kingdom

LU HUANG
Microbiology and Immunology, College of Veterinary Medicine,
Cornell University, Ithaca, New York

SCOTT J. HULTGREN
Department of Molecular Microbiology and Center for Women's Infectious
Disease Research (CWIDR), Washington University School of Medicine,
St. Louis, Missouri

RALPH R. ISBERG
Department of Molecular Biology and Microbiology, Tufts University School of
Medicine, Boston, Massachusetts

WILLIAM R. JACOBS, JR.
Department of Microbiology and Immunology, Albert Einstein College of
Medicine, Bronx, New York

JONATHAN C. KAGAN
Harvard Medical School and Division of Gastroenterology, Boston Children's
Hospital, Boston, Massachusetts

FRÉDÉRIC LANDMANN
CRBM, University of Montpellier, CNRS, Montpellier, France

YAN LI
Innate Immunity Unit, Immunology Department, Institut Pasteur, and INSERM
U1223, Paris, France

MIGUEL MANO
Functional Genomics and RNA-based Therapeutics Group, Center for
Neuroscience and Cell Biology (CNC), University of Coimbra, Coimbra,
Portugal

JOAN MECSAS
Department of Molecular Biology and Microbiology, Tufts University School of
Medicine, Boston, Massachusetts

KEIRA MELICAN
Swedish Medical Nanoscience Center, Karolinska Institutet, Stockholm, Sweden

THOMAS F. MEYER
Max Planck Institute for Infection Biology, Department of Molecular Biology,
Berlin, Germany

EVGENIYA V. NAZAROVA
Microbiology and Immunology, College of Veterinary Medicine,
Cornell University, Ithaca, New York

DORIAN OBINO
Pathogenesis of Vascular Infections, Institut Pasteur, INSERM, Paris, France

CHARLOTTE ODENDALL
Kings College, Department of Infectious Diseases, Guy's Hospital, London,
United Kingdom

NATALIE S. OMATTAGE
Department of Molecular Microbiology, Washington University School of
Medicine, St. Louis, Missouri

TITILAYO O. OMOTADE
Department of Microbial Pathogenesis, Yale University, New Haven,
Connecticut

KIM ORTH
Department of Molecular Biology, Department of Biochemistry, and Howard
Hughes Medical Institute, University of Texas Southwestern Medical Center,
Dallas, Texas

SOPHIE PALMER
Department of Medicine, University of Cambridge, Addenbrooke's Hospital,
Hills Road, Cambridge, United Kingdom

ANURA RAMBUKKANA
MRC Centre for Regenerative Medicine and Centre for Edinburgh Infectious
Diseases, University of Edinburgh, Edinburgh, United Kingdom

AGNETA RICHTER-DAHLFORS
Swedish Medical Nanoscience Center, Karolinska Institutet, Stockholm, Sweden

MARION ROTHER
Steinbeis Innovation, Berlin-Falkensee; Institute of Experimental Internal
Medicine, Otto von Guericke University Magdeburg, Magdeburg; and Max
Planck Institute for Infection Biology, Berlin, Germany

CRAIG R. ROY
Section of Microbial Pathogenesis, Yale University School of Medicine,
New Haven, Connecticut

THOMAS RUDEL
Department of Microbiology, Biocenter, University of Wuerzburg, Wuerzburg,
Germany

DAVID G. RUSSELL
Microbiology and Immunology, College of Veterinary Medicine,
Cornell University, Ithaca, New York

PHILIPPE J. SANSONETTI
Institut Pasteur, Unité de Pathogénie Microbienne Moléculaire, INSERM U1202,
and College de France, Paris, France

MARCELA DE SOUZA SANTOS
Department of Molecular Biology, University of Texas Southwestern Medical Center, Dallas, Texas

PAMELA SCHNUPF
Institut Imagine, Laboratory of Intestinal Immunity, INSERM UMR1163; Institut Necker Enfants Malade, Laboratory of Host-Microbiota Interaction, INSERM U1151; and Université Paris Descartes-Sorbonne, Paris, France

CAITLIN N. SPAULDING
Harvard University, School of Public Health, Boston, Massachusetts

ANNA SPIER
Institut Pasteur, UIBC; INSERM, U604; INRA, USC2020; and Bio Sorbonne Paris Cité, Université Paris Diderot, Paris, France

FABRIZIA STAVRU
Institut Pasteur, UIBC; INSERM, U604; INRA, USC2020; and CNRS, SNC 5101, Paris, France

VIRGINIE STÉVENIN
Institut Pasteur, Dynamics of Host-Pathogen Interactions Unit, Cell Biology and Infection Department, Paris, France

AGATHE SUBTIL
Institut Pasteur, Cell Biology of Microbial Infection, Paris, France

KEVIN O. TAMADONFAR
Department of Molecular Microbiology, Washington University School of Medicine, St. Louis, Missouri

ANA RITA TEIXEIRA DA COSTA
Max Planck Institute for Infection Biology, Department of Molecular Biology, Berlin, Germany

SANGEETA TIWARI
Department of Microbiology and Immunology, Albert Einstein College of Medicine, Bronx, New York

SÉBASTIEN TRIBOULET
Institut Pasteur, Cell Biology of Microbial Infection, Paris, France

AMY YEUNG
Wellcome Sanger Institute, Wellcome Genome Campus, Hinxton, Cambridge, United Kingdom

RIKE ZIETLOW
Max Planck Institute for Infection Biology, Department of Molecular Biology, Berlin, Germany

Preface

We wish to dedicate this book to Stanley Falkow, who has impressed and influenced so many of us. Dr. Falkow launched the molecular study of host-bacterial pathogen interactions in the late 1970s, capitalizing on his knowledge of plasmids, antibiotic resistance, and molecular biology, before including cell biology, anticipating what came to be called cellular microbiology. Since then, nearly four decades of intense work on a variety of pathogens has highlighted common concepts in intracellularity but also very diverse mechanisms underlying the various infections produced by bacteria.

In launching this book, we wanted to cover many aspects and mechanisms of cellular microbiology, but more importantly, we intended to show that cellular microbiology as a field has reached maturity, extending beyond the strictly cellular level to infections of various organs and tissues. Many model organisms (*Yersinia*, *Salmonella*, *Shigella*, and *Listeria*, among others) are foodborne pathogens, and tremendous progress has been achieved in deciphering how, when, and where bacteria interact with the gut. However, intestinal cells and the intestine are not the only cells and organs discussed in this book. There are also chapters on infections of the urogenital tract, the endothelial barriers, the nervous system, and the lungs. Progress in the latter two concern important public health infections produced by *Mycobacterium leprae* and *Mycobacterium tuberculosis*. These two bacteria, which were at first much more difficult to manipulate than *Escherichia coli*, are now genetically tractable, and their study can now benefit from all the techniques and approaches established with less fastidious bacteria.

To be complete, a book on intracellularity had to include subcellular microbiology, and several chapters cover a variety of topics including metabolism of infected cells, nuclear biology, and microRNAs in host-pathogen interactions. All facets of cellular physiology are targeted by pathogens, and their role in infection is now actively assessed.

A book dedicated to "bacterial intracellularity" had to also include endosymbionts and, in particular, *Wolbachia* and its intriguing biology, which influences the capacity of the insects (in particular, mosquitoes) that carry this organism to transmit important viral pathogens such as dengue, Zika, and chikungunya viruses. This chapter is particularly timely, as a large official release of mosquitoes carrying *Wolbachia* has just been completed in New Caledonia to limit virus transmission by decreasing the global competence of this vector system.

The cellular microbiology field started in the late 1980s with a particular focus on cytoskeletal structures and organelles targeted by intracellular pathogens, but studies rapidly spread to analyze the cell autonomous defense pathways. We are happy to have two important chapters reviewing a field of research that has led to many new concepts in immunology and, more specifically, in innate immunity.

Finally, techniques and technologies are constantly improving: four chapters dealing with imaging, "omics" systems biology, and mouse humanization highlight the rapid progress in developing techniques that are now or will soon be used in the next steps of the study of intracellularity.

We thank the many colleagues who agreed to write for us. We are particularly happy to have gathered so many great chapters written by internationally recognized experts. We are well aware that studying pathogens without taking into account the microorganisms and microbial assemblies that are present in their vicinity may appear somewhat reductionist. This was a considered decision, and we believe a discussion of bacterial pathogenesis in the framework of microbiotas and microbiomes should be the topic of another book.

We thank Ellie Tupper and Richard Sever for their enthusiasm and patience during what at some stages seemed an endless project!

Pascale Cossart
Craig R. Roy
Philippe Sansonetti

About the Editors

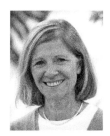

Pascale Cossart earned her masters degree at Georgetown University, Washington, DC. She then received her Ph.D. in Paris at the Institut Pasteur, where she now leads the Bacteria-Cell Interactions unit. After early studies in DNA-protein interactions, in 1986 she began investigating the molecular and cellular basis of infections by intracellular bacteria, taking as a model the bacterium *Listeria monocytogenes*. Her research has led to new concepts in infection biology as well as in cell biology and fundamental microbiology, including RNA-mediated regulation. Dr. Cossart is considered a pioneer in cellular microbiology. Her contributions have been recognized by several international awards and election to several academies including the National Academy of Sciences (2009) and the National Academy of Medicine (2014). In January 2016, she was named Secrétaire Perpétuel de l'Académie des Sciences, Paris.

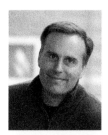

Craig R. Roy trained in the laboratory of Stanley Falkow at Stanford University, where his Ph.D. dissertation focused on the molecular mechanisms governing virulence in *Bordetella pertussis*. As a postdoctoral fellow in the laboratory of Ralph Isberg at Tufts University, he used cell biology to investigate *Legionella pneumophila* infection of macrophages. After a stint as assistant professor of Microbiology and Molecular Genetics at Stony Brook University, Dr. Roy helped found the new Department of Microbial Pathogenesis at Yale University in 1998. He is currently Waldemar Von Zedtwitz Professor of Microbial Pathogenesis and Immunobiology. Using multidisciplinary approaches, his laboratory has elucidated the mechanisms employed by intracellular pathogens to modulate vesicular transport and the host immune response against pathogens that reside in specialized organelles.

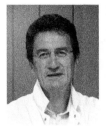 **Philippe Sansonetti** is professor and head of the Unité de Pathogénie Microbienne Moléculaire at the Pasteur Institute of Paris and chair of Microbiology and Infectious Diseases at the Collège de France. Professor Sansonetti qualified in medicine at the University of Paris in 1979. Following clinical work in France, he established his research career at Institut Pasteur in cellular microbiology and the pathogenesis of enteric infections, particularly *Shigella*, including vaccine development, and more recently the molecular cross-talks between microbiota and the gut epithelium. He is the recipient of numerous honors and awards including the Louis Jeantet Prize and a Howard Hughes Medical Institute Scholarship. He was awarded two successive ERC grants. He is currently Chief Editor of *EMBO Molecular Medicine* and a member of the French Academy of Science, the National Academy of Sciences (U.S.), and the Royal Society (UK).

Cellular Microbiology in the Study of Tissue and Organ Infections

I

Bacteria and Intracellularity
Edited by Pascale Cossart, Craig R. Roy, and Philippe Sansonetti
© 2019 American Society for Microbiology, Washington, DC
doi:10.1128/microbiolspec.BAI-0016-2019

Interaction between Intracellular Bacterial Pathogens and Host Cell Mitochondria

1

Anna Spier,[1,2,3,4] Fabrizia Stavru,[1,2,3,5] and Pascale Cossart[1,2,3]

INTRODUCTION

Mitochondria are dynamic organelles, which are fundamental to eukaryotic cell function. They originated from an endosymbiotic alphaproteobacterium of the genus *Rickettsia*, which was internalized by the ancestor of all eukaryotes (1). Consistent with this endosymbiotic event, mitochondria are surrounded by a double membrane and still share molecular and morphological features with prokaryotic cells, such as the ability to create energy in the form of ATP through aerobic respiration. To do so, mitochondria oxidize nutrients in a process termed oxidative phosphorylation, which involves the creation and harnessing of a membrane potential across the inner mitochondrial membrane, resulting in ATP synthesis.

Apart from energy production, mitochondria carry out essential steps of heme, iron-sulfur cluster, and amino acid biosynthesis as well as fatty acid oxidation and play an important role in calcium homeostasis and cell-autonomous innate immunity (2). In this context, mitochondria display antimicrobial activity through reactive oxygen species (ROS) production and through signaling. Mitochondrial innate immune signaling is mediated by the mitochondrial antiviral signaling protein (MAVS) and results in an interferon response (2, 3). Importantly, mitochondria also play a key role in apoptosis, as the intrinsic apoptosis pathway converges on mitochondrial outer membrane permeabilization (MOMP), which represents a point of no return. Mitochondrion-mediated apoptosis is highly regulated by members of the B cell lymphoma 2 (Bcl-2) protein family; proapoptotic BH3-only proteins are activated by intracellular stress signals, overcome the inhibitory effect of antiapoptotic Bcl-2 proteins, and enhance recruitment of Bcl2-associated X protein (Bax) and Bcl-2 antagonist or killer (Bak) to the mitochondrial outer membrane. There, Bax and Bak oligomerization results in MOMP and allows the release of cytochrome *c*, second mitochondrion-derived activator of caspases (SMAC), and Omi, promoting caspase activation and apoptosis (4).

Along with innate immune signaling and apoptosis, the highly dynamic morphology of mitochondria is one of the characteristics of the organelle that clearly differentiate it from most bacteria. Mitochondrial morphology is determined by a steady-state balance between the opposing events of fusion and fission, which are mediated by a set of dynamin-related GTPases. Mitofusin 1 (Mfn1) and mitofusin 2 (Mfn2) coordinate outer membrane fusion by homo- and heterotypic interactions, while optic atrophy 1 (Opa1) mediates fusion of the inner membrane. The current model for mitochondrial fission involves initial mitochondrial constriction through the endoplasmic reticulum (ER) and actin, followed by recruitment of dynamin-related protein 1 (Drp1) to its receptors on the mitochondrial outer membrane. There, Drp1 oligomerizes to form ring-like structures and mediates GTP-dependent mitochondrial fission in conjunction with dynamin 2 (5). Interestingly, Drp1-dependent mitochondrial fission is observed during apoptosis but is not strictly required for its progression (4). Depending on the cell type and functional status of mitochondria, they can adapt their morphology according to cellular energy demands (6) and move along cytoskeletal tracks with the help of molecular motors (7).

[1]Institut Pasteur, Unité des Interactions Bactéries-Cellules, Paris, France; [2]Institut National de la Santé et de la Recherche Médicale, U604, Paris, France; [3]Institut National de la Recherche Agronomique, USC2020, Paris, France; [4]Bio Sorbonne Paris Cité, Université Paris Diderot, Paris, France; [5]Centre National de la Recherche Scientifique, SNC 5101, France.

Owing to their central role in multiple cellular processes, mitochondria are an attractive target for pathogens. Modulation of mitochondrial functions can be advantageous for bacteria in terms of access to nutrients and/or evasion of the humoral immune system. Here, we explore the relationship between intracellular bacteria and host cell mitochondria, primarily focusing on the effect of the bacteria on mitochondrial morphology and manipulation of host cell death. Manipulation of cell death allows the bacteria to either preserve their intracellular niche by enhancing survival of the host cell or favor dissemination by inducing host cell death. We present examples of both cytosolic and intravacuolar pathogenic bacteria, including *Listeria monocytogenes*, *Shigella flexneri*, *Rickettsia* spp., *Legionella pneumophila*, *Mycobacterium tuberculosis*, *Salmonella enterica*, *Chlamydia* spp., and *Ehrlichia chaffeensis*. While cytosolic bacteria are able to directly interact with mitochondria and other organelles, intravacuolar pathogens are confined within a membrane-enclosed vacuole and employ specialized secretion systems to introduce effector proteins into the host cell cytoplasm that target mitochondria.

CYTOSOLIC BACTERIA

Listeria monocytogenes

The Gram-positive bacterium *L. monocytogenes* is a facultative intracellular pathogen causing the foodborne disease listeriosis, which mainly and most severely affects immunocompromised individuals. *L. monocytogenes* is capable of invading both phagocytic and nonphagocytic cells and employs the phospholipases PlcA and PlcB and the pore-forming toxin listeriolysin O (LLO) to escape the phagosome (8). Inside the cytosol, *L. monocytogenes* replicates and hijacks the host actin polymerization machinery in order to spread nonlytically to neighboring cells (9). Infection of epithelial cells with *L. monocytogenes* interferes with mitochondrial dynamics and induces a strong and rapid but transient fragmentation of the mitochondrial network at early time points of infection. The fragmentation is specific to virulent *L. monocytogenes*, and the secreted toxin LLO has been identified as the causative factor, but the exact mechanism remains to be elucidated. LLO appears not to localize to mitochondria, but rather oligomerizes and forms pores in the plasma membrane, causing a calcium influx, which is crucial for the induction of mitochondrial fission (10) (Fig. 1). Moreover, the *L. monocytogenes*-induced mitochondrial fragmentation is atypical, as it is independent of Opa1 and Drp1. Indeed, Drp1 dissociates from

mitochondria upon infection. On the other hand, the ER and actin, which both have been suggested as regulators of canonical mitochondrial fragmentation, play a role in this type of mitochondrial fission (11).

L. monocytogenes-induced mitochondrial fragmentation is not associated with apoptosis, as classical apoptotic markers such as cytochrome *c* release and Bax recruitment to mitochondria are absent. Nevertheless, LLO impacts mitochondrial function, since it causes a dissipation of the mitochondrial membrane potential as well as a drop in respiration activity and cellular ATP levels (10). Whether mitochondrial fragmentation directly impacts the host cell metabolic switch to glycolysis (12) remains speculative. As both the mitochondrial network morphology and ATP level recover within a few hours, mitochondria seem not to be terminally damaged upon infection. Interestingly, mitochondrial dynamics plays an important role in *L. monocytogenes* infection. It was shown that treatment with small interfering RNA favoring mitochondrial fusion augments the infection efficiency, whereas cells with fragmented mitochondria are less susceptible to *L. monocytogenes* infection. Based on these observations, it was proposed that *L. monocytogenes* targets mitochondria to temporarily impair mitochondrial functions in order to establish its replication niche (10). Subsequent studies showed that one of the mitochondrial functions, i.e., cell-autonomous innate immune signaling through MAVS, is not active during *L. monocytogenes* infection, and innate immune signaling is rather mediated by peroxisome-localized MAVS (13).

Shigella flexneri

S. flexneri is a Gram-negative bacterium which causes shigellosis, an inflammatory disease of the colon leading to tissue destruction, and a leading cause of diarrhea in the developing world. After crossing the colonic epithelium, the facultative intracellular pathogen infects both myeloid immune cells and intestinal epithelial cells. *S. flexneri* injects secreted effectors into the host cell by its type III secretion system (T3SS) to induce membrane ruffling, resulting in enterocyte invasion. The bacterium then rapidly escapes from the phagosome and proliferates in the cytosol, where it employs the host cell actin machinery for intracellular motility as well as for cell-to-cell spread (14). Interestingly, mitochondria were observed at bacterial invasion sites and appear to be entrapped in an actin meshwork induced by the bacterium (15). The authors of the study proposed a model in which an increase in mitochondrial calcium concentration would activate mitochondrial ATP production to locally provide ATP for further actin polymerization (15).

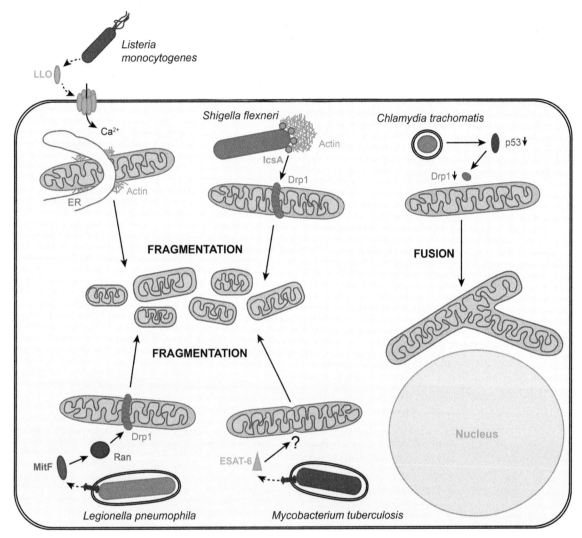

Figure 1 Strategies of intracellular bacteria to interfere with mitochondrial morphology. In epithelial cells, the secreted *L. monocytogenes* toxin LLO induces rapid mitochondrial fragmentation by pore formation in the plasma membrane, enabling calcium influx. Independent of Drp1 and Opa1, *L. monocytogenes*-induced mitochondrial fragmentation is of an atypical type; however, the ER and actin appear to play a regulatory role. The *S. flexneri* surface protein IcsA leads to Drp1-dependent mitochondrial fission in epithelial cells. Infecting macrophages, *L. pneumophila* induces mitochondrial fragmentation in macrophages by the secreted MitF, which activates Ran GTPase and triggers Drp1 recruitment. Infection of epithelial cells with *M. tuberculosis* leads to mitochondrial fission, induced by the bacterial pore-forming toxin ESAT-6. In contrast to the other bacteria shown here, *C. trachomatis* stabilizes the mitochondrial network; downregulating p53, the bacterium inhibits Drp1 expression and recruitment and prevents mitochondrial fragmentation.

At later time points of infection (3.5 h), *S. flexneri* infection induced mitochondrial fission, which was dependent on Drp1 (16). Another study reported local mitochondrial fragmentation in the context of counteracting host cell defense through septin cages. Septin cages have been described to reduce infection by actin-polymerizing bacteria, targeting them to autophagosomes, thus limiting both their motility and dissemination (17). Whereas mitochondrial recruitment to *S. flexneri* contributes to the formation of septin cages, local mitochondrial fission induced by the bacterial surface protein IcsA (Fig. 1) has been shown to prevent septin cage formation (18).

At the functional level, *S. flexneri* has been found to cause a dissipation of the mitochondrial membrane potential and a decrease in the cellular ATP levels by around 50%, correlating with *S. flexneri*-induced necrotic cell death in both epithelial cells (19) and macrophages (20). In epithelial cells, necrosis is counterbalanced by the bacterium, inducing Nod1 signaling. This signaling activates the prosurvival nuclear factor κB (NF-κB) signaling pathway, which in turn inhibits the BNIP3-CypD-dependent opening of the mitochondrial permeability transition pore, a crucial player in the induction of necrosis (19).

Rickettsia spp.

Rickettsia species are Gram-negative obligate intracellular bacteria and are further classified into two major antigenically defined groups, the typhus group and the spotted fever group. *Rickettsia prowazekii* represents the prototype of the typhus group and is transmitted by lice to humans, causing epidemic typhus. *Rickettsia rickettsii* and *Rickettsia conorii* belong to the spotted fever group and are the causative agents of Rocky Mountain spotted fever and Mediterranean spotted fever, respectively. *R. prowazekii*, *R. rickettsii*, and *R. conorii* preferentially infect vascular endothelial cells lining small and medium-sized blood vessels. After entering the host cell via induced phagocytosis, the bacteria rapidly escape the phagosome and replicate in the cytoplasm (21, 22). It has been shown that *R. prowazekii* and several spotted fever group species import the host mitochondrial protein VDAC1 (voltage-dependent anion-selective channel 1), which localizes to contact sites between inner and outer bacterial membranes and appears to be functional. The authors suggested that a primitive protein import mechanism hijacking mitochondrial proteins underlies the obligate endosymbiotic lifestyle of rickettsiae (23, 24). In order to maintain the endothelial cell as a bacterial replication niche, *R. rickettsii* suppresses apoptosis by activation of the prosurvival protein NF-κB (25). By regulating levels and localization of pro- and antiapoptotic Bcl2-family proteins, *R. rickettsii* furthermore maintains mitochondrial integrity and inhibits the activation of caspases 8 and 9 (26, 27).

VACUOLAR BACTERIA

Legionella pneumophila

L. pneumophila is a facultative intracellular bacterium infecting a wide range of hosts, ranging from amoebae to humans. In humans, *L. pneumophila* replicates in alveolar macrophages and causes Legionnaires' disease, a serious pulmonary infection. Inside the host cell, the Gram-negative bacterium resides inside an *L. pneumophila*-containing vacuole (LCV) and is able to evade fusion with the endosome. To manipulate host functions and allow bacterial replication, *L. pneumophila* injects more than 200 bacterial proteins into host cells via a type IV secretion system (T4SS) (28). It has been reported that 30% of LCVs associate with mitochondria as early as 15 min after infection, and the proportion increases to up to 65% after 1 h of infection (29). A close proximity of mitochondria to LCVs was also shown in *L. pneumophila*-infected amoebae (30).

In contrast to these data, more recent time-lapse imaging analyses failed to highlight a stable association of mitochondria with LCVs in *Drosophila* S2 cells (31) or in human primary macrophages (32). The latter study identified transient and highly dynamic mitochondrion-LCV contacts with virulent or avirulent (T4SS-deficient) strains (32). Escoll and colleagues further demonstrated that *L. pneumophila* induces mitochondrial fragmentation without induction of host cell apoptosis at 6 h postinfection (32). Indeed, previous studies had already proposed that *L. pneumophila* inhibits apoptosis, as the number of apoptotic cells remains stable despite effective bacterial replication (33). The secreted bacterial effectors SdhA (34) and SidF were later shown to prevent apoptosis. While the mode of SdhA action remains elusive, SidF mediates apoptotic resistance by specifically interacting with the proapoptotic Bcl-2 proteins BNIP3 and Bcl-rambo (35).

The bacterial factor inducing mitochondrial fragmentation upon *L. pneumophila* infection has been identified and termed mitochondrial fragmentation factor (MitF). MitF is a T4SS-secreted effector that was shown to promote Drp1-dependent mitochondrial fragmentation through a yet-to-be-discovered mechanism involving the nuclear transport factors Ran and Ran-binding protein B2 (RanBP2) as host targets of MitF (Fig. 1). Furthermore, *L. pneumophila*-induced mitochondrial fragmentation correlates with an alteration of the host cell energy metabolism by impairing mitochondrial respiration, leading to reduced mitochondrial ATP production and a decrease in ATP levels. Simultaneously, host cell glycolysis is upregulated and was shown to favor *L. pneumophila* intracellular replication, while mitochondrial respiration appears to be dispensable (32). In line with these findings, it was reported that the secreted *L. pneumophila* mitochondrial carrier protein LncP is not crucial for bacterial proliferation, even though it is targeted to the mitochondrial inner membrane, where it transports ATP from the matrix to the intermembrane space (36).

Mycobacterium tuberculosis

M. tuberculosis is the causative agent of tuberculosis, an infectious disease affecting approximately one-third of the world's population asymptomatically and leading to 1.8 million deaths annually (37). A facultative intracellular bacterium, *M. tuberculosis* colonizes primarily human monocytes and macrophages, where it replicates in a specialized phagosomal compartment. By preventing the fusion of the phagosome with lysosomes and inhibiting phagosomal acidification, *M. tuberculosis* preserves its intracellular niche and replicates. Eventually, *M. tuberculosis* induces necrosis of the host cell in order to spread to neighboring cells. The initiation of apoptosis is therefore considered a defense strategy of host cells to restrict *M. tuberculosis* spreading, as apoptotic cells maintain their contents inside and are cleared by phagocytes (38). In agreement with this hypothesis, infection of macrophages with an avirulent *M. tuberculosis* strain induces apoptosis at a higher level than infection with a virulent strain (39). Consistently, infection with virulent *M. tuberculosis* has been shown to upregulate antiapoptotic proteins such as Bcl-2 (40) and myeloid cell leukemia 1 (Mcl-1) (41). Regarding the interaction of *M. tuberculosis* and mitochondria, recent studies focused on mitochondrial implication in cell death modulation. Chen and colleagues correlated the primarily induced cell death in macrophages with mitochondrial membrane perturbations. While both virulent and avirulent strains lead to transient MOMP and cytochrome *c* release, only the virulent strain causes significantly more mitochondrial permeability transition at early infection time points (6 h). As a consequence, the virulent strain rapidly triggers necrosis, whereas the avirulent strain induces apoptosis only 48 h after infection (42).

Metabolomic profiling on aqueous tissue extracts suggested that *M. tuberculosis* infection in mice leads to an upregulation of host cell glycolysis (80), consistent with previous findings reporting mitochondrial damage (42, 43). In contrast, Jamwal and colleagues observed an increased mitochondrial membrane potential in cells infected with the virulent strain (44). Furthermore, the authors analyzed the mitochondrial response to infection at the proteomic level, revealing infection-induced upregulation of the mitochondrial protein VDAC2 (44), which appears to prevent apoptosis by keeping the proapoptotic protein Bak inactive (45).

Studies on the effect of *M. tuberculosis* infection on mitochondrial morphology are controversial. While one study described mitochondrial swelling and a reduction of the mitochondrial matrix density in J744 macrophages infected with virulent and avirulent *M. tubercu-* losis (43), another study reported different mitochondrial phenotypes and activities depending on the virulence of the strain. Upon infection with virulent H37Rv, monocytic THP-1 cells display elongated mitochondria with an increased electron density and augmented activity; in contrast, cells infected with the avirulent H37Ra strain appear to have less electron-dense mitochondria, which are considered nonfunctional (44). Infection of alveolar epithelial cells with a virulent strain caused mitochondrial fragmentation and aggregation in the perinuclear region at late time points of infection (48 h). The pore-forming toxin ESAT-6 has been proposed as the virulence factor responsible for this effect, as its absence prevents mitochondrial fragmentation and aggregation (46) (Fig. 1).

Salmonella enterica

S. enterica is a foodborne Gram-negative facultative intracellular bacterium causing gastroenteritis. To establish infection, *S. enterica* manipulates host cell functions through a plethora of secreted effector proteins. These effectors are secreted through two T3SSs and contribute to the very early steps of infection by inducing membrane ruffling, which mediates pathogen uptake into nonphagocytic host cells, where *S. enterica* then persists in a vacuole (47). In order to ensure bacterial survival and replication within epithelial cells, *S. enterica* remodels the vacuole to prevent its fusion with lysosomes (48) and inhibits host cell apoptosis. In recent years, *Salmonella* outer protein B (SopB) and fimbrial protein subunit A (FimA) have been identified as two secreted bacterial effector proteins which interfere with mitochondrial functions such as ROS production and apoptosis. SopB binds to cytosolic tumor necrosis factor receptor-associated factor 6 (TRAF6) and delays its mitochondrial recruitment, which causes decreased generation of mitochondrial ROS. In addition to this, Bax translocation to mitochondria and pore formation are inhibited, and induction of apoptosis by cytochrome *c* release is prevented (49). On the other hand, the soluble form of the pilus protein FimA targets mitochondria, where it binds to the outer mitochondrial membrane protein VDAC1. This results in a tight association between VDAC1 and the mitochondrial hexokinases, suppressing the integration of the pore-forming protein Bax into the outer mitochondrial membrane and the release of cytochrome *c* (50). Two mechanisms thus converge to prevent cytochrome *c* release from mitochondria in *S. enterica*-infected cells. Another effector, called *Salmonella* outer protein A (SopA), has been reported to localize to mitochondria (51). SopA was lately described as interacting with two host E3 ubiquitin ligases, TRIM56 and TRIM65, inducing an innate immune response involving MAVS activation and characterized by enhanced interferon beta signaling (52).

In contrast to *S. enterica* infection in epithelial cells, *S. enterica* infection induces programmed cell death in macrophages. In this context, Hernandez and colleagues proposed that the effector SipB localizes to mitochondria and disrupts mitochondrial morphology, causing swelling and loss of cristae integrity, triggering mitochondrial disruption and resulting in a caspase 1-independent and autophagy-mediated cell death (53).

Chlamydia spp.

The genus *Chlamydia* comprises three Gram-negative bacterial species, which are pathogenic to humans: *Chlamydia trachomatis*, *C. pneumoniae*, and *C. psittaci*. *C. trachomatis* is one of the most common sexually transmitted bacteria and causes trachoma, a severe eye infection that can lead to blindness. *C. pneumoniae* and *C. psittaci* are associated with respiratory infections such as pneumonia. The obligate intracellular *Chlamydia* species exhibit a characteristic biphasic life cycle with two distinct developmental forms. The infectious elementary bodies (EBs) attach to epithelial cells and are taken up by phagocytosis. Inside host cells, EBs reside inside membrane-bound inclusions, where they differentiate into metabolically active reticulate bodies (RBs). RBs proliferate by binary fission and undergo maturation to again form infectious EBs, which are released upon host cell lysis in order to infect new cells (54). Several *Chlamydia* species have been shown to prevent host cell apoptosis by acting on mitochondria (55). Upon *C. trachomatis* and *C. pneumoniae* infection, the chlamydial protease-like activity factor induces the degradation of proapoptotic BH3-only proteins, such as Bim, Puma, and Bad, thereby suppressing cytochrome *c* release from mitochondria and mediating cellular resistance to apoptosis (56, 57).

In terms of energy supply, *Chlamydia* species have been described as "energy parasites," as they depend on the import of host cell ATP and metabolites (58, 59). In agreement with this hypothesis, chlamydial infections influence localization and morphology of mitochondria, presumably to obtain ATP and metabolites. By employing electron microscopy, Masumoto identified a tight association of *C. psittaci* with mitochondria, supporting the former biochemical observations. Mitochondrial association occurred approximately 12 h postinfection, at the time when RBs start to replicate (60).

Interestingly, although all *Chlamydia* species possess genes encoding ATP transporters, the recruitment of mitochondria to the inclusion is unique to *C. psittaci* and was not observed for *C. trachomatis* or *C. pneumoniae* (61). Instead, *C. trachomatis* stabilizes the mitochondrial network upon infection-induced stress in order to preserve the mitochondrial ATP production capacity. To do so, *C. trachomatis* prevents Drp1-mediated mitochondrial fragmentation by downregulating p53 (62), a known regulator of Drp1 expression (63) (Fig. 1), and apoptosis. Mitochondrial morphology affects *C. trachomatis* infection, and cells with fragmented mitochondria display decreased infection levels (62). Liang and colleagues demonstrated a dependency of *C. trachomatis* EBs on mitochondrial energy production in epithelial cells; however, the authors also showed that later during infection, *C. trachomatis* RBs rely only to a limited extent on mitochondrial ATP and employ a sodium gradient to produce energy (64). In contrast to *C. trachomatis* infection, *C. pneumoniae* infection causes mitochondrial dysfunction characterized by mitochondrial hyperpolarization, increased ROS generation, and the induction of a metabolic switch to host cell glycolysis. Consistently, impairment of mitochondrial function enhances growth of *C. pneumoniae* inclusions (65).

Ehrlichia chaffeensis

E. chaffeensis is an obligate intracellular bacterium which causes the tick-borne disease human monocytic ehrlichiosis. This Gram-negative pathogen infects and proliferates inside monocytes and macrophages, where it resides inside vacuoles and forms characteristic mulberry-like bacterial aggregates, which are referred to as morulae. The first evidence that mitochondria play an important role for *E. chaffeensis* infection was reported by Popov and colleagues; they observed mitochondria closely associated with bacteria-containing morulae in infected macrophages (67). Functional studies of the interaction revealed that *E. chaffeensis* infection does not cause a change in the mitochondrial membrane potential; however, it reduces mitochondrial DNA synthesis and transcription of mitochondrial genes (68). These observations suggest that *E. chaffeensis* inhibits mitochondrial activity. Surprisingly, a screen in *Drosophila melanogaster* identified seven mitochondrion-associated genes whose mutation results in increased resistance to infection (69). A key process in *E. chaffeensis* pathogenicity is the secretion of effector proteins, which allow evasion of bacterial killing by preventing lysosomal degradation and inhibiting apoptosis, thereby preserving the bacterial replication niche (66). For example, *E. chaffeensis* secretes the bacterial effector ECH0825, which localizes to mitochondria and inhibits Bax-induced apoptosis. It has been furthermore proposed that ECH0825 prevents ROS-induced cellular stress and apoptosis by upregulating mitochondrial manganese superoxide dismutase (70). Transcriptional profiling of cells infected with *E. chaffeensis* revealed the induction of the antiapoptotic protein NF-κB and of the Bcl2 proteins Bcl2A1 and Mcl-1 as well as repression of the proapoptotic proteins Bik and BNIP3 (71).

CONCLUSIONS

In this chapter, we summarize several findings illustrating the importance of mitochondria during bacterial infection, involving the manipulation of mitochondrial morphology and function or the recruitment of mitochondria to the infection site. While viruses induce either

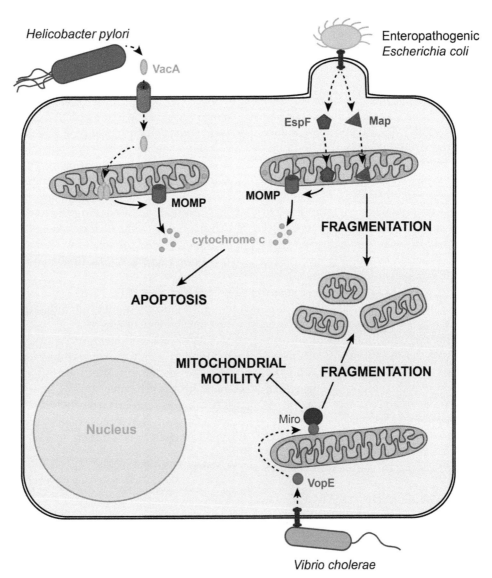

Figure 2 Relationship between extracellular bacteria and host cell mitochondria. The extracellular bacterium *H. pylori* secretes VacA, a pore-forming toxin, which localizes to the mitochondrial inner membrane and induces MOMP, resulting in apoptosis. EPEC interferes with mitochondrial morphology and function by the secretion of the effector proteins Map and EspF. Both proteins localize to the mitochondrial matrix, where Map leads to mitochondrial fragmentation and EspF induces MOMP and subsequent apoptosis. *V. cholerae* secreted VopE is a GTPase-activating protein that inactivates Miro at mitochondria, causing mitochondrial fragmentation and inhibiting kinesin-dependent mitochondrial motility. Movement is represented by dashed arrows, while solid arrows indicate induction.

mitochondrial fission or fusion (72), to date, bacterial infections seem to mainly induce mitochondrial fission. Although such fission appears to proceed either via the classical, Drp1-dependent fission pathway (*S. flexneri* and *L. pneumophila*) or through an atypical, Drp1-independent pathway (*L. monocytogenes*), fragmentation of the mitochondrial network may represent a common bacterial strategy to impact different mitochondrial functions, or a cellular stress response. Strikingly, mitochondrial morphology can impact the success of infection; cells with fragmented mitochondria display a reduced rate of infection by both *L. monocytogenes* and *C. trachomatis*.

Several bacteria use a similar mechanism to interfere with mitochondrial morphology and function, relying on secreted bacterial effectors. These effectors induce changes in mitochondrial structure, dynamics, and functionality which allow bacteria to preserve their replicative niche. Many of the bacterial effectors target Bcl-2 family members by modulating their expression and activity in order to suppress apoptosis. Several secreted effectors that affect mitochondrial morphology and function are pore-forming toxins, and pore formation is essential for their effects. While *L. monocytogenes* enables calcium influx through pores in the plasma membrane formed by the secreted toxin LLO (Fig. 1), vacuolating cytotoxin A (VacA) injected by extracellular *Helicobacter pylori* localizes to mitochondria and has been shown to form pores in the inner mitochondrial membrane, inducing a loss of the mitochondrial membrane potential and apoptosis (73, 74) (Fig. 2). In contrast, the exact mechanism by which the pore-forming toxin ESAT-6 from *M. tuberculosis* affects mitochondria remains speculative (Fig. 1). Other secreted bacterial effectors rely on different mechanisms to induce mitochondrial fission: for example, *L. pneumophila* MitF indirectly triggers Drp1 oligomerization to cause mitochondrial fragmentation (Fig. 1).

Several extracellular bacteria also secrete effectors that target mitochondrial dynamics and function through diverse mechanisms. The extracellular bacterium *Vibrio cholerae* secretes a GTPase-activating protein (VopE), which promotes mitochondrial fragmentation and prevents kinesin-dependent mitochondrial motility (Fig. 2). Thereby, VopE inhibits mitochondrial perinuclear clustering and MAVS-dependent innate immune responses (75). Enteropathogenic *Escherichia coli* (EPEC) effector proteins mitochondria-associated protein (Map) and EPEC-secreted protein F (EspF) display yet another way of targeting mitochondria, as they localize to the mitochondrial matrix and act from within (Fig. 2). While both proteins disrupt the mitochondrial membrane potential,

EspF has been shown to trigger apoptosis (76), while Map causes mitochondrial fragmentation and might work in an antiapoptotic fashion and control other mitochondrion-regulated cellular processes (77, 78).

Another way by which bacteria affect mitochondrial morphology is through the recruitment of mitochondria. This has been observed for several cytosolic and intravacuolar bacteria, which thereby presumably benefit from mitochondrion-derived ATP or other metabolites. An extreme example of a bacterium that may benefit from mitochondrial functions or metabolites is the alphaproteobacterium "*Candidatus* Midichloria mitochondrii," which invades mitochondria of tick ovarian cells (79).

Bacterial infection can affect not only mitochondrial morphology but also the host cell energy metabolism. In *L. pneumophila* infection, mitochondrial fragmentation correlates with a decrease in mitochondrial respiration. A similar scenario might apply to *L. monocytogenes* infection. Interestingly, although *C. pneumoniae* infection causes mitochondrial hyperpolarization and increased ROS production, it also triggers host cell glycolysis. Reprogramming of the host cell energy metabolism has also been reported for other intracellular bacteria, such as *L. monocytogenes* and *M. tuberculosis*. In contrast, *Francisella tularensis* infection was found to inhibit glycolysis in macrophages (81). However, the link between mitochondria and these infection-induced metabolic changes remains largely unknown.

The complex interactions between bacteria and mitochondria summarized here highlight the importance of this organelle in infection. Future studies will shed more light on the mechanisms by which bacteria affect mitochondria and afford a better understanding of the specific roles that mitochondria play during different stages of bacterial infection.

Citation. Spier A, Stavru F, Cossart P. 2019. Interaction between intracellular bacterial pathogens and host cell mitochondria. Microbiol Spectrum 7(2):BAI-0016-2019.

References

1. **Roger AJ, Muñoz-Gómez SA, Kamikawa R.** 2017. The origin and diversification of Mitochondria. *Curr Biol* **27:** R1177–R1192.

2. **Nunnari J, Suomalainen A.** 2012. Mitochondria: in sickness and in health. *Cell* **148:**1145–1159.

3. **Seth RB, Sun L, Ea C-K, Chen ZJ.** 2005. Identification and characterization of MAVS, a mitochondrial antiviral signaling protein that activates NF-kappaB and IRF 3. *Cell* **122:**669–682.

4. **Tait SWG, Green DR.** 2010. Mitochondria and cell death: outer membrane permeabilization and beyond. *Nat Rev Mol Cell Biol* **11:**621–632.

5. **Pagliuso A, Cossart P, Stavru F.** 2018. The ever-growing complexity of the mitochondrial fission machinery. *Cell Mol Life Sci* **75**:355–374.

6. **Wai T, Langer T.** 2016. Mitochondrial dynamics and metabolic regulation. *Trends Endocrinol Metab* **27**:105–117.

7. **Mishra P, Chan DC.** 2014. Mitochondrial dynamics and inheritance during cell division, development and disease. *Nat Rev Mol Cell Biol* **15**:634–646.

8. **Hamon MA, Ribet D, Stavru F, Cossart P.** 2012. Listeriolysin O: the Swiss army knife of *Listeria. Trends Microbiol* **20**:360–368.

9. **Kocks C, Gouin E, Tabouret M, Berche P, Ohayon H, Cossart P.** 1992. *L. monocytogenes*-induced actin assembly requires the *actA* gene product, a surface protein. *Cell* **68**:521–531.

10. **Stavru F, Bouillaud F, Sartori A, Ricquier D, Cossart P.** 2011. *Listeria monocytogenes* transiently alters mitochondrial dynamics during infection. *Proc Natl Acad Sci USA* **108**:3612–3617.

11. **Stavru F, Palmer AE, Wang C, Youle RJ, Cossart P.** 2013. Atypical mitochondrial fission upon bacterial infection. *Proc Natl Acad Sci USA* **110**:16003–16008.

12. **Gillmaier N, Götz A, Schulz A, Eisenreich W, Goebel W.** 2012. Metabolic responses of primary and transformed cells to intracellular *Listeria monocytogenes. PLoS One* **7**:e52378.

13. **Odendall C, Dixit E, Stavru F, Bierne H, Franz KM, Durbin AF, Boulant S, Gehrke L, Cossart P, Kagan JC.** 2014. Diverse intracellular pathogens activate type III interferon expression from peroxisomes. *Nat Immunol* **15**:717–726.

14. **Killackey SA, Sorbara MT, Girardin SE.** 2016. Cellular aspects of *Shigella* pathogenesis: focus on the manipulation of host cell processes. *Front Cell Infect Microbiol* **6**:38.

15. **Tran Van Nhieu G, Kai Liu B, Zhang J, Pierre F, Prigent S, Sansonetti P, Erneux C, Kuk Kim J, Suh PG, Dupont G, Combettes L.** 2013. Actin-based confinement of calcium responses during *Shigella* invasion. *Nat Commun* **4**:1567.

16. **Lum M, Morona R.** 2014. Dynamin-related protein Drp1 and mitochondria are important for *Shigella flexneri* infection. *Int J Med Microbiol* **304**:530–541.

17. **Mostowy S, Bonazzi M, Hamon MA, Tham TN, Mallet A, Lelek M, Gouin E, Demangel C, Brosch R, Zimmer C, Sartori A, Kinoshita M, Lecuit M, Cossart P.** 2010. Entrapment of intracytosolic bacteria by septin cage-like structures. *Cell Host Microbe* **8**:433–444.

18. **Sirianni A, Krokowski S, Lobato-Márquez D, Buranyi S, Pfanzelter J, Galea D, Willis A, Culley S, Henriques R, Larrouy-Maumus G, Hollinshead M, Sancho-Shimizu V, Way M, Mostowy S.** 2016. Mitochondria mediate septin cage assembly to promote autophagy of *Shigella. EMBO Rep* **17**:1029–1043.

19. **Carneiro LAM, Travassos LH, Soares F, Tattoli I, Magalhaes JG, Bozza MT, Plotkowski MC, Sansonetti PJ, Molkentin JD, Philpott DJ, Girardin SE.** 2009. *Shigella* induces mitochondrial dysfunction and cell death in nonmyeloid cells. *Cell Host Microbe* **5**:123–136.

20. **Koterski JF, Nahvi M, Venkatesan MM, Haimovich B.** 2005. Virulent *Shigella flexneri* causes damage to mitochondria and triggers necrosis in infected human monocyte-derived macrophages. *Infect Immun* **73**:504–513.

21. **Sahni SK, Rydkina E.** 2009. Host-cell interactions with pathogenic *Rickettsia* species. *Future Microbiol* **4**:323–339.

22. **Martinez JJ, Cossart P.** 2004. Early signaling events involved in the entry of *Rickettsia conorii* into mammalian cells. *J Cell Sci* **117**:5097–5106.

23. **Emelyanov VV, Vyssokikh MY.** 2006. On the nature of obligate intracellular symbiosis of rickettsiae—*Rickettsia prowazekii* cells import mitochondrial porin. *Biochemistry (Mosc)* **71**:730–735.

24. **Emelyanov VV.** 2009. Mitochondrial porin VDAC 1 seems to be functional in rickettsial cells. *Ann N Y Acad Sci* **1166**:38–48.

25. **Clifton DR, Goss RA, Sahni SK, van Antwerp D, Baggs RB, Marder VJ, Silverman DJ, Sporn LA.** 1998. NF-κB-dependent inhibition of apoptosis is essential for host cell survival during *Rickettsia rickettsii* infection. *Proc Natl Acad Sci USA* **95**:4646–4651.

26. **Joshi SG, Francis CW, Silverman DJ, Sahni SK.** 2003. Nuclear factor κB protects against host cell apoptosis during *Rickettsia rickettsii* infection by inhibiting activation of apical and effector caspases and maintaining mitochondrial integrity. *Infect Immun* **71**:4127–4136.

27. **Joshi SG, Francis CW, Silverman DJ, Sahni SK.** 2004. NF-kappaB activation suppresses host cell apoptosis during *Rickettsia rickettsii* infection via regulatory effects on intracellular localization or levels of apoptogenic and anti-apoptotic proteins. *FEMS Microbiol Lett* **234**:333–341.

28. **Newton HJ, Ang DKY, van Driel IR, Hartland EL.** 2010. Molecular pathogenesis of infections caused by *Legionella pneumophila. Clin Microbiol Rev* **23**:274–298.

29. **Horwitz MA.** 1983. Formation of a novel phagosome by the Legionnaires' disease bacterium (*Legionella pneumophila*) in human monocytes. *J Exp Med* **158**:1319–1331.

30. **Newsome AL, Baker RL, Miller RD, Arnold RR.** 1985. Interactions between *Naegleria fowleri* and *Legionella pneumophila. Infect Immun* **50**:449–452.

31. **Sun EW, Wagner ML, Maize A, Kemler D, Garland-Kuntz E, Xu L, Luo ZQ, Hollenbeck PJ.** 2013. *Legionella pneumophila* infection of *Drosophila* S2 cells induces only minor changes in mitochondrial dynamics. *PLoS One* **8**:e62972.

32. **Escoll P, Song OR, Viana F, Steiner B, Lagache T, Olivo-Marin JC, Impens F, Brodin P, Hilbi H, Buchrieser C.** 2017. *Legionella pneumophila* modulates mitochondrial dynamics to trigger metabolic repurposing of infected macrophages. *Cell Host Microbe* **22**:302–316.E7.

33. **Derré I, Isberg RR.** 2004. Macrophages from mice with the restrictive Lgn1 allele exhibit multifactorial resistance to *Legionella pneumophila. Infect Immun* **72**:6221–6229.

34. **Laguna RK, Creasey EA, Li Z, Valtz N, Isberg RR.** 2006. A *Legionella pneumophila*-translocated substrate that is required for growth within macrophages and protection from host cell death. *Proc Natl Acad Sci USA* **103**:18745–18750.

35. **Banga S, Gao P, Shen X, Fiscus V, Zong W-X, Chen L, Luo Z-Q.** 2007. *Legionella pneumophila* inhibits macrophage apoptosis by targeting pro-death members of the Bcl2 protein family. *Proc Natl Acad Sci USA* **104:** 5121–5126.

36. **Dolezal P, Aili M, Tong J, Jiang JH, Marobbio CM, Lee SF, Schuelein R, Belluzzo S, Binova E, Mousnier A, Frankel G, Giannuzzi G, Palmieri F, Gabriel K, Naderer T, Hartland EL, Lithgow T.** 2012. *Legionella pneumophila* secretes a mitochondrial carrier protein during infection. *PLoS Pathog* 8:e1002459. *CORRECTION PLoS Pathog* 8: 10.1371/annotation/5039541e-b48a-4cfc-84b1-21566e311-a62. *CORRECTION PLoS Pathog* 8:10.1371/annotation/ ee7c807b-032c-4d1f-b5ac-0f6620a2ef24.

37. **Corbett EL, Watt CJ, Walker N, Maher D, Williams BG, Raviglione MC, Dye C.** 2003. The growing burden of tuberculosis: global trends and interactions with the HIV epidemic. *Arch Intern Med* **163:**1009–1021.

38. **Dubey RK.** 2016. Assuming the role of mitochondria in mycobacterial infection. *Int J Mycobacteriol* 5:379–383.

39. **Keane J, Balcewicz-Sablinska MK, Remold HG, Chupp GL, Meek BB, Fenton MJ, Kornfeld H.** 1997. Infection by *Mycobacterium tuberculosis* promotes human alveolar macrophage apoptosis. *Infect Immun* 65:298–304.

40. **Zhang J, Jiang R, Takayama H, Tanaka Y.** 2005. Survival of virulent *Mycobacterium tuberculosis* involves preventing apoptosis induced by Bcl-2 upregulation and release resulting from necrosis in J774 macrophages. *Microbiol Immunol* 49:845–852.

41. **Sly LM, Hingley-Wilson SM, Reiner NE, McMaster WR.** 2003. Survival of *Mycobacterium tuberculosis* in host macrophages involves resistance to apoptosis dependent upon induction of antiapoptotic Bcl-2 family member Mcl-1. *J Immunol* 170:430–437.

42. **Chen M, Gan H, Remold HG.** 2006. A mechanism of virulence: virulent *Mycobacterium tuberculosis* strain H37Rv, but not attenuated H37Ra, causes significant mitochondrial inner membrane disruption in macrophages leading to necrosis. *J Immunol* 176:3707–3716.

43. **Abarca-Rojano E, Rosas-Medina P, Zamudio-Cortéz P, Mondragón-Flores R, Sánchez-García FJ.** 2003. *Mycobacterium tuberculosis* virulence correlates with mitochondrial cytochrome c release in infected macrophages. *Scand J Immunol* 58:419–427.

44. **Jamwal S, Midha MK, Verma HN, Basu A, Rao KVS, Manivel V.** 2013. Characterizing virulence-specific perturbations in the mitochondrial function of macrophages infected with *Mycobacterium tuberculosis*. *Sci Rep* 3:1328.

45. **Cheng EH-Y, Sheiko TV, Fisher JK, Craigen WJ, Korsmeyer SJ.** 2003. VDAC2 inhibits BAK activation and mitochondrial apoptosis. *Science* 301:513–517.

46. **Fine-Coulson K, Giguère S, Quinn FD, Reaves BJ.** 2015. Infection of A549 human type II epithelial cells with *Mycobacterium tuberculosis* induces changes in mitochondrial morphology, distribution and mass that are dependent on the early secreted antigen, ESAT-6. *Microbes Infect* 17:689–697.

47. **Cossart P, Sansonetti PJ.** 2004. Bacterial invasion: the paradigm of enteroinvasive pathogens. *Science* 304:242–248.

48. **Eng SK, Pusparajah P, Ab Mutalib NS, Ser HL, Chan KG, Lee LH.** 2015. *Salmonella*: a review on pathogenesis, epidemiology and antibiotic resistance. *Front Life Sci* 8:284–293.

49. **Ruan H, Zhang Z, Tian L, Wang S, Hu S, Qiao JJ.** 2016. The *Salmonella* effector SopB prevents ROS-induced apoptosis of epithelial cells by retarding TRAF6 recruitment to mitochondria. *Biochem Biophys Res Commun* 478: 618–623.

50. **Sukumaran SK, Fu NY, Tin CB, Wan KF, Lee SS, Yu VC.** 2010. A soluble form of the pilus protein FimA targets the VDAC-hexokinase complex at mitochondria to suppress host cell apoptosis. *Mol Cell* 37:768–783.

51. **Layton AN, Brown PJ, Galyov EE.** 2005. The *Salmonella* translocated effector SopA is targeted to the mitochondria of infected cells. *J Bacteriol* 187:3565–3571.

52. **Kamanova J, Sun H, Lara-Tejero M, Galán JE.** 2016. The *Salmonella* effector protein SopA modulates innate immune responses by targeting TRIM E3 ligase family members. *PLoS Pathog* 12:e1005552.

53. **Hernandez LD, Pypaert M, Flavell RA, Galán JE.** 2003. A *Salmonella* protein causes macrophage cell death by inducing autophagy. *J Cell Biol* 163:1123–1131.

54. **Elwell C, Mirrashidi K, Engel J.** 2016. *Chlamydia* cell biology and pathogenesis. *Nat Rev Microbiol* 14:385–400.

55. **Fischer SF, Harlander T, Vier J, Häcker G.** 2004. Protection against CD95-induced apoptosis by chlamydial infection at a mitochondrial step. *Infect Immun* 72: 1107–1115.

56. **Fischer SF, Vier J, Kirschnek S, Klos A, Hess S, Ying S, Häcker G.** 2004. *Chlamydia* inhibit host cell apoptosis by degradation of proapoptotic BH3-only proteins. *J Exp Med* 200:905–916.

57. **Fan T, Lu H, Hu H, Shi L, McClarty GA, Nance DM, Greenberg AH, Zhong G.** 1998. Inhibition of apoptosis in chlamydia-infected cells: blockade of mitochondrial cytochrome *c* release and caspase activation. *J Exp Med* 187:487–496.

58. **Moulder JW.** 1962. Structure and chemical composition of isolated particles. *Ann N Y Acad Sci* 98:92–99.

59. **Hatch TP, Al-Hossainy E, Silverman JA.** 1982. Adenine nucleotide and lysine transport in *Chlamydia psittaci*. *J Bacteriol* 150:662–670.

60. **Matsumoto A.** 1981. Isolation and electron microscopic observations of intracytoplasmic inclusions containing *Chlamydia psittaci*. *J Bacteriol* 145:605–612.

61. **Matsumoto A, Bessho H, Uehira K, Suda T.** 1991. Morphological studies of the association of mitochondria with chlamydial inclusions and the fusion of chlamydial inclusions. *J Electron Microsc (Tokyo)* 40:356–363.

62. **Chowdhury SR, Reimer A, Sharan M, Kozjak-Pavlovic V, Eulalio A, Prusty BK, Fraunholz M, Karunakaran K, Rudel T.** 2017. *Chlamydia* preserves the mitochondrial network necessary for replication via microRNA-dependent inhibition of fission. *J Cell Biol* 216:1071–1089.

63. **Li J, Donath S, Li Y, Qin D, Prabhakar BS, Li P.** 2010. miR-30 regulates mitochondrial fission through targeting p53 and the dynamin-related protein-1 pathway. *PLoS Genet* 6:e1000795. *CORRECTION PLoS Genet* 6:10.

1371/annotation/4050116d-8daa-4b5a-99e9-34cdd13-f6a26.

64. Liang P, Rosas-Lemus M, Patel D, Fang X, Tuz K, Juárez O. 2018. Dynamic energy dependency of *Chlamydia trachomatis* on host cell metabolism during intracellular growth: role of sodium-based energetics in chlamydial ATP generation. *J Biol Chem* **293**:510–522.

65. Käding N, Kaufhold I, Müller C, Szaszák M, Shima K, Weinmaier T, Lomas R, Conesa A, Schmitt-Kopplin P, Rattei T, Rupp J. 2017. Growth of *Chlamydia pneumoniae* is enhanced in cells with impaired mitochondrial function. *Front Cell Infect Microbiol* **7**:499.

66. Rikihisa Y. 2015. Molecular pathogenesis of *Ehrlichia chaffeensis* infection. *Annu Rev Microbiol* **69**:283–304.

67. Popov VL, Chen S-M, Feng H-M, Walker DH. 1995. Ultrastructural variation of cultured *Ehrlichia chaffeensis*. *J Med Microbiol* **43**:411–421.

68. Liu Y, Zhang Z, Jiang Y, Zhang L, Popov VL, Zhang J, Walker DH, Yu XJ. 2011. Obligate intracellular bacterium *Ehrlichia* inhibiting mitochondrial activity. *Microbes Infect* **13**:232–238.

69. Von Ohlen T, Luce-Fedrow A, Ortega MT, Ganta RR, Chapes SK. 2012. Identification of critical host mitochondrion-associated genes during *Ehrlichia chaffeensis* infections. *Infect Immun* **80**:3576–3586.

70. Liu H, Bao W, Lin M, Niu H, Rikihisa Y. 2012. *Ehrlichia* type IV secretion effector ECH0825 is translocated to mitochondria and curbs ROS and apoptosis by upregulating host MnSOD. *Cell Microbiol* **14**:1037–1050.

71. Zhang JZ, Sinha M, Luxon BA, Yu XJ. 2004. Survival strategy of obligately intracellular *Ehrlichia chaffeensis*: novel modulation of immune response and host cell cycles. *Infect Immun* **72**:498–507.

72. Khan M, Syed GH, Kim SJ, Siddiqui A. 2015. Mitochondrial dynamics and viral infections: a close nexus. *Biochim Biophys Acta* **1853**(10 Pt B):2822–2833.

73. Willhite DC, Blanke SR. 2004. *Helicobacter pylori* vacuolating cytotoxin enters cells, localizes to the mitochondria, and induces mitochondrial membrane permeability changes correlated to toxin channel activity. *Cell Microbiol* **6**:143–154.

74. Foo JH, Culvenor JG, Ferrero RL, Kwok T, Lithgow T, Gabriel K. 2010. Both the p33 and p55 subunits of the *Helicobacter pylori* VacA toxin are targeted to mammalian mitochondria. *J Mol Biol* **401**:792–798.

75. Suzuki M, Danilchanka O, Mekalanos JJ. 2014. *Vibrio cholerae* T3SS effector VopE modulates mitochondrial dynamics and innate immune signaling by targeting Miro GTPases. *Cell Host Microbe* **16**:581–591.

76. Nougayrède JP, Donnenberg MS. 2004. Enteropathogenic *Escherichia coli* EspF is targeted to mitochondria and is required to initiate the mitochondrial death pathway. *Cell Microbiol* **6**:1097–1111.

77. Kenny B, Jepson M. 2000. Targeting of an enteropathogenic *Escherichia coli* (EPEC) effector protein to host mitochondria. *Cell Microbiol* **2**:579–590.

78. Papatheodorou P, Domańska G, Öxle M, Mathieu J, Selchow O, Kenny B, Rassow J. 2006. The enteropathogenic *Escherichia coli* (EPEC) Map effector is imported into the mitochondrial matrix by the TOM/Hsp70 system and alters organelle morphology. *Cell Microbiol* **8**:677–689.

79. Sassera D, Beninati T, Bandi C, Bouman EAP, Sacchi L, Fabbi M, Lo N. 2006. 'Candidatus Midichloria mitochondrii', an endosymbiont of the tick *Ixodes ricinus* with a unique intramitochondrial lifestyle. *Int J Syst Evol Microbiol* **56**:2535–2540.

80. Shin JH, Yang JY, Jeon BY, Yoon YJ, Cho SN, Kang YH, Ryu DH, Hwang GS. 2011. ^{1}H NMR-based metabolomic profiling in mice infected with *Mycobacterium tuberculosis*. *J Proteome Res* **10**:2238–2247.

81. Wyatt EV, Diaz K, Griffin AJ, Rassmussen JA, Crane DD, Jones BD, Bosio CM. 2016. Metabolic reprogramming of host cells by virulent *Francisella tularensis* for optimal replication and modulation of inflammation. *J Immunol* **196**:4227–4236.

Bacteria and Intracellularity
Edited by Pascale Cossart, Craig R. Roy, and Philippe Sansonetti
© 2019 American Society for Microbiology, Washington, DC
doi:10.1128/microbiolspec.BAI-0023-2019

Shigella Pathogenesis: New Insights through Advanced Methodologies

2

Pamela Schnupf[1] and Philippe J. Sansonetti[2]

SHIGELLA AND SHIGELLOSIS

Shigella spp. are diarrheal pathogens closely related to *Escherichia coli*. They are named after Kiyoshi Shiga, who in 1898 identified its most virulent member, *Shigella dysenteriae*, as the causative agent of bacillary dysentery, also known as shigellosis (1). *Shigella* spp. are Gram-negative, non-spore-forming, facultative anaerobic bacilli that in humans and other primates cause diarrheal disease by invading the colonic epithelium. Spreading of the infection is generally limited to the intestinal lining, where it leads to colonic inflammation, mucosal ulceration, and a loss in intestinal barrier function. Shigellae are transmitted through the fecal-oral route or through ingestion of contaminated food and water. In most cases, *Shigella* spp. cause a self-limiting disease that can be effectively treated by oral rehydration or antibiotics, although a steady increase in the number of shigellosis cases caused by antibiotic-resistant *Shigella* strains has become a growing concern (2, 3). Shigellosis can be fatal in the very young and in infected individuals who are immunocompromised or do not have access to adequate medical treatment.

Clinical symptoms of shigellosis range from mild watery diarrhea to a bloody mucoid diarrhea accompanied by painful abdominal cramps and fever. The range of clinical symptoms is related to both the immune status of the host and the causative *Shigella* species, which differ in the presence of some critical virulence factors, including Shiga toxin. A major complication in infants and children is toxic megalocolon, while after clearance of the infection, other possible complications include hemolytic-uremic syndrome, characterized by renal failure, low platelet and red blood cell levels, and a 35% fatality rate, as well as postreactive arthritis, where

patients may suffer from chronic arthritis of the joints for years after the shigellosis episode (4).

Shigella has a very low infectious dose, estimated to be 10 to 100 bacteria, and *Shigella* remains a major public health concern with an estimated 165 million cases occurring worldwide every year, including up to 100,000 deaths, particularly in children under 5 years of age (5, 6). The occurrence of shigellosis is largely restricted to developing countries where limited availability of clean drinking water and poor hygiene foster disease transmission and malnutrition contributes to disease severity. A vaccine for *Shigella* has not been licensed, partly due to the large repertoire of *Shigella* serotypes that need to be targeted in order for the vaccine to be globally effective (6).

The genus *Shigella* is composed of four species: *S. dysenteriae*, *S. flexneri*, *S. boydii*, and *S. sonnei*. Each species represents a different serogroup (A through D, respectively) and is composed of multiple (15 to 20) serotypes, except for *S. sonnei*, which has only one (4). The large number of serotypes reflects the extensive variability in the composition, modification, and number of repeats of its lipopolysaccharide (LPS) O antigen, a major *Shigella* antigenic target of the humoral response of the host. *Shigella* spp. are endemic in a number of tropical and subtropical regions. Globally, *S. boydii* and *S. dysenteriae* are the least common agents of shigellosis, but they remain endemic in South Asia and sub-Saharan Africa, while *S. sonnei* is the most prevalent *Shigella* species linked to diarrheal disease in industrialized countries and an important cause of traveler's diarrhea (7). At 60% of all cases, *S. flexneri* is the most common cause of shigellosis worldwide. It is also the most widely studied *Shigella* species. *In vitro* and

[1]Institut Imagine, Laboratory of Intestinal Immunity, INSERM UMR1163; Institut Necker Enfants Malades, Laboratory of Host-Microbiota Interaction, INSERM U1151; and Université Paris Descartes-Sorbonne, 75006 Paris, France; [2]Institut Pasteur, Unité de Pathogénie Microbienne Moléculaire, INSERM U1202, and College de France, Paris, France.

in vivo studies, in combination with clinical observations, have led to a detailed description of *S. flexneri* pathogenesis (3).

THE *SHIGELLA* INFECTIOUS CYCLE

Virulence of *Shigella* requires its type III secretion system (T3SS), a needle-like molecular syringe anchored in the bacterial cell wall. Activation of the T3SS occurs through contact of the needle tip with the host plasma membrane, resulting in the formation of a direct channel between the bacterial and host cytoplasm. *Shigella* injects a large number of bacterial effectors through this syringe to subvert many different host cell processes and to facilitate infection and dissemination.

To invade the host, *Shigella* must first withstand the physiochemical conditions encountered through its transit of the digestive system and cross the mucus layer of the colon. *Shigella* then traverses the colonic epithelial barrier through M (microfold) cells of the specialized epithelium overlying lymphoid follicles (Fig. 1). M cells deliver *Shigella* to the basolateral side of the epithelium, where the bacteria are phagocytosed by antigen-presenting cells such as macrophages and dendritic cells residing within or near the M cell pocket. *Shigella*

rapidly lyses the phagosomal compartment of the macrophage in a T3SS-dependent manner, and after limited replication in the cytosol, escapes the macrophage through activation of a lytic inflammatory cell death called pyroptosis. Macrophage pyroptosis, a process actively promoted by *Shigella*, is accompanied by caspase-l-mediated proteolytic activation and subsequent secretion of the proinflammatory cytokines interleukin 1β (IL-1β) and IL-18. Lytic cell death of infected macrophages releases *Shigella* at the basolateral side of colonic epithelial cells. *Shigella* interacts with host cell proteins found at the basolateral side of epithelial cells and forces its uptake into epithelial cells by inducing epithelial cell macropinocytosis. Invasion depends on the T3SS and a first wave of effectors to subvert the host cell cytoskeleton and mediate vacuolar escape.

Once in the cytosol, *Shigella* replicates and uses actin-based motility to escape host cell innate defenses such as autophagy and to spread to neighboring cells. Lysis of the double membrane of secondary phagosomes formed by *Shigella* physically pushing into neighboring epithelial cells again releases *Shigella* into its replicative niche, the host cell cytosol. Cytosolic replication of *Shigella* is also facilitated through the injection of a second wave of T3SS effectors that function to damp the host

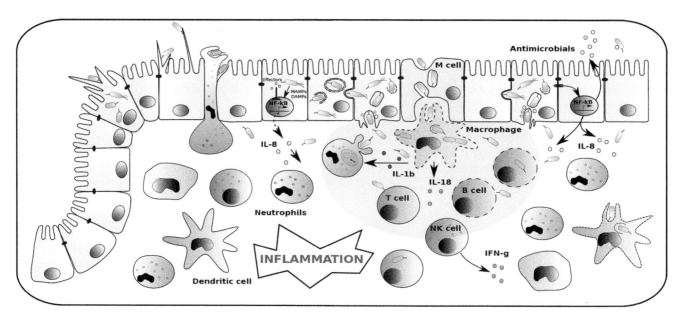

Figure 1 *Shigella* pathogenesis. *Shigella* infects the colonic epithelium at the follicle-associated epithelium and near the opening of colonic crypts. Invasion of M cells leads to *Shigella* transcytosis and release of *Shigella* at the basolateral side of the epithelium. *Shigella* can be taken up by macrophages and dendritic cells, which subsequently undergo pyroptosis, stimulating inflammation through the release of IL-1β and IL-18, which recruit neutrophils and activate innate defenses. *Shigella* also efficiently invades the basolateral side of the colonic epithelium from the lamina propria to reach its major replicative niche and the epithelial cell cytosol and propagate infection through cell-to-cell spread.

inflammatory response, promote host cell survival, and counteract antimicrobial processes. This ensures the integrity of its cytosolic niche and favorable conditions for replication and continued dissemination.

Although the inflammatory response is antagonized by *Shigella* effectors in infected epithelial cells, neighboring bystander cells actively participate in the inflammatory process by secreting the neutrophil chemoattractant IL-8 (8). Release of IL-8 from epithelial cells, in addition to release of the proinflammatory cytokines IL-1β and IL-18 by pyroptotic macrophages, fosters inflammation, the recruitment and activation of immune cells, including natural killer (NK) cells and particularly neutrophils, and antimicrobial defenses. Transmigration of neutrophils to the luminal side participates in the destabilization of the epithelial barrier and provides a means for luminal *Shigella* to translocate to the basolateral side. The host inflammatory response thereby can facilitate *Shigella* dissemination.

However, *Shigella* has devised numerous strategies to inhibit the host inflammatory response, subvert host innate immune responses, and maintain its privileged cytosolic replicative niche in order to prolong survival in the host. Ultimately, however, inflammation and neutrophil-mediated killing of *Shigella* lead to clearance of the infection. Neutrophils are particularly important in *Shigella* containment and resolution of infection, as they are more resistant than macrophages to *Shigella*-mediated cell death and can kill *Shigella* through phagocytosis, production of reactive oxygen species, and release of microbicidal molecules from their granules (degranulation) (9). In addition, *Shigella* induces neutrophil extracellular traps, whereby neutrophil death is accompanied by the release of nuclear chromatin and bactericidal proteins to immobilize and kill *Shigella* (10). Notably, *Shigella* also uses its T3SS and effectors to block the host from mounting an efficient adaptive immune response not only by suppressing innate immune response but also by directly targeting and subverting host processes of B and T cells.

SHIGELLA T3SS AND T3SS EFFECTORS

The T3SS apparatus and the majority of the ~30 T3SS effectors secreted by the T3SS are encoded on a large (~200-kb) virulence plasmid (Fig. 2) (11). Genes encoding the structural components of the T3SS apparatus, effectors involved in cellular invasion, and the main transcriptional regulators VirB and MxiE are located in a 31-kb pathogenicity island termed the entry region (12). Conversely, effectors whose genes are scattered throughout the plasmid are generally involved in

postinvasion processes. Expression of the T3SS and its effectors is under tight control of a regulatory network that responds to environmental cues encountered during transit through the host. The major trigger for the expression of the T3SS apparatus and the first wave of effectors involved in the host cell invasion is a shift to 37°C. Other factors that affect virulence gene expression are pH, osmolarity, and iron availability (3). A shift to 37°C induces the transcription of the transcriptional activator VirF, leading to the expression of IcsA, an adhesin and the actin nucleator required for cytosolic actin-based motility, as well as the transcription factor VirB. VirB, in turn, induces transcription of structural components of the T3SS apparatus (*mxi-spa* genes), effectors that mediate bacterial entry, and some additional effectors (3). A second wave of effectors, under the control of MxiE, is transcriptionally induced upon activation of the T3SS (Fig. 2A).

The T3SS is composed of a basal body spanning both the inner and outer bacterial membrane, a long needle-like structure that protrudes from the bacterium and a tip complex composed of the translocators IpaB and IpaD (Fig. 2B). The needle is composed of repeating MxiH subunits and has been resolved to a striking precision of 0.4 Å using a combination of cryo-electron microscopy and solid-state nuclear magnetic resonance (13). The high resolution obtained through this hybrid approach, together with alanine scanning mutagenesis of MxiH and effector translocation studies (14), supports a model whereby the translocation of unfolded effector proteins through the T3SS needle lumen is mediated by effector interactions with side chains of several luminal MxiH amino acids (K79 and K72) while interaction with the D73 side chain regulates substrate release from the needle together with the translocators at the needle tip.

Three-dimensional reconstruction of transmission electron microcopy images of the T3SS needle tip revealed IpaD to be a homopentamer at the needle tip with the distal domain in an elongated conformation that controls the stepwise assembly of the tip complex (Fig. 2B) (15). Bile salt recognition leads to conformational changes in IpaD and promotes the recruitment of the hydrophobic IpaB effector distal to IpaD (16). IpaD and IpaB keep the needle complex in an "off" state so that deletion of either IpaD or IpaB renders the T3SS constitutively active or in a perpetual "on" state. Activation of the T3SS is achieved through the interaction of the needle tip complex with cholesterol and lipid rafts of the host plasma membrane (17, 18); although activation can be artificially induced through the addition of the dye Congo red. T3SS activation involves

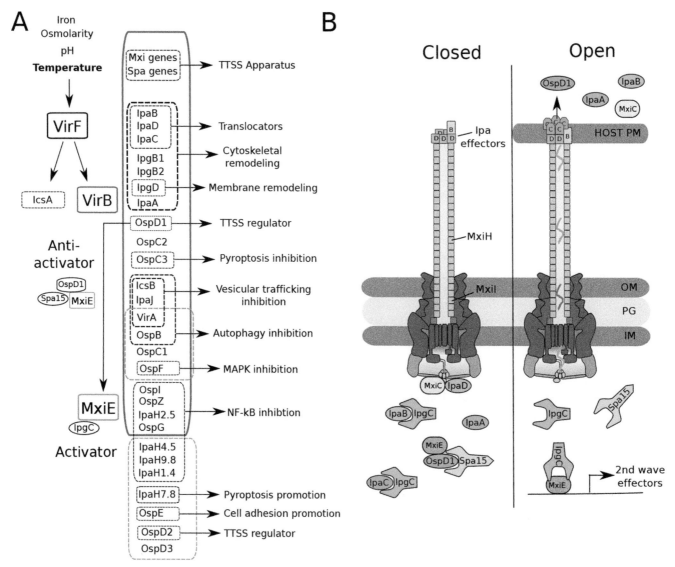

Figure 2 *Shigella* T3SS and effectors. (**A**) Expression of the T3SS apparatus and its effectors is regulated by a number of environmental factors that, through the transcription factor VirF, control the expression of the transcription factor VirB, which controls the expression of the T3SS apparatus and the first wave of effectors. Upon activation of the T3SS apparatus, MxiE is released from its inhibition and stimulates the transcription of the second wave of effectors. (**B**) When the T3SS is closed, first-wave effectors are stored in the bacterial cytoplasm with or without chaperones, while the gatekeeper MxiC and the translocator proteins IpaB and IpaD at the T3SS tip prevent effector secretion. Upon activation of the T3SS, effectors are secreted into the host cell cytosol, and expression of second-wave effectors is mediated by MxiE in complex with IpgC. IM, inner membrane; OM, outer membrane; PM, plasma membrane.

structural changes in IpaB, recruitment of the hydrophobic effector IpaC, their secretion, and the insertion of an IpaB-IpaC pore into the host membrane. Successful pore formation and opening of the T3SS lead to the secretion of MxiC, an effector that serves as a gatekeeper protein through direct interaction with IpaD to ensure that translocon proteins (IpaD, IpaB, and IpaC) are secreted before effectors (19). Removal of MxiC allows injection of the first wave of VirB-dependent *Shigella* effectors that are prestored in the bacterial cytoplasm and many of which are associated with their chaperone until the T3SS is activated (11).

Upon activation, secretion of IpaB and IpaC frees up their chaperone, IpgC, while secretion of OspD1 dissociates OspD1 from its chaperone Spa15 and the transcriptional activator MxiE, alleviating inhibition of MxiE by OspD1 (20). MxiE is free to interact with its coactivator IpgC, newly liberated from its interaction of IpaB and IpaC, to form an active MxiE-IpgC complex. The MxiE-IpgC complex drives transcription of "second-wave" effectors involved in subverting host immune responses, host innate defenses, and host cell death pathways (Fig. 2A). In addition, MxiE further upregulates expression of some VirB-regulated effectors containing an MxiE recognition sequence (called the MxiE box) as part of their promoters.

The highly coordinated and hierarchical regulatory network that controls the synthesis of the T3SS and its effectors maximizes energy usage and ensures controlled release of effectors in time and space. This was recently investigated using a novel transcription-based secretion activity reporter in combination with fluorescence recovery after photobleaching (21). In this system, control of green fluorescent protein synthesis was placed downstream of the MxiE-regulated promoter of the second-wave effector IpaH7.8 and thereby served as a visual reporter for MxiE activity and a surrogate for T3SS activity during infection. The secretion activity reporter revealed tight control of T3SS activity during infection whereby the T3SS is active upon entry, shut off during cytosolic growth, and reactivated when bacteria form protrusions into neighboring cells for cell-to-cell spread.

Functional screening using a novel bottom-up, reductionist approach of heterologous expression of the *Shigella* T3SS and individual effectors in *E. coli* recently identified OspD2 as a T3SS regulator that limits effector secretion during cytosolic growth (22). By limiting VirA secretion, OspD2 functionally reduces epithelial cell death fostered by VirA-mediated calpain activation (23). In addition, T3SS shutdown during cytosolic growth allows the resynthesis and storage of effectors required for phagosomal lysis and facilitates escape from the secondary vacuole during cell-to-cell spread (21).

Shigella effectors and virulence factors exhibit various biochemical activities to subvert host cell processes. These include phosphorylation, dephosphorylation, deamination, demyristoylation, stimulation of GTP hydrolysis of small GTPases, promotion of GDP-GTP exchange of small GTPases, and ubiquitination. Polyubiquitination generally leads to degradation of the tagged protein by host proteasomes, although ubiquitination can also function in host cell signaling, transcriptional regulation, DNA damage control, and membrane trafficking. Ubiquitination is a recurring feature in the subversion of

the host by *Shigella*, mainly because *Shigella* codes for a large IpaH effector family composed of five plasmid-encoded members and seven chromosome-encoded paralogs (24). IpaHs contain an N-terminal leucine-rich repeat domain involved in specific binding to target proteins and a C-terminal region with E3 ubiquitin ligase activity that mediates the ubiquitination of a bound target protein and subsequent ubiquitin-dependent degradation by host proteasomes (25, 26).

SHIGELLA OVERCOMES THE PHYSICOCHEMICAL BARRIERS OF THE HOST AND THE GUT MICROBIOTA TO REACH THE COLONIC EPITHELIUM

Shigella infects the colonic epithelium but first needs to overcome multiple barriers to reach the epithelial surface. For one, *Shigella* has to compete with the resident microbiota and overcome the microbiota-mediated colonization resistance. Streptomycin treatment, and thus reduction in the resident microbiota, facilitates *Shigella* infection (27), but how the resident microbiota restricts *Shigella* infection remains somewhat unclear. Microbiota-mediated colonization resistance can be either indirect, by the stimulation of host defenses such as antimicrobial peptides, or direct, by, for example, the secretion of small-molecule inhibitors such as colicins to kill phylogenetically related strains, scavenging of essential nutrients, or contact-dependent injection of toxins through the T6SS. To be competitive in the interbacterial war of the microbiota, *Shigella* has been described to resist colicins, through modulation of the O-antigen chain length of its LPS, as well as to itself produce colicins to kill competing bacterial strains (2). In addition, some *Shigella* spp., such as *S. sonnei*, code for a T6SS that provides a competitive advantage over T6SS-deficient strains to infect the host (28).

To prime itself for infection and activate its own defenses, *Shigella* also senses environmental changes specific to the host as it transits through the intestine. *Shigella* survives the acid environment of the stomach through an effective acid resistance system (3, 29). In the small intestine, *Shigella* becomes primed for adhesion through the presence of bile salts. First, the surface protein IcsA, whose transcription is temperature dependent and is induced when *Shigella* enters the host, undergoes bile salt-dependent structural changes that lead to enhanced polar adhesion of *Shigella* to epithelial cells (30). In addition, the transcription of the effectors OspE1 and -2 is induced by bile salts and leads to an OspE1/2-mediated increase in cellular adhesion (31). In the colon, *Shigella* secretes mucinases to facilitate their crossing of the mucus layer in order the reach the epithelial surface. There, oxygen sensing plays an integral part in priming *Shigella* for infection. While strict anaerobes are largely restricted to the colon, where luminal oxygen concentrations are very low, oxygen concentrations are elevated at the epithelial surface due to diffusion of oxygen from the oxygenated epithelium. Oxygen levels remain highest at the epithelial surface, as oxygen diffusion may be limited by the thick mucus layer. While the transcription of the T3SS is inhibited under anaerobic conditions (32), *Shigella* senses the increased oxygen concentration at the epithelial surface to activate their T3SS and enhance invasion, thereby avoiding unnecessary activation of its T3SS when physically far from its cellular target (33).

SHIGELLA INVADES COLONOCYTES AND ELICITS HELP FROM THE HOST TO REACH THE EPITHELIUM

Once *Shigella* crosses the mucus layer, it reaches the colonic epithelium. This single-layer intestinal epithelium provides a physical barrier between the contents of the intestinal lumen and the immune system of the host and is a critical part of the host defense system. Tight junctions located near the apical side link neighboring epithelial cells together to form a fluid-impermeable barrier. However, regulated sampling of luminal contents does occur through specialized M cells of the follicle-associated epithelium (FAE) overlying Peyer's patches and smaller mucosal lymphoid tissues, such as cryptopatches, isolated lymphoid follicles, and colonic patches. Experiments in monkeys and morphological analysis of rectal biopsy samples from shigellosis patients identified the FAE of the colon as the first site targeted by *Shigella* (34, 35). More targeted analysis of *Shigella* interactions with the FAE of small intestinal Peyer's patches using rabbit ileal loop models supported the early interaction of *Shigella* with the FAE and specifically implicated M cells as the entry portal (36–38). These observations, together with the observation that *Shigella* invades the basolateral side of polarized colonocytes *in vitro* much more efficiently than the apical side, established M cells as the main entry portal of *Shigella*. However, the early steps of invasion are still not clear. The relatively recently developed colonic guinea pig infection model (39) has highlighted *Shigella*'s ability to also interact and invade the apical side of colonocytes. At the same time, *Shigella* infection of epithelial cells *in vitro* has provided interesting insights into the interaction of *Shigella* with the apical side of epithelial cells.

Shigella is nonflagellated and therefore does not use flagellum-mediated motility to either reach the colonic mucosa or carry out close interaction with the host epithelium. Instead, *Shigella* elicits the help of the host to reach the epithelial surface. Time-lapse video microscopy of *Shigella* infection of epithelial cells *in vitro* has revealed that *Shigella* can be captured by nanometer-width micropodial extensions resembling filopodia that extend from the epithelial cell body (40). Capture of *Shigella* triggers retraction of the filopodia, effectively bringing *Shigella* into close proximity to the cell body, where invasion can then proceed. Filopodium-mediated motility can be considered a pathogenic feature of *Shigella*, as it is dependent on the T3SS and particularly on a functional IpaB and IpaD tip complex. Thus, *Shigella* T3SS mutants are captured less often, and capture does not stimulate filopodial retraction. During infection of polarized colonocytes, these filopodial-capture events mostly occur at cell-cell junctions, and in addition to enhancing invasion efficiency, filopodial capture of *Shigella* facilitates the entry of multiple bacteria within one entry focus.

Filopodium-mediated capture by *Shigella* is enhanced by host cell signaling in response to *Shigella* infection through Ca^{2+}-mediated release of ATP via connexin hemichannels at the plasma membrane. ATP sensing then leads to Erk1/2 activation, which stimulates filopodium retraction through enhancement of actin retrograde flow (40). Measurements of stall forces for the retraction of single filopodia using optical tweezers suggests that interactions of only a limited number of *Shigella* T3SS with receptors on the filopodial tip is sufficient for a high retraction stall force of 10 pN (41). In comparison, a maximal stall force of 8 pN was reached with beads heavily coated with *Yersinia* invasin, a β1 integrin ligand.

In addition, it was recently shown that *Shigella* membrane proteins are targeted by human defensin 5 (HD5) and that this interaction promotes *Shigella* adhesion and invasion of colonocytes both *in vitro* and in several *in vivo* models (42). Enhanced attachment and invasion were specific to HD5 and did not occur with mouse cryptdins, leaving open the possibility that HD5-mediated infection participates in the narrow host range of *Shigella*. The investigation of the interaction and invasion of the apical side of colonocytes by *Shigella* has been facilitated by new *in vivo* and *ex vivo* models. Indeed, the analysis of *Shigella* invasion of the colon, the natural site of infection, was long hindered due to the lack of a suitable infection model. This limitation was recently overcome through the development of a guinea pig colonic infection model that largely recapitulates the disease phenotype in humans (39).

Although the guinea pig model generally suffers from a shortage of available reagents to interrogate the host immune response, infection with *Shigella* can be monitored using simple fluorescent markers of the actin cytoskeleton. Interrogation of *Shigella* infection of the guinea pig colon using advanced quantitative bioimaging and correlative light and electron microscopy revealed that *Shigella* preferentially associates with colonic crypts and invades colonocytes located at the crypt mouth while rarely reaching the base of the crypt, where stem cells are located in their protected niche (43). Similarly, *Shigella* is preferentially found at crypt openings during early interactions with human colonic explants (44). In the guinea pig model, *Shigella* infection of cryptoproximal colonocytes is followed by spreading of the bacteria within the epithelium and increasing levels of tissue destruction until the infection is controlled by the host immune system. As seen in human rectal biopsy samples, *Shigella* infection does not generally reach the level of the intestinal crypt, although shigellosis and the associated vascular lesions do lead to an increase in mitotic activity in the crypt (43). Under these circumstances, direct invasion of colonocytes near the crypt opening likely delays the interaction of *Shigella* with macrophages to a later time point in the infection process.

SHIGELLA LIKELY TRAVERSES THE COLONIC EPITHELIUM THROUGH M CELLS

M cells are part of the specialized epithelium overlying mucosa-associated lymphoid tissue, including cryptopatches, isolated lymphoid follicles, and Peyer's patches of the small intestine as well as colonic patches (45). These secondary lymphoid tissues are inductive sites for adaptive B and T cell immune responses against antigens found in the intestinal lumen. Compared to neighboring villus epithelial cells, the FAE is characterized by reduced levels of mucus, antimicrobial peptides, and fucosylation and a site more easily accessible to antigens and microbes. M cells are best characterized as part of the small intestinal Peyer's patches, as these are large and accessible lymphoid structures. Lymphoid tissues of the large intestine resemble Peyer's patches but are smaller and less discernible with fewer follicles and smaller germinal centers, the sites where B cells are activated, proliferate, switch immunoglobulin class, and increase immunoglobulin antigen affinity by somatic hypermutation. Small intestinal Peyer's patches instead bulge out of the intestinal wall, allowing easy identification, and therefore often serve as proxies for the interaction of microbes with lymphoid tissue.

M cells are involved in immunosurveillance by the host and are characterized by their lack of microvilli, an apical microfold structure, and a large pocket-like invagination on their basolateral side (45). These cells are thereby structured to mediate the controlled sampling of antigens and bacteria from the intestinal lumen and transcytose these to the basolateral side, where antigen-presenting cells such as macrophages and dendritic cells are strategically located in or near the M cell pocket to kill commensals and process antigens. Like other enteropathogenic bacteria, *Shigella* can hijack this specialized M cell portal to breach the protective intestinal barrier and gain access to the basolateral side of the epithelium.

In both the mouse and rabbit ileal loop models, *Shigella* invades M cells overlying Peyer's patches early during infection (36, 37, 46). Notably, little is still known about the interaction of *Shigella* with M cells, as this interaction remains to be investigated in detail on a cellular level. However, time course analysis coupled with transmission electron microscopy of rabbit ileal loops suggests that *Shigella* does not access the M cell cytosol but rather traverses M cells in endocytic vacuoles (36). *Shigella* transcytosis is not generally associated with significant cytotoxicity to the M cells and thus leaves the entry portal intact (36). After transcytosis, *Shigella* is captured by macrophages residing in the M cell pocket and in the subepithelial dome of the Peyer's patches. Macrophages are, however, largely unable to contain *Shigella* in the phagosomal compartment. Instead, *Shigella* reaches the macrophage cytosol and the macrophage undergoes pyroptotic death, allowing *Shigella* to escape to the lamina propria.

SHIGELLA ESCAPES MACROPHAGES BY INDUCING PYROPTOSIS

The main functions of macrophages are to detect and phagocytose microbes, to kill them, and to coordinate an inflammatory response to regain sterility. Due to their central role in clearing infections, pathogens have devised strategies to subvert them. Macrophages are used by some pathogens, such as *Listeria monocytogenes*, as replicative niches and Trojan horses to reach deeper tissues. *Listeria* therefore evolved to support macrophage survival in order to safeguard its replicative cytosolic niche. Unlike *Listeria*, *Shigella* does not generally disseminate into deeper tissues and instead aims to rapidly escape from the macrophage to reach and invade its preferred replicative niche, the colonic epithelium. *Shigella* escapes from macrophages by triggering and actively promoting pyroptotic macrophage death (Fig. 3) (47).

Pyroptosis is a highly inflammatory type of programmed cell death that links the detection of danger

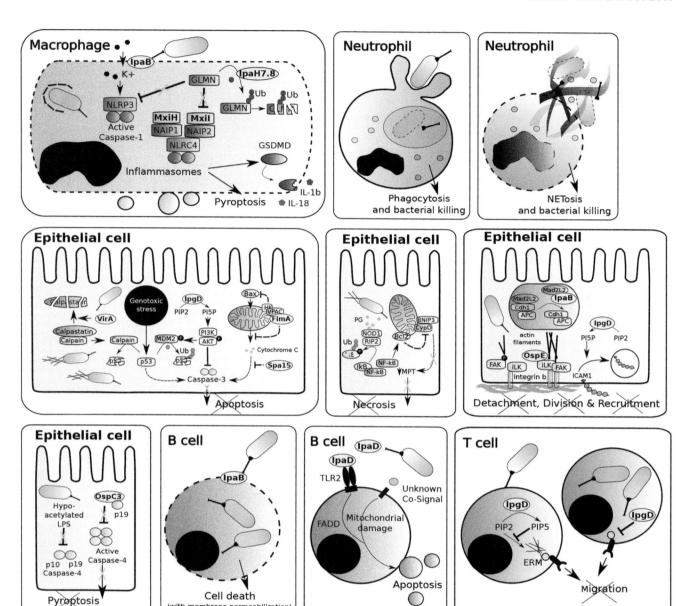

Figure 3 *Shigella* subversion of host cell survival, integrity, and function. *Shigella* produces numerous effectors that subvert various host cell processes to promote its virulence. Upon invasion of epithelial cells, numerous effectors function to protect the cytosolic replicative niche of *Shigella* by antagonizing host cell death (apoptosis, pyroptosis, and necrosis), promoting host cell integrity, and inhibiting the recruitment of neutrophils, which kill *Shigella*. Conversely, *Shigella* actively promotes host cell death in infected macrophages. For immune cells, *Shigella* mediates B cell death and the inhibition of T cell migration in infected and noninfected cells.

signals known as microbe-associated molecular patterns (MAMPs) and danger-associated molecular patterns (DAMPs) by cytosolic pattern recognition receptors (PRRs) to the release of proinflammatory cytokines and lytic cell death (48). Rupture of the infected cell in turn releases cytokines and DAMPs such as ATP and

DNA, which further augment the proinflammatory environment and lead to the recruitment of immune cells. Pyroptosis is therefore an antimicrobial response to intracellular pathogens activated when the host cell has been compromised and MAMPs are sensed in the host cell cytoplasm. It thereby serves to release the invading bacteria into the extracellular space, making them accessible for killing by the more bactericidal neutrophils while concomitantly alerting the immune system to the intruder.

Pyroptosis, like apoptosis, is mediated through the controlled activation of caspases, which are aspartate-specific cysteine proteases that cleave cellular targets to ultimately kill the cell (48, 49). Unlike apoptosis, a non-inflammatory programmed cell death, pyroptosis involves the activation of inflammatory caspases, such as caspase-1 and caspase-11 in mice and caspase-4 and -5 in humans. The canonical inflammasome is a multiprotein complex composed of activated PRRs and, depending on the PRR, the adaptor protein-associated speck-like protein and caspase-1, previously known as IL-1β-converting enzyme (50). Three types of cytosolic PRRs sense a wide variety of MAMPS: the nucleotide-binding oligomerization domain (NOD)-like receptor (NLR) family, the Aim2 (absent in melanoma 2)-like receptor family, and the retinoic acid-inducible gene-related I-like receptor family. Activation of a subset of these cytosolic PRRs leads to inflammasome formation and caspase-1 activation.

Direct sensing of bacterial compounds is achieved by Aim2, a bacterial double-stranded DNA sensor, and NLRC4/IPAF, a PRR coreceptor that links the recognition of conserved bacterial proteins such as flagella and T3SS rod and needle proteins by neuronal apoptosis inhibitory proteins (NAIPs) to caspase-1 activation. Conversely, indirect sensing of bacterial infection through sensing of pathogenicity patterns is achieved by NLRP1B, a sensor for the proteolytic activity of bacterial toxins (e.g., *Bacillus anthracis* lethal factor); by NLRP3, a PRR activated by a wide range of MAMPs and DAMPs that lead to host cell changes such as potassium efflux, production of reactive oxygen species, and lysosomal destabilization; and by pyrin, a sensor for the deactivation of a subset of small GTPases (RhoA, -B, and -C) involved in cytoskeleton regulation and a frequent target of bacterial effectors.

Upon its activation by the inflammasome, caspase-1 cleaves and activates the proinflammatory cytokines IL-1β and IL-18 and the cellular protein gasdermin D (49). Activated gasdermin D oligomerizes and forms pores in host membranes that allow the release of the proinflammatory cytokine IL-1β but eventually lead to water influx, cell swelling, host cell lysis, and release of the cellular contents. Gasdermin D-mediated host cell death can also be induced by the activation of caspase-11, or its human homolog, through direct sensing of the cytosolic hexa-acyl lipid A moiety of LPS. The secreted proinflammatory cytokines IL-1β and IL-18 bind to the IL-1 and related IL-18 receptors, respectively, to trigger

NF-κB- and mitogen-activated protein kinase (MAPK)-signaling pathways in a MyD88- and TRAF-dependent manner, leading to release of additional proinflammatory cytokines such as tumor necrosis factor alpha and IL-6. IL-1β also functions to recruit neutrophils and to stimulate a Th17 response, while IL-18 stimulates T and NK cells to produce gamma interferon, which enhances the antimicrobial activity of macrophages by inducing nitric oxide production.

In *Shigella*-infected macrophages, pyroptotic host cell death requires phagosomal escape of *Shigella* and is mediated by the NLRC4 inflammasome, with some contribution from the NLRP3 inflammasome (Fig. 3) (47, 51). *Shigella* first escapes the phagosome with the help of the pore-forming activity of the IpaC-IpaB translocon at the tip of the T3SS. Pore formation by IpaB allows influx of potassium, and phagosomal rupture releases vacuolar contents and results in membrane damage that may be recognized and serves to activate the NLRC4 inflammasome (47). In addition, during cytosolic replication, the T3SS rod and needle proteins MxiH and MxiI are sensed by NAIP1 and NAIP2 of the NLR family and activate NAIP-dependent NLRC4 inflammasomes, triggering caspase-1 activation and pyroptosis (52–55). *Shigella* LPS is also sensed by human caspase-4, exacerbating the pro-death response.

Notably, *Shigella* is not an innocent bystander in triggering macrophage cell death but actively promotes caspase-1 activation and pyroptosis, as the T3SS-secreted E3 ubiquitin ligase IpaH7.8 was shown to ubiquitinate glomulin, an inhibitor of NALP3/NLRC4 inflammasome activity, and target it for degradation by host proteasomes (26). Loss of glomulin inhibition leads to inflammasome activation and pyroptosis. Notably, in the absence of IpaH7.8, intranasal challenge of mice with *Shigella* leads to a reduction in macrophage cell death, reduced IL-1β production, and less extensive colonization. Thus, although pyroptosis serves as an antimicrobial defense mechanism of the host, *Shigella* actively promotes it and, at least in the early stages of the infection, uses it to its advantage. Pyroptosis of infected macrophages releases *Shigella* near the basolateral side of the epithelium, which *Shigella* invades to reach its replicative niche, the epithelial cell cytosol.

ADHESION AND FORCED ENTRY INTO NONPHAGOCYTIC HOST CELLS

Shigella interacts with several host receptors to adhere to epithelial cells and to favor insertion of the T3SS tip complex, which is required for epithelial cell invasion. The needle complex components IpaB, IpaC, and IpaD can bind $\alpha_5\beta_1$ integrins, and their overexpression in Chinese hamster ovary cells increases invasion efficiency of *Shigella* in these cells (56). In addition, IpaB can bind to CD44, a hyaluronic acid receptor, to mediate entry. Expression of CD44 in host cells increases *Shigella* adhesion, while treatment of CD44-expressing cells with a monoclonal antibody directed against CD44 decreases *Shigella* invasion (57). Both $\alpha_5\beta_1$ integrins and CD44 are surface receptors that interact with the extracellular matrix and, as expected, are located on the basolateral side of polarized epithelial cells, supporting a role for these receptors in the basolateral invasion of *Shigella*. *Shigella* may also use IcsA-mediated adhesion to a yet-undefined receptor to facilitate entry during basolateral invasion of epithelial cells.

Unlike *L. monocytogenes*, which induces a zipper-type uptake into epithelial cells, *Shigella* uses a trigger mechanism that results in extensive ruffle formation at the cell surface. Ruffle formation and invasion are mediated by a combination of changes in membrane tension, host cell signaling, and hijacking of the host actin cytoskeleton, although other cytoskeletal components, such as intermediate filaments, are also implicated. Cellular actin cytoskeletal rearrangements are largely regulated through p21 Rho-family small GTPases, including Rho, Rac, and Cdc42 GTPases. These master regulators of actin dynamics are molecular switches. In their GTP-bound "on" state, they activate a range of host factors to promote actin dynamics. When the intrinsic GTPase activity of the small GTPases is stimulated by GTPase-activating proteins (GAPs), GTP is hydrolyzed to GDP and renders the small GTPase in its "off" state. The replacement of GDP with GTP is then promoted by guanine nucleotide exchange factors. Through this cycling between the GTP- and GDP-bound states, these small GTPases drive actin dynamics.

Overall, *Shigella* promotes ruffle formation and entry by stimulating actin cytoskeleton remodeling and actin polymerization through a complex but coordinated process involving numerous effectors, including IpaC, IpaA, VirA, IpgD, and the guanine nucleotide exchange factors IpgB1 and IpgB2. Upon insertion into the host membrane, the C terminus of IpaC faces the cytoplasm and directly binds to the intermediate filaments vimentin and keratin 18 (58). The IpaC-vimentin interaction is necessary for stable docking of *Shigella* with the host cell membrane and a requirement for the secretion of effectors (58). The IpaC C terminus also stimulates actin polymerization and actin remodeling through Cdc42, Rac1, and the activation of the tyrosine kinase Src (59). The role of these host factors has been addressed through targeted inhibition in host cells. Thus, inhibi-

tion of Cdc42 blocks *Shigella*-induced membrane extensions and inhibition of Rac activity interferes with lamellae formation, while inhibition of the Src pathway blocks cellular extensions and *Shigella* engulfment and reduces entry by a factor of 10. Src activation by IpaC leads to the phosphorylation and activation of the actin-binding protein cortactin, which in turn interacts with the Arp2/3 complex and the Src-related tyrosine kinase CrK to stimulate actin polymerization and actin remodeling around the entry site.

IpaA is also a critical effector for entry, as an IpaA deletion mutant exhibits a 10-fold entry defect (60). IpaA regulates formation of actin protrusions and counteracts the uncontrolled formation of microspike structures induced by IpaC by promoting actin filament depolymerization (60). IpaA directly binds vinculin, a cytosolic actin-binding protein that is enriched in focal adhesions and links integrin adhesion molecules to the actin cytoskeleton (61). Binding of vinculin to the C-terminal domain of IpaA enhances vinculin affinity for F-actin, thereby partially capping the barbed end of actin filaments to inhibit monomer addition and promoting F-actin depolymerization. At the same time, IpaA promotes actin cytoskeletal rearrangements by targeting $\beta 1$ integrins and stimulating the GTPase activity of the small GTPase RhoA, rendering RhoA inactive. Through the ROCK (Rho-associated protein kinase)–myosin II pathway, this leads to stress fiber disassembly and the freeing up of actin for membrane ruffle formation.

IpgB1, like IpaC, stimulates Rac1 and Cdc42 activity and, by stabilizing them in their GTP-bound state, promotes ruffle formation in an Arp2/3 complex-dependent manner. In the absence of IpgB1, invasion is reduced twofold. In addition, VirA may indirectly destabilize microtubules to promote Rac1 activity (62, 63). In contrast to IpaA, IpgB2 stimulates actin nucleation and stress fiber formation by stimulating GDP-GTP exchange in RhoA. *Shigella* thereby targets stress fibers for disassembly and formation in a coordinated fashion to promote bacterial entry. Entry is also supported by the hydrolysis of phosphatidylinositol 4,5-bisphosphate [PI(4,5)P2] by the effector IpgD. This activity loosens the connection between cortical actin and the membrane to facilitate actin dynamics at the invasion site (64).

Entry is furthermore dependent on local calcium signaling induced by *Shigella* (65). T3SS translocators, likely through their pore-forming activity, stimulate the activity of host phospholipases C-β1 and C-γ1, leading to the production of InsP3 through the hydrolysis of PIP2. A local increase in InsP3 at the invasion site and its binding to recruited InsP3 receptors on the endoplasmic reticulum (ER) leads to an atypical and highly localized

Ca^{2+} response. Fluorescent recovery after photobleaching revealed that bacterially induced actin reorganization at the site of entry hinders diffusion of small molecules, thereby restricting diffusion of InsP3, enriching InsP3 receptors, and favoring sustained local Ca^{2+} increases that are of long (tens of seconds) duration, peaking 15 minutes after *Shigella* makes contact with the host cell (66). In addition, long-lasting local Ca^{2+} signals are promoted by hydrolysis of PI(4,5)P2 through IpgD, which effectively limits the substrate pool available to host phospholipases and thereby restricts the generation, and subsequent diffusion, of InsP3 (67). Low InsP3 diffusion curbs the release of Ca^{2+} stores from the ER, thereby also maintaining cell integrity by preventing Ca^{2+}-mediated disassembly of focal adhesions (67). These atypical local Ca^{2+} responses are critical for entry; more global Ca^{2+} responses with slower dynamics follow and, while not critical to entry, facilitate *Shigella* invasion by filopodial capture. *Shigella* mediates these atypical Ca^{2+} responses through IpgD.

PHAGOSOMAL ESCAPE OF *SHIGELLA FLEXNERI*

Shigella invasion of epithelial cells and phagosomal escape are difficult processes to investigate because they are rapid events that last less than 15 minutes. Phagosomal rupture is dependent on a functional T3SS and is facilitated by a number of *Shigella* effectors, including IpgB1, IpgB2, and IpgD, that each contribute a small amount to the efficiency of phagosomal lysis (68, 69). Small interfering RNA screens and advanced large-volume correlative light electron microscopy have recently yielded new insights into the invasion and phagosomal escape process of *Shigella* (68, 70). Despite the massive ruffling induced upon invasion, *Shigella* is found in a tight vacuole where the bacteria are in close contact with the phagosomal membrane. Ruffling leads to the formation of macropinosomes surrounding the entry site, but while macropinosomes take up fluid-phase markers, such as fluorescently labeled dextran, these markers are excluded from the *Shigella*-containing vacuole.

IpgD activity promotes ruffle formation and fosters the formation of macropinosomes and recruitment of the GTPase Rab11 to macropinosomes in the vicinity of bacterial entry (Fig. 4A) (70). Although Rab11 is not required for macropinosome formation, inhibition of Rab11 by expression of a dominant negative mutant delays vacuolar rupture and interferes with the entry process (70). How exactly Rab11 macropinosomes foster phagosomal lysis remains unclear. Rab11-positive macropinosomes come into direct contact with the *Shigella*-

containing vacuole but do not fuse or deliver fluid-phase markers to the phagosome (68). In nonphagocytic cells, macropinosomes recycle back to the plasma membrane with minimal interaction with the endosomal pathway and are not known to recruit Rab11, a marker of the endosomal recycling compartment. *Shigella* thereby triggers macropinosome formation but through the action of IpgD initiates a novel vesicular trafficking pathway that is dependent on the formation of modified macropinosomes to mediate phagosomal lysis.

SURVIVAL OF *SHIGELLA FLEXNERI* IN EPITHELIAL CELLS

Shigella uses the epithelial host cell cytosol as its main replicative niche and therefore has evolved mechanisms to escape host antimicrobial defenses and to safeguard its replicative niche from destruction. One major host defense mechanism that is activated and that *Shigella* must subvert in order to survive in host cells is autophagy (Fig. 4A) (71). Canonical autophagy involves around 40 autophagy-related proteins that act together in a multistep process to sequester cytoplasmic cargo, including large structures such as whole organelles, in newly generated double-membrane vacuoles. Autophagosomes mature along the endocytic pathway into autolysosomes, where lysosomal enzymes degrade their contents. The main function of this process is to recycle cellular components for the host cell and maintain cellular homeostasis.

A second critical role of autophagy is in cellular defense, whereby intracellular bacteria are targeted and delivered to autolysosomes for killing and degradation in a process termed xenophagy. During xenophagy, cytosolic bacteria are recognized by autophagy sensor proteins such as p62 and nuclear dot protein 52 (NDP52), which bind ubiquitinated proteins and the major autophagy marker LC3 to initiate autophagosome formation. Conversely, pathogens surrounded by phagosomal membranes may be targeted for lysosomal degradation by noncanonical autophagy that involves only a subset of the autophagy machinery, including the autophagy markers LC3 and Atg5. In this noncanonical pathway, phagosomes containing bacterial pathogens are distinguished by the host from endogenous vesicles through the detection of phagosomal membrane damage. Membrane damage associated with the insertion of the secretion system pores of the T3SS exposes the sugar-coated luminal side of the vacuole, which can be recognized by carbohydrate-binding proteins such as galectin-3 and galectin-8, leading to recruitment of autophagy-related proteins.

Shigella is susceptible to recognition by both the noncanonical and canonical autophagy pathways but coun-

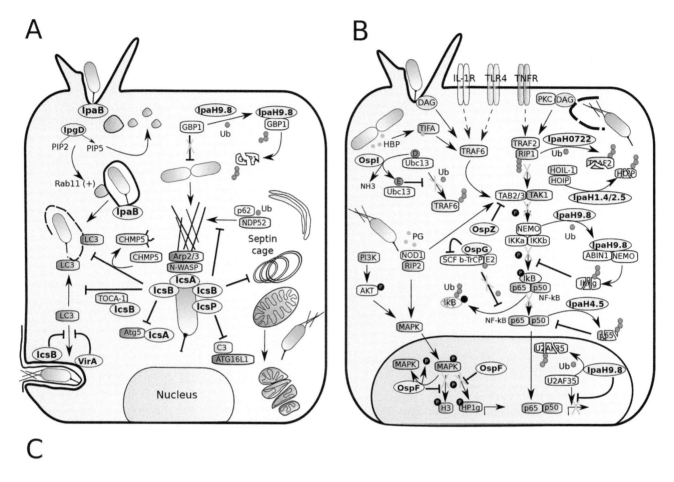

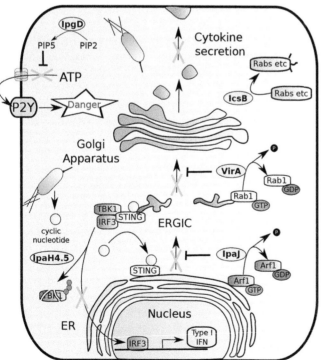

Figure 4 *Shigella* modulation of antimicrobial defenses and proinflammatory responses. (**A**) Numerous effectors have been linked to the evasion of autophagy during *Shigella* cytosolic growth and cell-to-cell spread to foster bacterial survival and propagation. The presence, replication, and spreading of *Shigella* are sensed by the cellular immune surveillance system of the host, which is linked to proinflammatory responses. *Shigella* actively counteracts the cellular proinflammatory response in epithelial cells through inhibition of key signaling pathways (**B**) and disruption of the vesicular trafficking pathways (**C**).

teracts autophagic capture through at least three effectors, IcsP, IcsB, and VirA (Fig. 4A). During initial entry, recognition of *Shigella* peptidoglycan by the cytosolic sensor NOD1 at the bacterial entry site leads to the recruitment of the autophagic factor ATG16L and stimulation of autophagy (72). In addition, *Shigella* induces a nutrient stress response that blocks mTOR signaling and leads to a stimulation of autophagy (73).

Before invasion, *Shigella* is susceptible to being recognized by the complement system, which leads to the coating of bacteria with split products of complement C3 (74). In the host cell cytosol, surface-deposited C3 targets bacteria for autophagy through a direct interaction with the autophagy marker ATG16L1 (74). *Shigella* subverts this process by the shedding of C3, in part, through the proteolytic activity of the surface protease IcsP (74). During invasion, phagosomal damage induced by the *Shigella* T3SS is recognized by galectin-3 and galectin-8, but *Shigella* escapes recruitment of the autophagic marker LC3 to the phagosome or phagosomal remnants by secreting IcsB (75). IcsB prevents LC3 and NDP52 targeting by binding to Toca-1 (transducer of CDC42-dependent actin assembly 1), a host protein necessary for efficient actin polymerization.

Biorthogonal chemical proteomic profiling, biochemical assays, and proteomic analysis using SILAC (stable isotope labelling with amino acids in cell culture) recently revealed IcsB to be an 18-carbon fatty acyltransferase catalyzing lysine N^{ε}-fatty acylation of up to 60 host proteins involved in the regulation of the actin cytoskeleton, membrane trafficking, cell-cell adherens junctions, endocytosis, and endosomal recycling (76). By stearoylating charged multivesicular body protein 5, a component of the ESCRT-III complex involved in endosomal membrane sorting, IcsB is thought to inhibit the development of the autophagic response (76).

Lysis of the phagosome allows *Shigella* access to cytosolic host factors, including those required for actin-based mobility, and enables *Shigella* to move within the cell and to ultimately reach new replicative niches in neighboring cells (77). Actin-based motility is mediated by surface-localized IcsA. IcsA acts as a mimic of the small GTPase Cdc42 to recruit neutral Wiskott-Aldrich syndrome protein, which binds actin monomers and activates the actin-related protein 2 (Arp2)–Arp3 complex to mediate actin polymerization. Arp2/Arp3 complex-mediated F-actin assembly and filament growth provide the propulsive force for *Shigella* to move in the cytosol, at speeds up to 26 µm/min, and induce membrane protrusions into neighboring cells for cell-to-cell spread. IcsP also mediates correct polar localization and cleavage of IcsA to facilitate directed motility and efficient spreading

(78), which primarily occurs at multicellular junctions involving components of the clathrin endocytic pathway (79). By hijacking the host cell cytoskeletal machinery, *Shigella* gains motility in the cytosol without itself having to invest into metabolically costly motility machinery, such as flagella, which could also be recognized as a MAMP and activate the host NLRC4 inflammasome. However, while subversion of the host cytoskeleton is an evolutionarily conserved mechanism used by pathogens to gain intracellular motility, it also triggers autophagic defense mechanisms that the pathogen then must try to counter to survive and replicate (Fig. 4A).

One way the host tries to target cytosolic *Shigella* to autophagy is through septins (80). These GTP-binding proteins are part of the cytoskeleton network, as they can form filaments that interact with cellular membranes, actin filaments, and microtubules (80). They are involved in several biological processes, including cell division, but also link the recognition of actin polymerization to the autophagic pathway. Septins are recruited to IcsA-mediated actin polymerization and form cages around cytosolic *Shigella*. Septin cages restrict *Shigella* movement and recruit the autophagic adaptors p62 and NDP52 to target *Shigella* for autophagic destruction (81). This process is antagonized by mitochondrial fragmentation through *Shigella* actin-mediated motility, as well as the effector IcsB, as wild-type cytosolic bacteria are only half as likely to show recruitment of these autophagic markers as an *icsB* mutant (82, 83). Notably, the evolutionary conservation of septin caging as an innate host defense that targets bacteria for autophagic destruction was demonstrated in a novel zebrafish *Shigella* infection model (84). In this model, as observed *in vitro* in mammalian cells, *Shigella* became trapped in p62-associated septin cages upon infection of the zebrafish, leading to p62 recruitment and autophagic restriction.

Besides the recognition of actin polymerization, the autophagic marker Atg5 directly recognizes the surface-localized protein IcsA. IcsB appears to antagonize this autophagic process by binding to IcsA, thereby masking the Atg5 recognition site and competitively inhibiting Atg5 binding to IcsA (83).

Shigella also uses the T3SS effector VirA to interfere with autophagy. Besides being important during the entry process (85), VirA counteracts autophagosome formation during cytosolic growth of *Shigella* by disrupting ER-to-Golgi vesicular trafficking. VirA activates the GTPase activity of the small GTPase Rab1, rendering Rab1 inactive and unable to direct vesicle traffic from the ER to the Golgi apparatus (86, 87). Finally, VirA and IcsB also have important functions in preventing autophagy by mediating phagosomal escape from the double-membrane phagosome formed during cell-to-cell spread. In the absence of VirA and/or IcsB, intercellular spreading is reduced as *Shigella* becomes impaired in escaping the secondary phagosome and becomes trapped in LC3-decorated phagosomes that mature to autolysosomes (88).

In addition to autophagy, *Shigella* replication and motility are further antagonized through guanylate-binding proteins (GBPs) (Fig. 4A) (89, 90). GBPs are induced by gamma interferon stimulation and mediate cell-autonomous antimicrobial defenses to a number of intracellular pathogens in a yet poorly characterized manner. However, during *Shigella* infection, IpaH9.8 specifically targets human GBP1 for ubiquitin-mediated degradation to promote *Shigella* replication and facilitate polymerization of host actin for actin-based motility.

MAINTENANCE OF THE EPITHELIAL CELL CYTOSOLIC REPLICATIVE NICHE

Aside from escaping the degradative autophagy system and spreading from cell to cell to extend its replicative niche, *Shigella* also needs to safeguard its cytosolic niche and uses several strategies to prevent host cell death (47). Since the infectious dose of *Shigella* can be as low as 10 to 100 bacteria, safeguarding its replicative niche is of particular importance early during the infection process in order to increase the bacterial load. *Shigella* evades host cell death by obstructing the activation of pro-death pathways and by activating pro-survival pathways (Fig. 3). The inhibition of epithelial cell death is impressive, as *Shigella* can replicate to high numbers (>100 bacteria) without lysing the epithelial cell, which is in stark contrast to the rapid cell death induced in macrophages.

As *Shigella* replicates in the epithelial cell cytosol, it is highly susceptible to recognition by cytosolic PRRs. One of the most abundant MAMPs, LPS, is recognized by human caspase-4 (caspase-11 in mice) and leads to pyroptotic host cell death. *Shigella*, however, limits recognition of its LPS during cytosolic growth by switching from a hexa-acylated LPS form, typically observed during growth in laboratory medium and highly stimulating for both TLR4 and caspase-11, to a tetra- and triacylated form, which is poorly recognized by these PRRs, upon cytosolic growth (91). In addition to the hypoacylation of its LPS, *Shigella* counteracts caspase-4 activity with the secretion of the late T3SS effector OspC3 (92). OspC3 binds to the p19 subunit of caspase-4 and thereby inhibits the assembly of the active caspase-4 tetramer, consisting of two p19 and two p10 subunits. In the absence of OspC3, *Shigella* infection leads to increased pyroptosis and enhanced IL-18 release by epi-

thelial cells *in vitro* and, in the *in vivo* guinea pig colon infection model, to greater cell death of the colonic mucosa and a reduction in colonizing bacteria compared to wild-type *Shigella* infection.

Shigella infection of epithelial cells also leads to host DNA damage, or genotoxic stress, which triggers the proapoptotic p53 pathway (23) (Fig. 3). This pathway is antagonized by the delivery of VirA during entry into epithelial cells. VirA binds to calpastatin, the inhibitor of calpain protease, and targets it for degradation, resulting in the activation of calpain and calpain-mediated p53 degradation. However, while calpain activation limits apoptotic host cell death during the early phase of *Shigella* infection, calpain activation during later stages promotes necrotic cell death. Strikingly, short hairpin RNA inhibition of calpain and live fluorescence video microscopy showed that in the absence of calpain, *Shigella* intracellular growth is impressively enhanced and cells resist lysis until the cells are literally bursting with bacteria (23). In addition to VirA, p53-mediated apoptosis is antagonized through the phosphoinositide phosphatase activity of IpgD. During bacterial entry, PI5P, liberated through IpgD activity on PI(4,5)P2, promotes the activation of the epidermal growth factor receptor and the downstream PI3-kinase/Akt pro-survival pathway (23, 93, 94). Akt activation inhibits p53 proapoptotic signaling through the phosphorylation and stabilization of Mdm2, an E3 ubiquitin ligase that, when activated, targets p53 for degradation.

The mitochondrion is another organelle affected by *Shigella*. Induction of mitochondrial permeability during infection releases cytochrome *c*, which is sensed by APAF-1, leading to the formation of the apoptosome, activation of caspase-9, and activation of the executioner caspase, caspase-3, resulting in apoptosis (95). *Shigella* antagonizes caspase-3-mediated apoptosis by FimA, Spa15m, and IpgD. FimA is a pilus protein that in the cytosol of infected cells antagonizes cytochrome *c* release and subsequent caspase-3 activation (96). By binding to the mitochondrial outer membrane protein VPAC, FimA strengthens the interaction of VPAC with hexokinase. This prevents hexokinase dissociation from the mitochondrial membrane, an event that triggers Bax translocation to the outer mitochondrial membrane, the formation of Bax/Bak mitochondrial outer membrane pores, loss of membrane integrity, and release of cytochrome *c*. Notably, however, *Shigella* does not have fimbriae, and FimA expression is questionable due to mutational inactivation across at least three phylogenetic groups (97).

Further down the pathway, *Shigella* inhibits caspase-3 activation in response to cytochrome *c* release and caspase-9 activation through the involvement of the T3SS chaperone Spa15, by a yet-unknown mechanism (98). In addition, secretion of the T3SS effector IpgD antagonizes caspase-3 activation again through the stimulation of the PI3-kinase/Akt pro-survival pathway (99). *Shigella* infection also leads to oxidative stress of the cell that triggers a mitochondrial permeability transition-dependent necrosis-like cell death through the signaling of the BH3-only protein BNIP3 and CypD (100). This cell death pathway is counterbalanced by the sensing of *Shigella* peptidoglycan and activation of the cytosolic PRR Nod1-mediated Rip2–IKKβ–NF-κB signaling cascade, which upregulates proinflammatory factors but also induces the expression of potent antiapoptotic factors, including Bcl-2. *Shigella* thereby uses the activation of pro-survival pathways to counteract necrotic and apoptotic cell death.

In addition to obstructing host cell death, *Shigella* also preserves its intracellular niche within the epithelial layer by promoting the adhesion of infected cells to the basement membrane and preventing cell division. To ensure adhesion, the *Shigella* T3SS effector OspE is recruited to focal adhesions, where it interacts with the integrin-like kinase ILK, reduces focal adhesion kinase phosphorylation, and increases surface β1 integrins (101). The OspE-ILK complex thereby promotes epithelial adhesion to the basal membrane by inhibiting focal adhesion disassembly (101, 102) (Fig. 3). To prevent division, and the accompanying reduction of adhesion to neighboring cells and the lamina propria, the *Shigella* effector IpaB can mediate cell cycle arrest by interfering with the binding of the anaphase-promoting complex inhibitor Mad2L2 to Cdh1 (103), which is part of the anaphase-promoting complex and is involved in preventing mitosis by suppressing mitotic cyclins needed to enter mitosis. Lack of binding of Mad2L2 to Cdh1 keeps Cdh1 constitutively active and prevents cells from undergoing mitosis. Additionally, the phosphatase activity of IpgD that generates PI5P favors the internalization and subsequent degradation of ICAM-1 in infected epithelial cells, thereby reducing the adhesion of neutrophils and the inflammation and tissue destruction associated with their recruitment (104).

Through these multiple mechanisms, *Shigella* safeguards its replicative niche and ensures sufficient time to replicate extensively in the host cell and to spread to neighboring cells.

REPLICATION OF *SHIGELLA* IN THE EPITHELIAL CELL CYTOSOL

Unlike intravacuolar pathogens, such as *Salmonella*, which need strategies to acquire nutrients in the phago-

somal compartment and to subvert the endomembrane system of the host to prevent the maturation of the phagosome into hostile and degradative lysosomal compartments, *Shigella* enters and replicates in what is considered a relatively nutrient-rich environment of the cytosol. Transcriptional profiling and global proteomic analysis of *Shigella* during cytosolic growth have given a good overview of the metabolic changes that accompany *Shigella* adaptation to the cytosolic replicative niche. In contrast to its extracellular growth, *Shigella* adapts to the low-oxygen environment of the epithelial cytosol by downregulating enzymes involved in oxidative respiration and increasing expression of enzymes involved in glycolysis and mixed-acid fermentation (105). *Shigella* also increases fructose and mannose importers as well as the dipeptide transporter DppA to scavenge nutrients from the host. Transcriptional profiling also suggests that the cytosolic environment of epithelial cells is not a particularly stressful environment as, at least in the *in vitro* system, *Shigella* does not upregulate stress response proteins, such as nitric oxide dioxygenase, during cytosolic growth compared to growth in broth (105).

A notable exception is iron stress. Due to the inherent toxicity of iron, the host limits intracellular iron concentrations and sequesters free iron by expressing iron-binding proteins. Iron is an essential micronutrient for *Shigella* growth, and *Shigella* can capture intracellular iron through multiple routes, including the expression of siderophores and uptake of heme or ferric and ferrous iron through dedicated iron transport systems, which *Shigella* upregulates in response to the low iron accessibility in the cytosolic milieu (106). However, overall, nutrients are not limiting for *Shigella* growth in the host cell cytosol, as *Shigella* maintains an extremely high growth rate during cytosolic growth, doubling around every 37 minutes, similar to what is seen in rich nutrient broth (107). Analysis of auxotrophic mutants of *Shigella* also indicates that *Shigella* has access to diverse amino acids in sufficient quantities, while availability of host fatty acids, purine nucleosides, and some amino acids, such as asparagine and proline, is limiting.

While *Shigella* obtains a substantial amount of biomass through uptake of nutrients, metabolite mass spectrometry using ^{13}C glucose isotype tracking revealed that *Shigella* derives its energy almost exclusively from pyruvate during cytosolic growth in HeLa cells (107). Pyruvate is a particularly abundant metabolite in HeLa cells, as these cancer cells mostly rely on glycolytic pathways rather than the oxidative tricarboxylic acid cycle for energy production. *Shigella* metabolizes pyruvate into acetate using the low-yield but high-speed acetate pathway. The acetate pathway is a typical pathway used during rapid growth under nutrient-rich conditions in *Enterobacteriaceae* because although it produces only one ATP per pyruvate molecule, it also uses only two enzymes and can therefore rapidly generate energy to sustain rapid growth. Infected host cells are therefore not compromised for energy output, as *Shigella* infection does not affect the host's main energy pathways. Rather, *Shigella* efficiently uses the waste product of the host energy production to power its replication.

Shigella infection of epithelial cells does, however, activate metabolic stress responses, as metabolic labeling of *de novo* protein synthesis shows a global shutdown of host protein synthesis, particularly early within the first two hours during infection (108). *Shigella* infection triggers the host amino acid starvation response whereby activation of the sensor kinase GCN2 (general control nonderepressible 2) leads to downstream phosphorylation of the master regulator eIF2α (eukaryotic initiation factor 2α) (73). Phosphorylated eIF2α blocks translation initiation on a global scale while selectively enhancing translation of the transcription factor ATF4, which together with ATF3 enhances transcription of stress-related genes involved in amino acid metabolism and protection against oxidative damage. Nutrient limitation is also sensed through the mechanistic target of rapamycin (mTOR) pathway and leads to its inhibition. Inhibition of the mTOR pathway during *Shigella* infection stimulates autophagy and contributes to the general inhibition of translation. To support the metabolic needs of its rapid replication, *Shigella* may benefit from the amino acid resources made available through the reduction in overall host translation and stress-induced stimulation of amino acid metabolism. However, *Shigella* also actively antagonizes the downregulation of the mTOR pathway through the secretion of the T3SS effector OspB (109). OspB acts early during infection by turning on the mTOR complex 1 through the scaffolding protein IQ motif-containing GAP1, possibly to prevent the activation of the autophagy pathway.

SHIGELLA-MEDIATED SUBVERSION OF HOST INFLAMMATORY RESPONSES

While inflammation can support *Shigella* virulence early during infection by facilitating *Shigella* invasion of the colonic epithelium, *Shigella* has devised multiple strategies to limit the inflammatory response of infected epithelial cells to promote its virulence. This includes targeted inhibition of factors involved in proinflammatory pathways, interference in transcriptional activation of proinflammatory cytokines, inhibition of the endomembrane

system required for cytokine secretion, and prevention of the release of endogenous danger signals (Fig. 4) (12).

Epithelial cells, similar to professional immune cells, are alerted to the presence of microbes through sensing of conserved MAMPs by various PRRs. Sensing of bacterial compounds in the extracellular environment is largely mediated by the membrane-anchored Toll-like receptor (TLR) family, while cytosolic sensing is mediated by cytosolic PRRs, including NOD1 and -2 and the family of NLRs. The host response to PRR activation depends on the type of PRR activated, its location, and the danger it represents (110). Thus, CpG activation of TLR9 on the apical side of differentiated epithelial cells leads to a cytoprotective and tolerogenic host response, while engagement of TLR9 located at the basolateral side leads to expression of proinflammatory genes, as it signals a breach in the epithelial barrier (111). In addition, sensing of the same MAMP by different receptors can lead to different host responses. For example, while sensing of extracellular LPS by membrane-bound TLR4 triggers the activation of two major proinflammatory pathways, NF-κB and MAPKs, cytosolic LPS is sensed by caspase-11 (and caspase-4 in humans), which leads to gasdermin D-mediated host cell lysis, potentially because the presence of a pathogen in the cytosol is a greater threat to the cell than sensing of the microbe extracellularly.

Extracellular and intracellular sensing of MAMPs is also intimately linked to the cellular response (112). Thus, TLR sensing, through for example TLR-3 or -4, activates the NF-κB pathway and leads to transcriptional upregulation and synthesis of IL-1β, IL-18, and caspase-1. Under these circumstances, whereby the host cell is first primed, activation of caspase-11 leads to pyroptotic host cell death, as gasdermin D-mediated membrane damage is sensed by the NLRP3 inflammasome and leads to caspase-1 activation and proteolytic activation of the proinflammatory cytokines IL-1β and IL-18.

The NF-κB and MAPK pathway are two major proinflammatory pathways activated by epithelial cells in response to PRR recognition, danger sensing, and cytokine stimulation. Both pathways use the activation of presynthesized transcriptional activators, allowing a rapid transcriptional response to harmful stimuli. The MAPK pathway involves the activation of MAPKs ERK, JNK, and p38 through a phosphorelay system of upstream kinases and the downstream activation of transcription factors. Conversely, the transcription factor NF-κB, composed of a p50 and p65 subunit in its canonical state, is maintained in an inactive state in the cytoplasm through direct interaction with the inhibitor IκBα. Phosphorylation of IκBα by the upstream IκB kinase (IKK), composed of the master regulator NEMO (also called IKKγ) and the catalytic heterodimer IKKα and IKKβ, targets IκBα for ubiquitination and degradation by host proteasomes, releasing NF-κB from its inhibition and freeing it to move into the nucleus to drive transcription of target genes.

Early during *Shigella* invasion, recognition of the bacterial MAMP diaminopimelic acid-containing peptidoglycan fragments by the PRR NOD1 drives a robust inflammatory response through the activation of the JNK MAPK pathway and a RIP2-dependent NF-κB activation (113, 114). NOD1-independent activation of NF-κB also occurs in response to sensing of DAMPs generated during *Shigella* invasion and phagosomal escape. Notably, later during infection, active replication of intracellular *Shigella* is sensed through the TRAF-interacting forkhead-associated protein A (TIFA)-dependent cytosolic surveillance pathway (Fig. 4B). The TIFA pathway senses cytosolic levels of the bacterial metabolite heptose-1,7-bisphosphate, a MAMP specific to Gram-negative-specific bacteria, leading to TIFA oligomerization, recruitment, and activation of the E3 ubiquitin ligase TRAF6 and NF-κB (115).

Attesting to the central role of NF-κB in host defense, *Shigella* employs at least nine effectors to inhibit the NF-κB pathway. *Shigella* effectors inhibit steps upstream of IKK activation, at the level of IKK and the NF-κB complex, and at the level of NF-κB transcription factor trafficking and target promoter binding, as well as downstream of NF-κB-mediated transcription (Fig. 4B).

During *Shigella* entry, the accumulation and liberation of diacylglycerol at the entry site are sensed as a danger signal and lead to TRAF6-dependent activation of NF-κB signaling. This pathway is inhibited by OspI, a glutamine deaminase, which targets UBC13, an E2 ubiquitin-conjugating enzyme (116, 117). Binding of OspI to UBC13-ubiquitin leads to deamination of UBC13 at Gln-100 and inactivation of its E2 activity. This prevents ubiquitination of TRAF6, which is necessary for the activation of NF-κB signaling. Lysis of the phagosomal membrane is also sensed by the host cell and leads to activation of the protein kinase C pathway, which activates NF-κB through TRAF2. This pathway is antagonized by IpaH0722, which targets TRAF2 for degradation by host proteasomes and thereby damps NF-κB activation (118). In addition, IpaH1.4 and IpaH2.5 ubiquitinate and target for proteasome degradation HOIP, a component of the linear ubiquitin chain assembly complex that generates Met1-linked linear ubiquitin chains involved in activating NF-κB signaling downstream of TRAF2 signaling (119).

The methyltransferase OspZ interferes with NF-κB signaling by modifying the zinc finger cysteines of TAK1-binding proteins 2 and 3 in order to prevent ubiquitin chain binding and subsequent NF-κB activation (120, 121). Conversely, IpaH9.8 is particularly important for blocking NF-κB activation through Nod1 sensing of *Shigella* peptidoglycan fragments. IpaH9.8 targets NEMO for degradation through its interaction with the IKK complex and ABIN-1, a ubiquitin-binding adaptor protein that further promotes NEMO degradation by stimulating NEMO polyubiquitination (122). Acting at the level of the NF-κB complex, the secreted kinase OspG prevents ubiquitination and subsequent degradation of phosphorylated IκBα by inhibiting the E3 ubiquitin ligase SCF^{b-TrCP} through its interaction with the ubiquitinated E2 ubiquitin-conjugating enzyme, which is part of the SCF^{b-TrCP} complex (123). OspG thereby inhibits NF-κB activation within the first hour of infection. In addition, IpaH4.5 interferes with NF-κB activation by targeting the p64 subunit of the NF-κB complex for ubiquitination and subsequent degradation (124).

In the nucleus, NF-κB-dependent and -independent transcription of proinflammatory genes is inhibited through several mechanisms involving OspF. OspF has a phosphothreonine lyase activity, a rare enzymatic activity that irreversibly dephosphorylates threonine through beta elimination (125). OspF specifically targets and inactivates MAPKs (Erk1/2 and p38), thereby preventing transcription of MAPK-dependent proinflammatory genes (126). OspF-mediated MAPK inactivation also inhibits NF-κB-mediated transcriptional activation through at least two epigenetic modifications downstream of MAPK activation. OspF indirectly reduces phosphorylation of histone H3 (H3pS10) and heterochromatin protein 1γ (HP1γS83) at proinflammatory target genes, including the IL-8 gene (127). Reduced phosphorylation of histone H3 and HP1γ promotes chromatin condensation and a transcriptionally inactive chromatin state, thereby preventing access of NF-κB to the gene promoters, leading to repression of proinflammatory-cytokine transcription. Notably, phosphoproteomics showed that OspF affects the phosphorylation status of several hundred host proteins, highlighting the extensive effect a single effector can have, directly and indirectly, on host signaling networks (128). In addition, IpaH9.8 interferes with proinflammatory gene activation at the posttranscriptional level (129). After nuclear translocation, IpaH9.8 interacts with the mRNA splicing factor U2AF^{35} and inhibits U2AF^{35}-mediated splicing reactions, resulting in reduced proinflammatory gene transcripts.

Vesicular trafficking, required for cytokine secretion, is also subverted by *Shigella* with the injection of the effectors IpaJ and VirA, and likely IcsB, as IcsB targets and modifies numerous host proteins involved in vesicular trafficking (76) (Fig. 4C). Vesicular trafficking is regulated by small GTPases of the Ras superfamily, such as Rabs and ADP-ribosylation factors (ARFs). These GTPases regulate successive steps in endomembrane trafficking from the ER to the Golgi apparatus and beyond, as well as endocytic trafficking, by mediating the formation, trafficking, and docking of vesicles from donor membranes to specific target membranes. IpaJ is a cysteine protease that preferentially cleaves N-myristoylated proteins but specifically targets ARFs, and notably ARF1, during infection. IpaJ cleavage of the myristoyl moiety from ARF1 irreversibly releases ARF1 from the Golgi membrane, inhibiting vesicular trafficking from the ER to the ER-Golgi intermediate compartments (ERGIC) (130). Conversely, as a GAP, VirA can interact with and inactivate many Rab GTPases, but through its preferred activity on Rab1, which localizes on the ERGIC, it mainly disrupts vesicular trafficking from the ERGIC to the Golgi (87). The activity of IpaJ, and to a lesser degree VirA, thereby leads to a striking fragmentation of the Golgi membrane.

Functionally, the disruption of vesicular trafficking during *Shigella* infection inhibits the general secretory pathway used to secrete cytokines and also interferes with the innate immune sensor STING (87, 130–132). STING senses the cytosolic presence of cyclic dinucleotides released from intracellular bacteria or generated from cytosolic double-stranded DNA by the nucleotidyl-transferase cyclic GMP-AMP synthase. Recognition of cyclic nucleotides by the ER transmembrane protein STING triggers its activation and relocation from the ER to the ERGIC, where it recruits TBK1 and the transcription factor IRF3 to initiate IRF3-mediated transcriptional activation of an antiviral interferon response. By interfering with ER-to-ERGIC vesicular trafficking, IpaJ effectively blocks type I interferon induction by STING in response to *Shigella* infection (131). In addition, *Shigella* interferes with TBK1-mediated immune activation with its effector IpaH4.5, which targets TBK1 for ubiquitination and proteasomal degradation (133).

A separate mechanism used by *Shigella* to limit inflammation is preventing the release of ATP by connexin hemichannels. Connexin hemichannels are gated pores formed at the plasma membrane through the assembly of six connexins into a ring structure. Connexin channels allow the flow of ions and signaling molecules either to the extracellular milieu in the case of hemichannels or between neighboring cells through the stacking of hemichannels at sites of cell-cell contact. Release of ATP into the extracellular environment by connexin hemichannels is sensed by the host as a danger signal and promotes inflammatory responses by binding to purinergic receptors

on both professional and nonprofessional immune cells. The rapid release of cellular ATP, the ubiquitous expression of ATP-sensing receptors, and a positive feedback loop of ATP release upon ATP sensing make extracellular ATP a highly potent immune mediator that rapidly amplifies the response to a local cellular insult.

Downstream signaling to ATP depends on the cell type, but in addition to enhancing filopodium formation, it includes phagocytosis and motility, the activation of NF-κB signaling, expression of adhesion molecules, induction of proinflammatory mediators, and activation of the NLRP3 inflammasome. ATP release is a common response of epithelial cells to challenge with enteric pathogens, but *Shigella* subverts this innate immune response and limits inflammation at the early stages of infection by injecting the T3SS effector IpgD (134). IpgD phosphatase activity on PI(4,5)P2 increases the levels of PI5P, which blocks hemichannel opening and ATP release in a poorly understood manner. However, as PI5P is a relatively rare lipid in the host cell, small changes in its cellular abundance may have a rapid and large impact.

The multiple mechanisms used by *Shigella* and the many host pathways targeted during infection of epithelial cells to limit inflammation clearly demonstrate the crucial role innate immune evasion plays in promoting infection.

SHIGELLA SUBVERTS HOST ADAPTIVE IMMUNITY

In recent years, evasion of acquired immune cell responses and function has become an exciting new area of investigation, driven by new methods and applications of new technologies. The main portal of entry for *Shigella* during its crossing of the epithelial barrier is the specialized lymphoid follicle-associated epithelium, bringing *Shigella* into early contact with both innate and acquired immune cells. At the same time, *Shigella* can migrate to the draining mesenteric lymph nodes using the host lymphatic system. In these secondary lymphoid tissues, *Shigella* encounters not only macrophages but also dendritic cells (DCs), B cells, and T cells. DCs are specialized antigen-presenting cells that stimulate T cell responses, while both DCs and T cells support B cell responses, including memory B cell responses. Shigellosis is characterized by massive T and B cell death in rectal biopsy samples and by poor long-lived B cell immunity, requiring multiple infections for the host to become more resistant to infection. *Shigella* is therefore effective in inhibiting the generation of long-lived immunity and likely does this through several mechanisms.

Shigella interactions with DCs are similar to those of macrophages, whereby invasion leads to pyroptotic host cell death, limiting DC-mediated immune activation, while the interaction of *Shigella* with B and T cells has only recently been highlighted. In *in vivo* models, *Shigella* has been demonstrated to invade both T and B cells, while *in vitro*, *Shigella* is capable of invading B cells and activated, but not unactivated, T cells (44, 135, 136). Real-time two-photon microscopy of popliteal lymph nodes after footpad inoculation with *Shigella* showed that *Shigella* invasion of CD4$^+$ T cells arrested T cell migration, while T cell mobility patterns were also dramatically affected independently of *Shigella* invasion (136).

Mechanistic insights were unraveled *in vitro*, where *Shigella* inhibited T cell motility towards a chemokine attractant in an IpgD-dependent manner (135). IpgD injected into T cells hydrolyzed PIP2 and reduced the pool of PIP2 at the plasma membrane, leading to a reduction in phosphorylated active ezrin, radixin, and myosin proteins, which are important for the early steps of cell cortex organization during T cell polarization in response to a chemokine stimulus, effectively impairing T cell function (Fig. 3). Notably, a FACS (fluorescence-activated cell sorting)-based analysis of a FRET (fluorescence resonance energy transfer) pair-based approach for monitoring effector injection revealed that IpgD can be injected into activated T cells and can inhibit T cell migration in the absence of invasion (135). In this assay, activated T cells are loaded with the FRET pair CCF4 and then challenged with *Shigella* in the presence of cytochalasin D, a drug that inhibits actin polymerization and prevents invasion. T3SS-dependent injection of an IpgD–β-lactamase fusion construct into T cells is then monitored through the shift in fluorescent emission upon β-lactamase cleavage of CCF4 in the host cytosol. Inhibition of T cell migration may interfere with T-cell-mediated immunity by preventing T cell interactions with DCs and B cells and thereby preventing priming of an effective protective response. Notably, improvements in the sensitivity of this *in vitro* reporter system, coupled to the use single-cell FACS imaging, suggests that injection of effectors in the absence of invasion is the main mechanism *Shigella* uses to target T cells (137).

Conversely, *Shigella* interactions with B cells lead to both necrotic and apoptotic cell death depending on the interaction pattern (44). While invasion of B cells leads to necrotic cell death, noninfected B cells primarily undergo apoptosis. During apoptosis, B cells are first sensitized via a yet-unidentified bacterial cosignal, leading to upregulation of TLR2, which recognizes the *Shigella* translocator protein IpaD, a novel TLR2 ligand, and triggers apoptosis. Induction of B cell death in both invaded and noninvaded cells antagonizes antibody-mediated immune responses and likely contributes to the poor priming of B cell immunity to *Shigella* infection.

THE COMPLEXITY OF *SHIGELLA* PATHOGENESIS

The pathogenesis of *Shigella* is a highly complex and multifaceted process at the tissue, cellular, and molecular levels, underscored by the multitude of effectors *Shigella* uses to subvert host processes. However, the context of timing and cell specificity are also important considerations. Thus, *Shigella* benefits from inflammation early during infection and actively promotes the proinflammatory pyroptosis of macrophages while using a multitude of effectors to damp the host inflammatory responses in epithelial cells. Having evolved to utilize the host cell cytosol as its main replicative niche, *Shigella* targets numerous host cell processes to ensure its own survival and the integrity of the infected cell. These host cell processes may be targeted by a single effector or by many, and an effector may have one or multiple cellular targets or an enzymatic activity that can affect a wide range of processes. In addition, while most investigations have centered on elucidating effector function in infected cells, recent advances in our understanding of interaction of *Shigella* with cells of the adaptive immune system have already highlighted the role that some *Shigella* effectors can play independently of cell invasion to subvert host cell function. This new "kiss and run" model adds an additional layer of complexity to the study of *Shigella* pathogenesis and, like many other areas of *Shigella* pathogenesis, has strongly benefited from the development of novel methods and new techniques.

Acknowledgments. We apologize to investigators whose work on Shigella pathogenesis was not included in the review or only cited through other reviews due to space limitations. We thank Mariana Ferrari and Nathalie Sauvonnet for critical reading of the manuscript. Work in the group of P.S. is supported by Gates Foundation Grand Challenge grant OPP1141322, while P.J.S. is a Howard Hughes International Scholar and supported by the ERC Advance grant DECRYPT (339579).

Citation. Schnupf P, Sansonetti PJ. 2019. *Shigella* pathogenesis: new insights through advanced methodologies. Microbiol Spectrum 7(2):BAI-0023-2019.

References

1. **Trofa AF, Ueno-Olsen H, Oiwa R, Yoshikawa M.** 1999. Dr. Kiyoshi Shiga: discoverer of the dysentery bacillus. *Clin Infect Dis* 29:1303–1306.

2. **Anderson M, Sansonetti PJ, Marteyn BS.** 2016. Shigella diversity and changing landscape: insights for the twenty-first century. *Front Cell Infect Microbiol* 6:45.

3. **Schroeder GN, Hilbi H.** 2008. Molecular pathogenesis of Shigella spp.: controlling host cell signaling, invasion,

and death by type III secretion. *Clin Microbiol Rev* **21:** 134–156.

4. **Muthuirulandi Sethuvel DP, Devanga Ragupathi NK, Anandan S, Veeraraghavan B.** 2017. Update on: *Shigella* new serogroups/serotypes and their antimicrobial resistance. *Lett Appl Microbiol* **64:**8–18.

5. **Kotloff KL, Riddle MS, Platts-Mills JA, Pavlinac P, Zaidi AKM.** 2018. Shigellosis. *Lancet* **391:**801–812.

6. **Hosangadi D, Smith PG, Giersing BK.** 2017. Considerations for using ETEC and *Shigella* disease burden estimates to guide vaccine development strategy. *Vaccine* S0264-410X(17)31343-9.

7. **Kotloff KL, Nataro JP, Blackwelder WC, Nasrin D, Farag TH, Panchalingam S, Wu Y, Sow SO, Sur D, Breiman RF, Faruque AS, Zaidi AK, Saha D, Alonso PL, Tamboura B, Sanogo D, Onwuchekwa U, Manna B, Ramamurthy T, Kanungo S, Ochieng JB, Omore R, Oundo JO, Hossain A, Das SK, Ahmed S, Qureshi S, Quadri F, Adegbola RA, Antonio M, Hossain MJ, Akinsola A, Mandomando I, Nhampossa T, Acácio S, Biswas K, O'Reilly CE, Mintz ED, Berkeley LY, Muhsen K, Sommerfelt H, Robins-Browne RM, Levine MM.** 2013. Burden and aetiology of diarrhoeal disease in infants and young children in developing countries (the Global Enteric Multicenter Study, GEMS): a prospective, case-control study. *Lancet* **382:**209–222.

8. **Kasper CA, Sorg I, Schmutz C, Tschon T, Wischnewski H, Kim ML, Arrieumerlou C.** 2010. Cell-cell propagation of NF-κB transcription factor and MAP kinase activation amplifies innate immunity against bacterial infection. *Immunity* **33:**804–816.

9. **Raqib R, Ekberg C, Sharkar P, Bardhan PK, Zychlinsky A, Sansonetti PJ, Andersson J.** 2002. Apoptosis in acute shigellosis is associated with increased production of Fas/Fas ligand, perforin, caspase-1, and caspase-3 but reduced production of Bcl-2 and interleukin-2. *Infect Immun* **70:**3199–3207.

10. **Brinkmann V, Reichard U, Goosmann C, Fauler B, Uhlemann Y, Weiss DS, Weinrauch Y, Zychlinsky A.** 2004. Neutrophil extracellular traps kill bacteria. *Science* **303:**1532–1535.

11. **Parsot C.** 2009. Shigella type III secretion effectors: how, where, when, for what purposes? *Curr Opin Microbiol* **12:**110–116.

12. **Mattock E, Blocker AJ.** 2017. How do the virulence factors of *Shigella* work together to cause disease? *Front Cell Infect Microbiol* **7:**64.

13. **Demers J-P, Habenstein B, Loquet A, Kumar Vasa S, Giller K, Becker S, Baker D, Lange A, Sgourakis NG.** 2014. High-resolution structure of the *Shigella* type-III secretion needle by solid-state NMR and cryo-electron microscopy. *Nat Commun* **5:**4976.

14. **Dohlich K, Zumsteg AB, Goosmann C, Kolbe M.** 2014. A substrate-fusion protein is trapped inside the type III secretion system channel in *Shigella flexneri. PLoS Pathog* **10:**e1003881.

15. **Epler CR, Dickenson NE, Bullitt E, Picking WL.** 2012. Ultrastructural analysis of IpaD at the tip of the nascent

MxiH type III secretion apparatus of *Shigella flexneri. J Mol Biol* **420:**29–39.

16. **Barta ML, Guragain M, Adam P, Dickenson NE, Patil M, Geisbrecht BV, Picking WL, Picking WD.** 2012. Identification of the bile salt binding site on IpaD from *Shigella flexneri* and the influence of ligand binding on IpaD structure. *Proteins* **80:**935–945.

17. **van der Goot FG, Tran Van Nhieu G, Allaoui A, Sansonetti P, Lafont F.** 2004. Rafts can trigger contact-mediated secretion of bacterial effectors via a lipid-based mechanism. *J Biol Chem* **279:**47792–47798.

18. **Hayward RD, Cain RJ, McGhie EJ, Phillips N, Garner MJ, Koronakis V.** 2005. Cholesterol binding by the bacterial type III translocon is essential for virulence effector delivery into mammalian cells. *Mol Microbiol* **56:** 590–603.

19. **Roehrich AD, Bordignon E, Mode S, Shen D-K, Liu X, Pain M, Murillo I, Martinez-Argudo I, Sessions RB, Blocker AJ.** 2017. Steps for *Shigella* gatekeeper protein MxiC function in hierarchical type III secretion regulation. *J Biol Chem* **292:**1705–1723.

20. **Parsot C, Ageron E, Penno C, Mavris M, Jamoussi K, d'Hauteville H, Sansonetti P, Demers B.** 2005. A secreted anti-activator, OspD1, and its chaperone, Spa15, are involved in the control of transcription by the type III secretion apparatus activity in *Shigella flexneri. Mol Microbiol* **56:**1627–1635.

21. **Campbell-Valois F-X, Schnupf P, Nigro G, Sachse M, Sansonetti PJ, Parsot C.** 2014. A fluorescent reporter reveals on/off regulation of the *Shigella* type III secretion apparatus during entry and cell-to-cell spread. *Cell Host Microbe* **15:**177–189.

22. **Mou X, Souter S, Du J, Reeves AZ, Lesser CF.** 2018. Synthetic bottom-up approach reveals the complex interplay of *Shigella* effectors in regulation of epithelial cell death. *Proc Natl Acad Sci USA* **115:** 6452–6457.

23. **Bergounioux J, Elisee R, Prunier A-L, Donnadieu F, Sperandio B, Sansonetti P, Arbibe L.** 2012. Calpain activation by the *Shigella flexneri* effector VirA regulates key steps in the formation and life of the bacterium's epithelial niche. *Cell Host Microbe* **11:**240–252.

24. **Ashida H, Sasakawa C.** 2016. *Shigella* IpaH family effectors as a versatile model for studying pathogenic bacteria. *Front Cell Infect Microbiol* **5:**100.

25. **Rohde JR, Breitkreutz A, Chenal A, Sansonetti PJ, Parsot C.** 2007. Type III secretion effectors of the IpaH family are E3 ubiquitin ligases. *Cell Host Microbe* **1:**77–83.

26. **Ashida H, Sasakawa C.** 2017. Bacterial E3 ligase effectors exploit host ubiquitin systems. *Curr Opin Microbiol* **35:**16–22.

27. **Martino MC, Rossi G, Martini I, Tattoli I, Chiavolini D, Phalipon A, Sansonetti PJ, Bernardini ML.** 2005. Mucosal lymphoid infiltrate dominates colonic pathological changes in murine experimental shigellosis. *J Infect Dis* **192:**136–148.

28. **Anderson MC, Vonaesch P, Saffarian A, Marteyn BS, Sansonetti PJ.** 2017. *Shigella sonnei* encodes a func-

tional T6SS used for interbacterial competition and niche occupancy. *Cell Host Microbe* 21:769–776.e3.

29. Yang G, Wang L, Wang Y, Li P, Zhu J, Qiu S, Hao R, Wu Z, Li W, Song H. 2015. *hfq* regulates acid tolerance and virulence by responding to acid stress in *Shigella flexneri*. *Res Microbiol* 166:476–485.

30. Brotcke Zumsteg A, Goosmann C, Brinkmann V, Morona R, Zychlinsky A. 2014. IcsA is a *Shigella flexneri* adhesin regulated by the type III secretion system and required for pathogenesis. *Cell Host Microbe* 15:435–445.

31. Faherty CS, Redman JC, Rasko DA, Barry EM, Nataro JP. 2012. *Shigella flexneri* effectors OspE1 and OspE2 mediate induced adherence to the colonic epithelium following bile salts exposure. *Mol Microbiol* 85:107–121.

32. Vergara-Irigaray M, Fookes MC, Thomson NR, Tang CM. 2014. RNA-seq analysis of the influence of anaerobiosis and FNR on *Shigella flexneri*. *BMC Genomics* 15:438.

33. Marteyn B, West NP, Browning DF, Cole JA, Shaw JG, Palm F, Mounier J, Prévost M-C, Sansonetti P, Tang CM. 2010. Modulation of *Shigella* virulence in response to available oxygen in vivo. *Nature* 465:355–358.

34. Sansonetti PJ, Arondel J, Fontaine A, d'Hauteville H, Bernardini ML. 1991. *Omp*B (osmo-regulation) and *ics*A (cell-to-cell spread) mutants of *Shigella flexneri*: vaccine candidates and probes to study the pathogenesis of shigellosis. *Vaccine* 9:416–422.

35. Mathan MM, Mathan VI. 1991. Morphology of rectal mucosa of patients with shigellosis. *Rev Infect Dis* 13 (Suppl 4):S314–S318.

36. Sansonetti PJ, Arondel J, Cantey JR, Prévost MC, Huerre M. 1996. Infection of rabbit Peyer's patches by *Shigella flexneri*: effect of adhesive or invasive bacterial phenotypes on follicle-associated epithelium. *Infect Immun* 64:2752–2764.

37. Wassef JS, Keren DF, Mailloux JL. 1989. Role of M cells in initial antigen uptake and in ulcer formation in the rabbit intestinal loop model of shigellosis. *Infect Immun* 57:858–863.

38. Perdomo OJ, Cavaillon JM, Huerre M, Ohayon H, Gounon P, Sansonetti PJ. 1994. Acute inflammation causes epithelial invasion and mucosal destruction in experimental shigellosis. *J Exp Med* 180:1307–1319.

39. Shim D-H, Suzuki T, Chang S-Y, Park S-M, Sansonetti PJ, Sasakawa C, Kweon M-N. 2007. New animal model of shigellosis in the guinea pig: its usefulness for protective efficacy studies. *J Immunol* 178:2476–2482.

40. Romero S, Grompone G, Carayol N, Mounier J, Guadagnini S, Prevost M-C, Sansonetti PJ, Tran Van Nhieu GT. 2011. ATP-mediated Erk1/2 activation stimulates bacterial capture by filopodia, which precedes *Shigella* invasion of epithelial cells. *Cell Host Microbe* 9:508–519.

41. Romero S, Quatela A, Bornschlögl T, Guadagnini S, Bassereau P, Tran Van Nhieu G. 2012. Filopodium retraction is controlled by adhesion to its tip. *J Cell Sci* 125:4999–5004. *ERRATUM J Cell Sci* 125:5587.

42. Xu D, Liao C, Zhang B, Tolbert WD, He W, Dai Z, Zhang W, Yuan W, Pazgier M, Liu J, Yu J, Sansonetti PJ, Bevins CL, Shao Y, Lu W. 2018. Human enteric α-defensin 5 promotes *Shigella* infection by enhancing bacterial adhesion and invasion. *Immunity* 48:1233–1244.e6.

43. Arena ET, Campbell-Valois F-X, Tinevez J-Y, Nigro G, Sachse M, Moya-Nilges M, Nothelfer K, Marteyn B, Shorte SL, Sansonetti PJ. 2015. Bioimage analysis of *Shigella* infection reveals targeting of colonic crypts. *Proc Natl Acad Sci USA* 112:E3282–E3290.

44. Nothelfer K, Arena ET, Pinaud L, Neunlist M, Mozeleski B, Belotserkovsky I, Parsot C, Dinadayala P, Burger-Kentischer A, Raqib R, Sansonetti PJ, Phalipon A. 2014. B lymphocytes undergo TLR2-dependent apoptosis upon *Shigella* infection. *J Exp Med* 211:1215–1229.

45. Miller H, Zhang J, Kuolee R, Patel GB, Chen W. 2007. Intestinal M cells: the fallible sentinels? *World J Gastroenterol* 13:1477–1486.

46. Jensen VB, Harty JT, Jones BD. 1998. Interactions of the invasive pathogens *Salmonella typhimurium*, *Listeria monocytogenes*, and *Shigella flexneri* with M cells and murine Peyer's patches. *Infect Immun* 66:3758–3766.

47. Ashida H, Kim M, Sasakawa C. 2014. Manipulation of the host cell death pathway by *Shigella*. *Cell Microbiol* 16:1757–1766.

48. Jorgensen I, Miao EA. 2015. Pyroptotic cell death defends against intracellular pathogens. *Immunol Rev* 265:130–142.

49. Shi J, Gao W, Shao F. 2017. Pyroptosis: gasdermin-mediated programmed necrotic cell death. *Trends Biochem Sci* 42:245–254.

50. Storek KM, Monack DM. 2015. Bacterial recognition pathways that lead to inflammasome activation. *Immunol Rev* 265:112–129.

51. Hermansson A-K, Paciello I, Bernardini ML. 2016. The orchestra and its maestro: *Shigella*'s fine-tuning of the inflammasome platforms. *Curr Top Microbiol Immunol* 397:91–115.

52. Suzuki S, Franchi L, He Y, Muñoz-Planillo R, Mimuro H, Suzuki T, Sasakawa C, Núñez G. 2014. *Shigella* type III secretion protein MxiI is recognized by Naip2 to induce Nlrc4 inflammasome activation independently of Pkcδ. *PLoS Pathog* 10:e1003926.

53. Miao EA, Mao DP, Yudkovsky N, Bonneau R, Lorang CG, Warren SE, Leaf IA, Aderem A. 2010. Innate immune detection of the type III secretion apparatus through the NLRC4 inflammasome. *Proc Natl Acad Sci USA* 107:3076–3080.

54. Yang J, Zhao Y, Shi J, Shao F. 2013. Human NAIP and mouse NAIP1 recognize bacterial type III secretion needle protein for inflammasome activation. *Proc Natl Acad Sci USA* 110:14408–14413.

55. Rayamajhi M, Zak DE, Chavarria-Smith J, Vance RE, Miao EA. 2013. Cutting edge: mouse NAIP1 detects the type III secretion system needle protein. *J Immunol* 191:3986–3989.

56. Watarai M, Funato S, Sasakawa C. 1996. Interaction of Ipa proteins of *Shigella flexneri* with α5β1 integrin promotes entry of the bacteria into mammalian cells. *J Exp Med* **183**:991–999.

57. Skoudy A, Mounier J, Aruffo A, Ohayon H, Gounon P, Sansonetti P, Tran Van Nhieu G. 2000. CD44 binds to the *Shigella* IpaB protein and participates in bacterial invasion of epithelial cells. *Cell Microbiol* **2**:19–33.

58. Russo BC, Stamm LM, Raaben M, Kim CM, Kahoud E, Robinson LR, Bose S, Queiroz AL, Herrera BB, Baxt LA, Mor-Vaknin N, Fu Y, Molina G, Markovitz DM, Whelan SP, Goldberg MB. 2016. Intermediate filaments enable pathogen docking to trigger type 3 effector translocation. *Nat Microbiol* **1**:16025.

59. Tran Van Nhieu G, Caron E, Hall A, Sansonetti PJ. 1999. IpaC induces actin polymerization and filopodia formation during *Shigella* entry into epithelial cells. *EMBO J* **18**:3249–3262.

60. Tran Van Nhieu G, Ben-Ze'ev A, Sansonetti PJ. 1997. Modulation of bacterial entry into epithelial cells by association between vinculin and the *Shigella* IpaA invasin. *EMBO J* **16**:2717–2729.

61. Izard T, Tran Van Nhieu G, Bois PRJ. 2006. *Shigella* applies molecular mimicry to subvert vinculin and invade host cells. *J Cell Biol* **175**:465–475.

62. Yoshida S, Handa Y, Suzuki T, Ogawa M, Suzuki M, Tamai A, Abe A, Katayama E, Sasakawa C. 2006. Microtubule-severing activity of *Shigella* is pivotal for intercellular spreading. *Science* **314**:985–989.

63. Germane KL, Ohi R, Goldberg MB, Spiller BW. 2008. Structural and functional studies indicate that *Shigella* VirA is not a protease and does not directly destabilize microtubules. *Biochemistry* **47**:10241–10243.

64. Niebuhr K, Giuriato S, Pedron T, Philpott DJ, Gaits F, Sable J, Sheetz MP, Parsot C, Sansonetti PJ, Payrastre B. 2002. Conversion of PtdIns(4,5)P(2) into PtdIns(5)P by the *S. flexneri* effector IpgD reorganizes host cell morphology. *EMBO J* **21**:5069–5078.

65. Bonnet M, Tran Van Nhieu G. 2016. How *Shigella* utilizes Ca(2+) jagged edge signals during invasion of epithelial cells. *Front Cell Infect Microbiol* **6**:16.

66. Tran Van Nhieu G, Kai Liu B, Zhang J, Pierre F, Prigent S, Sansonetti P, Erneux C, Kuk Kim J, Suh P-G, Dupont G, Combettes L. 2013. Actin-based confinement of calcium responses during *Shigella* invasion. *Nat Commun* **4**:1567.

67. Sun CH, Wacquier B, Aguilar DI, Carayol N, Denis K, Boucherie S, Valencia-Gallardo C, Simsek C, Erneux C, Lehman A, Enninga J, Arbibe L, Sansonetti P, Dupont G, Combettes L, Tran Van Nhieu G. 2017. The *Shigella* type III effector IpgD recodes Ca^{2+} signals during invasion of epithelial cells. *EMBO J* **36**:2567–2580.

68. Weiner A, Mellouk N, Lopez-Montero N, Chang Y-Y, Souque C, Schmitt C, Enninga J. 2016. Macropinosomes are key players in early *Shigella* invasion and vacuolar escape in epithelial cells. *PLoS Pathog* **12**:e1005602.

69. High N, Mounier J, Prévost MC, Sansonetti PJ. 1992. IpaB of *Shigella flexneri* causes entry into epithelial cells and escape from the phagocytic vacuole. *EMBO J* **11**:1991–1999.

70. Mellouk N, Weiner A, Aulner N, Schmitt C, Elbaum M, Shorte SL, Danckaert A, Enninga J. 2014. *Shigella* subverts the host recycling compartment to rupture its vacuole. *Cell Host Microbe* **16**:517–530.

71. Krokowski S, Mostowy S. 2016. Interactions between *Shigella flexneri* and the autophagy machinery. *Front Cell Infect Microbiol* **6**:17.

72. Travassos LH, Carneiro LAM, Ramjeet M, Hussey S, Kim Y-G, Magalhães JG, Yuan L, Soares F, Chea E, Le Bourhis L, Boneca IG, Allaoui A, Jones NL, Nuñez G, Girardin SE, Philpott DJ. 2010. Nod1 and Nod2 direct autophagy by recruiting ATG16L1 to the plasma membrane at the site of bacterial entry. *Nat Immunol* **11**:55–62.

73. Tattoli I, Sorbara MT, Vuckovic D, Ling A, Soares F, Carneiro LAM, Yang C, Emili A, Philpott DJ, Girardin SE. 2012. Amino acid starvation induced by invasive bacterial pathogens triggers an innate host defense program. *Cell Host Microbe* **11**:563–575.

74. Sorbara MT, Foerster EG, Tsalikis J, Abdel-Nour M, Mangiapane J, Sirluck-Schroeder I, Tattoli I, van Dalen R, Isenman DE, Rohde JR, Girardin SE, Philpott DJ. 2018. Complement C3 drives autophagy-dependent restriction of cyto-invasive bacteria. *Cell Host Microbe* **23**:644–652.e5.

75. Baxt LA, Goldberg MB. 2014. Host and bacterial proteins that repress recruitment of LC3 to *Shigella* early during infection. *PLoS One* **9**:e94653.

76. Liu W, Zhou Y, Peng T, Zhou P, Ding X, Li Z, Zhong H, Xu Y, Chen S, Hang HC, Shao F. 2018. N$^\varepsilon$-fatty acylation of multiple membrane-associated proteins by *Shigella* IcsB effector to modulate host function. *Nat Microbiol* **3**:996–1009.

77. Agaisse H. 2016. Molecular and cellular mechanisms of *Shigella flexneri* dissemination. *Front Cell Infect Microbiol* **6**:29.

78. Monack DM, Theriot JA. 2001. Actin-based motility is sufficient for bacterial membrane protrusion formation and host cell uptake. *Cell Microbiol* **3**:633–647.

79. Fukumatsu M, Ogawa M, Arakawa S, Suzuki M, Nakayama K, Shimizu S, Kim M, Mimuro H, Sasakawa C. 2012. *Shigella* targets epithelial tricellular junctions and uses a noncanonical clathrin-dependent endocytic pathway to spread between cells. *Cell Host Microbe* **11**:325–336.

80. Torraca V, Mostowy S. 2016. Septins and bacterial infection. *Front Cell Dev Biol* **4**:127.

81. Mostowy S, Sancho-Shimizu V, Hamon MA, Simeone R, Brosch R, Johansen T, Cossart P. 2011. p62 and NDP52 proteins target intracytosolic *Shigella* and *Listeria* to different autophagy pathways. *J Biol Chem* **286**:26987–26995.

82. Sirianni A, Krokowski S, Lobato-Márquez D, Buranyi S, Pfanzelter J, Galea D, Willis A, Culley S, Henriques R, Larrouy-Maumus G, Hollinshead M, Sancho-Shimizu V, Way M, Mostowy S. 2016. Mitochondria mediate septin cage assembly to promote autophagy of *Shigella*. *EMBO Rep* **17**:1029–1043.

83. Ogawa M, Yoshimori T, Suzuki T, Sagara H, Mizushima N, Sasakawa C. 2005. Escape of intracellular *Shigella* from autophagy. *Science* 307:727–731.

84. Mostowy S, Boucontet L, Mazon Moya MJ, Sirianni A, Boudinot P, Hollinshead M, Cossart P, Herbomel P, Levraud J-P, Colucci-Guyon E. 2013. The zebrafish as a new model for the in vivo study of *Shigella flexneri* interaction with phagocytes and bacterial autophagy. *PLoS Pathog* 9:e1003588.

85. Uchiya K, Tobe T, Komatsu K, Suzuki T, Watarai M, Fukuda I, Yoshikawa M, Sasakawa C. 1995. Identification of a novel virulence gene, *virA*, on the large plasmid of *Shigella*, involved in invasion and intercellular spreading. *Mol Microbiol* 17:241–250.

86. Huang J, Brumell JH. 2014. Bacteria-autophagy interplay: a battle for survival. *Nat Rev Microbiol* 12:101–114.

87. Dong N, Zhu Y, Lu Q, Hu L, Zheng Y, Shao F. 2012. Structurally distinct bacterial TBC-like GAPs link Arf GTPase to Rab1 inactivation to counteract host defenses. *Cell* 150:1029–1041.

88. Campbell-Valois F-X, Sachse M, Sansonetti PJ, Parsot C. 2015. Escape of actively secreting *Shigella flexneri* from ATG8/LC3-positive vacuoles formed during cell-to-cell spread is facilitated by IcsB and VirA. *mBio* 6:e02567-14.

89. Li P, Jiang W, Yu Q, Liu W, Zhou P, Li J, Xu J, Xu B, Wang F, Shao F. 2017. Ubiquitination and degradation of GBPs by a *Shigella* effector to suppress host defence. *Nature* 551:378–383.

90. Piro AS, Hernandez D, Luoma S, Feeley EM, Finethy R, Yirga A, Frickel EM, Lesser CF, Coers J. 2017. Detection of cytosolic *Shigella flexneri* via a C-terminal triple-arginine motif of GBP1 inhibits actin-based motility. *mBio* 8:e01979-17.

91. Paciello I, Silipo A, Lembo-Fazio L, Curcurù L, Zumsteg A, Noël G, Ciancarella V, Sturiale L, Molinaro A, Bernardini ML. 2013. Intracellular *Shigella* remodels its LPS to dampen the innate immune recognition and evade inflammasome activation. *Proc Natl Acad Sci USA* 110:E4345–E4354. CORRECTION *Proc Natl Acad Sci USA* 110:20843.

92. Kobayashi T, Ogawa M, Sanada T, Mimuro H, Kim M, Ashida H, Akakura R, Yoshida M, Kawalec M, Reichhart J-M, Mizushima T, Sasakawa C. 2013. The *Shigella* OspC3 effector inhibits caspase-4, antagonizes inflammatory cell death, and promotes epithelial infection. *Cell Host Microbe* 13:570–583.

93. Mayo LD, Donner DB. 2001. A phosphatidylinositol 3-kinase/Akt pathway promotes translocation of Mdm2 from the cytoplasm to the nucleus. *Proc Natl Acad Sci USA* 98:11598–11603.

94. Ramel D, Lagarrigue F, Pons V, Mounier J, Dupuis-Coronas S, Chicanne G, Sansonetti PJ, Gaits-Iacovoni F, Tronchère H, Payrastre B. 2011. *Shigella flexneri* infection generates the lipid PI5P to alter endocytosis and prevent termination of EGFR signaling. *Sci Signal* 4:ra61.

95. Bhola PD, Letai A. 2016. Mitochondria—judges and executioners of cell death sentences. *Mol Cell* 61:695–704.

96. Sukumaran SK, Fu NY, Tin CB, Wan KF, Lee SS, Yu VC. 2010. A soluble form of the pilus protein FimA targets the VDAC-hexokinase complex at mitochondria to suppress host cell apoptosis. *Mol Cell* 37:768–783.

97. Bravo V, Puhar A, Sansonetti P, Parsot C, Toro CS. 2015. Distinct mutations led to inactivation of type 1 fimbriae expression in *Shigella* spp. *PLoS One* 10:e0121785.

98. Faherty CS, Maurelli AT. 2009. Spa15 of *Shigella flexneri* is secreted through the type III secretion system and prevents staurosporine-induced apoptosis. *Infect Immun* 77:5281–5290.

99. Pendaries C, Tronchère H, Arbibe L, Mounier J, Gozani O, Cantley L, Fry MJ, Gaits-Iacovoni F, Sansonetti PJ, Payrastre B. 2006. PtdIns5P activates the host cell PI3-kinase/Akt pathway during *Shigella flexneri* infection. *EMBO J* 25:1024–1034.

100. Carneiro LAM, Travassos LH, Soares F, Tattoli I, Magalhaes JG, Bozza MT, Plotkowski MC, Sansonetti PJ, Molkentin JD, Philpott DJ, Girardin SE. 2009. *Shigella* induces mitochondrial dysfunction and cell death in nonmyeloid cells. *Cell Host Microbe* 5:123–136.

101. Kim M, Ogawa M, Fujita Y, Yoshikawa Y, Nagai T, Koyama T, Nagai S, Lange A, Fässler R, Sasakawa C. 2009. Bacteria hijack integrin-linked kinase to stabilize focal adhesions and block cell detachment. *Nature* 459:578–582.

102. Miura M, Terajima J, Izumiya H, Mitobe J, Komano T, Watanabe H. 2006. OspE2 of *Shigella sonnei* is required for the maintenance of cell architecture of bacterium-infected cells. *Infect Immun* 74:2587–2595.

103. Iwai H, Kim M, Yoshikawa Y, Ashida H, Ogawa M, Fujita Y, Muller D, Kirikae T, Jackson PK, Kotani S, Sasakawa C. 2007. A bacterial effector targets Mad2L2, an APC inhibitor, to modulate host cell cycling. *Cell* 130:611–623.

104. Boal F, Puhar A, Xuereb J-M, Kunduzova O, Sansonetti PJ, Payrastre B, Tronchère H. 2016. PI5P triggers ICAM-1 degradation in *Shigella*-infected cells, thus dampening immune cell recruitment. *Cell Reports* 14:750–759.

105. Pieper R, Fisher CR, Suh M-J, Huang S-T, Parmar P, Payne SM. 2013. Analysis of the proteome of intracellular *Shigella flexneri* reveals pathways important for intracellular growth. *Infect Immun* 81:4635–4648.

106. Payne SM, Wyckoff EE, Murphy ER, Oglesby AG, Boulette ML, Davies NML. 2006. Iron and pathogenesis of *Shigella*: iron acquisition in the intracellular environment. *Biometals* 19:173–180.

107. Kentner D, Martano G, Callon M, Chiquet P, Brodmann M, Burton O, Wahlander A, Nanni P, Delmotte N, Grossmann J, Limenitakis J, Schlapbach R, Kiefer P, Vorholt JA, Hiller S, Bumann D. 2014. *Shigella* reroutes host cell central metabolism to obtain high-flux nutrient supply for vigorous intracellular growth. *Proc Natl Acad Sci USA* 111:9929–9934.

108. Vonaesch P, Campbell-Valois F-X, Dufour A, Sansonetti PJ, Schnupf P. 2016. *Shigella flexneri* modulates stress granule composition and inhibits stress granule aggregation. *Cell Microbiol* 18:982–997.

109. Lu R, Herrera BB, Eshleman HD, Fu Y, Bloom A, Li Z, Sacks DB, Goldberg MB. 2015. *Shigella* effector OspB activates mTORC1 in a manner that depends on IQGAP1 and promotes cell proliferation. *PLoS Pathog* 11:e1005200.

110. Yu S, Gao N. 2015. Compartmentalizing intestinal epithelial cell toll-like receptors for immune surveillance. *Cell Mol Life Sci* 72:3343–3353.

111. Lee J, Mo J-H, Katakura K, Alkalay I, Rucker AN, Liu Y-T, Lee H-K, Shen C, Cojocaru G, Shenouda S, Kagnoff M, Eckmann L, Ben-Neriah Y, Raz E. 2006. Maintenance of colonic homeostasis by distinctive apical TLR9 signalling in intestinal epithelial cells. *Nat Cell Biol* 8:1327–1336.

112. He Y, Hara H, Núñez G. 2016. Mechanism and regulation of NLRP3 inflammasome activation. *Trends Biochem Sci* 41:1012–1021.

113. Girardin SE, Tournebize R, Mavris M, Page AL, Li X, Stark GR, Bertin J, DiStefano PS, Yaniv M, Sansonetti PJ, Philpott DJ. 2001. CARD4/Nod1 mediates NF-κB and JNK activation by invasive *Shigella flexneri*. *EMBO Rep* 2:736–742.

114. Killackey SA, Sorbara MT, Girardin SE. 2016. Cellular aspects of *Shigella* pathogenesis: focus on the manipulation of host cell processes. *Front Cell Infect Microbiol* 6:38.

115. Gaudet RG, Guo CX, Molinaro R, Kottwitz H, Rohde JR, Dangeard A-S, Arrieumerlou C, Girardin SE, Gray-Owen SD. 2017. Innate recognition of intracellular bacterial growth is driven by the TIFA-dependent cytosolic surveillance pathway. *Cell Reports* 19:1418–1430.

116. Sanada T, Kim M, Mimuro H, Suzuki M, Ogawa M, Oyama A, Ashida H, Kobayashi T, Koyama T, Nagai S, Shibata Y, Gohda J, Inoue J, Mizushima T, Sasakawa C. 2012. The *Shigella flexneri* effector OspI deamidates UBC13 to dampen the inflammatory response. *Nature* 483:623–626.

117. Nishide A, Kim M, Takagi K, Himeno A, Sanada T, Sasakawa C, Mizushima T. 2013. Structural basis for the recognition of Ubc13 by the *Shigella flexneri* effector OspI. *J Mol Biol* 425:2623–2631.

118. Ashida H, Nakano H, Sasakawa C. 2013. *Shigella* IpaH0722 E3 ubiquitin ligase effector targets TRAF2 to inhibit PKC-NF-κB activity in invaded epithelial cells. *PLoS Pathog* 9:e1003409.

119. de Jong MF, Liu Z, Chen D, Alto NM. 2016. *Shigella flexneri* suppresses NF-κB activation by inhibiting linear ubiquitin chain ligation. *Nat Microbiol* 1:16084.

120. Zhang Y, Mühlen S, Oates CV, Pearson JS, Hartland EL. 2016. Identification of a distinct substrate-binding domain in the bacterial cysteine methyltransferase effectors NleE and OspZ. *J Biol Chem* 291:20149–20162.

121. Newton HJ, Pearson JS, Badea L, Kelly M, Lucas M, Holloway G, Wagstaff KM, Dunstone MA, Sloan J, Whisstock JC, Kaper JB, Robins-Browne RM, Jans DA, Frankel G, Phillips AD, Coulson BS, Hartland EL. 2010. The type III effectors NleE and NleB from enteropathogenic *E. coli* and OspZ from *Shigella* block nuclear translocation of NF-κB p65. *PLoS Pathog* 6:e1000898.

122. Ashida H, Kim M, Schmidt-Supprian M, Ma A, Ogawa M, Sasakawa C. 2010. A bacterial E3 ubiquitin ligase IpaH9.8 targets NEMO/IKKγ to dampen the host NF-κB-mediated inflammatory response. *Nat Cell Biol* 12:66–73.

123. Kim DW, Lenzen G, Page A-L, Legrain P, Sansonetti PJ, Parsot C. 2005. The *Shigella flexneri* effector OspG interferes with innate immune responses by targeting ubiquitin-conjugating enzymes. *Proc Natl Acad Sci USA* 102:14046–14051.

124. Wang F, Jiang Z, Li Y, He X, Zhao J, Yang X, Zhu L, Yin Z, Li X, Wang X, Liu W, Shang W, Yang Z, Wang S, Zhen Q, Zhang Z, Yu Y, Zhong H, Ye Q, Huang L, Yuan J. 2013. *Shigella flexneri* T3SS effector IpaH4.5 modulates the host inflammatory response via interaction with NF-κB p65 protein. *Cell Microbiol* 15:474–485.

125. Li H, Xu H, Zhou Y, Zhang J, Long C, Li S, Chen S, Zhou J-M, Shao F. 2007. The phosphothreonine lyase activity of a bacterial type III effector family. *Science* 315:1000–1003.

126. Arbibe L, Kim DW, Batsche E, Pedron T, Mateescu B, Muchardt C, Parsot C, Sansonetti PJ. 2007. An injected bacterial effector targets chromatin access for transcription factor NF-kappaB to alter transcription of host genes involved in immune responses. *Nat Immunol* 8:47–56.

127. Harouz H, Rachez C, Meijer BM, Marteyn B, Donnadieu F, Cammas F, Muchardt C, Sansonetti P, Arbibe L. 2014. *Shigella flexneri* targets the HP1γ subcode through the phosphothreonine lyase OspF. *EMBO J* 33:2606–2622.

128. Schmutz C, Ahrné E, Kasper CA, Tschon T, Sorg I, Dreier RF, Schmidt A, Arrieumerlou C. 2013. Systems-level overview of host protein phosphorylation during *Shigella flexneri* infection revealed by phosphoproteomics. *Mol Cell Proteomics* 12:2952–2968.

129. Okuda J, Toyotome T, Kataoka N, Ohno M, Abe H, Shimura Y, Seyedarabi A, Pickersgill R, Sasakawa C. 2005. *Shigella* effector IpaH9.8 binds to a splicing factor U2AF(35) to modulate host immune responses. *Biochem Biophys Res Commun* 333:531–539.

130. Burnaevskiy N, Fox TG, Plymire DA, Ertelt JM, Weigele BA, Selyunin AS, Way SS, Patrie SM, Alto NM. 2013. Proteolytic elimination of N-myristoyl modifications by the *Shigella* virulence factor IpaJ. *Nature* 496:106–109.

131. Dobbs N, Burnaevskiy N, Chen D, Gonugunta VK, Alto NM, Yan N. 2015. STING activation by translocation from the ER is associated with infection and autoinflammatory disease. *Cell Host Microbe* 18:157–168.

132. Mounier J, Boncompain G, Senerovic L, Lagache T, Chrétien F, Perez F, Kolbe M, Olivo-Marin J-C, Sansonetti PJ, Sauvonnet N. 2012. *Shigella* effector IpaB-induced cholesterol relocation disrupts the Golgi complex and recycling network to inhibit host cell secretion. *Cell Host Microbe* 12:381–389.

133. Zheng Z, Wei C, Guan K, Yuan Y, Zhang Y, Ma S, Cao Y, Wang F, Zhong H, He X. 2016. Bacterial E3 ubiquitin ligase IpaH4.5 of *Shigella flexneri* targets TBK1 to dampen the host antibacterial response. *J Immunol* 196:1199–1208.

134. Puhar A, Tronchère H, Payrastre B, Tran Van Nhieu GTV, Sansonetti PJ. 2013. A *Shigella* effector dampens inflammation by regulating epithelial release of danger signal ATP through production of the lipid mediator PtdIns5P. *Immunity* **39**:1121–1131.

135. Konradt C, Frigimelica E, Nothelfer K, Puhar A, Salgado-Pabón W, di Bartolo V, Scott-Algara D, Rodrigues CD, Sansonetti PJ, Phalipon A. 2011. The *Shigella flexneri* type three secretion system effector IpgD inhibits T cell migration by manipulating host phosphoinositide metabolism. *Cell Host Microbe* **9**:263–272.

136. Salgado-Pabón W, Celli S, Arena ET, Nothelfer K, Roux P, Sellge G, Frigimelica E, Bousso P, Sansonetti PJ, Phalipon A. 2013. *Shigella* impairs T lymphocyte dynamics in vivo. *Proc Natl Acad Sci USA* **110**: 4458–4463.

137. Pinaud L, Samassa F, Porat Z, Ferrari ML, Belotserkovsky I, Parsot C, Sansonetti PJ, Campbell-Valois F-X, Phalipon A. 2017. Injection of T3SS effectors not resulting in invasion is the main targeting mechanism of *Shigella* toward human lymphocytes. *Proc Natl Acad Sci USA* **114**:9954–9959.

Bacteria and Intracellularity
Edited by Pascale Cossart, Craig R. Roy, and Philippe Sansonetti
© 2019 American Society for Microbiology, Washington, DC
doi:10.1128/microbiolspec.BAI-0004-2019

The Interplay between *Salmonella enterica* Serovar Typhimurium and the Intestinal Mucosa during Oral Infection

3

Annika Hausmann[1] and Wolf-Dietrich Hardt[1]

INTRODUCTION

Bacterial pathogens typically target specific host tissues. The interaction between host and pathogen is a complex process that differs from cell to cell (1). It strongly depends on the targeted organ and the pathogen itself. Organs are composed of multiple cell types that may cooperate in antimicrobial defense. While earlier work focused on the role of immune cells, it is becoming increasingly clear that non-hematopoietic cells can also serve as key orchestrators of defense. Pathogens employ a combination of virulence factors in order to ensure nutrient supply, avoid killing by innate defenses, and actively manipulate the host in order to establish infection and fuel transmission (2). Deciphering virulence factor function during actual infection of an animal host therefore holds the key to understanding the infection process.

Cell culture models are useful tools for in-depth analysis of individual host-pathogen interactions in a controlled system. They are frequently used to demonstrate the disease- and infection-promoting capacity of certain virulence factors. However, tissue culture assays cannot discern whether such interactions are indeed relevant during infection of a whole organism. Often, the complex structure of organs with their particular tissue architecture and interaction between cell types cannot be mimicked in a cell culture dish. Therefore, robust animal models are indispensable for translatable insights into the reciprocal relationship between a pathogen's virulence factors and the host.

The intestine is a particularly interesting organ for studies of host-pathogen interactions. As a barrier tissue, it forms the interface between the sterile compartment of the host's body and the gut luminal environment, which is home to a large variety of microorganisms. This microbiota colonizes the intestinal lumen and engages in a symbiotic relationship with the host, contributing to nutrient uptake (3) and shaping of the immune system (4, 5). Moreover, the occupation of the intestinal niche by the microbiota prevents pathogen growth in the gut lumen (dubbed "colonization resistance") (6, 7). In spite of these beneficial effects, the microbiota shares conserved molecules with pathogenic bacteria, creating a critical detection problem for the gut tissue. Pathogens are regularly ingested, requiring immune surveillance of the intestine to avoid infections. However, no immune response is mounted against commensals in healthy individuals (8). Thus, the intestine provides a fascinating system to study how the delicate balance of peaceful cohabitation with the commensal microbiota is maintained and how specific defense against pathogen attack is achieved (9).

Salmonella enterica serovar Typhimurium represents a major health issue. As one of the top causes of diarrheal disease burden worldwide (10), this foodborne pathogen usually causes self-limiting gastroenteritis accompanied by fever, abdominal pain, and nausea. In children, the elderly, and immunocompromised persons, infection with *S.* Typhimurium can even be life-threatening (11). *S.* Typhimurium is a versatile pathogen for the study of host-pathogen interactions. It is able to cope with the host response and even exploits defense mechanisms to its own advantage.

[1]Institute of Microbiology, D-BIOL ETH Zurich, Zurich, Switzerland.

Several animal models exist for studying *Salmonella* diarrhea (11). Seminal insights into disease pathology and key pathogen virulence factors were gained in opium-treated guinea pigs (12) and calves (13). The calf gastro-enteritis model parallels disease symptoms in humans, making it relevant for translation (14, 15). More recently, the field has shifted to mouse models (16), which also mimic the disease. Importantly, these mouse models offer several technical advantages for mechanistic research, including genetically homogeneous host strains, a plethora of knockout models, and immunological methods for analysis (17).

S. Typhimurium infection in streptomycin-pretreated mice is a model for nontyphoidal *Salmonella* diarrhea. In this model, colonization resistance is alleviated by streptomycin (16, 18, 19). This leads to efficient colonization of the intestinal lumen within 4 to 6 h after intragastric inoculation. The disease is characterized by strong inflammation of the cecal mucosa, expulsion of infected epithelial cells, and the recruitment of neutrophils and NK cells (16). The robust disease induction in this model allows a detailed analysis of the underlying mechanisms, including function of the virulence factors in tissue invasion. It makes it possible to study innate defenses protecting the gut, like host responses that mount the characteristic gut inflammation and pathogen clearance by microbiota regrowth, as well as O-antigen-specific secretory IgA at the end of an acute infection (20).

Here, we briefly describe the infection cycle of *S.* Typhimurium in the streptomycin-pretreated mouse model and focus on physical, chemical, and immunological defenses limiting the infection. Further, we discuss how *S.* Typhimurium adapts and exploits these mechanisms for the establishment of an infection and efficient transmission.

INFECTION KINETICS OF *S.* TYPHIMURIUM IN THE STREPTOMYCIN-PRETREATED MOUSE MODEL

In the streptomycin mouse model, the cecum is well established as the major site of *S.* Typhimurium invasion (16). So far, it is not well understood why *S.* Typhimurium preferentially targets this site of the murine intestine. We speculate that this might be due to its particular anatomical features (e.g., low flow rate of the content of this dead-end side arm of the gut), metabolite availability, or environmental signals that trigger virulence factor expression. Nevertheless, around 2 h after intragastric inoculation, *S.* Typhimurium reaches the murine cecum and grows to a density of 10^9 bacteria per gram of cecal content within the next 4 to 6 h (16, 21).

By 8 to 12 h, *S.* Typhimurium invasion into the mucosa yields pathogen densities of $>10^6$ bacteria per gram of cecal tissue. Three mechanisms have been suggested to drive this tissue invasion: (i) active invasion of intestinal epithelial cells (IECs) by *S.* Typhimurium (classical pathway), (ii) uptake by phagocytes sampling the intestinal lumen (alternative pathway), and (iii) uptake of *S.* Typhimurium by M cells. The latter occurs mainly in the Peyer's patches of the small intestine and possibly in the cecal patch at the tip of the cecum. We do not discuss this in detail but describe the former two mechanisms, which explain the infection of the cecal absorptive mucosa.

Active IEC invasion via the classical pathway is promoted by type III secretion system 1 (TTSS-1), encoded by *Salmonella* pathogenicity island 1 (SPI-1), the *sii* adhesin, and the flagella (22–24) (Fig. 1). The expression of SPI-1 occurs in response to environmental signals in the intestinal lumen, which induce a regulatory feed-forward loop, ensuring that the invasion machinery is "trigger ready" before the pathogen actually reaches the gut epithelium.

Flagella mediate bacterial motility. During orogastric *S.* Typhimurium infection, they are crucial for active swimming toward the intestinal epithelium as well as for attachment to IECs (17, 24–27). Importantly, flagella are coexpressed with TTSS-1 (28). TTSS-1 is a needle-like complex, which allows injection of a virulence factor cocktail (effector proteins) into the cytosol of the host cell (29, 30). In the host cellular cytosol, these effector proteins trigger cytoskeletal rearrangements and bacterial uptake. SipA, SopB, SopE, and SopE2 cooperate to induce Rho GTPase activation and Arp2/3-dependent rearrangements of the actin cytoskeleton (31, 32). This process is well characterized in HeLa cells, where it leads to a membrane ruffle-dependent uptake of the bacterial cell (33, 34). Similar observations were made during M-cell invasion in the murine small intestine and in classical orogastric infection experiments in opium-treated guinea pigs (12). These ruffles are thought to facilitate *S.* Typhimurium entry into epithelial cells and thereby contribute to initiation of intestinal inflammation as well as penetration into deeper layers of the mucosal tissue (23, 35, 36) (Fig. 1).

S. Typhimurium mutants lacking a functional TTSS-1 apparatus (e.g., Δ*invG* mutants) rely on sampling by phagocytes from the intestinal lumen to breach the epithelial barrier (alternative pathway) (Fig. 1) (37). It is likely that classical and alternative pathways operate in parallel during infections with wild-type *S.* Typhimurium.

Once taken up by the host cell, *S.* Typhimurium resides within a *Salmonella*-containing vacuole (SCV)

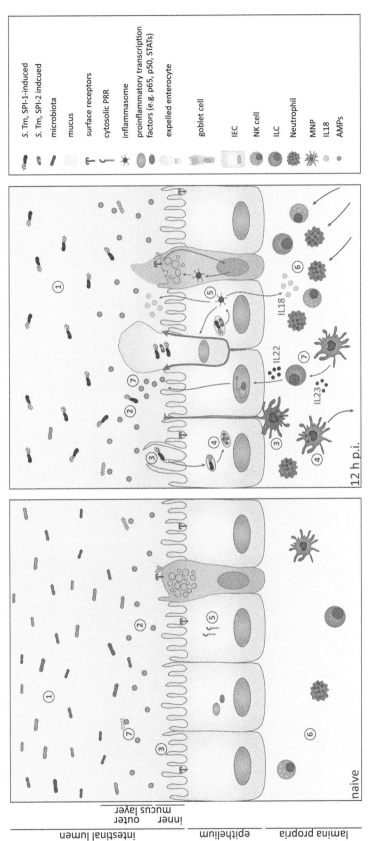

Figure 1 Innate defense mechanisms in naive and *S.* Typhimurium (12 h)-infected intestinal mucosa. For efficient infection, *S.* Typhimurium has to overcome several mucosal defense mechanisms. This comprises occupation of the intestinal niche by the microbiota (1) and breaching of the mucus layer (2), the epithelium (3), and physical barriers between the intestinal lumen and the sterile lamina propria (LP) (4, 5). Recognition of intracellular bacteria by PRRs leads to recruitment of immune cells (6) that are able to efficiently kill bacteria and the induction of increased AMP production via immune cells (7). TLR, Toll-like receptor; ILC, innate lymphoid cell; MNP, mononuclear phagocyte; p.i., postinfection.

(Fig. 1). The SCV is an endosomal compartment that is actively modified by the bacterium. Early SCV biogenesis is controlled mainly by TTSS-1 (36, 38–41). Throughout the maturation process, acidification of the SCV leads to SPI-2-mediated induction of TTSS-2 (Fig. 2), which contributes to later stages of SCV maintenance. SPI-1 and SPI-2 effectors (e.g., SipA, SopB, SopE, SpiC, SipC, and SifA) stabilize the SCV membrane and control SCV fusion with the endocytic pathway of the host cell (42). Accordingly, SCVs display altered surface markers compared to classical lysosomes. They are positive for LAMP1 (lysosome-associated membrane protein 1) and vATPase but lack cathepsins and mannose 6-phosphate receptors (42).

SPI-2 can promote intracellular replication and survival of *S.* Typhimurium by controlling the fusion of lysosomes with the SCV, suppression of inducible nitric oxide synthase- and NADPH oxidase-induced bactericidal effects, and inhibition of apoptosis. This is well established in macrophages *in vitro* and *in vivo* but may also be relevant for *S.* Typhimurium growth within other cell types *in vivo* (43–45).

SPI-1 expression is downregulated immediately after host cell invasion. However, in HeLa cells, its expression may resume after 6 h of infection (46). This reinduction goes along with an induction of flagellar gene expression and might also happen *in vivo* (47). The switch to an invasive phenotype is specifically observed in HeLa cells

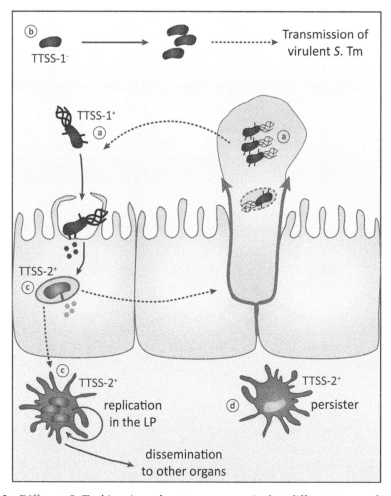

Figure 2 Different *S.* Typhimurium phenotypes are required at different stages of infection. (a) TTSS-1⁺, flagellum positive, TTSS-2⁻, required for active invasion of host cells; (b) TTSS-1⁺, flagellum negative *in vitro* (109), TTSS-2⁻, fast growing, ensures transmission; (c) TTSS-1⁻, flagellum negative, TTSS-2⁺, fast growing, intracellular survival; (d) TTSS-1⁻, flagellum negative, TTSS-2⁺, slow growing, antibiotic tolerance (persisters). LP, lamina propria.

(not in bone marrow-derived macrophages [BMDMs]) and strongly correlates with cytosolic escape from the SCV and hyperreplication in the nutrient-rich cytosol (46, 48, 49). In line with this, HeLa cells infected with *sifA* mutants—which lack a main stabilizer of the SCV membrane—harbor high loads of cytosolic S. Typhimurium already at early stages of the infection. BMDMs, in contrast, are not permissive for cytosolic hyperreplication of S. Typhimurium (50), which might be due to different pattern recognition receptor (PRR) expression schemes in these two cell types (e.g., caspase-11 [Casp11]; see below).

These fluctuations in SPI-1 gene expression in epithelial cells might represent a cycle of invasion, replication, expulsion, and reinfection that could also take place in the intestinal mucosa of infected mice. S. Typhimurium might make use of the protected niche of the SCV to adapt to an intracellular lifestyle. It switches on TTSS-2 in enterocytes and replicates moderately within these cells. Escape from the SCV appears to be detected by the chemosensors of the NLR (Nod-like receptor)-family caspase recruitment domain-containing protein 4 (NLRC4) inflammasome, leading to expulsion of infected enterocytes into the gut lumen (see below) (Fig. 1 and 2). Back in the lumen, TTSS-1 and flagella may ideally prepare the S. Typhimurium cell for the next round of enterocyte invasion (21, 47, 49). Clearly, this hypothesis can only be tested *in vivo*, when the pathogen faces the multilayered architecture of the intestinal defenses.

INNATE MUCOSAL DEFENSE MECHANISMS

Mucus Layer

In mice, the main structural component of the mucus layer is MUC2, a gel-forming mucin that is produced by goblet cells residing in the intestinal epithelium (51). It has been thoroughly characterized in the murine colon, where it is organized in two layers. The inner layer close to the epithelial cells is around 50 m thick, viscous, dense in MUC2, and devoid of bacteria. The outer, loose layer is around 100 μm thick, populated, and slowly degraded by some specialized commensals. Together, the two mucus layers act as a protective filter which keeps bacteria at a distance while allowing free diffusion of amino acids, sugars, and small molecular compounds (52, 53).

Muc2−/− mice are unable to produce a mucus layer. They remain healthy if held under germfree conditions. Upon colonization with a pathogen-free microbiota, bacteria can be found in direct contact with the epithelium. Under these conditions, the mice develop colitis by 7 weeks of age and are predisposed to colon cancer (52).

This underlines the importance of mucus for the maintenance of intestinal homeostasis in the context of a commensal microbiota. Interestingly, the dense mucus layer seems to be mainly of importance in the colon and the stomach, as the mucus in the small intestine is organized discontinuously in clouds between the villi (53). To date, little is known about the organization of the cecal mucus. This is of particular interest, as pathogens like S. Typhimurium preferentially attack this site, at least in mouse models of diarrheal disease.

A recent study showed that the colonic epithelium is equipped with sentinel goblet cells located at the top of the crypts. These cells recognize pathogen-associated molecular patterns (PAMPs) of bacterial intruders in the inner mucus layer via Toll-like receptors and the NLR family pyrin domain-containing 6 (NLRP6) inflammasome. They react by signaling via gap junctions to induce coordinated mucus secretion, pushing the intruding bacteria away from the epithelial surface (54, 55) (Fig. 1). Furthermore, mucus secretion is triggered by gamma interferon (IFN-γ) signaling, which is abundant during mucosal S. Typhimurium infection (56, 57). This indicates that the mucus architecture and its shielding functions are tuned in response to defined stimuli.

Antimicrobial Peptides

Another factor in the maintenance of intestinal microbial homeostasis and the defense against pathogens is antimicrobial peptides (AMPs). IECs express several different AMPs, including defensins, cathelicidins, lipocalin-2, and the lectin family RegIII. Low levels of AMPs are expressed under homeostatic conditions and are thought to promote homeostasis by maintaining a favorable microbiota composition and by preventing microbiota penetration of the epithelial barrier (58, 59). Lipocalin-2 and the RegIII lectins are strongly induced upon bacterial infection (60–62). This is mediated at least in part by intestinal dendritic cells, which sense microbial products (e.g., flagellin) and elicit a signaling cascade involving interleukin 23 (IL-23), mucosal innate lymphoid cells, and IL-22, a strong inducer of AMP production in IECs (63) (Fig. 1). Thus, the AMP-mediated chemical barrier is tunable in response to infection.

AMPs play main roles in the defense against a variety of intestinal pathogens (64–68). However, in some cases, AMP production can also promote, instead of preventing, disease. In oral S. Typhimurium infections, RegIIIβ delays remission from acute S. Typhimurium enterocolitis by suppressing the regrowth of certain microbiota species, especially some *Bacteroides* spp. (60). While S. Typhimurium is resistant to RegIIIβ and lipocalin-2

(60, 61), key members of the microbiota are highly susceptible. Thus, by eliciting an antibacterial response program, the host keeps the intestinal niche open for *S*. Typhimurium by depleting the resident microbiota.

PRR-Mediated Expulsion of Infected Enterocytes

The intestinal epithelium separates the gut luminal microbes from the sterile compartments of the gut mucosa. IECs are equipped with PRRs that recognize conserved structures on microbes. This includes Toll-like receptors recognizing extracellular or vacuolar microbes and microbial products as well as inflammasomes detecting cytoplasmic insults.

Inflammasomes are an important element of the innate immune system (69). The cytosolic PRRs recognize conserved microbial structures or cellular damage. Recognition events typically activate downstream caspases, promote cytokine release, and elicit a specific type of cell death termed pyroptosis (69). The NLR-family apoptosis inhibitory protein (NAIP)/NLRC4 inflammasome detects flagella (70, 71) and subunits of the TTSS-1 apparatus (72, 73). NLRP1 and the pyrin inflammasome detect bacterial toxins (74, 75), the Aim2 (absent in melanoma 2) inflammasome is sensitive to double-stranded DNA in the cytosol (76, 77), and NLRP3 is activated upon recognition of microbial stimuli and/or cellular damage (78). Cytosolic binding of lipopolysaccharide (LPS) by Casp11 leads to noncanonical induction of pyroptosis and induces Casp1 activation via indirect activation of NLRP3 (79). Thus, inflammasomes mount a defense in response to cytoplasmic evidence of infection.

For many years, *S*. Typhimurium host cell invasion has been studied in epithelial cell line models, which show highly aberrant patterns of inflammasome expression (80). In contrast, inflammasome research has focused on BMDMs. Thus, it had remained largely unclear whether inflammasomes may protect the intestinal mucosa. Recent studies revealed a major role of inflammasomes in the defense of IECs against *S*. Typhimurium. In streptomycin-pretreated mice, defects in the NLRC4 inflammasome lead to 100-fold-increased pathogen loads in the cecal epithelium. This effect partially depends on Casp1 and relies on the expulsion of infected enterocytes from the epithelium (21, 81).

Observations in mice infected with *S*. Typhimurium suggest that infected enterocytes are expelled from the epithelium and undergo cell death in the intestinal lumen (21, 82). The dependence of infected-IEC expulsion on the NLRC4 inflammasome was recently verified by an elegant genetic reconstitution of NLRC4 specifically in IECs of *S*. Typhimurium-infected or FlaTox-treated

mice (81). FlaTox is a bioengineered AB toxin. The *Legionella pneumophila* flagellin (FlaA), a strong stimulator of the NAIP/NLRC4 inflammasome, is fused to the N-terminal domain of *Bacillus anthracis* lethal factor (LFn). In combination with the anthrax protective antigen channel, FlaA is delivered into the cytosol. FlaTox can be used for sterile activation of the NLRC4 inflammasome (83). This is highly elegant, as it avoids confounding effects elicited by the innate immune recognition of other bacterial factors present when infecting with pathogen cells. In FlaTox-treated mice, NLRC4 was confirmed as the key inducer of the enterocyte expulsion defense. In this system, activated IECs lost plasma membrane integrity before being expelled into the gut lumen. Nevertheless, in spite of epithelium-wide NLRC4 activation, the epithelial layer remained intact for at least 60 minutes, as voids left by enterocyte expulsion were sealed by neighboring IECs, which form actin "purse strings" around the expelled enterocyte (81).

FlaTox treatment was also used to specifically analyze downstream signaling of NLRC4 activation in the cecal mucosa of mice. This study revealed two parallel downstream signaling pathways. One pathway involves Casp1, gasdermin D, secretion of the proinflammatory cytokine IL-18, and a pyroptosis-like enterocyte cell death. The parallel pathway requires an apoptosis-associated speck-like protein containing a caspase recruitment domain (ASC) and Casp8 and elicits expulsion via an apoptosis-like enterocyte cell death with little IL-18 release. The key role of Casp8 was later verified by enterocyte-specific ablation (84). Moreover, this work identified a modulating function of receptor-interacting serine/threonine-protein kinase 3 (RipK3) and mixed-lineage kinase domain-like protein (MLKL), suggesting that Casp8, RipK3, and MLKL cooperate in defining whether apoptosis or necroptosis dominates this second enterocyte cell death pathway upon NLRC4 activation.

In BMDMs, the binding of cytosolic LPS by Casp11 induces noncanonical inflammasome activation, resulting in pyroptosis (79). Whether this Casp11-mediated cell death of infected cells plays a role in IECs, however, remains controversial. Several studies tested the importance of Casp11 in the context of epithelial *S*. Typhimurium infection and found contradictory results (21, 82). Sellin et al. (21) showed that Casp11 plays no role in the control of cecal tissue loads in *S*. Typhimurium infection, whereas Knodler and colleagues (82) observed increased pathogen loads in the cecal tissue at 7 days of infection. To conclusively interpret these data, further experiments assessing the initial 24 h after infection in littermate-controlled experimental settings will be of great value.

Generally, it appears that Casp11—at least in BMDMs—confers resistance against cytosolic bacteria, like the naturally cytosolic pathogen *Burkholderia thailandensis*, as well as the cytosolic escaper mutants of *S.* Typhimurium (Δ*sifA* mutants) and *L. pneumophila* (Δ*sdhA* mutants) (85). Interestingly, the cytosolic pathogen *Francisella novicida* has a tetra-acylated lipid A (which is not detected by Casp11), instead of penta- or hexa-acylated lipid A, which binds to Casp11. This might represent a mechanism of immune evasion for this naturally cytosolic bacterium (86). However, it remains unclear whether LPS recognition by inflammasomes contributes to epithelial defense and whether stealthy LPS modifications might offer ways to avoid recognition.

In conclusion, NLRC4-driven defenses reduce pathogen loads in the gut tissue by eliciting caspase-mediated expulsion of infected enterocytes. The role of Casp11 in this process is not fully understood. In parallel, the NLRC4-mediated response induces profound proinflammatory signals which recruit granulocytes, mature NK cells, macrophages, and dendritic cells to clear remaining pathogens from the gut tissue (21, 80, 87). Which downstream signaling pathways (via Casp1 or via Casp8; death by pyroptosis, necroptosis, or apoptosis) dominate the defense against *S.* Typhimurium remains an important topic for further work.

DOWNSTREAM ELICITATION OF OVERT MUCOSAL INFLAMMATION

Besides expulsion of infected enterocytes, assembly of the NAIP/NLRC4 inflammasome leads to activation and secretion of IL-1β and IL-18. Both cytokines are produced as inactive precursors (pro-IL-1β and pro-IL-18) that are activated upon cleavage by Casp1 and Casp11. IL-18 secretion by IECs is mainly regulated at the protein level (88). This cytokine is constantly produced and secreted at low levels by IECs during homeostatic conditions. IL-1β, in contrast, seems to be further regulated on a transcriptional level, leading to a specific upregulation of *Il1b* mRNA levels in response to exposure to microbial stimuli (21). The contribution of IECs to IL-1β secretion is thought to be minor (55, 89). Nevertheless, the infected mucosa features elevated levels of both IL-18 and IL-1β. Whereas IL-1β is dispensable for the mounting of inflammation at early time points after oral *S.* Typhimurium infection, IL-18 is crucial for induction of inflammation within the first 12 h after oral infection (Fig. 1) (87). This IL-18-mediated inflammation was shown to require Casp1 (most likely within IECs), with a contribution of immune cells in the intestinal mucosa (80, 87).

IL-18 recruits neutrophils and mature natural killer (NK) cells into the cecal lamina propria (Fig. 1). NK cells express perforin, which plays a major role in the swift induction of mucosal inflammation. Interestingly, this IL-18-mediated NK cell-elicited mucosal inflammation is not required for the control of local or systemic bacterial loads in the first 12 h of infection. This indicates that the early host response against oral *S.* Typhimurium infection relies mainly on the NAIP/NLRC4-mediated expulsion of infected IECs, not the recruited phagocytes (21, 80, 87). Strikingly, the induction of mucosal inflammation seems to have, during early infection, no obvious benefit for the host. In contrast, it might even hinder pathogen clearance at later stages of the infection cycle by contributing to antimicrobial responses that repress regrowth of the microbiota (59–61, 90).

The inflamed mucosa also attracts neutrophils via IL-18 and IL-1β, most likely through induction of chemokines. Neutrophils play an important role in limiting pathogen loads both in the mucosa as well as in the intestinal lumen at later stages of infection (87, 91). Pathogen clearance by neutrophils is mediated indirectly (via cytokine-mediated recruitment of further phagocytes) and directly via phagocytosis and intracellular killing of pathogens (87). Macrophages contribute to pathogen phagocytosis. In the case of pathogens like *Chromobacterium violaceum* and *S.* Typhimurium, these infected macrophages tend to undergo pyroptosis, thus forming pore-induced intracellular traps. These traps retain surviving bacteria and are taken up by neutrophils, which kill the entrapped bacteria in an NADPH oxidase-dependent way (92, 93). This is well established for systemic infection. However, it remains to be shown whether this mechanism also contributes to pathogen clearance from the *S.* Typhimurium-infected gut tissue.

Inflammatory processes in the mucosa are to some extent self-sustained. The remission after antibiotic treatment of *S.* Typhimurium intestinal infection is slowed by IFN-γ signaling, a prominent by-product of mucosal inflammation (90). Treatment of *S.* Typhimurium-infected mice with ciprofloxacin eliminates pathogen cells from the intestinal lumen within a few hours. However, a small antibiotic-tolerant fraction of bacteria (persisters) remains in the mucosal tissue and in the mesenteric lymph nodes (Fig. 2) (94, 95). This may further prolong IFN-γ-driven defenses in the mucosal tissue, slowing the clearance of granulocytes from the gut and inhibiting the polarization of lamina propria phagocytes toward a homeostatic phenotype (90). Overall, such prolonged signaling slows remission and might contribute to gastrointestinal disorders after intestinal infections and increase susceptibility to subsequent infections (96).

AVOIDING RECOGNITION BY MODULATING THE HOST'S INNATE IMMUNE RESPONSE

Coevolution tends to result in a delicate adaptation of pathogens to their hosts (2). *S.* Typhimurium provides one well-studied example of complementary adaptations to avoid innate immune defenses, i.e., the downregulation of PAMPs and the expression of virulence factors disrupting innate immune signaling (Table 1). The latter approach appears to be common to many pathogenic bacteria (Table 2). This was recently reviewed in detail (97). Here, we present a few examples to illustrate the finely tuned interplay between *Salmonella* virulence factors and the host immune response as well as its role in promoting virulence of the bacterium.

As described above, *S.* Typhimurium relies on certain virulence factors to initiate gut tissue invasion. Flagella and TTSS-1 are required for efficient invasion of IECs (Fig. 1 and 2). These two molecular complexes are conserved structures that are associated with many pathogenic bacteria. IECs are well equipped with specific receptors for recognition of exactly these PAMPs. In consequence, the expression of flagella and TTSS-1 in the early phase of infection not only leads to efficient

host invasion but also elicits inflammatory defenses. IECs employ inflammasome sensors to specifically detect *S.* Typhimurium virulence factors which are needed by the pathogen to infect these cells (80, 98). This creates a dilemma for the pathogen between dependence on virulence factor expression and recognition of those factors by the immune system of the host.

This recognition problem might explain why several enteropathogenic bacteria employ TTSS effector proteins to inhibit the host's innate immune response (Tables 1 and 2). Common targets are found in the NF-κB and cell death pathways, which are tightly interlinked to regulate survival versus death and which elicit (or avoid) the production and release of proinflammatory cytokines (99). The NF-κB pathway is a major proinflammatory pathway, to which a variety of stimuli converge inside host cells. RelA and RelB are the main NF-κB transcription factors. They are sequestered in the cytosol of the naive cell and translocate to the nucleus for induction of proinflammatory target genes upon stimulation (100). Indeed, *S.* Typhimurium expresses a variety of effector proteins targeting the NF-κB signaling pathway (Table 1). One striking example is the effector proteins PipA, GogA, and GtgA, which are injected into host cells via TTSS-1

Table 1 *S.* Typhimurium virulence factors that modulate the host immune response

Effector(s)	Target molecule(s)	Target pathway(s)[a]	Type of interaction	Outcome of interaction	System	Reference(s)
SseK1, SseK3	FADD, TRADD	TNF-α-induced NF-κB signaling	Inactivation by arginine-GlcNAcylation	Inhibition of necroptosis (apoptosis not affected)	*In vitro*	117
AvrA	IκBa, MKK4, MKK7	NF-κB, JNK, MAPK signaling	Inactivation by acetylation	Anti-inflammatory and antiapoptotic	*In vitro, in vivo*	118, 119
GogB	Scf ubiquitin ligase complex (Skp1, FBOX22)	IκB degradation and MAPK signaling	Inhibition	Anti-inflammatory	*In vitro, in vivo*	120
SpvC	ERK, p38, JNK	MAPK	Phosphothreonine lyase, inhibition	Anti-inflammatory	*In vitro, in vivo*	121–124
SseL	IκBa?	NF-κB signaling, autophagy	Inactivation by deubiquitination	Anti-inflammatory	*In vitro, in vivo*	125–127
SspH1	PKN1	NF-κB signaling	Inhibition by E3 ubiquitin ligation	Anti-inflammatory	*In vitro*	128–130
SpvD	Xpo2	NF-κB nuclear translocation	Inhibition of importin-mediated nuclear import, deconjugation	Anti-inflammatory	*In vitro*, small *in vivo* effect	131
PipA, GogA, GtgA	RelA and RelB, redundant	NF-κB signaling	Inhibition	Anti-inflammatory	*In vitro, in vivo*	101
SopB	NLRC4 inflammasome pathway?	Inflammasome activation	Inhibition	Anti-inflammatory	*In vitro*	132
SopA	TRIM56 and TRIM65	IFN-β signaling	HECT-like E3 ligase, stimulation	Proinflammatory	*In vitro*	133–136

[a]TNF-α, tumor necrosis factor alpha; MAPK, mitogen-activated protein kinase.

Table 2 Examples of host response-modulating virulence factors of a variety of pathogenic bacteria

Effector	Target molecule	Target pathway	Type of interaction	Outcome of interaction	System	Organism	Reference(s)
YopM	Pyrin inflammasome	Pyrin inflammasome	Inhibition	Anti-inflammatory	*In vivo*	*Yersinia*	137, 138
YopH	IL-18 secretion	Inflammasome downstream signaling	Inhibition	Anti-inflammatory	*In vitro*	*Yersinia*	89
NleF	Casp4, -8, -9	Caspase-mediated cell death	Inhibition	Antiapoptotic	*In vitro*	*Escherichia coli*	139
OspC3	Casp4	Caspase-mediated cell death	Inhibition	Antiapoptotic	*In vivo* (guinea pig)	*Shigella*	140
IpaH9.8	NEMO	NF-κB signaling	Promotes ubiquitination of NEMO	Anti-inflammatory	*In vitro*	*Shigella*	141
NleB1	FADD	Casp8-mediated cell death	Inhibition	Antiapoptotic	*In vivo*	*Citrobacter rodentium*	142–145

and/or TTSS-2. They redundantly block the NF-κB signaling pathway by cleaving RelA and RelB. Interestingly, these NF-κB transcription factors are targeted directly inside the nucleus. This implies that a short triggering of proinflammatory downstream mechanisms is permitted. After one cycle of induction, the inflammatory response is shut down by PipA, GogA, and GtgA. This reduces gut tissue pathology and prevents an overwhelming immune response. In contrast, an *S.* Typhimurium mutant lacking PipA, GogA, and GtgA elicits more pronounced enteropathy and host death (101). Future work will need to address the question of whether PipA, GogA, and GtgA block NF-κB signaling in infected enterocytes (and may delay their demise) or in lamina propria phagocytes.

Numerous additional *S.* Typhimurium TTSS effectors exist and may well contribute to damping the host's mucosal innate response (Table 1). However, demonstrating their *in vivo* function might be challenging, for several reasons. Due to redundant activities, it will be necessary to test mutants with reduced effector protein repertoires in a trial-and-error type of approach. Also, fine-tuning of the mouse infection model will be crucial to decipher immune modulation during particular steps of the gut tissue infection process. It should be noted that the classical streptomycin mouse model might be suboptimal, as invading pathogen loads increase very sharply by 6 to 10 h of infection, which leads to extensive inflammation (and may cover up more subtle TTSS effector phenotypes) by 10 to 12 h of infection (16). More benign gut infection kinetics, as observed in mice with a low-complexity gut microbiota, might help to resolve this issue (25). Finally, it remains unclear whether some *S.* Typhimurium TTSS effectors work only in specific hosts. This is particularly pressing, as *S.* Typhimurium is a broad-host-range pathogen and new epidemic clones emerge in its zoonotic animal reservoirs, i.e., chickens, swine, and cattle.

S. Typhimurium transmission via the fecal-oral route is more efficient the longer the host is viable and mobile while shedding high loads of the pathogen. Thus, the pathogen employs a sophisticated regulatory machinery to ideally promote its spread in the host population by induction of early inflammation and tight control of the immune response by bacterial virulence factors to avoid overwhelming disease (2, 102).

DIFFERENT VIRULENCE PHENOTYPES ARE REQUIRED AT EACH STEP OF GUT TISSUE INFECTION

A second adaptation to achieve successful gut infection resides in the tight regulation of virulence factor gene expression. Numerous studies have established an elaborate network of transcriptional and posttranscriptional controls that allow the pathogen to identify its exact location within the host and to trigger the appropriate virulence factors for survival in that niche and/or to prepare the next step of the infection process (103–105). This creates pathogen cells with quite distinct virulence gene expression patterns at the different sites in the host.

In the gut lumen, the pathogen forms (at least) two distinct phenotypes, TTSS-1⁺ and TTSS-1⁻ (Fig. 2). According to the division-of-labor hypothesis proposed by Diard et al. (106), both phenotypes play a key role in the life cycle of *S.* Typhimurium. The TTSS-1⁺ phenotype expresses flagella (to reach the epithelium), the invasion-mediating TTSS-1 apparatus, and a cocktail of TTSS-1 effector proteins to be deployed as soon as the pathogen docks at an epithelial cell. This mediates invasion of the host cell (46, 106–110) (Fig. 2). The TTSS-1$^+$ population is poised to invade the epithelium and triggers pronounced inflammation. However, the expression of TTSS-1 is associated with a reduced growth rate due to fitness costs (106, 109). In contrast, the TTSS-1$^-$ population does not express TTSS-1, remains in the gut lumen, and blooms in the milieu of the infected gut (Fig. 2). This stabilizes S. Typhimurium virulence by preventing overgrowth of avirulent mutants that spontaneously emerge from the S. Typhimurium population during infection. These mutants are genetically unable to express the TTSS-1$^+$ phenotype and are fast-growing. This represents an advantage in the inflamed gut of infected hosts but a major disadvantage upon transmission to the next host, as these mutants are unable to trigger inflammation on their own (111, 112). The fast-growing TTSS-1$^-$ phenotype therefore keeps avirulent mutants at bay by competing against them for the same niche in the gut. This is thought to ensure the transmission of virulent genotypes upon chronic infection (106, 111) (Fig. 2).

After arrival in the gut tissue, most S. Typhimurium cells switch off TTSS-1 and flagellar gene expression and trigger TTSS-2 expression instead (Fig. 2). This may partially help to avoid stimulation of the NLRC4 inflammasome. TTSS-2 effector proteins may help to further damp such innate immune responses and promote intracellular survival (23). Interestingly, some of the tissue-resident S. Typhimurium cells reinitiate TTSS-1 and flagellar gene expression (47), probably in preparation for reinvasion of the epithelium. Other S. Typhimurium cells appear to enter a slow-growing state of persistence (TTSS-1$^-$ TTSS-2$^+$; some populations may also feature no or low TTSS-2 expression; extremely slow growth) (Fig. 2), which creates a tissue-lodged pathogen reservoir that can survive antibiotic therapy for >10 days and reseed the host's gut lumen as soon as the therapy is discontinued (94, 95, 112). Yet another S. Typhimurium phenotype (TTSS-1$^-$ TTSS-2$^+$; fast growth) forms inside phagocytes and may promote pathogen growth in the lamina propria, boosting dissemination to other organs upon migration of infected cells to systemic sites (35, 37, 43, 95, 113).

Owing to the multitude of different phagocyte populations that take up S. Typhimurium in the gut tissue (35, 37), the time dependence of SCV maturation, and the different defenses faced within particular host cells, the spectrum of stimuli and of the resulting S. Typhimurium phenotypes is likely much more diverse than depicted in Fig. 2 (114, 115). Phenotypic heterogeneity

and the cooperation between different pathogen subpopulations are likely of key importance for disease progression, pathogen blooms in the infected gut, and successful transmission within the host population.

DISCUSSION AND OUTLOOK

S. Typhimurium faces a variety of challenges and environments during the infection cycle. A cardinal dilemma is created by the host's innate immune system, which detects key virulence factors essential for infection. The pathogen employs two general strategies to avoid elimination, i.e., controlling the innate immune response and stage-specific adaptation of the gene expression profile, leading to phenotypic heterogeneity of the infecting population.

The host response against S. Typhimurium infection is similarly multifaceted. Different cell types within the infected tissue cooperate to fight the infection. As described above, gut epithelial cells emerge as central players in this defense. Indeed, the epithelium-intrinsic expulsion of infected enterocytes is the most potent host defense mechanism during the first 12 to 18 h of oral S. Typhimurium infection identified so far. On top of that, complex interaction networks as well as the development of organotypic features like the mucus layer require the interplay of different cell types in a specific microenvironment, creating a major challenge for in vitro culture.

Taken together, the available data show that in the early phase of gut tissue invasion by S. Typhimurium, there seems to be (i) a need for expression of certain virulence factors required for invasion and (ii) initiation of an inflammatory host response by factors crucial for or supportive of invasion. This host response is quite effective and reduces pathogen tissue loads as much as 100-fold. However, this defense is not purely beneficial for the host, as it imposes tissue damage, delays remission of the inflamed mucosa, fuels gut luminal pathogen blooms, and suppresses regrowth of the microbiota, thereby allowing prolonged inhabitation of the intestinal lumen by the pathogen (6, 20, 60, 90). In conclusion, inflammation triggered by the bacterium is a double-edged sword, at least in the case of well-adapted pathogens like S. Typhimurium.

The complexity of the system highlights the importance of analyzing host-pathogen interactions in vivo in the organs of an infected host. Cell culture models have great value for detailed analysis of molecular signaling mechanisms. However, immortalized cell lines are unlikely to represent a realistic model for short-lived IECs. Intestinal organoids (116) might serve as a more realistic model, especially for studies focusing on cell death. Nevertheless, the relevance of mechanisms discovered *in vitro* can be fully verified only in animal models.

Real-time analysis of the interaction between host and pathogen is facilitated by the usage of genetically modified bacteria. Fluorescent reporters can be used to monitor localization or gene expression by the bacterium during different stages of infection (21, 136), as a readout for replication (94), or as probes for environmental conditions such as oxygen levels (146), reactive oxygen species (147), or pH (148). In combination with intravital microscopy, these fluorescent reporters provide a powerful tool to decipher real-time dynamics of host-pathogen interaction (144). In the future, epitope-tag surface display might further expand the repertoire of techniques for scrutinizing the heterogeneity of the pathogen-host interaction at the single cell level (149). Finally, barcoded strains in combination with mathematical modeling allow the analysis of population dynamics and determination of bottlenecks throughout the infection (95). The combination of single-cell approaches with population dynamics has great potential.

For comparability and interpretability of *in vivo* data, the use of littermate controls in S. Typhimurium infections is crucial, as the microbiota composition can influence S. Typhimurium infection kinetics (17). This will be of particular importance when the new gnotobiotic mouse models are used; these permit slow gut luminal pathogen growth and realistic stimulation kinetics of the host's defenses. Such models may hold the key for deciphering the *in vivo* function of the numerous S. Typhimurium virulence factors.

Acknowledgments. We are grateful to Médéric Diard, Markus Furter, Stefan Fattinger, and Ersin Gül for helpful comments and discussions. Work in W.D.H.'s laboratory relevant to this review is supported by the Swiss National Science Foundation (SNF 310030_53074 and 310030B_173338).

Citation. Hausmann A, Hardt W-D. 2019. The interplay between *Salmonella enterica* serovar Typhimurium and the intestinal mucosa during oral infection. Microbiol Spectrum 7 (2):BAI-0004-2019.

References

1. Avital G, Avraham R, Fan A, Hashimshony T, Hung DT, Yanai I. 2017. scDual-Seq: mapping the gene regulatory program of *Salmonella* infection by host and pathogen single-cell RNA-sequencing. *Genome Biol* 18:200.

2. Diard M, Hardt W-D. 2017. Evolution of bacterial virulence. *FEMS Microbiol Rev* 41:679–697.

3. Samuel BS, Gordon JI. 2006. A humanized gnotobiotic mouse model of host-archaeal-bacterial mutualism. *Proc Natl Acad Sci USA* 103:10011–10016.

4. Gomez de Agüero M, Ganal-Vonarburg SC, Fuhrer T, Rupp S, Uchimura Y, Li H, Steinert A, Heikenwalder M, Hapfelmeier S, Sauer U, McCoy KD, Macpherson AJ. 2016. The maternal microbiota drives early postnatal innate immune development. *Science* 351:1296–1302.

5. Macpherson AJ, de Agüero MG, Ganal-Vonarburg SC. 2017. How nutrition and the maternal microbiota shape the neonatal immune system. *Nat Rev Immunol* 17:508–517.

6. Stecher B, Hardt W-D. 2008. The role of microbiota in infectious disease. *Trends Microbiol* 16:107–114.

7. Stecher B, Robbiani R, Walker AW, Westendorf AM, Barthel M, Kremer M, Chaffron S, Macpherson AJ, Buer J, Parkhill J, Dougan G, von Mering C, Hardt W-D. 2007. *Salmonella enterica* serovar Typhimurium exploits inflammation to compete with the intestinal microbiota. *PLoS Biol* 5:2177–2189.

8. Corridoni D, Chapman T, Ambrose T, Simmons A. 2018. Emerging mechanisms of innate immunity and their translational potential in inflammatory bowel disease. *Front Med (Lausanne)* 5:32.

9. Mowat AM, Agace WW. 2014. Regional specialization within the intestinal immune system. *Nat Rev Immunol* 14:667–685.

10. Kirk MD, Pires SM, Black RE, Caipo M, Crump JA, Devleesschauwer B, Döpfer D, Fazil A, Fischer-Walker CL, Hald T, Hall AJ, Keddy KH, Lake RJ, Lanata CF, Torgerson PR, Havelaar AH, Angulo FJ. 2015. World Health Organization estimates of the global and regional disease burden of 22 foodborne bacterial, protozoal, and viral diseases, 2010: a data synthesis. *PLoS Med* 12: e1001921. CORRECTION *PLoS Med* 12:e1001940.

11. Tsolis RM, Xavier MN, Santos RL, Bäumler AJ. 2011. How to become a top model: impact of animal experimentation on human *Salmonella* disease research. *Infect Immun* 79:1806–1814.

12. Takeuchi A. 1967. Electron microscope studies of experimental *Salmonella* infection. I. Penetration into the intestinal epithelium by *Salmonella typhimurium*. *Am J Pathol* 50:109–136.

13. Schmitt CK, Ikeda JS, Darnell SC, Watson PR, Bispham J, Wallis TS, Weinstein DL, Metcalf ES, O'Brien AD. 2001. Absence of all components of the flagellar export and synthesis machinery differentially alters virulence of *Salmonella enterica* serovar Typhimurium in models of typhoid fever, survival in macrophages, tissue culture invasiveness, and calf enterocolitis. *Infect Immun* 69: 5619–5625.

14. Tsolis RM, Adams LG, Ficht TA, Bäumler AJ. 1999. Contribution of *Salmonella typhimurium* virulence factors to diarrheal disease in calves. *Infect Immun* 67:4879–4885.

15. Wray C, Sojka WJ. 1978. Experimental *Salmonella typhimurium* infection in calves. *Res Vet Sci* 25:139–143.

16. Barthel M, Hapfelmeier S, Quintanilla-Martínez L, Kremer M, Rohde M, Hogardt M, Pfeffer K, Rüssmann H, Hardt W-D. 2003. Pretreatment of mice with streptomycin provides a *Salmonella enterica* serovar Typhimurium colitis model that allows analysis of both pathogen and host. *Infect Immun* 71:2839–2858.

17. Kaiser P, Diard M, Stecher B, Hardt W-D. 2012. The streptomycin mouse model for *Salmonella* diarrhea: functional analysis of the microbiota, the pathogen's virulence factors, and the host's mucosal immune response. *Immunol Rev* 245:56–83.

18. Bohnhoff M, Miller CP. 1962. Enhanced susceptibility to *Salmonella* infection in streptomycin-treated mice. *J Infect Dis* 111:117–127.

19. Bohnhoff M, Drake BL, Miller CP. 1954. Effect of streptomycin on susceptibility of intestinal tract to experimental Salmonella infection. *Proc Soc Exp Biol Med* 86:132–137.

20. Wotzka SY, Nguyen BD, Hardt W-D. 2017. *Salmonella* Typhimurium diarrhea reveals basic principles of enteropathogen infection and disease-promoted DNA exchange. *Cell Host Microbe* 21:443–454.

21. Sellin ME, Müller AA, Felmy B, Dolowschiak T, Diard M, Tardivel A, Maslowski KM, Hardt W-D. 2014. Epithelium-intrinsic NAIP/NLRC4 inflammasome drives infected enterocyte expulsion to restrict *Salmonella* replication in the intestinal mucosa. *Cell Host Microbe* 16:237–248.

22. Gerlach RG, Jäckel D, Stecher B, Wagner C, Lupas A, Hardt W-D, Hensel M. 2007. Salmonella pathogenicity island 4 encodes a giant non-fimbrial adhesin and the cognate type 1 secretion system. *Cell Microbiol* 9:1834–1850.

23. Hapfelmeier S, Stecher B, Barthel M, Kremer M, Müller AJ, Heikenwalder M, Stallmach T, Hensel M, Pfeffer K, Akira S, Hardt W-D. 2005. The *Salmonella* pathogenicity island (SPI)-2 and SPI-1 type III secretion systems allow *Salmonella* serovar Typhimurium to trigger colitis via MyD88-dependent and MyD88-independent mechanisms. *J Immunol Baltim Md* 174:1675–1685.

24. Stecher B, Barthel M, Schlumberger MC, Haberli L, Rabsch W, Kremer M, Hardt W-D. 2008. Motility allows *S.* Typhimurium to benefit from the mucosal defence. *Cell Microbiol* 10:1166–1180.

25. Maier L, Vyas R, Cordova CD, Lindsay H, Schmidt TSB, Brugiroux S, Periaswamy B, Bauer R, Sturm A, Schreiber F, von Mering C, Robinson MD, Stecher B, Hardt W-D. 2013. Microbiota-derived hydrogen fuels *Salmonella typhimurium* invasion of the gut ecosystem. *Cell Host Microbe* 14:641–651.

26. Stecher B, Hapfelmeier S, Müller C, Kremer M, Stallmach T, Hardt W-D. 2004. Flagella and chemotaxis are required for efficient induction of *Salmonella enterica* serovar Typhimurium colitis in streptomycin-pretreated mice. *Infect Immun* 72:4138–4150.

27. Wangdi T, Lee C-Y, Spees AM, Yu C, Kingsbury DD, Winter SE, Hastey CJ, Wilson RP, Heinrich V, Bäumler AJ. 2014. The Vi capsular polysaccharide enables *Salmonella enterica* serovar Typhi to evade microbe-guided neutrophil chemotaxis. *PLoS Pathog* 10:e1004306.

28. Golubeva YA, Sadik AY, Ellermeier JR, Slauch JM. 2012. Integrating global regulatory input into the *Salmonella* pathogenicity island 1 type III secretion system. *Genetics* 190:79–90.

29. Galán JE, Waksman G. 2018. Protein-injection machines in bacteria. *Cell* 172:1306–1318.

30. Galán JE, Lara-Tejero M, Marlovits TC, Wagner S. 2014. Bacterial type III secretion systems: specialized nanomachines for protein delivery into target cells. *Annu Rev Microbiol* 68:415–438.

31. Hardt WD, Chen LM, Schuebel KE, Bustelo XR, Galán JE. 1998. *S. typhimurium* encodes an activator of Rho GTPases that induces membrane ruffling and nuclear responses in host cells. *Cell* 93:815–826.

32. Srikanth CV, Mercado-Lubo R, Hallstrom K, McCormick BA. 2011. *Salmonella* effector proteins and host-cell responses. *Cell Mol Life Sci* 68:3687–3697.

33. Zhou D, Mooseker MS, Galán JE. 1999. An invasion-associated *Salmonella* protein modulates the actin-bundling activity of plastin. *Proc Natl Acad Sci USA* 96:10176–10181.

34. Zhou D, Mooseker MS, Galán JE. 1999. Role of the *S. typhimurium* actin-binding protein SipA in bacterial internalization. *Science* 283:2092–2095.

35. Müller AJ, Kaiser P, Dittmar KEJ, Weber TC, Haueter S, Endt K, Songhet P, Zellweger C, Kremer M, Fehling H-J, Hardt W-D. 2012. *Salmonella* gut invasion involves TTSS-2-dependent epithelial traversal, basolateral exit, and uptake by epithelium-sampling lamina propria phagocytes. *Cell Host Microbe* 11:19–32.

36. Zhang K, Riba A, Nietschke M, Torow N, Repnik U, Pütz A, Fulde M, Dupont A, Hensel M, Hornef M. 2018. Minimal SPI1-T3SS effector requirement for *Salmonella* enterocyte invasion and intracellular proliferation in vivo. *PLoS Pathog* 14:e1006925.

37. Hapfelmeier S, Müller AJ, Stecher B, Kaiser P, Barthel M, Endt K, Eberhard M, Robbiani R, Jacobi CA, Heikenwalder M, Kirschning C, Jung S, Stallmach T, Kremer M, Hardt W-D. 2008. Microbe sampling by mucosal dendritic cells is a discrete, MyD88-independent step in Δ*invG S.* Typhimurium colitis. *J Exp Med* 205:437–450.

38. Knodler LA, Steele-Mortimer O. 2005. The *Salmonella* effector PipB2 affects late endosome/lysosome distribution to mediate Sif extension. *Mol Biol Cell* 16:4108–4123.

39. Knodler LA, Vallance BA, Hensel M, Jäckel D, Finlay BB, Steele-Mortimer O. 2003. *Salmonella* type III effectors PipB and PipB2 are targeted to detergent-resistant microdomains on internal host cell membranes. *Mol Microbiol* 49:685–704.

40. Kreibich S, Emmenlauer M, Fredlund J, Rämö P, Münz C, Dehio C, Enninga J, Hardt W-D. 2015. Autophagy proteins promote repair of endosomal membranes damaged by the *Salmonella* type three secretion system 1. *Cell Host Microbe* 18:527–537.

41. Steele-Mortimer O, Brumell JH, Knodler LA, Méresse S, Lopez A, Finlay BB. 2002. The invasion-associated type III secretion system of *Salmonella enterica* serovar Typhimurium is necessary for intracellular proliferation and vacuole biogenesis in epithelial cells. *Cell Microbiol* 4:43–54.

42. Steele-Mortimer O. 2008. The *Salmonella*-containing vacuole: moving with the times. *Curr Opin Microbiol* 11:38–45.

43. Hensel M, Shea JE, Gleeson C, Jones MD, Dalton E, Holden DW. 1995. Simultaneous identification of bacterial virulence genes by negative selection. *Science* 269: 400–403.

44. Shea JE, Hensel M, Gleeson C, Holden DW. 1996. Identification of a virulence locus encoding a second type III secretion system in *Salmonella typhimurium*. *Proc Natl Acad Sci USA* 93:2593–2597.

45. Waterman SR, Holden DW. 2003. Functions and effectors of the *Salmonella* pathogenicity island 2 type III secretion system. *Cell Microbiol* 5:501–511.

46. Hautefort I, Thompson A, Eriksson-Ygberg S, Parker ML, Lucchini S, Danino V, Bongaerts RJM, Ahmad N, Rhen M, Hinton JCD. 2008. During infection of epithelial cells *Salmonella enterica* serovar Typhimurium undergoes a time-dependent transcriptional adaptation that results in simultaneous expression of three type 3 secretion systems. *Cell Microbiol* 10:958–984.

47. Laughlin RC, Knodler LA, Barhoumi R, Payne HR, Wu J, Gomez G, Pugh R, Lawhon SD, Bäumler AJ, Steele-Mortimer O, Adams LG. 2014. Spatial segregation of virulence gene expression during acute enteric infection with *Salmonella enterica* serovar Typhimurium. *mBio* 5:e00946-13.

48. Brumell JH, Tang P, Zaharik ML, Finlay BB. 2002. Disruption of the *Salmonella*-containing vacuole leads to increased replication of *Salmonella enterica* serovar typhimurium in the cytosol of epithelial cells. *Infect Immun* 70:3264–3270.

49. Knodler LA, Vallance BA, Celli J, Winfree S, Hansen B, Montero M, Steele-Mortimer O. 2010. Dissemination of invasive *Salmonella* via bacterial-induced extrusion of mucosal epithelia. *Proc Natl Acad Sci USA* 107: 17733–17738.

50. Thurston TLM, Matthews SA, Jennings E, Alix E, Shao F, Shenoy AR, Birrell MA, Holden DW. 2016. Growth inhibition of cytosolic *Salmonella* by caspase-1 and caspase-11 precedes host cell death. *Nat Commun* 7:13292.

51. Johansson MEV, Hansson GC. 2016. Immunological aspects of intestinal mucus and mucins. *Nat Rev Immunol* 16:639–649.

52. Johansson MEV, Phillipson M, Petersson J, Velcich A, Holm L, Hansson GC. 2008. The inner of the two Muc2 mucin-dependent mucus layers in colon is devoid of bacteria. *Proc Natl Acad Sci USA* 105:15064–15069.

53. Johansson MEV, Ambort D, Pelaseyed T, Schütte A, Gustafsson JK, Ermund A, Subramani DB, Holmén-Larsson JM, Thomsson KA, Bergström JH, van der Post S, Rodriguez-Piñeiro AM, Sjövall H, Bäckström M, Hansson GC. 2011. Composition and functional role of the mucus layers in the intestine. *Cell Mol Life Sci* 68:3635–3641.

54. Birchenough GMH, Nyström EEL, Johansson MEV, Hansson GC. 2016. A sentinel goblet cell guards the colonic crypt by triggering Nlrp6-dependent Muc2 secretion. *Science* 352:1535–1542.

55. Wlodarska M, Thaiss CA, Nowarski R, Henao-Mejia J, Zhang J-P, Brown EM, Frankel G, Levy M, Katz MN, Philbrick WM, Elinav E, Finlay BB, Flavell RA. 2014. NLRP6 inflammasome orchestrates the colonic host-microbial interface by regulating goblet cell mucus secretion. *Cell* 156:1045–1059.

56. Klose CSN, Kiss EA, Schwierzeck V, Ebert K, Hoyler T, d'Hargues Y, Göppert N, Croxford AL, Waisman A, Tanriver Y, Diefenbach A. 2013. A T-bet gradient controls the fate and function of CCR6-RORγt+ innate lymphoid cells. *Nature* 494:261–265.

57. Songhet P, Barthel M, Stecher B, Müller AJ, Kremer M, Hansson GC, Hardt W-D. 2011. Stromal IFN-γR-signaling modulates goblet cell function during *Salmonella* Typhimurium infection. *PLoS One* 6:e22459.

58. Cullen TW, Schofield WB, Barry NA, Putnam EE, Rundell EA, Trent MS, Degnan PH, Booth CJ, Yu H, Goodman AL. 2015. Antimicrobial peptide resistance mediates resilience of prominent gut commensals during inflammation. *Science* 347:170–175.

59. Miki T, Okada N, Hardt W-D. 2018. Inflammatory bactericidal lectin RegIIIβ: friend or foe for the host? *Gut Microbes* 9:179–187.

60. Miki T, Goto R, Fujimoto M, Okada N, Hardt W-D. 2017. The bactericidal lectin RegIIIβ prolongs gut colonization and enteropathy in the streptomycin mouse model for *Salmonella* diarrhea. *Cell Host Microbe* 21: 195–207.

61. Raffatellu M, George MD, Akiyama Y, Hornsby MJ, Nuccio S-P, Paixao TA, Butler BP, Chu H, Santos RL, Berger T, Mak TW, Tsolis RM, Bevins CL, Solnick JV, Dandekar S, Bäumler AJ. 2009. Lipocalin-2 resistance confers an advantage to *Salmonella enterica* serotype Typhimurium for growth and survival in the inflamed intestine. *Cell Host Microbe* 5:476–486.

62. Stelter C, Käppeli R, König C, Krah A, Hardt W-D, Stecher B, Bumann D. 2011. *Salmonella*-induced mucosal lectin RegIIIβ kills competing gut microbiota. *PLoS One* 6:e20749.

63. Kinnebrew MA, Buffie CG, Diehl GE, Zenewicz LA, Leiner I, Hohl TM, Flavell RA, Littman DR, Pamer EG. 2012. Interleukin 23 production by intestinal CD103 +CD11b+ dendritic cells in response to bacterial flagellin enhances mucosal innate immune defense. *Immunity* 36: 276–287.

64. Brandl K, Plitas G, Schnabl B, DeMatteo RP, Pamer EG. 2007. MyD88-mediated signals induce the bactericidal lectin RegIII gamma and protect mice against intestinal *Listeria monocytogenes* infection. *J Exp Med* 204: 1891–1900.

65. Dessein R, Gironella M, Vignal C, Peyrin-Biroulet L, Sokol H, Secher T, Lacas-Gervais S, Gratadoux J-J, Lafont F, Dagorn J-C, Ryffel B, Akira S, Langella P, Nùñez G, Sirard J-C, Iovanna J, Simonet M, Chamaillard M. 2009. Toll-like receptor 2 is critical for induction of Reg3 beta expression and intestinal clearance of *Yersinia pseudotuberculosis*. *Gut* 58:771–776.

66. Loonen LMP, Stolte EH, Jaklofsky MTJ, Meijerink M, Dekker J, van Baarlen P, Wells JM. 2014. REG3γ-deficient mice have altered mucus distribution and increased mucosal inflammatory responses to the microbiota

and enteric pathogens in the ileum. *Mucosal Immunol* **7:** 939–947.

67. Miki T, Hardt W-D. 2013. Outer membrane permeabilization is an essential step in the killing of gram-negative bacteria by the lectin RegIIIβ. *PLoS One* **8:**e69901.

68. Zheng Y, Valdez PA, Danilenko DM, Hu Y, Sa SM, Gong Q, Abbas AR, Modrusan Z, Ghilardi N, de Sauvage FJ, Ouyang W. 2008. Interleukin-22 mediates early host defense against attaching and effacing bacterial pathogens. *Nat Med* **14:**282–289.

69. Broz P, Dixit VM. 2016. Inflammasomes: mechanism of assembly, regulation and signalling. *Nat Rev Immunol* **16:**407–420.

70. Franchi L, Amer A, Body-Malapel M, Kanneganti T-D, Ozören N, Jagirdar R, Inohara N, Vandenabeele P, Bertin J, Coyle A, Grant EP, Núñez G. 2006. Cytosolic flagellin requires Ipaf for activation of caspase-1 and interleukin 1β in salmonella-infected macrophages. *Nat Immunol* **7:**576–582.

71. Miao EA, Alpuche-Aranda CM, Dors M, Clark AE, Bader MW, Miller SI, Aderem A. 2006. Cytoplasmic flagellin activates caspase-1 and secretion of interleukin 1β via Ipaf. *Nat Immunol* **7:**569–575.

72. Kofoed EM, Vance RE. 2011. Innate immune recognition of bacterial ligands by NAIPs determines inflammasome specificity. *Nature* **477:**592–595.

73. Zhao Y, Yang J, Shi J, Gong Y-N, Lu Q, Xu H, Liu L, Shao F. 2011. The NLRC4 inflammasome receptors for bacterial flagellin and type III secretion apparatus. *Nature* **477:**596–600.

74. Boyden ED, Dietrich WF. 2006. Nalp1b controls mouse macrophage susceptibility to anthrax lethal toxin. *Nat Genet* **38:**240–244.

75. Xu H, Yang J, Gao W, Li L, Li P, Zhang L, Gong Y-N, Peng X, Xi JJ, Chen S, Wang F, Shao F. 2014. Innate immune sensing of bacterial modifications of Rho GTPases by the Pyrin inflammasome. *Nature* **513:**237–241.

76. Fernandes-Alnemri T, Yu J-W, Juliana C, Solorzano L, Kang S, Wu J, Datta P, McCormick M, Huang L, McDermott E, Eisenlohr L, Landel CP, Alnemri ES. 2010. The AIM2 inflammasome is critical for innate immunity to *Francisella tularensis*. *Nat Immunol* **11:** 385–393.

77. Rathinam VAK, Jiang Z, Waggoner SN, Sharma S, Cole LE, Waggoner L, Vanaja SK, Monks BG, Ganesan S, Latz E, Hornung V, Vogel SN, Szomolanyi-Tsuda E, Fitzgerald KA. 2010. The AIM2 inflammasome is essential for host defense against cytosolic bacteria and DNA viruses. *Nat Immunol* **11:**395–402.

78. Muñoz-Planillo R, Kuffa P, Martínez-Colón G, Smith BL, Rajendiran TM, Núñez G. 2013. K⁺ efflux is the common trigger of NLRP3 inflammasome activation by bacterial toxins and particulate matter. *Immunity* **38:** 1142–1153.

79. Kayagaki N, Warming S, Lamkanfi M, Vande Walle L, Louie S, Dong J, Newton K, Qu Y, Liu J, Heldens S, Zhang J, Lee WP, Roose-Girma M, Dixit VM. 2011. Non-canonical inflammasome activation targets caspase-11. *Nature* **479:**117–121.

80. Sellin ME, Müller AA, Hardt W-D. 2018. Consequences of epithelial inflammasome activation by bacterial pathogens. *J Mol Biol* **430:**193–206.

81. Rauch I, Deets KA, Ji DX, von Moltke J, Tenthorey JL, Lee AY, Philip NH, Ayres JS, Brodsky IE, Gronert K, Vance RE. 2017. NAIP-NLRC4 inflammasomes coordinate intestinal epithelial cell expulsion with eicosanoid and IL-18 release via activation of caspase-1 and -8. *Immunity* **46:**649–659.

82. Knodler LA, Crowley SM, Sham HP, Yang H, Wrande M, Ma C, Ernst RK, Steele-Mortimer O, Celli J, Vallance BA. 2014. Noncanonical inflammasome activation of caspase-4/caspase-11 mediates epithelial defenses against enteric bacterial pathogens. *Cell Host Microbe* **16:** 249–256.

83. von Moltke J, Trinidad NJ, Moayeri M, Kintzer AF, Wang SB, van Rooijen N, Brown CR, Krantz BA, Leppla SH, Gronert K, Vance RE. 2012. Rapid induction of inflammatory lipid mediators by the inflammasome in vivo. *Nature* **490:**107–111.

84. Hefele M, Stolzer I, Ruder B, He G-W, Mahapatro M, Wirtz S, Neurath MF, Günther C. 2018. Intestinal epithelial caspase-8 signaling is essential to prevent necroptosis during *Salmonella* Typhimurium induced enteritis. *Mucosal Immunol* **11:**1191–1202.

85. Aachoui Y, Leaf IA, Hagar JA, Fontana MF, Campos CG, Zak DE, Tan MH, Cotter PA, Vance RE, Aderem A, Miao EA. 2013. Caspase-11 protects against bacteria that escape the vacuole. *Science* **339:**975–978.

86. Hagar JA, Powell DA, Aachoui Y, Ernst RK, Miao EA. 2013. Cytoplasmic LPS activates caspase-11: implications in TLR4-independent endotoxic shock. *Science* **341:** 1250–1253.

87. Müller AA, Dolowschiak T, Sellin ME, Felmy B, Verbree C, Gadient S, Westermann AJ, Vogel J, LeibundGut-Landmann S, Hardt WD. 2016. An NK cell perforin response elicited via IL-18 controls mucosal inflammation kinetics during *Salmonella* gut infection. *PLoS Pathog* **12:**e1005723.

88. Harrison OJ, Srinivasan N, Pott J, Schiering C, Krausgruber T, Ilott NE, Maloy KJ. 2015. Epithelial-derived IL-18 regulates Th17 cell differentiation and Foxp3⁺ Treg cell function in the intestine. *Mucosal Immunol* **8:**1226–1236.

89. Thinwa J, Segovia JA, Bose S, Dube PH. 2014. Integrin-mediated first signal for inflammasome activation in intestinal epithelial cells. *J Immunol* **193:**1373–1382.

90. Dolowschiak T, Mueller AA, Pisan LJ, Feigelman R, Felmy B, Sellin ME, Namineni S, Nguyen BD, Wotzka SY, Heikenwalder M, von Mering C, Mueller C, Hardt W-D. 2016. IFN-γ hinders recovery from mucosal inflammation during antibiotic therapy for *Salmonella* gut infection. *Cell Host Microbe* **20:**238–249.

91. Maier L, Diard M, Sellin ME, Chouffane E-S, Trautwein-Weidner K, Periaswamy B, Slack E, Dolowschiak T, Stecher B, Loverdo C, Regoes RR, Hardt W-D. 2014. Granulocytes impose a tight bottleneck upon the gut luminal pathogen population during *Salmonella typhimurium* colitis. *PLoS Pathog* **10:** e1004557. CORRECTION *PLoS Pathog* **11:**e1005047.

92. Jorgensen I, Lopez JP, Laufer SA, Miao EA. 2016. IL-1β, IL-18, and eicosanoids promote neutrophil recruitment to pore-induced intracellular traps following pyroptosis. *Eur J Immunol* 46:2761–2766.

93. Jorgensen I, Zhang Y, Krantz BA, Miao EA. 2016. Pyroptosis triggers pore-induced intracellular traps (PITs) that capture bacteria and lead to their clearance by efferocytosis. *J Exp Med* 213:2113–2128.

94. Claudi B, Spröte P, Chirkova A, Personnic N, Zankl J, Schürmann N, Schmidt A, Bumann D. 2014. Phenotypic variation of *Salmonella* in host tissues delays eradication by antimicrobial chemotherapy. *Cell* 158: 722–733.

95. Kaiser P, Slack E, Grant AJ, Hardt W-D, Regoes RR. 2013. Lymph node colonization dynamics after oral *Salmonella* Typhimurium infection in mice. *PLoS Pathog* 9:e1003532.

96. Yang WH, Heithoff DM, Aziz PV, Sperandio M, Nizet V, Mahan MJ, Marth JD. 2017. Recurrent infection progressively disables host protection against intestinal inflammation. *Science* 358:eaao5610.

97. Pinaud L, Sansonetti PJ, Phalipon A. 2018. Host cell targeting by enteropathogenic bacteria T3SS effectors. *Trends Microbiol* 26:266–283.

98. Rauch I, Tenthorey JL, Nichols RD, Al Moussawi K, Kang JJ, Kang C, Kazmierczak BI, Vance RE. 2016. NAIP proteins are required for cytosolic detection of specific bacterial ligands in vivo. *J Exp Med* 213:657–665.

99. Blaser H, Dostert C, Mak TW, Brenner D. TNF and ROS crosstalk in inflammation. *Trends Cell Biol* 26: 249–261.

100. Mitchell S, Vargas J, Hoffmann A. 2016. Signaling via the NFκB system. *Wiley Interdiscip Rev Syst Biol Med* 8:227–241.

101. Sun H, Kamanova J, Lara-Tejero M, Galán JE. 2016. A Family of *Salmonella* type III secretion effector proteins selectively targets the NF-κB signaling pathway to preserve host homeostasis. *PLoS Pathog* 12:e1005484.

102. Lawley TD, Bouley DM, Hoy YE, Gerke C, Relman DA, Monack DM. 2008. Host transmission of *Salmonella enterica* serovar Typhimurium is controlled by virulence factors and indigenous intestinal microbiota. *Infect Immun* 76:403–416.

103. Kröger C, Colgan A, Srikumar S, Händler K, Sivasankaran SK, Hammarlöf DL, Canals R, Grissom JE, Conway T, Hokamp K, Hinton JCD. 2013. An infection-relevant transcriptomic compendium for *Salmonella enterica* serovar Typhimurium. *Cell Host Microbe* 14:683–695.

104. Saini S, Ellermeier JR, Slauch JM, Rao CV. 2010. The role of coupled positive feedback in the expression of the SPI1 type three secretion system in *Salmonella*. *PLoS Pathog* 6:e1001025. CORRECTION *PLoS Pathog* 6.

105. Westermann AJ, Förstner KU, Amman F, Barquist L, Chao Y, Schulte LN, Müller L, Reinhardt R, Stadler PF, Vogel J. 2016. Dual RNA-seq unveils noncoding RNA functions in host-pathogen interactions. *Nature* 529: 496–501.

106. Diard M, Garcia V, Maier L, Remus-Emsermann MNP, Regoes RR, Ackermann M, Hardt W-D. 2013. Stabili-

107. Ackermann M, Stecher B, Freed NE, Songhet P, Hardt W-D, Doebeli M. 2008. Self-destructive cooperation mediated by phenotypic noise. *Nature* 454:987–990.

108. Schlumberger MC, Müller AJ, Ehrbar K, Winnen B, Duss I, Stecher B, Hardt W-D. 2005. Real-time imaging of type III secretion: *Salmonella* SipA injection into host cells. *Proc Natl Acad Sci USA* 102:12548–12553.

109. Sturm A, Heinemann M, Arnoldini M, Benecke A, Ackermann M, Benz M, Dormann J, Hardt W-D. 2011. The cost of virulence: retarded growth of *Salmonella* Typhimurium cells expressing type III secretion system 1. *PLoS Pathog* 7:e1002143.

110. Winnen B, Schlumberger MC, Sturm A, Schüpbach K, Siebenmann S, Jenny P, Hardt W-D. 2008. Hierarchical effector protein transport by the *Salmonella* Typhimurium SPI-1 type III secretion system. *PLoS One* 3:e2178.

111. Diard M, Hardt W-D. 2017. Basic processes in *Salmonella*-host interactions: within-host evolution and the transmission of the virulent genotype. *Microbiol Spectr* 5:MTBP-0012-2016.

112. Diard M, Sellin ME, Dolowschiak T, Arnoldini M, Ackermann M, Hardt W-D. 2014. Antibiotic treatment selects for cooperative virulence of *Salmonella typhimurium*. *Curr Biol* 24:2000–2005.

113. Carden SE, Walker GT, Honeycutt J, Lugo K, Pham T, Jacobson A, Bouley D, Idoyaga J, Tsolis RM, Monack D. 2017. Pseudogenization of the secreted effector gene sseI confers rapid systemic dissemination of *S.* Typhimurium ST313 within migratory dendritic cells. *Cell Host Microbe* 21:182–194.

114. Bumann D, Cunrath O. 2017. Heterogeneity of *Salmonella*-host interactions in infected host tissues. *Curr Opin Microbiol* 39:57–63.

115. Kreibich S, Hardt W-D. 2015. Experimental approaches to phenotypic diversity in infection. *Curr Opin Microbiol* 27:25–36.

116. Sato T, Vries RG, Snippert HJ, van de Wetering M, Barker N, Stange DE, van Es JH, Abo A, Kujala P, Peters PJ, Clevers H. 2009. Single Lgr5 stem cells build crypt-villus structures in vitro without a mesenchymal niche. *Nature* 459:262–265.

117. Günster RA, Matthews SA, Holden DW, Thurston TLM. 2017. SseK1 and SseK3 type III secretion system effectors inhibit NF-κB signaling and necroptotic cell death in *Salmonella*-infected macrophages. *Infect Immun* 85:e00010-17.

118. Collier-Hyams LS, Zeng H, Sun J, Tomlinson AD, Bao ZQ, Chen H, Madara JL, Orth K, Neish AS. 2002. Cutting edge: salmonella AvrA effector inhibits the key proinflammatory, anti-apoptotic NF-kappa B pathway. *J Immunol* 169:2846–2850.

119. Ye Z, Petrof EO, Boone D, Claud EC, Sun J. 2007. *Salmonella* effector AvrA regulation of colonic epithelial cell inflammation by deubiquitination. *Am J Pathol* 171: 882–892.

120. Pilar AVC, Reid-Yu SA, Cooper CA, Mulder DT, Coombes BK. 2012. GogB is an anti-inflammatory

zation of cooperative virulence by the expression of an avirulent phenotype. *Nature* 494:353–356.

effector that limits tissue damage during *Salmonella* infection through interaction with human FBXO22 and Skp1. *PLoS Pathog* 8:e1002773.

121. Haneda T, Ishii Y, Shimizu H, Ohshima K, Iida N, Danbara H, Okada N. 2012. *Salmonella* type III effector SpvC, a phosphothreonine lyase, contributes to reduction in inflammatory response during intestinal phase of infection. *Cell Microbiol* 14:485–499.

122. Li H, Xu H, Zhou Y, Zhang J, Long C, Li S, Chen S, Zhou J-M, Shao F. 2007. The phosphothreonine lyase activity of a bacterial type III effector family. *Science* 315:1000–1003.

123. Mazurkiewicz P, Thomas J, Thompson JA, Liu M, Arbibe L, Sansonetti P, Holden DW. 2008. SpvC is a *Salmonella* effector with phosphothreonine lyase activity on host mitogen-activated protein kinases. *Mol Microbiol* 67:1371–1383.

124. Zhu Y, Li H, Long C, Hu L, Xu H, Liu L, Chen S, Wang D-C, Shao F. 2007. Structural insights into the enzymatic mechanism of the pathogenic MAPK phosphothreonine lyase. *Mol Cell* 28:899–913.

125. Le Negrate G, Faustin B, Welsh K, Loeffler M, Krajewska M, Hasegawa P, Mukherjee S, Orth K, Krajewski S, Godzik A, Guiney DG, Reed JC. 2008. *Salmonella* secreted factor L deubiquitinase of *Salmonella typhimurium* inhibits NF-κB, suppresses IκBα ubiquitination and modulates innate immune responses. *J Immunol* 180:5045–5056.

126. Mesquita FS, Thomas M, Sachse M, Santos AJM, Figueira R, Holden DW. 2012. The *Salmonella* deubiquitinase SseL inhibits selective autophagy of cytosolic aggregates. *PLoS Pathog* 8:e1002743.

127. Mesquita FS, Holden DW, Rolhion N. 2013. Lack of effect of the *Salmonella* deubiquitinase SseL on the NF-κB pathway. *PLoS One* 8:e53064.

128. Haraga A, Miller SI. 2003. A *Salmonella enterica* serovar typhimurium translocated leucine-rich repeat effector protein inhibits NF-κB-dependent gene expression. *Infect Immun* 71:4052–4058.

129. Haraga A, Miller SI. 2006. A *Salmonella* type III secretion effector interacts with the mammalian serine/threonine protein kinase PKN1. *Cell Microbiol* 8:837–846.

130. Keszei AFA, Tang X, McCormick C, Zeqiraj E, Rohde JR, Tyers M, Sicheri F. 2014. Structure of an SspH1-PKN1 complex reveals the basis for host substrate recognition and mechanism of activation for a bacterial E3 ubiquitin ligase. *Mol Cell Biol* 34:362–373.

131. Rolhion N, Furniss RCD, Grabe G, Ryan A, Liu M, Matthews SA, Holden DW. 2016. Inhibition of nuclear transport of NF-B p65 by the *Salmonella* type III secretion system effector SpvD. *PLoS Pathog* 12:e1005653.

132. Hu G-Q, Song P-X, Chen W, Qi S, Yu S-X, Du C-T, Deng X-M, Ouyang H-S, Yang Y-J. 2017. Critical [*sic*] role for *Salmonella* effector SopB in regulating inflammasome activation. *Mol Immunol* 90:280–286. *CORRIGENDUM Mol Immunol* 105:283.

133. Diao J, Zhang Y, Huibregtse JM, Zhou D, Chen J. 2008. Crystal structure of SopA, a *Salmonella* effector protein

mimicking a eukaryotic ubiquitin ligase. *Nat Struct Mol Biol* 15:65–70.

134. Fiskin E, Bhogaraju S, Herhaus L, Kalayil S, Hahn M, Dikic I. 2017. Structural basis for the recognition and degradation of host TRIM proteins by *Salmonella* effector SopA. *Nat Commun* 8:14004.

135. Kamanova J, Sun H, Lara-Tejero M, Galán JE. 2016. The *Salmonella* effector protein SopA modulates innate immune responses by targeting TRIM E3 ligase family members. *PLoS Pathog* 12:e1005552.

136. Zhang Y, Higashide WM, McCormick BA, Chen J, Zhou D. 2006. The inflammation-associated *Salmonella* SopA is a HECT-like E3 ubiquitin ligase. *Mol Microbiol* 62:786–793.

137. Chung LK, Park YH, Zheng Y, Brodsky IE, Hearing P, Kastner DL, Chae JJ, Bliska JB. 2016. The *Yersinia* virulence factor YopM hijacks host kinases to inhibit type III effector-triggered activation of the pyrin inflammasome. *Cell Host Microbe* 20:296–306.

138. Ratner D, Orning MPA, Proulx MK, Wang D, Gavrilin MA, Wewers MD, Alnemri ES, Johnson PF, Lee B, Mecsas J, Kayagaki N, Goguen JD, Lien E. 2016. The *Yersinia pestis* effector YopM inhibits pyrin inflammasome activation. *PLoS Pathog* 12:e1006035.

139. Blasche S, Mörtl M, Steuber H, Siszler G, Nisa S, Schwarz F, Lavrik I, Gronewold TMA, Maskos K, Donnenberg MS, Ullmann D, Uetz P, Kögl M. 2013. The *E. coli* effector protein NleF is a caspase inhibitor. *PLoS One* 8:e58937.

140. Kobayashi T, Ogawa M, Sanada T, Mimuro H, Kim M, Ashida H, Akakura R, Yoshida M, Kawalec M, Reichhart J-M, Mizushima T, Sasakawa C. 2013. The *Shigella* OspC3 effector inhibits caspase-4, antagonizes inflammatory cell death, and promotes epithelial infection. *Cell Host Microbe* 13:570–583.

141. Ashida H, Kim M, Schmidt-Supprian M, Ma A, Ogawa M, Sasakawa C. 2010. A bacterial E3 ubiquitin ligase IpaH9.8 targets NEMO/IKKgamma to dampen the host NF-κB-mediated inflammatory response. *Nat Cell Biol* 12:66–73.

142. El Qaidi S, Chen K, Halim A, Siukstaite L, Rueter C, Hurtado-Guerrero R, Clausen H, Hardwidge PR. 2017. NleB/SseK effectors from *Citrobacter rodentium*, *Escherichia coli*, and *Salmonella enterica* display distinct differences in host substrate specificity. *J Biol Chem* 292:11423–11430.

143. Li S, Zhang L, Yao Q, Li L, Dong N, Rong J, Gao W, Ding X, Sun L, Chen X, Chen S, Shao F. 2013. Pathogen blocks host death receptor signalling by arginine GlcNAcylation of death domains. *Nature* 501:242–246.

144. Pearson JS, Giogha C, Ong SY, Kennedy CL, Kelly M, Robinson KS, Lung TWF, Mansell A, Riedmaier P, Oates CVL, Zaid A, Mühlen S, Crepin VF, Marches O, Ang C-S, Williamson NA, O'Reilly LA, Bankovacki A, Nachbur U, Infusini G, Webb AI, Silke J, Strasser A, Frankel G, Hartland EL. 2013. A type III effector antagonizes death receptor signalling during bacterial gut infection. *Nature* 501:247–251.

145. Scott NE, Giogha C, Pollock GL, Kennedy CL, Webb AI, Williamson NA, Pearson JS, Hartland EL. 2017. The bacterial arginine glycosyltransferase effector NleB preferentially modifies Fas-associated death domain protein (FADD). *J Biol Chem* **292:**17337–17350.

146. Nomata J, Hisabori T. 2018. Development of heme protein based oxygen sensing indicators. *Sci Rep* **8**(1):11849.

147. Schürmann N, Forrer P, Casse O, Li J, Felmy B, Burgener A-V, Ehrenfeuchter N, Hardt W-D, Recher M, Hess C, Tschan-Plessl A, Khanna N, Bumann D. 2017. Myeloperoxidase targets oxidative host attacks to Salmonella and prevents collateral tissue damage. *Nat Microbiol* **2:**16268.

148. Morimoto YV, Kami-ike N, Miyata T, Kawamoto A, Kato T, Namba K, Minamino T. 2016. High-resolution pH imaging of living bacterial cells to detect local pH differences. *mBio* **7:**e01911–16.

149. Curkić I, Schütz M, Oberhettinger P, Diard M, Claassen M, Linke D, Hardt W-D. 2016. Epitope-tagged autotransporters as single-cell reporters for gene expression by a Salmonella Typhimurium wbaP mutant. *PloS One* **11:** e0154828.

Bacteria and Intracellularity
Edited by Pascale Cossart, Craig R. Roy, and Philippe Sansonetti
© 2019 American Society for Microbiology, Washington, DC
doi:10.1128/microbiolspec.BAI-0013-2019

New Age Strategies To Reconstruct Mucosal Tissue Colonization and Growth in Cell Culture Systems

4

Alyssa C. Fasciano,[1,2] Joan Mecsas,[1] and Ralph R. Isberg[1]

INTRODUCTION: THE STUDY OF HOST-PATHOGEN INTERACTIONS IN CULTURE

With the current understanding that microbes play a large role in shaping human physiology, there has been renewed interest in the study of host-microbe interactions. Much of our present knowledge of host-pathogen interactions has resulted from studies with animal models or cultured immortalized cell lines that attempt to reproduce specific events during host-microbe interactions (1). Underlying these strategies is the goal of reproducing the important events that occur during human disease. The closest approximation to human infection has been animal infections using model organisms such as the mouse, to attempt to generate a system with complexity and biological functions similar to those of humans. Unfortunately, many important pathogens do not readily colonize or establish disease in common mammalian models, and the response to infection does not always recapitulate the human response (2, 3). A particularly confounding problem is that the infection site is often inaccessible in the animal, interfering with the ability to perform manipulations in real time or to make direct observations at the microscopic level.

As an alternative to performing infections in animals, an entire subfield of microbiology has matured over the past 30 years that involves direct interrogation of microbial interactions with cultured mammalian cells (4). This has allowed access to the infection site and improved visualization of the host-pathogen interface. This strategy also has resulted in great advances in our understanding of how mammalian cell processes are manipulated by microbes (5, 6), but there are several shortcomings to this approach. First, microbial interactions in the host are often complex, with diverse subsets of both immune and nonimmune cells interfacing with the microorganism simultaneously or in rapid succession. Most cell culture systems, in contrast, include only one cell type and therefore are unable to represent these complex interactions. Secondly, microbial interactions often involve targeting epithelial or other cells that have topological constraints with defined polarity (7). Most cell culture systems involve monolayers of immortalized cells, which lack these constraints. Finally, cell culture systems often use immortalized cells, which can behave quite differently from primary cells in the host (8).

To overcome some of these shortcomings, a few immortalized epithelial cell lines can be grown as confluent monolayers with tight junctions on Transwell filters, which has allowed the generation of defined apical and basal surfaces of the monolayer (9–11). These systems also have shortcomings, as they lack other biophysical properties and the three-dimensional (3D) structure of the particular organ system that they are trying to represent (12). One strategy to solve this problem has been to perform primary culture of cells from model mammals, such as the mouse or rat, but again, this raises the problem of species differences in trying to reproduce events that take place in the human host (13). Thus, primary cells from various human organs have been harvested and cultured *in vitro* but have to be used for very short periods, as the tissues often deteriorate in culture (14). The lack of a system that fully represents the intricacy of the human body has left an incomplete understanding of what occurs during infection with a pathogen.

Recent technological advances in propagating human tissue long-term in culture have provided exciting ave-

---

[1]Department of Molecular Biology and Microbiology, Tufts University School of Medicine, Boston, MA; [2]Program in Immunology, Sackler School of Biomedical Sciences, Tufts University School of Medicine, Boston, MA.

nues for the study of host-pathogen interactions. Particularly exciting is the use of organoids, which are 3D structures that can be derived from a variety of tissue types and include many of the cell types relevant to their tissue (15). Since they are derived from pluripotent stem cells or adult tissue stem cells, they maintain their capacity for self-renewal and self-organization into structures that mimic the given organ (15). Furthermore, engineering advances have improved the methods used for cell culture, allowing the inclusion of additional biophysical tissue features, such as flow and mechanical stresses. These exciting new developments will likely provide a path for culturing organoids under physiologically relevant conditions and could prove to be invaluable for the study of host-pathogen interactions. In this chapter, we address recent advances in *ex vivo* models for the analysis of host-microbe interactions in various mucosal tissues.

DEVELOPMENT OF INTESTINAL ORGANOIDS

In 2009, two groups developed methods for long-term culture of primary mouse intestinal cells from single Lgr5$^+$ stem cells or stem cells originating from crypts that could recapitulate intestinal differentiation (16, 17). The LGR5 gene had recently been identified as a marker for multipotent intestinal stem cells that give rise to all intestinal cell types (18). Prior to these discoveries, methods to develop long-term culture of primary cells had uniformly failed, and attempts to induce cultured primary cells to mimic intestinal villi and crypt morphology were unsuccessful. Supplying stem cells with proper growth factors resulted in the formation of 3D structures, termed organoids, that maintain stem cell quality and therefore could self-renew *in vitro* for long-term culture (19). Removal of stem cell-promoting factors resulted in differentiation of the organoids to exhibit the main cell types found in the intestine, including enterocytes, Paneth cells, goblet cells, and enteroendocrine cells (19). These methods were also applied to human tissue from the colon for the culture of colonoids and have since been applied to other regions of the gastrointestinal tract from both diseased and healthy tissues (19). Perhaps one of the most exciting aspects of these cells is that they can be isolated from human patients during very common standard procedures, such as colonoscopies, allowing diverse patient populations to be analyzed as well as providing important tools directed toward studying human genetic diseases.

Another method to establish long-term human intestinal cell culture involves the culture of human pluripotent stem cells (hPSCs), and the resulting 3D structures are of-ten termed human intestinal organoids (HIOs) (20–22). Thus, to distinguish the origin of the derived tissue, the organoids previously described that are derived from intestinal Lgr5$^+$ stem cells are now often termed human intestinal enteroids (HIEs). Organoids developed from hPSCs contain an epithelial layer and a mesenchymal layer and are more like fetal tissue, and therefore, they may be particularly useful for studies of intestinal development (21). Both enteroids and organoids maintain physiological properties of the intestine, such as functional ion transport via absorption and secretion (23) and peptide transport (21). They also maintain intestinal structure as they self-assemble into stem cell-containing proliferative zones and differentiated zones (21). Altogether, the development of these human "mini-intestines" has opened the door for the study of intestinal development, pathogenesis, and host-pathogen interactions.

USE OF INTESTINAL ORGANOIDS FOR THE STUDY OF HOST-PATHOGEN INTERACTIONS

Organoids as 3D Structures and 2D Monolayers

One of the primary complications of analyzing pathogen interaction with organoids is that their multicellular 3D structure results in topological constraints. There is an opportunity cost, because organoids allow new analysis strategies, in that the 3D cellular structures can mimic a miniorgan in structural topology and function. However, as the apical side of the epithelium faces the lumen of the structure, microorganisms must be microinjected into the organoid to allow contact with the relevant cells (24) (Fig. 1). In this fashion, Leslie and coworkers have used HIOs to analyze bacterial interactions. They have shown that the anaerobe *Clostridioides* (formerly *Clostridium*) *difficile* can colonize the lumen of these structures and cause damage to epithelium due to the secretion of clostridial Tcd toxins (25). Therefore, the luminal environment is of sufficiently low oxygen tension to allow survival and expression of toxin genes by an anaerobe. The Spence group also took advantage of the fact that the culture of HIOs allows researchers to study the interaction between immature stem cells and microbiota components to determine how microbes affect host epithelial development. To this end, HIOs were microinjected with nonpathogenic *Escherichia coli* to study the initial colonization of the microbes (26). Colonization promoted antimicrobial responses, such as the production of inflammatory cytokines as well as mucin production, under conditions in which the epithelial barrier integrity

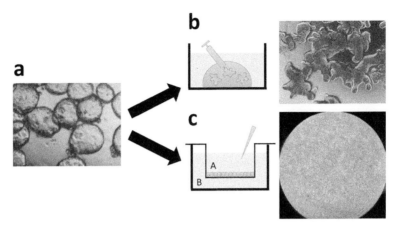

Figure 1 Methods for using intestinal organoids to study host-pathogen interactions. (**a**) Image of undifferentiated intestinal cysts containing stem cells. (**b**) (Left) Cysts can be differentiated in Matrigel and used for microinjection with bacteria. (Right) Image of differentiated enteroids. (**c**) (Left) Cysts can be broken up enzymatically with trypsin, seeded on Transwell filters, and differentiated into a polarized monolayer with an apical side (A) and a basolateral side (B). Microbes can be added to the apical side using a pipette. (Right) Apical surface of the monolayer. All images were taken with a 4× objective lens on an optical microscope.

was maintained. This system could provide key tools to interrogate events linked to microbial control of intestinal epithelial cell development.

To facilitate infection of the apical side of the intestine, enteroids grown as 3D cultures can be broken up into single cells and seeded onto Transwell filters (27) (Fig. 1). In this model, the enteroids form a polarized monolayer with defined apical and basolateral surfaces. Importantly, the monolayers contain differentiated cell types found in the intestine, and a mucus layer covers the apical surface. Pathogenic strains of *E. coli* adhere to both ileal and rectal epithelial monolayers, indicating that this model is amenable to the study of host-pathogen interactions (27). Furthermore, enterohemorrhagic *E. coli* preferentially colonizes differentiated monolayers rather than undifferentiated monolayers, which may be due to the presence of mucin on the differentiate monolayers, a target of enterohemorrhagic *E. coli* during infection (28). Transmission scanning electron microscopy images of the colonoid monolayers reveal typical attaching and effacing lesions that are associated with the natural infection of the human intestine. Thus, the monolayers provide a useful tool for visualization of early events during host-pathogen interactions.

Organoids as a Model for Pathogens That Are Difficult To Culture

Studies of enteric viruses have been hindered by the lack of good models, with the consequence that there is a lack of effective intervention therapies. For example, human noroviruses do not replicate to high levels when cultured with transformed intestinal cell lines (29, 30) and do not readily infect animal models (31). To determine if enteroids can be used for culturing norovirus, human norovirus strains were isolated from stool filtrates and used to infect jejunum-derived monolayers (32). Using the HIE model, human norovirus strains of the GII.4 genotype, which cause the majority of norovirus disease worldwide, replicate to high titers. Other relevant clinical strains require pretreatment of the enteroid cultures with bile in order to replicate. Since replication can be detected, this system can be exploited to test the efficacy of viral neutralization techniques by subjecting HIEs to norovirus strains that have undergone heat inactivation or gamma irradiation (32). In addition, HIOs have been found to express histo-blood group antigens which can bind human noroviruses, although replication is not as robust as that seen in the HIE model (33). Differences in replication levels between the models may be due to the differentiation state of the enterocytes; however, taken together, these results demonstrate that each system holds promise for analyzing various aspects of norovirus infection.

Similar approaches using both organoids and enteroids have been taken to study rotavirus replication. Replication of clinical isolates of rotavirus in HIOs was shown to reach levels 10 times that in the conventional monkey cell line MA104 (34). This study provided evidence that organoids could be used as a model for achieving rotavirus replication and studying rotavirus infection. Using HIEs as a model for rotavirus infection, the same group found that human rotavirus can replicate in enteroids derived from all three sections of the small intestine (35). 3D enteroids were shown to swell and expand in response to rotavirus infection or treatment with rotaviral enterotoxin, likely representing fluid movement to the lumen, which occurs during a diarrheal episode. This indicates that enteroids can be used to study pathophysiological features of infection. In more recent work, rotavirus infection was shown to induce the type III interferon (IFN) response by HIEs, although this is ineffective at blocking viral replication in this system (36). In contrast, viral growth can be restricted when the HIEs are treated with exogenous type I IFNs. Enteroids have also been used to test the effectiveness of the anti-rotavirus activity of IFN-α and ribavirin (37). The effect of these antivirals is variable among different patient strains of enteroids and is less effective than when immortalized cells are used as model hosts. Since this result more closely relates to clinical outcomes of the antivirals, it suggests that enteroids can be used to evaluate drug efficacy, possibly on a person-by-person basis.

Investigating Intestinal Tropism

Organoids can also be used to determine cell type tropism or differences between the intestinal segments, which is impossible with immortalized cell lines that lack the segment specificity and cellular diversity found in the intestine (38). Using differentiated ileum enteroids, the respiratory adenovirus HAdV-5p primarily infects intestinal goblet cells, but interestingly, this cellular preference is not a feature of the enteric serotype HAdV-41p (39). Similarly, goblet cells are resistant to the enterovirus echovirus 11, but enteroendocrine cells are permissive for this virus (40). Rotavirus infection of HIOs shows tropism for replication in enterocytes as well as mesenchymal cells (34).

Intestinal enteroids, derived from the duodenum, jejunum, ileum, and colon of three patients and infected with multiple pathogenic strains of enteroaggregative E. coli (EAEC), demonstrated the remarkable tropism of the pathogen (41). There are five patterns of aggregative adherence of EAEC to these tissues, which can be seen to occur in both a segment-specific and a host-specific manner. Minimal diffuse adherence to the jejunum occurs across all donors and among the adherent EAEC strains. Total adherence to the duodenum, ileum, and colon varies among donors but is consistently robust in the duodenum. Adherence to the ileum occurs in a stacked-brick pattern, whereas adherence to the colon is mesh-like. The pattern of adherence to the duodenum is more dependent on the donor and occurs in sheet-like or microcolony patterns. Thus, enteroids provide the potential for studying host variability and intestinal tropism.

Incorporation of Immune Cells

The immune system is an essential component of the host response to infection, but organoid and enteroid cultures do not include immune cells. Therefore, there have been efforts to include immune components in enteroid cultures, especially in the context of studying host-pathogen interactions. HIOs have been cocultured with human neutrophils prior to microinjection with the Shiga toxin-producing E. coli O157:H7 strain or a commensal E. coli strain (42). In response to infection with O157:H7, neutrophils migrate to the lumen of the enteroids to a greater extent than in enteroids harboring the commensal strain (42). To develop an enteroid-macrophage coculture model, Transwell filters with human enteroid monolayers have been constructed that allow human macrophages derived from human peripheral blood monocytes to be seeded on the basolateral side (43). During apical infection with enteropathogenic E. coli or enterotoxigenic E. coli, macrophages extend projections through to the apical side, decreasing the recovery of enterotoxigenic E. coli relative to culture without macrophages (43). The addition of immune components is critical to understanding the host response to infection, so continuing to develop ways to increase cellular complexity in these models will contribute to a fuller understanding of the events that occur at the interface of infection.

Use of Gastric Organoids To Study Host-Pathogen Interactions

The stomach is composed of two main regions, the corpus and the antrum, that each harbor specialized cell types. The corpus contains parietal cells (which secrete acid), chief cells (which aid in digestion), surface mucous pit cells, mucous neck cells, and endocrine cells, while the antrum contains few parietal or chief cells but has mucous pit cells, endocrine cells, and basal gland cells (which secrete mucus) (44). Recently, methods for culturing intestinal organoids were applied to the development of organoids from the stomach, from both induced PSCs (iPSCs) and human gastric glands that contain self-renewing stem cells, making gastric organoids the first long-term primary human cell culture system for gastric tissue (45–48). The organoids from each stomach region express the distinct gastric cell types and can form typical gland and pit organization (45, 47, 48).

Gastric organoids have proved useful for studying infection by Helicobacter pylori (45–49), a bacterium that causes inflammation of the stomach epithelium and is known to be a major risk factor for the occurrence of peptic ulcers and gastric cancers. Interestingly, H. pylori colonizes the stem and progenitor cell-containing gland region of microinjected gastric organoids and can induce epithelial cell proliferation, a tantalizing finding given the association between *H. pylori* infection and stomach adenocarcinoma (45, 47). *H. pylori* infection can also be supported by 2D monolayers of polarized epithelium derived from gastric organoids, leading to upregulation of host inflammatory response genes (48). Gastric organoids will likely be valuable not only for investigating host-pathogen interactions but also for investigating links between infection-generated tissue damage and long-term gastric disease.

ENGINEERING ADVANCES THAT HAVE IMPROVED THE INVESTIGATION OF HOST-PATHOGEN INTERACTIONS

Organs-on-a-Chip

A promising area of research for the application of host-pathogen interactions is the development of microfluidic devices, termed organs-on-a-chip, which have been reviewed extensively by Bhatia and Ingber (50). In this approach, human cells from a given organ are seeded into a chamber and subjected to continuous flow, with additional mechanical forces that mimic physiological organ conditions. These devices are exciting because they provide opportunities to increase assay complexity and provide a mimic for tissues subjected to hydrostatic forces. For instance, the devices can include multiple chambers that are separated by a porous membrane that is seeded with cells on each side, providing a tissue-tissue interface. Alternatively, they can consist of multiple chips seeded with cells from different organs that connect with each other. These multiorgan models have great potential for studying how infections propagate between organs.

Lung-on-a-chip for the study of respiratory pathogens

The lungs and respiratory tract, like the digestive system, are topologically exterior mucosal tissues and are therefore subject to pathogenic and environmental insults from inhaled respiratory droplets. The lungs consist of highly structured conducting airways and alveoli. The epithelium of the conducting airway is made of ciliated, goblet, basal, and other secretory cells, while the epithelium of the alveoli is made of alveolar type I and type II cells (51). Underlying smooth muscle cells, fibroblasts, and immune cells also contribute to the overall architecture of the lung (51). Due to the complexity of the lung and the various cell types that contribute to proper lung function, the lung has not been well mimicked *in vitro*. The recent development of lung-on-a-chip devices pro-

vides an opportunity to recreate various features of the lung microenvironment, including the simultaneous culture of multiple cell types and cyclic breathing forces. Furthermore, development of lung organoids from the different regions of the lung has allowed studies with defined lung cell types whose responses are functionally more similar to *in vivo* responses than those of immortalized cell lines. As these models have only recently been described, they have been underutilized for the study of host-pathogen interactions but have great potential.

A lung-on-a-chip model, developed by Huh et al., includes two chambers separated by an extracellular-matrix-coated porous membrane (52). The upper chamber is seeded with immortalized airway epithelial cells and interfaces with air, while the opposite side of the membrane facing the lower chamber is seeded with human pulmonary microvascular endothelial cells and exposed to culture media. To mimic the pressures that occur during normal breathing, the device includes additional chambers connected to a vacuum that when activated reproduces the forces of breathing on the epithelium. Interestingly, when tumor necrosis factor alpha is added to the upper chamber to mimic an inflammatory stimulus, the epithelium induces a change in the endothelium, resulting in an increase in surface expression of ICAM-1. Neutrophils flowing through the lower endothelial chamber, representing the vasculature, adhere to ICAM-1 and migrate through the endothelium and across the epithelium. This exciting system should provide an excellent model for the study of host-pathogen interactions to examine the immune response to infection.

Several laboratories have developed lung-on-a-chip models for studying airway diseases such as asthma and chronic obstructive pulmonary disease (COPD) (53, 54). In addition, differentiated primary human airway epithelial cells have been seeded into a microfluidic model at the air-liquid interface and subjected to a pollen extract challenge (55). The basolateral flowthrough can be collected through the fluidics system, allowing secretion of the inflammatory marker interleukin 8 (IL-8) by epithelial cells to be measured in response to pollen, again providing evidence that this system provides the potential for novel analyses of the immune response and the mechanisms of disease.

Excitingly, methods have been described creating lung organoids from isolated stem cells from various regions of the lungs or from iPSCs (reviewed by Barkauskas et al. [56]). While these lung organoids are still new and being functionally explored, a few groups have used them for the study of virus infection. Lung organoids developed from pluripotent stem cells can be infected with respiratory syncytial virus, a virus that causes respiratory illness in very young children (57). After 2 days, infected cells begin to swell, detach from the epithelium, and are shed into the lumen of the organoid, a pathological response seen in humans during disease. Furthermore, in a different study, human lung organoids derived from adult patient tissues were demonstrated to be infected with various strains of enterovirus 71, a virus that infects the gastrointestinal and respiratory tracts (58). The virus replicates in lung organoids in a strain-dependent manner. The successes with both the lung-on-a-chip model and the lung organoids indicate that combining these two technologies has the potential to broaden our knowledge of host-pathogen interactions in the lungs, to further evaluate the effect of drugs on tissues and infections, and to study pathogenesis of long-term infectious and noninfectious diseases in the lung.

Gut-on-a-chip

Taking advantage of the microfluidics systems that have recently been developed to model the lung, the Ingber group created a gut-on-a-chip in which the top chamber of the microfluidics device is seeded with Caco-2 cells, an immortalized human intestinal cell line (59). This model supports peristalsis movements and flow, important physiological forces that contribute to the intestinal microenvironment and are essential for maintaining proper epithelial barrier function (60). Compared to the static Transwell filter system, which results in a flat monolayer of Caco-2 cells, the microfluidics chamber with flow results in the formation of a taller monolayer of cells that are columnar, more closely mimicking *in vivo* conditions (59). Also, due to flow, the chip model supports the growth, but not overgrowth, of *Lactobacillus rhamnosus* GG, which improves the barrier function of the epithelial layer, as assessed by transepithelial electrical resistance, a measurement of the resistance between the sides of the chip. The Caco-2 cells under flow conditions form villus-like structures with defined proliferative and basal regions with cells that express intestinal markers (61).

To study the intestinal epithelial response during chronic inflammation, human peripheral blood mononuclear cells added to the lower chamber of the gut-on-a-chip model allow recruitment of white blood cells to the underlying lamina propria to be mimicked (62). In the absence of underlying immune cells, addition of a nonpathogenic strain of *E. coli* causes no barrier dysfunction. In the presence of peripheral blood mononuclear cells, however, addition of the commensal leads to disruption of the monolayer barrier, as detected by transepithelial electrical resistance measurement, suggesting that the presence of chronic inflammation promotes epithe-

lial injury, as may occur during inflammatory bowel diseases. Thus, the chip model could be useful for studying how the interplay between the immune system and the microbiome contributes to disease pathology during conditions of chronic inflammation.

The chip model has also been used to study the epithelial response to the enteric pathogen coxsackievirus B1 with loss of villus morphology detected by immunofluorescence after 24 hours postinfection (63). Coxsackievirus B1 can infect these monolayers both apically (via inoculation in the top chamber of the microfluidic device) and basolaterally (via inoculation in the bottom chamber). Interestingly, virions and inflammatory cytokines are released apically under both infection conditions. Future modifications to the gut-on-a-chip model, such as the inclusion of immune cells, mesenchymal cells, and/or nerve cells, would improve the physiological relevance to the human intestine and make it a more robust model for the study of host-pathogen interactions (64).

Combining Engineering Technologies With Enteroids

There have been recent exciting efforts to combine engineering technologies with intestinal organoids to create microenvironments that more closely represent the actual human intestine and exceed the capabilities of static 2D cell culture. The Kaplan group has developed an *in vitro* silk-based 3D scaffold model of the intestine that is cylindrical and consists of a hollow lumen for the seeding of intestinal cells and a porous bulk that can support intestinal myofibroblasts (65) (Fig. 2). Using immortalized intestinal cell lines to seed the lumen, this tissue model exhibits luminal mucus secretion and oxygen levels similar to those seen under *in vivo* conditions and could support *C. difficile* growth, toxin production, and epithelial damage (65, 66). Connecting the 3D scaffolds to a bioreactor perfusion system allows the incorporation of luminal flow, induction of peristalsis-like contractions, and tunable oxygen levels (67). The addition of flow and peristalsis is essential for mimicking the microenvironment of the intestine, which works to constantly clear luminal contents. Furthermore, the 3D scaffold model has since been seeded with cells from human intestinal enteroids, resulting in monolayers that express a dense brush border of microvilli, markers of the four major intestinal cell types, and digestive enzyme production (68). This provides evidence that the silk-based scaffolding model can support and sustain growth and differentiation of a polarized monolayer of intestinal epithelium derived from enteroids. The design of these scaffolds could be modified to include immune

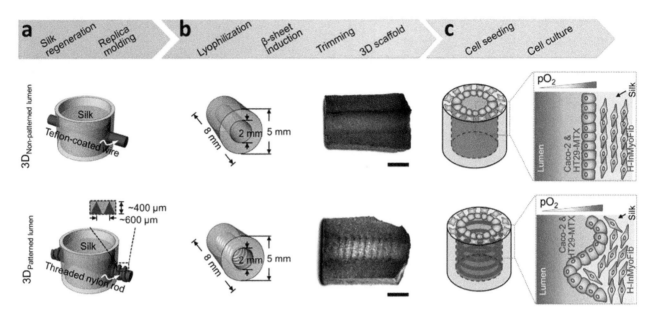

Figure 2   Method for development of a 3D silk scaffold to model human intestines. Reprinted from reference 65 under the CC BY 4.0 license.

cells on the basolateral side and to further mimic physiological conditions present during initial infection.

The Ingber group has improved the gut-on-a-chip with the development of the intestine chip, in which Caco-2 cells have been replaced with enteroids (69) (Fig. 3). By seeding human intestinal duodenum enteroid fragments on the intestine chip and subjecting the device to continuous flow, Kasendra et al. have demonstrated that villus-like structures can be formed that extend out from a polarized epithelium (69). Further, compared to human duodenum, cells grown in the intestine chip model are closer in gene expression profile to the human duodenum than to the cultured enteroids from which the chips were derived (69). They also increased the complexity of the

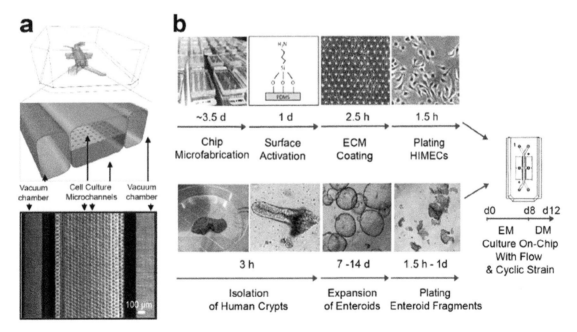

Figure 3   Method for development of the intestine chip using enteroids to model human intestines. Reprinted from reference 69 under the CC BY 4.0 license.

microenvironment by seeding primary human intestinal microvascular endothelial cells in the chip model on the opposite surface from the intestinal enteroids in the lower chamber of the device. The inclusion of these cells results in enhanced confluency of the enteroid layer. This is a promising model that can now be applied to the study of host-pathogen interactions.

CONCLUSIONS

Researchers have barely skimmed the surface of the usefulness of organoids, but these promising studies demonstrate that organoids can be used for a variety of biomedical applications, including infectious disease modeling, pathogenesis, and drug testing. One of the most exciting aspects of this approach is the ability to derive organoids from different patients with distinct genetic backgrounds exposed to different microbiota populations, providing great potential for patient-specific therapies and personalized medicine. The development of organoids is a monumental step forward in terms of having a long-term culture system of nontransformed cells that have many of the properties of the cell types found in the respective tissue. However, many challenges remain, as organoids lack many players that affect the physiology of disease, such as immune cells, microbiota, and stromal cells, as well as distinct tissue forces and fluid flow. Modeling the interplay between of all these features and a pathogen is essential for a complete understanding of pathophysiology of a given disease. Therefore, the advancement of engineering technologies will further harness the great power of organoids through the development of innovative ways to incorporate human parameters into robust culture systems, with the ultimate goal of improving human health.

Acknowledgments. We thank our collaborators and members of our laboratories for useful discussions. A.C.F. was supported by NIAID T32 AI007077, J.M. was supported by NIAID U19 AI131126 and NIAID R21 AI12809, and R.R.I. was supported by NIAID R01 AI110684.

Citation. Fasciano AC, Mecsas J, Isberg RR. 2019. New Age strategies to reconstruct mucosal tissue colonization and growth in cell culture systems. Microbiol Spectrum 7(2):BAI-0013-2019.

References

1. Falkow S. 2004. Molecular Koch's postulates applied to bacterial pathogenicity—a personal recollection 15 years later. *Nat Rev Microbiol* 2:67–72.

2. Mestas J, Hughes CC. 2004. Of mice and not men: differences between mouse and human immunology. *J Immunol* 172:2731–2738.

3. Rall GF, Lawrence DM, Patterson CE. 2000. The application of transgenic and knockout mouse technology for the study of viral pathogenesis. *Virology* 271:220–226.

4. Falkow S, Isberg RR, Portnoy DA. 1992. The interaction of bacteria with mammalian cells. *Annu Rev Cell Biol* 8:333–363.

5. Cossart P. 1997. Host/pathogen interactions. Subversion of the mammalian cell cytoskeleton by invasive bacteria. *J Clin Invest* 99:2307–2311.

6. Falkow S. 1991. Bacterial entry into eukaryotic cells. *Cell* 65:1099–1102.

7. Kazmierczak BI, Mostov K, Engel JN. 2001. Interaction of bacterial pathogens with polarized epithelium. *Annu Rev Microbiol* 55:407–435.

8. Sun H, Chow EC, Liu S, Du Y, Pang KS. 2008. The Caco-2 cell monolayer: usefulness and limitations. *Expert Opin Drug Metab Toxicol* 4:395–411.

9. Hidalgo IJ, Raub TJ, Borchardt RT. 1989. Characterization of the human colon carcinoma cell line (Caco-2) as a model system for intestinal epithelial permeability. *Gastroenterology* 96:736–749.

10. Grainger CI, Greenwell LL, Lockley DJ, Martin GP, Forbes B. 2006. Culture of Calu-3 cells at the air interface provides a representative model of the airway epithelial barrier. *Pharm Res* 23:1482–1490.

11. McCormick BA. 2003. The use of transepithelial models to examine host-pathogen interactions. *Curr Opin Microbiol* 6:77–81.

12. Abbott A. 2003. Cell culture: biology's new dimension. *Nature* 424:870–872.

13. Evans GS, Flint N, Somers AS, Eyden B, Potten CS. 1992. The development of a method for the preparation of rat intestinal epithelial cell primary cultures. *J Cell Sci* 101:219–231.

14. Honegger P. 2001. Overview of cell and tissue culture techniques. *Curr Protoc Pharmacol* Chapter 12:Unit 12 1.

15. Lancaster MA, Knoblich JA. 2014. Organogenesis in a dish: modeling development and disease using organoid technologies. *Science* 345:1247125.

16. Ootani A, Li X, Sangiorgi E, Ho QT, Ueno H, Toda S, Sugihara H, Fujimoto K, Weissman IL, Capecchi MR, Kuo CJ. 2009. Sustained in vitro intestinal epithelial culture within a Wnt-dependent stem cell niche. *Nat Med* 15:701–706.

17. Sato T, Vries RG, Snippert HJ, van de Wetering M, Barker N, Stange DE, van Es JH, Abo A, Kujala P, Peters PJ, Clevers H. 2009. Single Lgr5 stem cells build crypt-villus structures in vitro without a mesenchymal niche. *Nature* 459:262–265.

18. Barker N, van Es JH, Kuipers J, Kujala P, van den Born M, Cozijnsen M, Haegebarth A, Korving J, Begthel H, Peters PJ, Clevers H. 2007. Identification of stem cells in small intestine and colon by marker gene Lgr5. *Nature* 449:1003–1007.

19. Sato T, Stange DE, Ferrante M, Vries RG, Van Es JH, Van den Brink S, Van Houdt WJ, Pronk A, Van Gorp J, Siersema PD, Clevers H. 2011. Long-term expansion of epithelial organoids from human colon, adenoma, adeno-

carcinoma, and Barrett's epithelium. *Gastroenterology* **141**: 1762–1772.

20. McCracken KW, Howell JC, Wells JM, Spence JR. 2011. Generating human intestinal tissue from pluripotent stem cells in vitro. *Nat Protoc* **6**:1920–1928.

21. Spence JR, Mayhew CN, Rankin SA, Kuhar MF, Vallance JE, Tolle K, Hoskins EE, Kalinichenko VV, Wells SI, Zorn AM, Shroyer NF, Wells JM. 2011. Directed differentiation of human pluripotent stem cells into intestinal tissue in vitro. *Nature* **470**:105–109.

22. Sinagoga KL, Wells JM. 2015. Generating human intestinal tissues from pluripotent stem cells to study development and disease. *EMBO J* **34**:1149–1163.

23. Foulke-Abel J, In J, Yin J, Zachos NC, Kovbasnjuk O, Estes MK, de Jonge H, Donowitz M. 2016. Human enteroids as a model of upper small intestinal ion transport physiology and pathophysiology. *Gastroenterology* **150**:638–649.e8.

24. Hill DR, Huang S, Tsai YH, Spence JR, Young VB. 2017. Real-time measurement of epithelial barrier permeability in human intestinal organoids. *J Vis Exp* **2017**:e56960.

25. Leslie JL, Huang S, Opp JS, Nagy MS, Kobayashi M, Young VB, Spence JR. 2015. Persistence and toxin production by *Clostridium difficile* within human intestinal organoids result in disruption of epithelial paracellular barrier function. *Infect Immun* **83**:138–145.

26. Hill DR, Huang S, Nagy MS, Yadagiri VK, Fields C, Mukherjee D, Bons B, Dedhia PH, Chin AM, Tsai YH, Thodla S, Schmidt TM, Walk S, Young VB, Spence JR. 2017. Bacterial colonization stimulates a complex physiological response in the immature human intestinal epithelium. *eLife* **6**:e29132.

27. VanDussen KL, Marinshaw JM, Shaikh N, Miyoshi H, Moon C, Tarr PI, Ciorba MA, Stappenbeck TS. 2015. Development of an enhanced human gastrointestinal epithelial culture system to facilitate patient-based assays. *Gut* **64**:911–920.

28. In J, Foulke-Abel J, Zachos NC, Hansen AM, Kaper JB, Bernstein HD, Halushka M, Blutt S, Estes MK, Donowitz M, Kovbasnjuk O. 2016. Enterohemorrhagic *Escherichia coli* reduce mucus and intermicrovillar bridges in human stem cell-derived colonoids. *Cell Mol Gastroenterol Hepatol* **2**:48–62.e3.

29. Duizer E, Schwab KJ, Neill FH, Atmar RL, Koopmans MP, Estes MK. 2004. Laboratory efforts to cultivate noroviruses. *J Gen Virol* **85**:79–87.

30. Papafragkou E, Hewitt J, Park GW, Greening G, Vinjé J. 2013. Challenges of culturing human norovirus in three-dimensional organoid intestinal cell culture models. *PLoS One* **8**:e63485.

31. Wobus CE, Thackray LB, Virgin HW IV. 2006. Murine norovirus: a model system to study norovirus biology and pathogenesis. *J Virol* **80**:5104–5112.

32. Ettayebi K, Crawford SE, Murakami K, Broughman JR, Karandikar U, Tenge VR, Neill FH, Blutt SE, Zeng XL, Qu L, Kou B, Opekun AR, Burrin D, Graham DY, Ramani S, Atmar RL, Estes MK. 2016. Replication of human noroviruses in stem cell-derived human enteroids. *Science* **353**: 1387–1393.

33. Zhang D, Tan M, Zhong W, Xia M, Huang P, Jiang X. 2017. Human intestinal organoids express histo-blood group antigens, bind norovirus VLPs, and support limited norovirus replication. *Sci Rep* **7**:12621.

34. Finkbeiner SR, Zeng XL, Utama B, Atmar RL, Shroyer NF, Estes MK. 2012. Stem cell-derived human intestinal organoids as an infection model for rotaviruses. *mBio* **3**: e00159-12.

35. Saxena K, Blutt SE, Ettayebi K, Zeng XL, Broughman JR, Crawford SE, Karandikar UC, Sastri NP, Conner ME, Opekun AR, Graham DY, Qureshi W, Sherman V, Foulke-Abel J, In J, Kovbasnjuk O, Zachos NC, Donowitz M, Estes MK. 2016. Human intestinal enteroids: a new model to study human rotavirus infection, host restriction, and pathophysiology. *J Virol* **90**:43–56.

36. Saxena K, Simon LM, Zeng XL, Blutt SE, Crawford SE, Sastri NP, Karandikar UC, Ajami NJ, Zachos NC, Kovbasnjuk O, Donowitz M, Conner ME, Shaw CA, Estes MK. 2017. A paradox of transcriptional and functional innate interferon responses of human intestinal enteroids to enteric virus infection. *Proc Natl Acad Sci USA* **114**:E570–E579.

37. Yin Y, Bijvelds M, Dang W, Xu L, van der Eijk AA, Knipping K, Tuysuz N, Dekkers JF, Wang Y, de Jonge J, Sprengers D, van der Laan LJ, Beekman JM, Ten Berge D, Metselaar HJ, de Jonge H, Koopmans MP, Peppelenbosch MP, Pan Q. 2015. Modeling rotavirus infection and antiviral therapy using primary intestinal organoids. *Antiviral Res* **123**:120–31.

38. Middendorp S, Schneeberger K, Wiegerinck CL, Mokry M, Akkerman RD, van Wijngaarden S, Clevers H, Nieuwenhuis EE. 2014. Adult stem cells in the small intestine are intrinsically programmed with their location-specific function. *Stem Cells* **32**:1083–1091.

39. Holly MK, Smith JG. 2018. Adenovirus infection of human enteroids reveals interferon sensitivity and preferential infection of goblet cells. *J Virol* **92**:e00250-18.

40. Drummond CG, Bolock AM, Ma C, Luke CJ, Good M, Coyne CB. 2017. Enteroviruses infect human enteroids and induce antiviral signaling in a cell lineage-specific manner. *Proc Natl Acad Sci USA* **114**:1672–1677.

41. Rajan A, Vela L, Zeng XL, Yu X, Shroyer N, Blutt SE, Poole NM, Carlin LG, Nataro JP, Estes MK, Okhuysen PC, Maresso AW. 2018. Novel segment- and host-specific patterns of enteroaggregative *Escherichia coli* adherence to human intestinal enteroids. *mBio* **9**:e02419-17.

42. Karve SS, Pradhan S, Ward DV, Weiss AA. 2017. Intestinal organoids model human responses to infection by commensal and Shiga toxin producing *Escherichia coli*. *PLoS One* **12**:e0178966.

43. Noel G, Baetz NW, Staab JF, Donowitz M, Kovbasnjuk O, Pasetti MF, Zachos NC. 2017. A primary human macrophage-enteroid co-culture model to investigate mucosal gut physiology and host-pathogen interactions. *Sci Rep* **7**:45270. ERRATUM *Sci Rep* **7**:46790.

44. Willet SG, Mills JC. 2016. Stomach organ and cell lineage differentiation: from embryogenesis to adult homeostasis. *Cell Mol Gastroenterol Hepatol* **2**:546–559.

45. Bartfeld S, Bayram T, van de Wetering M, Huch M, Begthel H, Kujala P, Vries R, Peters PJ, Clevers H. 2015.

In vitro expansion of human gastric epithelial stem cells and their responses to bacterial infection. *Gastroenterology* **148**:126–136 e6.

46. Bartfeld S, Clevers H. 2015. Organoids as model for infectious diseases: culture of human and murine stomach organoids and microinjection of *Helicobacter pylori*. *J Vis Exp* (105).

47. McCracken KW, Catá EM, Crawford CM, Sinagoga KL, Schumacher M, Rockich BE, Tsai YH, Mayhew CN, Spence JR, Zavros Y, Wells JM. 2014. Modelling human development and disease in pluripotent stem-cell-derived gastric organoids. *Nature* **516**:400–404.

48. Schlaermann P, Toelle B, Berger H, Schmidt SC, Glanemann M, Ordemann J, Bartfeld S, Mollenkopf HJ, Meyer TF. 2016. A novel human gastric primary cell culture system for modelling *Helicobacter pylori* infection in vitro. *Gut* **65**:202–213.

49. Huang JY, Sweeney EG, Sigal M, Zhang HC, Remington SJ, Cantrell MA, Kuo CJ, Guillemin K, Amieva MR. 2015. Chemodetection and destruction of host urea allows *Helicobacter pylori* to locate the epithelium. *Cell Host Microbe* **18**:147–156.

50. Bhatia SN, Ingber DE. 2014. Microfluidic organs-on-chips. *Nat Biotechnol* **32**:760–772.

51. Franks TJ, Colby TV, Travis WD, Tuder RM, Reynolds HY, Brody AR, Cardoso WV, Crystal RG, Drake CJ, Engelhardt J, Frid M, Herzog E, Mason R, Phan SH, Randell SH, Rose MC, Stevens T, Serge J, Sunday ME, Voynow JA, Weinstein BM, Whitsett J, Williams MC. 2008. Resident cellular components of the human lung: current knowledge and goals for research on cell phenotyping and function. *Proc Am Thorac Soc* **5**:763–766.

52. Huh D, Matthews BD, Mammoto A, Montoya-Zavala M, Hsin HY, Ingber DE. 2010. Reconstituting organ-level lung functions on a chip. *Science* **328**:1662–1668.

53. Benam KH, Novak R, Nawroth J, Hirano-Kobayashi M, Ferrante TC, Choe Y, Prantil-Baun R, Weaver JC, Bahinski A, Parker KK, Ingber DE. 2016. Matched-comparative modeling of normal and diseased human airway responses using a microengineered breathing lung chip. *Cell Syst* **3**:456–466.E4.

54. Benam KH, Villenave R, Lucchesi C, Varone A, Hubeau C, Lee HH, Alves SE, Salmon M, Ferrante TC, Weaver JC, Bahinski A, Hamilton GA, Ingber DE. 2016. Small airway-on-a-chip enables analysis of human lung inflammation and drug responses in vitro. *Nat Methods* **13**:151–157.

55. Blume C, Reale R, Held M, Millar TM, Collins JE, Davies DE, Morgan H, Swindle EJ. 2015. Temporal monitoring of differentiated human airway epithelial cells using microfluidics. *PLoS One* **10**:e0139872.

56. Barkauskas CE, Chung MI, Fioret B, Gao X, Katsura H, Hogan BL. 2017. Lung organoids: current uses and future promise. *Development* **144**:986–997.

57. Chen YW, Huang SX, de Carvalho ALRT, Ho SH, Islam MN, Volpi S, Notarangelo LD, Ciancanelli M, Casanova JL, Bhattacharya J, Liang AF, Palermo LM, Porotto M, Moscona A, Snoeck HW. 2017. A three-dimensional model of human lung development and disease from pluripotent stem cells. *Nat Cell Biol* **19**:542–549.

58. van der Sanden SMG, Sachs N, Koekkoek SM, Koen G, Pajkrt D, Clevers H, Wolthers KC. 2018. Enterovirus 71 infection of human airway organoids reveals VP1-145 as a viral infectivity determinant. *Emerg Microbes Infect* **7**:84.

59. Kim HJ, Huh D, Hamilton G, Ingber DE. 2012. Human gut-on-a-chip inhabited by microbial flora that experiences intestinal peristalsis-like motions and flow. *Lab Chip* **12**:2165–2174.

60. Gayer CP, Basson MD. 2009. The effects of mechanical forces on intestinal physiology and pathology. *Cell Signal* **21**:1237–1244.

61. Kim HJ, Ingber DE. 2013. Gut-on-a-chip microenvironment induces human intestinal cells to undergo villus differentiation. *Integr Biol* **5**:1130–1140.

62. Kim HJ, Li H, Collins JJ, Ingber DE. 2016. Contributions of microbiome and mechanical deformation to intestinal bacterial overgrowth and inflammation in a human gut-on-a-chip. *Proc Natl Acad Sci USA* **113**:E7–E15.

63. Villenave R, Wales SQ, Hamkins-Indik T, Papafragkou E, Weaver JC, Ferrante TC, Bahinski A, Elkins CA, Kulka M, Ingber DE. 2017. Human gut-on-a-chip supports polarized infection of coxsackie B1 virus in vitro. *PLoS One* **12**:e0169412.

64. Bein A, Shin W, Jalili-Firoozinezhad S, Park MH, Sontheimer-Phelps A, Tovaglieri A, Chalkiadaki A, Kim HJ, Ingber DE. 2018. Microfluidic organ-on-a-chip models of human intestine. *Cell Mol Gastroenterol Hepatol* **5**:659–668.

65. Chen Y, Lin Y, Davis KM, Wang Q, Rnjak-Kovacina J, Li C, Isberg RR, Kumamoto CA, Mecsas J, Kaplan DL. 2015. Robust bioengineered 3D functional human intestinal epithelium. *Sci Rep* **5**:13708.

66. Shaban L, Chen Y, Fasciano AC, Lin Y, Kaplan DL, Kumamoto CA, Mecsas J. 2018. A 3D intestinal tissue model supports *Clostridioides difficile* germination, colonization, toxin production and epithelial damage. *Anaerobe* **50**:85–92.

67. Zhou W, Chen Y, Roh T, Lin Y, Ling S, Zhao S, Lin JD, Khalil N, Cairns DM, Manousiouthakis E, Tse M, Kaplan DL. 2018. Multifunctional bioreactor system for human intestine tissues. *ACS Biomater Sci Eng* **4**:231–239.

68. Chen Y, Zhou W, Roh T, Estes MK, Kaplan DL. 2017. In vitro enteroid-derived three-dimensional tissue model of human small intestinal epithelium with innate immune responses. *PLoS One* **12**:e0187880.

69. Kasendra M, Tovaglieri A, Sontheimer-Phelps A, Jalili-Firoozinezhad S, Bein A, Chalkiadaki A, Scholl W, Zhang C, Rickner H, Richmond CA, Li H, Breault DT, Ingber DE. 2018. Development of a primary human small intestine-on-a-chip using biopsy-derived organoids. *Sci Rep* **8**:2871.

Bacteria and Intracellularity
Edited by Pascale Cossart, Craig R. Roy, and Philippe Sansonetti
© 2019 American Society for Microbiology, Washington, DC
doi:10.1128/microbiolspec.BAI-0010-2019

The Many Faces of Bacterium-Endothelium Interactions during Systemic Infections

5

Dorian Obino[1] and Guillaume Duménil[1]

THE ENDOTHELIUM AS A SITE OF BACTERIAL INFECTIONS

The endothelium is the layer of endothelial cells lining the inner surface of blood vessels, which span the entire body and ensure the distribution of blood throughout the organism (1). It is estimated that the human body contains a staggering 100,000 km of blood vessels, more than twice the earth's circumference (2). Therefore, a bacterium reaching the circulation is engaged in a network of huge proportions. Moreover, a pathogen traveling through the circulatory system does not encounter a homogeneous environment, as an important feature of the vascular network is its diversity. Although endothelial cells are present in all vessels, the organization of the vessel wall, which is formed by three layers—the tunica intima, media, and adventitia (from the vessel lumen outward)—is different among different vessel types and different organs (3). Vessels can be first differentiated by the complex extracellular matrix layers surrounding them. For instance, elastic arteries such as the aorta are surrounded by 50 elastic layers, providing them with unique mechanical properties (3). Second, the cellular content is also different according to vessel type; the walls of arteries and veins contain a layer of smooth muscle cells that gives them the capacity to relax or constrict in response to vasoactive molecules (4). An additional level of complexity in the network stems from the fact that larger vessels, veins or arteries, are themselves vascularized by smaller vessels, the vasa vasorum (5).

Although endothelial cells are a constituent of all vessels, they themselves possess different properties depending on their anatomical location, in particular in the case of capillaries. The lumens of continuous capillaries, which are the most common, are lined with an uninterrupted layer of endothelial cells. Fenestrated capillaries, typically present in glomeruli of the kidney, are laced with 50- to 80-nm openings, thus giving them different permeability properties. In the liver, sinusoidal capillaries contain numerous holes that can reach several micrometers in diameter and could in principle allow objects such as bacteria to escape the circulation (6). Also, particularly relevant to infection, sinusoidal capillaries host a large number of Kupffer cells, phagocytic cells that constantly filter particulate matter, including bacteria, from the blood (7). Finally, the heart, a central element of the circulation network and also a potential site of infection, displays a specialized endothelium referred to as the endocardium. In contrast to the endothelium, the endocardium is composed of three juxtaposed layers that ensure (i) its physical anchorage to the surface of the myocardium (the heart muscle); (ii) its mechanoelastic properties, allowing its adaptation to the heart contraction and relaxation cycles; and (iii) its low permeability, thanks to a sealed monolayer of endothelial cells (8).

Although it is usually viewed as a static structure, the design of the blood vessel network is dynamic, in particular in the case of the smaller vessels, first during development but also following wound healing, cancer development, ischemia, or infection (9, 10). During development, vasculogenesis supports the establishment of the arteries and the veins, which transport the blood from and back to the heart, respectively (11). An additional mechanism, referred to as angiogenesis, gives rise to smaller vessels, such as blood capillaries a few micrometers in diameter, which deliver oxygen and nutrients to the body's tissues. These vessels elongate from endothelial sprouts emanating from preexisting ves-

[1]Pathogenesis of Vascular Infections, Institut Pasteur, INSERM, Paris, France.

sels and invade nonvascularized areas (12). Of note, capillaries are also able to interconnect through anastomosis, a process resulting in the fusion of two capillary growing ends (13). Therefore, pathogens reaching the circulation encounter a complex, diverse, and dynamic network.

CELLULAR JUNCTIONS AS THE GATEKEEPERS OF THE ENDOTHELIAL BARRIER

Through the fine control of vessel permeability, intercellular junctions within the endothelium are at the heart of the maintenance of vascular integrity, thus ensuring the proper barrier function of the endothelium (14). Among the two main types of endothelial cell-cell junctions, adherens junctions are ubiquitous, whereas tight junctions are mainly located in endothelial barriers with a very high selectivity (15). This is the case for the blood-brain barrier, where tight junctions ensure charge- and size-selective exchanges between the cerebral vasculature and the central nervous system (16), thus participating in the protection of the brain parenchyma from bacterial invasion, for instance. The main component of adherens junctions is the intercellular adhesion molecule vascular endothelial cadherin (VE-cadherin). VE-cadherin proteins expressed at the surface of neighboring endothelial cells engage their extracellular domain within homotypic interactions that are stabilized by extracellular calcium (17), thus ensuring the sealing of the endothelium. PECAM-1 (platelet-endothelial cell adhesion molecule 1) also participates in the structural integrity of adherens junctions (18). Intracellularly, VE-cadherin is linked to the actin cytoskeleton through its interactions with α-, β-, γ-, and p120-catenin (19) (Fig. 1). In contrast, tight junctions are made by the homophilic interaction of cell adhesion molecules such as claudins, occludin, and junction adhesion molecules, which are connected to the actin cytoskeleton through the proteins zonula occludens 1, 2, and 3 (Fig. 1).

Because of their importance, the establishment and maintenance of cell-to-cell junctions are tightly controlled. One of the best illustrations of such regulation is the modulation of vessel permeability by the vascular endothelial growth factor (VEGF) (20, 21). Its binding to VEGF receptor 2 induces an increase in intracellular calcium levels, leading to the subsequent activation of Src family kinases, mitogen-activated protein kinases, phosphatidylinositol 3-kinase, and protein kinase G (21, 22). This mainly results in (i) the remodeling of the actin cytoskeleton through the activation of the small GTPase RhoA; (ii) the activation of myosin light-chain

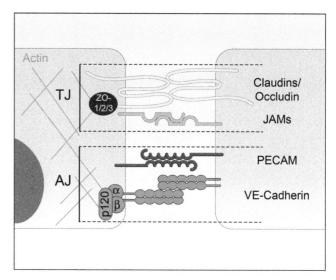

Figure 1 Schematic representation of the two main types of intercellular junctions within the endothelium. Adherens junctions (AJ) are made by the homophilic interaction of VE-cadherin and PECAM (also known as CD31). In contrast, claudins, occludin, and proteins from the junctional adhesion molecule (JAM) family are involved in establishing tight junctions. Connection with the actin cytoskeleton is ensured by proteins of the catenin family (alpha-, beta-, and p120-catenin) in the case of adherens junctions and by proteins from the zonula occludens family (ZO-1, -2, and -3) in the case of tight junctions.

kinase, which favors actomyosin contractility; (iii) the destabilization of integrin-mediated adhesion to the extracellular matrix; and (iv) the phosphorylation of VE-cadherin and its internalization, thus loosening cell-cell junctions (23). Together, these events contribute to increasing endothelial permeability. In contrast, the activation of other small GTPases, such as Rac-1 and Cdc42, protects the barrier function of the endothelium by stabilizing intercellular junctions and the cortical actin cytoskeleton (24). Therefore, the fine regulation of the interface between intercellular junctions and the actin cytoskeleton plays a crucial role in regulating endothelial integrity.

Strikingly, certain pathogens have the ability to overcome the physical barrier imposed by the endothelium from the outside in and/or vice versa to exit the vascular lumen and reach specific organs. Pathogenic bacteria can reach the circulation by accessing the vascular lumen through microabrasions within the skin or mucosa but also through insect bites (25–27). Once bacteria are in the circulatory system, bacterial adhesion to the endothelium is a frequent starting point for infection (28–30). Bacteria then either divert the host cell actin cytoskeleton to induce their internalization and transcytosis, leading to the passage of live bacteria through endothelial cells (31–35), or remain extracellular and interfere with the assembly of intercellular junctions, facilitating their paracellular passage (36). Hence, bacterial interaction with the endothelium often leads to the alteration of vascular integrity, which might be at the origin of vascular leaks, bacterial dissemination within the surrounding tissues, and/or organ dysfunction.

By using different examples of infection, we illustrate the many faces of bacterium-endothelium interactions and the subsequent perturbations of specific vascular functions in the particular environment of the blood circulation.

ALTERATION OF VASCULAR INTEGRITY UPON INFECTION BY *RICKETTSIA*

Rickettsiae that cause spotted fevers are among the best-characterized examples of pathogenic bacteria that have vascular tropism and disturb endothelial functions. Members of the genus *Rickettsia* are obligate intracellular vector-borne pathogens mainly transmitted by tick bites and triggering diverse diseases, such as typhus and spotted fever (27). Endothelial cells of the peripheral circulation represent the main target of *Rickettsia* species belonging to the spotted fever group (27, 37, 38) (Fig. 2). *Rickettsia* adhesion to the endothelial surface is mediated by the expression of the outer membrane proteins OmpA and OmpB (39) and their interaction with endothelial integrins, such as the $\alpha_2\beta_1$ integrin (40). This induces a rapid and efficient internalization of the adherent bacteria within a few minutes after the initial contact. Internalization occurs through a mechanism called induced phagocytosis, which is at the crossroads between phagocytosis and endocytosis (41, 42) and involves clathrin and caveolin-2, two canonical proteins of the endocytic pathway (43).

Adhesion of *Rickettsia* to endothelial cells also leads to a drastic remodeling of the actin cytoskeleton within the host cells that not only facilitates bacterial entry but also contributes to bacterial movement and spreading

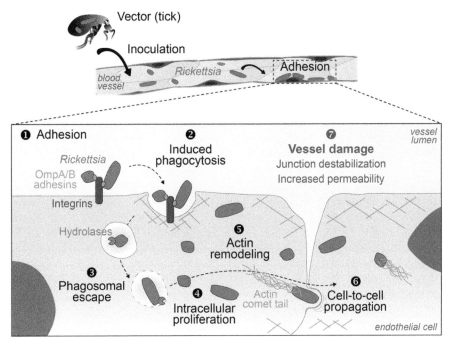

Figure 2 Infection of the endothelium by *Rickettsia*. Following bacterial inoculation into the lumen of blood vessels, *Rickettsia* adheres at the surface of the endothelium through the surface expression of OmpA and OmpB. Binding of OmpA and -B to cell surface integrins induces the phagocytosis of bacteria and the remodeling of the cellular actin cytoskeleton. Then, hemolysin C- and/or phospholipase D-expressing bacteria escape phagosomal vesicles, proliferate intracellularly, and utilize cellular components, such as actin monomers and nutrients, to assemble actin comet tails, which support bacterial movement and cell-to-cell spreading. Both actin cytoskeleton remodeling and bacterial propagation participate in damaging infected vessels, including the destabilization of cellular junctions responsible for the increase in vessel permeability.

within the endothelium. Endothelial cell surface-binding bacteria locally regulate actin rearrangements by recruiting the Arp2/3 actin-nucleating complex and activating Cdc42 and kinases of the Src family to support bacterial internalization within phagosomal vesicles (44). The expression of the pore-forming proteins hemolysin C and phospholipase D by *Rickettsia* allows the bacteria to escape phagosomes and access the host cell cytosol (45–47), where nutrients and energy are available to support their growth (48). Within infected cells, *Rickettsia* also uses proteins from the actin cytoskeleton to propel and disseminate within adjacent endothelial cells. *Rickettsia* assembles polar actin tails made of unbranched parallel actin filaments, which help intracellular bacterial movement (49). The precise machinery allowing bacteria to assemble these actin comet tails remains under debate. Whereas the involvement of RickA, a WASP family protein omolog encoded by *Rickettsia*, in Arp2/3-mediated actin polymerization *in vitro* favors a mechanism of tail assembly relying on Arp2/3 activity (50, 51), Arp2/3 was not found to associate with *Rickettsia* actin tails (52, 53). An alternative hypothesis suggests that the bacterial protein Sca2 might participate in assembling actin tails through a formin-like mechanism (54, 55).

The infection of endothelial cells by *Rickettsia* leads to the activation of the endothelium, which is associated with the upregulation and secretion of a plethora of cytokines and chemokines, collectively referred to as rickettsial vasculitis (56). Interestingly, *Rickettsia* has developed different strategies to counteract immune responses and optimize its intracellular residence. First, *Rickettsia* has the ability to escape phagosomal vesicles before their fusion with lysosomes, hindering their degradation by the lysosomal content (47). Moreover, the bacterium activates the antiapoptotic NF-κB signaling pathway within infected cells (57–60), thus balancing the killing of these cells mediated by the recruitment of CD8 T cells (61).

Importantly, *Rickettsia* also damages the endothelium by altering the assembly of endothelial intercellular junctions, most probably by disturbing the actin cytoskeleton (62), as well as by inducing an oxidative stress within infected cells that contributes to cell death (63, 64). Therefore, rickettsial infections lead to endothelial cell activation and dysfunction, including an alteration of the vascular integrity that results in the increase in vascular permeability and is consistent with the pathophysiology of *Rickettsia*-induced vascular leaks (56, 65). Despite alterations in vascular integrity, rickettsial infections are not associated with subsequent dissemination to other organs, such as the brain as in the case of meningitis-causing pathogens.

VASCULAR COLONIZATION AND BLOOD-BRAIN BARRIER CROSSING BY *NEISSERIA MENINGITIDIS*

A limited number of pathogenic bacteria have developed mechanisms allowing them to cross the blood-brain barrier, most often triggering bacterial meningitis, a high-fatality-rate disease (66). A hallmark feature of the clinical manifestations of bacterial meningitis is the presence of the pathogenic bacterium within the cerebrospinal fluid (CSF), where it triggers the inflammation of the meninges and the recruitment of immune cells within the CSF (66, 67). Since the bacterium is also found in the bloodstream, the most prevalent view is that the bacterium breaches the blood-CSF barrier to reach the CSF. However, because the anatomical site at which crossing occurs is not known, we refer instead to crossing of the blood-brain barrier to be more inclusive.

With significant socioeconomic and geographic variations, *N. meningitidis*, *Streptococcus pneumoniae*, and *Haemophilus influenzae* type b are the most frequent causative agents of bacterial meningitis in adults and children. Of note, while neonatal meningitis is mainly triggered by group B *Streptococcus*, *Listeria monocytogenes*, and *Escherichia coli* K1 (68), immunocompromised patients frequently develop *Mycobacterium tuberculosis* or nontyphoid *Salmonella* meningitis (69, 70). Despite their heterogeneity, common features in the mechanisms used by these pathogenic bacteria to cross the blood-brain barrier can be observed (for a review, see reference 71).

Recent studies have pointed to the importance of a process called vascular colonization during *N. meningitidis* infections and probably during meningitis (72). This bacterium has the ability to adhere to the endothelial surface and proliferate in the form of bacterial aggregates that eventually fill the lumens of small vessels of 10 to 50 m in diameter (Fig. 3). A recent study showed that this colonization process is facilitated by the honey-like viscous liquid properties of the bacterial aggregates, which allow them to adapt to the complex morphology of the vasculature upon proliferation (73). Adhesion to the endothelium likely contributes to immune evasion, as this prevents phagocytosis from Kupffer cells in the liver. Histological analysis of postmortem samples reveals large bacterial aggregates in the brain vessels, suggesting that vascular colonization could promote crossing of the blood-brain barrier by concentrating a high number of bacteria at specific sites and by altering endothelial cell physiology (74). The combined effect of vessel occlusion due to bacterial accumulation and the activation of the coagulation cascade (75) might participate in altering endothelium integrity.

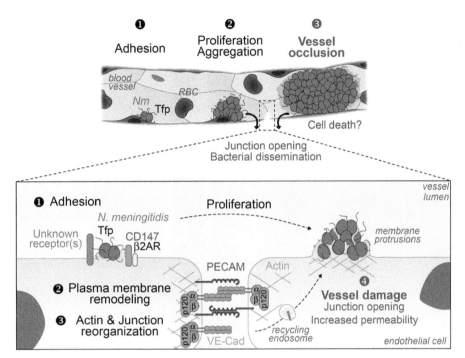

Figure 3 Vascular colonization by *N. meningitidis*. Once in the bloodstream, *N. meningitidis* adheres to the endothelium thanks to the surface expression of Tfp. While proliferating, and owing to their autoaggregative property, bacteria form a tight microcolony at the surface of the endothelium, which ultimately leads to the congestion of the colonized vessel. Bacterial adhesion at the surface of endothelial cells induces a drastic remodeling of the host cell plasma membrane that forms membrane protrusions that interdigitate within the bacterial aggregate. In addition, pilus interaction with endothelial cell surface receptors, such as CD147 or β2-adrenergic receptor (β2AR), induces the reorganization of the actin cytoskeleton and intercellular junctions by recruiting their components underneath the microcolony. Together, these events are proposed to destabilize intercellular junctions, resulting in an increase in vessel permeability. *Nm*, *N. meningitidis*; RBC, red blood cell; Cad, cadherin.

Alternatively, *in vitro* studies have identified specific signaling pathways triggered by *N. meningitidis*, which lead to the opening of intercellular junctions within the cerebral endothelium. Meningococcal adhesion to the host cells is mediated by their expression of type IV pili (Tfp) (76), which engage host cell surface receptors, such as CD147 and β2-adrenergic receptor (77, 78). While proliferating at the surface of infected endothelial cells, thus forming bacterial aggregates, meningococci induce the remodeling of the host cell plasma membrane (79, 80) (Fig. 3). Associated with their aggregation capacity, plasma membrane protrusions infiltrating meningococcal microcolonies were shown to enhance the mechanical cohesion of the microcolony, thus allowing them to resist blood flow-induced shear stress (81).

Interestingly, although the cortical actin network is strongly reorganized below the bacterial colonies (82), the active contribution of the host cells has been shown to be dispensable in *N. meningitidis*-mediated plasma membrane remodeling. The actin cytoskeleton or even the intracellular ATP is not necessary for the Tfp-induced plasma membrane reorganization (80, 81). Rather, it is the adhesion of the plasma membrane along type IV pili nanofibers that triggers the formation of the protrusions by a physical process termed one-dimensional wetting (83). In a second step, this process is associated with the activation of small GTPases such as Cdc42 (cell division cycle protein 42) and Rac1, along with the local recruitment of proteins of the polarity complex, including PAR3 (partitioning-defective 3), PAR6, and protein kinase C-ζ (PKC-ζ), as well as the branched-actin nucleating complex Arp2/3. On the other hand, by mistargeting recycling endosomes, meningococci induce the accumulation of junctional proteins, such as VE-cadherin, underneath bacterial aggregates, a process shown to weaken intercellular junctions and increase blood-brain barrier permeability, thus facilitating meningococcal dissemination within the cerebral tissues and the CSF (83). These elaborate mechanisms illustrate the panoply of strategies enabling patho-genic bacteria to alter the endothelial barrier.

ALTERATION OF THE ENDOCARDIUM AND ENDOCARDITIS

Infective endocarditis (IE) is a bacterial infection of the cardiac endothelium. The hallmark of IE is the coloniza-tion and destruction of the cardiac valves by pathogenic bacteria following local endothelial injury or inflamma-tion (84, 85) (for a review, see reference 86). Although the causative agent of such a disease varies greatly ac-cording to geographic zone, most cases of IE result from *Staphylococcus aureus*, *Enterococcus* species, or *Strep-tococcus* species, including *Streptococcus gallolyticus* (87, 88).

The pathologic cascade begins after formation of ster-ile lesions on the cardiac valve endothelium of unclear origin that lead to the exposure of the extracellular ma-trix. This triggers the formation of a platelet- and fibrin-rich thrombus, considered a hot spot for the adhesion of bacteria in the circulatory system (89) (Fig. 4). Alterna-tively, bacterial adhesion can occur at the surface of in-flamed endothelium, a process facilitated by the local upregulation of cell surface adhesion molecules, such as β1 integrins (90). From the bacterial side, adhesion is me-diated by the surface expression of extracellular matrix-targeting adhesins, such as fibronectin-binding proteins

(91, 92). Adherent bacteria proliferate locally and form a vegetation, a biofilm-like structure where aggregated bac-teria are mixed with extracellular matrix proteins, clot components, and/or immune cells (93). As the vegetation matures, the adjacent endothelial cells are exposed, thus driving the propagation of the local inflammation and cell death and ultimately leading to the destruction of the infected valves, which requires surgical replacement (94). However, this mechanism probably does not entirely ac-count for IE induced by intracellular bacteria such as *Bartonella* species or *S. aureus*, which rely instead on the secretion of exoenzymes and toxins to mediate their pathogenic effects (95) and for which the host immune response might play an important role (96). Although *Bartonella* species have been described in relatively rare cases of human endocarditis (97, 98) with a preferential localization at the aortic valve (99), these bacteria are mostly known for their involvement in angioproliferative syndromes.

ANGIOPROLIFERATION DURING *BARTONELLA* INFECTIONS

As mentioned earlier, angiogenesis supports the forma-tion of new blood vessels from preexisting ones (12). In-terestingly, this process can be diverted by pathogenic bacteria and especially *Bartonella henselae* (for a review, see reference 100). *Bartonella* spp. are Gram-negative

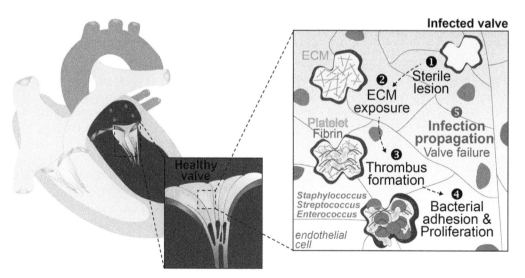

Figure 4 The stepwise process leading to endocarditis. The appearance of sterile lesions (most often of unknown origin) on the heart valvular endothelium leads to the exposure of the underlying extracellular matrix (ECM). This in turn triggers the formation of a thrombus —characterized by the local deposition of platelets and fibrin at the surface of the damaged endothelium—that favors bacterial adhesion. While bacteria proliferate and spread, the val-vular endothelium becomes more and more damaged, eventually leading to the failure of the valve and the need for its surgical replacement.

organisms found in domestic and wild mammals with a tropism for red blood cells and endothelial cells (100, 101). While in healthy individuals, *B. henselae* infections cause benign cat scratch diseases (102), in immunocompromised patients, these infections can trigger a vasoproliferative syndrome resulting in the formation of tumor-like nodules in the skin, known as cutaneous bacillary angiomatosis (100). This results from the ability of *B. henselae* to invade endothelial cells and trigger their proliferation and migration (103, 104), together with the recruitment of macrophages, monocytes, and polymorphonuclear neutrophils (105, 106) (Fig. 5).

Interestingly, similar to *N. meningitidis* microcolonies, *B. henselae* also forms plasma membrane-associated bacterial aggregates that either remain at the surface of or are internalized in infected endothelial cells (106). Two actin-dependent mechanisms of bacterial internalization within endothelial cells have been described (107, 108): the first one is reminiscent of the previously described bacterium-induced phagocytosis and allows the relatively fast entry of *Bartonella* into perinuclear phagosomes (109). The second mechanism, lasting for up to 24 hours, allows the slow internalization of small *B. henselae* aggregates within large vacuoles, referred to as invasomes (107). Of note, similarly to the protective mechanisms developed by *Rickettsia* to promote their survival during their intracellular residence, *Bartonella* is able to inhibit key steps of the apoptosis program induced upon cell infections (110).

Although not fully understood, the proliferation of infected endothelial cells is in part supported by bacterial proteins that are translocated within the host cells through the VirB-VirD4 type IV secretion system encoded by *Bartonella* (111, 112). In addition, several reports have shown that macrophages, locally recruited upon endothelial cell infection, participate in the pathological angiogenesis induced by *Bartonella*. Indeed, macrophages are well-known producers of proangiogenic factors upon activation (113). *In vitro*, macrophages have been shown to support endothelial proliferation through the secretion of VEGF in response to *B. henselae* infection (114, 115), thus suggesting that macrophages are involved in a paracrine loop that enhances *Bartonella*-mediated vasoproliferation (116).

SYSTEMIC IMPLICATIONS OF VASCULAR INFECTIONS

Under steady-state conditions, except for normal transitory bacteremia, the vascular organ is thought to be

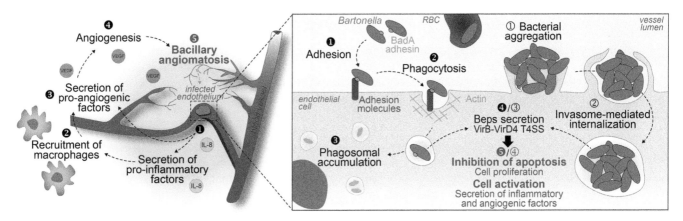

Figure 5 *Bartonella*-induced angioproliferation. Interactions of *Bartonella* with the endothelium can occur at the single-bacterium level through bacterial expression of the *Bartonella* adhesin A (BadA) protein. This triggers the phagocytosis of the cell surface-bound bacteria and results in their perinuclear accumulation within phagosomes. Similarly to *N. meningitidis*, *Bartonella* also forms aggregates that are internalized through a slower process within large vacuoles, referred to as invasomes. In both cases, the VirB-VirD4 type IV secretion system-dependent cytoplasmic release of *Bartonella* effector proteins (Beps) by intravesicular bacteria promotes the proliferation and activation of the infected endothelial cells. This results in the secretion by the endothelium of proinflammatory (e.g., IL-8) and proangiogenic (e.g., VEGF) factors. As a consequence, cells from the innate immunity system, including neutrophils and macrophages, are locally recruited to fight the infection. Activated macrophages locally secrete VEGF, thus reinforcing the proangiogenic microenvironment. Combined with the bacterium-mediated endothelial cell proliferation, this particular environment promotes angiogenesis that ultimately leads to the local accumulation of new blood capillaries and the formation of bacillary angiomatosis lesions. RBC, red blood cell.

sterile (26). Therefore, it possesses robust mechanisms to recognize circulating pathogens and trigger innate and/or adaptive immune responses (117, 118). Similarly to immune cells specialized in pathogen recognition, endothelial cells express chemokine receptors, such as CXCR-1, -2, and -4 (119, 120), as well as pattern recognition receptors, such as Toll-like receptors and NOD-like receptors (121, 122). They have also been shown to secrete proinflammatory molecules, such as the cytokines interleukin 1 (IL-1) and IL-8 (123–125), and to respond to bacterial lipopolysaccharide, tumor necrosis factor alpha, and gamma interferon by signaling through the canonical proinflammatory NF-κB pathway (126). Hence, the endothelium possesses an array of tools allowing the recognition of pathogenic microorganisms and the recruitment of cells from the innate immune system in order to clear blood-circulating pathogens.

Of particular interest, endothelial cells also participate in mounting adaptive immune responses, since they can act as antigen-presenting cells (127). The hallmark of antigen-presenting cells is their expression of major histocompatibility complex class II (MHC-II) molecules, allowing them to present extracellular antigens to T cells (128). Whereas quiescent endothelial cells express basal levels of MHC-II molecules (129), they possess the capacity to upregulate their expression upon activation (130), providing them with the ability to present antigenic determinants to T cells and rapidly initiate pathogen-specific immune responses. Therefore, endothelial cells are equipped to recognize pathogenic microorganisms, locally attract cells of the innate immunity system, and serve as a link to trigger adaptive immune responses in order to efficiently fight invaders (for a review, see reference 131).

Although invasion of the endothelium by bacteria leads to the activation of the immune system, in the absence of appropriate treatments or when the body fails to clear the pathogens, it may evolve toward an uncontrolled and systemic infection. Indeed, the constant release of damage-associated molecular patterns by invading bacteria and/or injured endothelium leads to the imbalance of various body systems, including the overstimulation of immune cells through Toll-like receptors and the complement pathway (132), as well as the exacerbated production of cytokines, referred to as the cytokine storm (133). Together with a persistent bacteremia, this systemic inflammatory response syndrome is the hallmark of sepsis (134, 135).

Paradoxically, a common feature of sepsis is its association with a form of immune suppression occurring after the unregulated inflammation (132, 136). While not fully understood, sepsis is marked by the severe depletion of T and B cells, as well as dendritic cells, which all show an enhanced proapoptotic activity (137, 138). In addition, in patients suffering from sepsis, a bias in the ratio of regulatory T cells to effector T cells is often observed (138, 139). The latter also show a reduced ability to produce cytokines, a feature known as T cell exhaustion (140), most probably due to dysregulations in the PD1 (programmed cell death 1)-PD1 ligand 1 axis (141), owing to the exacerbated cytokine production.

In addition, sepsis frequently affects the coagulation pathway: ranging from the formation of small thrombi to the manifestation of disseminated intravascular coagulation, which corresponds to the coagulation of the blood throughout the entire body; coagulopathies are one of the major complications in sepsis and are extensively reviewed elsewhere (142, 143). Nevertheless, it is worth mentioning that perturbation of the coagulation pathway occurs early during sepsis and first results from the activation of the endothelium in response to the cytokine storm, thus favoring the local deposition of fibrin at the surface of the vessel walls (133).

Alternatively, endotoxins derived from Gram-negative bacteria, such as lipopolysaccharide, can trigger in an NF-κB-dependent manner both the secretion and the surface expression of tissue factor by endothelial cells and circulatory blood cells. By forming a complex with activated coagulation factor VII, tissue factor becomes a highly potent procoagulant molecule (144, 145). In both scenarios, thrombus formation in turn leads to the activation of the endothelial cell surface protease-activated receptor 1, which signals through the small GTPase RhoA to disassemble actin filaments and induce VE-cadherin internalization, hence affecting the stability of intercellular junctions and the integrity of the vascular endothelium (118). As a consequence, vessels become leaky, blood pressure decreases, and proteins from the endothelial extracellular matrix, such as collagen, are exposed to the vessel contents, which further activates platelet aggregation and fibrin formation (118, 143). Multiorgan failure is often associated with the late phases of disseminated intravascular coagulation, which results from microvascular thrombosis and poor tissue perfusion (146, 147).

CONCLUDING REMARKS

Bacterial infections taking place in the circulatory system are particularly problematic because of the specific alterations they cause to the circulation, possibly affecting the entire body. According to the specific site of infection and the properties of the different pathogens, a complex set of interactions takes place during these infections. Blood vessels are highly diverse, with broad ranges of size and structure, and each pathogen has a set of virulence factors that alter blood vessel function in specific ways. As a result, clinical manifestations are also very different. However, despite this diversity, the endothelium is at the center of these infectious processes, and a limited number of endothelial functions are targeted in these infectious contexts: the integrity of the vasculature and its permeability, but also its inflammatory and coagulation status. More research is needed on host-pathogen interactions during these systemic infections and on endothelial cell biology to better treat these infections.

Acknowledgments. We acknowledge Daria Bonazzi and Paul Kennouche for critical reading of the manuscript. D.O. was supported by a Pasteur-Roux postdoctoral fellowship from the Institut Pasteur. Funding was obtained from the European Research Council (ERC VIP consolidator grant) and the Integrative Biology of Emerging Infectious Diseases (IBEID) laboratory of excellence (ANR-10-LABX-62) to G.D.

Citation. Obino D, Duménil G. 2019. The many faces of bacterium-endothelium interactions during systemic infections. Microbiol Spectrum 7(2):BAI-0010-2019.

References

1. **Lerman A, Burnett JC Jr.** 1992. Intact and altered endothelium in regulation of vasomotion. *Circulation* **86** (Suppl):III12–III19.

2. **Sender R, Fuchs S, Milo R.** 2016. Revised estimates for the number of human and bacteria cells in the body. *PLoS Biol* **14**:e1002533.

3. **Pugsley MK, Tabrizchi R.** 2000. The vascular system. An overview of structure and function. *J Pharmacol Toxicol Methods* **44**:333–340.

4. **Brozovich FV, Nicholson CJ, Degen CV, Gao YZ, Aggarwal M, Morgan KG.** 2016. Mechanisms of vascular smooth muscle contraction and the basis for pharmacologic treatment of smooth muscle disorders. *Pharmacol Rev* **68**:476–532.

5. **Galili O, Herrmann J, Woodrum J, Sattler KJ, Lerman LO, Lerman A.** 2004. Adventitial vasa vasorum heterogeneity among different vascular beds. *J Vasc Surg* **40**:529–535.

6. **Sarin H.** 2010. Physiologic upper limits of pore size of different blood capillary types and another perspective on the dual pore theory of microvascular permeability. *J Angiogenes Res* **2**:14.

7. **Bilzer M, Roggel F, Gerbes AL.** 2006. Role of Kupffer cells in host defense and liver disease. *Liver Int* **26**:1175–1186.

8. **Harris IS, Black BL.** 2010. Development of the endocardium. *Pediatr Cardiol* **31**:391–399.

9. **Carmeliet P.** 2003. Angiogenesis in health and disease. *Nat Med* **9**:653–660.

10. **Zecchin A, Kalucka J, Dubois C, Carmeliet P.** 2017. How endothelial cells adapt their metabolism to form vessels in tumors. *Front Immunol* **8**:1750.

11. **Risau W, Flamme I.** 1995. Vasculogenesis. *Annu Rev Cell Dev Biol* **11**:73–91.

12. **Risau W.** 1997. Mechanisms of angiogenesis. *Nature* **386**:671–674.

13. **Diaz-Santana A, Shan M, Stroock AD.** 2015. Endothelial cell dynamics during anastomosis in vitro. *Integr Biol* **7**:454–466.

14. **Komarova Y, Malik AB.** 2010. Regulation of endothelial permeability via paracellular and transcellular transport pathways. *Annu Rev Physiol* **72**:463–493.

15. **Hawkins BT, Davis TP.** 2005. The blood-brain barrier/neurovascular unit in health and disease. *Pharmacol Rev* **57**:173–185.

16. **Daneman R, Prat A.** 2015. The blood-brain barrier. *Cold Spring Harb Perspect Biol* **7**:a020412.

17. **Rudini N, Dejana E.** 2008. Adherens junctions. *Curr Biol* **18**:R1080–R1082.

18. **Privratsky JR, Newman PJ.** 2014. PECAM-1: regulator of endothelial junctional integrity. *Cell Tissue Res* **355**:607–619.

19. **Hartsock A, Nelson WJ.** 2008. Adherens and tight junctions: structure, function and connections to the actin cytoskeleton. *Biochim Biophys Acta* **1778**:660–669.

20. **Bates DO, Harper SJ.** 2002. Regulation of vascular permeability by vascular endothelial growth factors. *Vascul Pharmacol* **39**:225–237.

21. **Bates DO.** 2010. Vascular endothelial growth factors and vascular permeability. *Cardiovasc Res* **87**:262–271.

22. **Wu HM, Huang Q, Yuan Y, Granger HJ.** 1996. VEGF induces NO-dependent hyperpermeability in coronary venules. *Am J Physiol* **271**:H2735–H2739.

23. **Aghajanian A, Wittchen ES, Allingham MJ, Garrett TA, Burridge K.** 2008. Endothelial cell junctions and the regulation of vascular permeability and leukocyte transmigration. *J Thromb Haemost* **6**:1453–1460.

24. **Popoff MR, Geny B.** 2009. Multifaceted role of Rho, Rac, Cdc42 and Ras in intercellular junctions, lessons from toxins. *Biochim Biophys Acta* **1788**:797–812.

25. **Round H, Kirkpatrick HJ, Hails CG.** 1936. Further investigations on bacteriological infections of the mouth (section of odontology). *Proc R Soc Med* **29**:1552–1556.

26. **Cobe HM.** 1954. Transitory bacteremia. *Oral Surg Oral Med Oral Pathol* **7**:609–615.

27. **Snowden J, Bhimji SS.** 2018. *Rickettsial Infection.* Stat Pearls, Treasure Island, FL.

28. **Stins MF, Prasadarao NV, Ibric L, Wass CA, Luckett P, Kim KS.** 1994. Binding characteristics of S fimbriated *Escherichia coli* to isolated brain microvascular endothelial cells. *Am J Pathol* **145**:1228–1236.

29. **Greiffenberg L, Goebel W, Kim KS, Weiglein I, Bubert A, Engelbrecht F, Stins M, Kuhn M.** 1998. Interaction of *Listeria monocytogenes* with human brain microvascular endothelial cells: InlB-dependent invasion, long-term intracellular growth, and spread from macrophages to endothelial cells. *Infect Immun* **66**:5260–5267.

30. **Sheen TR, Ebrahimi CM, Hiemstra IH, Barlow SB, Peschel A, Doran KS.** 2010. Penetration of the blood-brain barrier by *Staphylococcus aureus*: contribution of

membrane-anchored lipoteichoic acid. *J Mol Med (Berl)* **88**:633–639.

31. Stins MF, Badger J, Sik Kim K. 2001. Bacterial invasion and transcytosis in transfected human brain microvascular endothelial cells. *Microb Pathog* **30**:19–28.

32. Jain SK, Paul-Satyaseela M, Lamichhane G, Kim KS, Bishai WR. 2006. *Mycobacterium tuberculosis* invasion and traversal across an in vitro human blood-brain barrier as a pathogenic mechanism for central nervous system tuberculosis. *J Infect Dis* **193**:1287–1295.

33. Nikulin J, Panzner U, Frosch M, Schubert-Unkmeir A. 2006. Intracellular survival and replication of *Neisseria meningitidis* in human brain microvascular endothelial cells. *Int J Med Microbiol* **296**:553–558.

34. Prasadarao NV, Wass CA, Stins MF, Shimada H, Kim KS. 1999. Outer membrane protein A-promoted actin condensation of brain microvascular endothelial cells is required for *Escherichia coli* invasion. *Infect Immun* **67**:5775–5783.

35. Das A, Asatryan L, Reddy MA, Wass CA, Stins MF, Joshi S, Bonventre JV, Kim KS. 2001. Differential role of cytosolic phospholipase A2 in the invasion of brain microvascular endothelial cells by *Escherichia coli* and *Listeria monocytogenes*. *J Infect Dis* **184**:732–737.

36. Dumenil G. 2011. Revisiting the extracellular lifestyle. *Cell Microbiol* **13**:1114–1121.

37. Olano JP. 2005. Rickettsial infections. *Ann N Y Acad Sci* **1063**:187–196.

38. Walker DH, Ismail N. 2008. Emerging and re-emerging rickettsioses: endothelial cell infection and early disease events. *Nat Rev Microbiol* **6**:375–386.

39. Li H, Walker DH. 1998. rOmpA is a critical protein for the adhesion of *Rickettsia rickettsii* to host cells. *Microb Pathog* **24**:289–298.

40. Hillman RD Jr, Baktash YM, Martinez JJ. 2013. OmpA-mediated rickettsial adherence to and invasion of human endothelial cells is dependent upon interaction with α2β1 integrin. *Cell Microbiol* **15**:727–741.

41. Walker TS, Winkler HH. 1978. Penetration of cultured mouse fibroblasts (L cells) by *Rickettsia prowazeki* [sic]. *Infect Immun* **22**:200–208.

42. Walker TS. 1984. Rickettsial interactions with human endothelial cells in vitro: adherence and entry. *Infect Immun* **44**:205–210.

43. Chan YG, Cardwell MM, Hermanas TM, Uchiyama T, Martinez JJ. 2009. Rickettsial outer-membrane protein B (rOmpB) mediates bacterial invasion through Ku70 in an actin, c-Cbl, clathrin and caveolin 2-dependent manner. *Cell Microbiol* **11**:629–644.

44. Martinez JJ, Cossart P. 2004. Early signaling events involved in the entry of *Rickettsia conorii* into mammalian cells. *J Cell Sci* **117**:5097–5106.

45. Radulovic S, Troyer JM, Beier MS, Lau AO, Azad AF. 1999. Identification and molecular analysis of the gene encoding *Rickettsia typhi* hemolysin. *Infect Immun* **67**:6104–6108.

46. Renesto P, Dehoux P, Gouin E, Touqui L, Cossart P, Raoult D. 2003. Identification and characterization of a phospholipase D-superfamily gene in rickettsiae. *J Infect Dis* **188**:1276–1283.

47. Whitworth T, Popov VL, Yu XJ, Walker DH, Bouyer DH. 2005. Expression of the *Rickettsia prowazekii pld* or *tlyC* gene in *Salmonella enterica* serovar Typhimurium mediates phagosomal escape. *Infect Immun* **73**:6668–6673.

48. Walker DH, Valbuena GA, Olano JP. 2003. Pathogenic mechanisms of diseases caused by *Rickettsia*. *Ann N Y Acad Sci* **990**:1–11.

49. Heinzen RA. 2003. Rickettsial actin-based motility: behavior and involvement of cytoskeletal regulators. *Ann N Y Acad Sci* **990**:535–547.

50. Jeng RL, Goley ED, D'Alessio JA, Chaga OY, Svitkina TM, Borisy GG, Heinzen RA, Welch MD. 2004. A *Rickettsia* WASP-like protein activates the Arp2/3 complex and mediates actin-based motility. *Cell Microbiol* **6**:761–769.

51. Gouin E, Egile C, Dehoux P, Villiers V, Adams J, Gertler F, Li R, Cossart P. 2004. The RickA protein of *Rickettsia conorii* activates the Arp2/3 complex. *Nature* **427**:457–461.

52. Gouin E, Gantelet H, Egile C, Lasa I, Ohayon H, Villiers V, Gounon P, Sansonetti PJ, Cossart P. 1999. A comparative study of the actin-based motilities of the pathogenic bacteria *Listeria monocytogenes*, *Shigella flexneri* and *Rickettsia conorii*. *J Cell Sci* **112**:1697–1708.

53. Harlander RS, Way M, Ren Q, Howe D, Grieshaber SS, Heinzen RA. 2003. Effects of ectopically expressed neuronal Wiskott-Aldrich syndrome protein domains on *Rickettsia rickettsii* actin-based motility. *Infect Immun* **71**:1551–1556.

54. Haglund CM, Choe JE, Skau CT, Kovar DR, Welch MD. 2010. *Rickettsia* Sca2 is a bacterial formin-like mediator of actin-based motility. *Nat Cell Biol* **12**:1057–1063.

55. Kleba B, Clark TR, Lutter EI, Ellison DW, Hackstadt T. 2010. Disruption of the *Rickettsia rickettsii* Sca2 autotransporter inhibits actin-based motility. *Infect Immun* **78**:2240–2247.

56. Sahni SK, Narra HP, Sahni A, Walker DH. 2013. Recent molecular insights into rickettsial pathogenesis and immunity. *Future Microbiol* **8**:1265–1288.

57. Sporn LA, Sahni SK, Lerner NB, Marder VJ, Silverman DJ, Turpin LC, Schwab AL. 1997. *Rickettsia rickettsii* infection of cultured human endothelial cells induces NF-κB activation. *Infect Immun* **65**:2786–2791.

58. Sahni SK, Van Antwerp DJ, Eremeeva ME, Silverman DJ, Marder VJ, Sporn LA. 1998. Proteasome-independent activation of nuclear factor κB in cytoplasmic extracts from human endothelial cells by *Rickettsia rickettsii*. *Infect Immun* **66**:1827–1833.

59. Clifton DR, Goss RA, Sahni SK, van Antwerp D, Baggs RB, Marder VJ, Silverman DJ, Sporn LA. 1998. NF-κB-dependent inhibition of apoptosis is essential for host cell survival during *Rickettsia rickettsii* infection. *Proc Natl Acad Sci USA* **95**:4646–4651.

60. Walker DH. 2007. Rickettsiae and rickettsial infections: the current state of knowledge. *Clin Infect Dis* **45**(Suppl 1):S39–S44.

61. Walker DH, Olano JP, Feng HM. 2001. Critical role of cytotoxic T lymphocytes in immune clearance of rickettsial infection. *Infect Immun* **69**:1841–1846.

62. Valbuena G, Walker DH. 2005. Changes in the adherens junctions of human endothelial cells infected with spotted fever group rickettsiae. *Virchows Arch* **446**:379–382.

63. Santucci LA, Gutierrez PL, Silverman DJ. 1992. *Rickettsia rickettsii* induces superoxide radical and superoxide dismutase in human endothelial cells. *Infect Immun* **60**:5113–5118.

64. Eremeeva ME, Silverman DJ. 1998. Effects of the antioxidant alpha-lipoic acid on human umbilical vein endothelial cells infected with *Rickettsia rickettsii*. *Infect Immun* **66**:2290–2299.

65. Schmaier AH, Srikanth S, Elghetany MT, Normolle D, Gokhale S, Feng HM, Walker DH. 2001. Hemostatic/fibrinolytic protein changes in C3H/HeN mice infected with *Rickettsia conorii*—a model for Rocky Mountain spotted fever. *Thromb Haemost* **86**:871–879.

66. Doran KS, Fulde M, Gratz N, Kim BJ, Nau R, Prasadarao N, Schubert-Unkmeir A, Tuomanen EI, Valentin-Weigand P. 2016. Host-pathogen interactions in bacterial meningitis. *Acta Neuropathol* **131**:185–209.

67. Brandtzaeg P, van Deuren M. 2012. Classification and pathogenesis of meningococcal infections. *Methods Mol Biol* **799**:21–35.

68. Thigpen MC, Whitney CG, Messonnier NE, Zell ER, Lynfield R, Hadler JL, Harrison LH, Farley MM, Reingold A, Bennett NM, Craig AS, Schaffner W, Thomas A, Lewis MM, Scallan E, Schuchat A, Emerging Infections Programs Network. 2011. Bacterial meningitis in the United States, 1998-2007. *N Engl J Med* **364**:2016–2025.

69. Békondi C, Bernede C, Passone N, Minssart P, Kamalo C, Mbolidi D, Germani Y. 2006. Primary and opportunistic pathogens associated with meningitis in adults in Bangui, Central African Republic, in relation to human immunodeficiency virus serostatus. *Int J Infect Dis* **10**:387–395.

70. Fernández Guerrero ML, Ramos JM, Núñez A, Cuenca M, de Górgolas M. 1997. Focal infections due to non-typhi *Salmonella* in patients with AIDS: report of 10 cases and review. *Clin Infect Dis* **25**:690–697.

71. van Sorge NM, Doran KS. 2012. Defense at the border: the blood-brain barrier versus bacterial foreigners. *Future Microbiol* **7**:383–394.

72. Melican K, Michea Veloso P, Martin T, Bruneval P, Duménil G. 2013. Adhesion of *Neisseria meningitidis* to dermal vessels leads to local vascular damage and purpura in a humanized mouse model. *PLoS Pathog* **9**:e1003139.

73. Bonazzi D, Lo Schiavo V, Machata S, Djafer-Cherif I, Nivoit P, Manriquez V, Tanimoto H, Husson J, Henry N, Chaté H, Voituriez R, Duménil G. 2018. Intermittent pili-mediated forces fluidize *Neisseria meningitidis* aggregates promoting vascular colonization. *Cell* **174**:143–155.e16.

74. Mairey E, Genovesio A, Donnadieu E, Bernard C, Jaubert F, Pinard E, Seylaz J, Olivo-Marin JC, Nassif X,

Duménil G. 2006. Cerebral microcirculation shear stress levels determine *Neisseria meningitidis* attachment sites along the blood-brain barrier. *J Exp Med* **203**:1939–1950.

75. Faust SN, Levin M, Harrison OB, Goldin RD, Lockhart MS, Kondaveeti S, Laszik Z, Esmon CT, Heyderman RS. 2001. Dysfunction of endothelial protein C activation in severe meningococcal sepsis. *N Engl J Med* **345**:408–416.

76. Imhaus AF, Duménil G. 2014. The number of *Neisseria meningitidis* type IV pili determines host cell interaction. *EMBO J* **33**:1767–1783.

77. Bernard SC, Simpson N, Join-Lambert O, Federici C, Laran-Chich MP, Maïssa N, Bouzinba-Ségard H, Morand PC, Chretien F, Taouji S, Chevet E, Janel S, Lafont F, Coureuil M, Segura A, Niedergang F, Marullo S, Couraud PO, Nassif X, Bourdoulous S. 2014. Pathogenic *Neisseria meningitidis* utilizes CD147 for vascular colonization. *Nat Med* **20**:725–731.

78. Maïssa N, Covarelli V, Janel S, Durel B, Simpson N, Bernard SC, Pardo-Lopez L, Bouzinba-Ségard H, Faure C, Scott MGH, Coureuil M, Morand PC, Lafont F, Nassif X, Marullo S, Bourdoulous S. 2017. Strength of *Neisseria meningitidis* binding to endothelial cells requires highly-ordered CD147/β_2-adrenoceptor clusters assembled by alpha-actinin-4. *Nat Commun* **8**:15764.

79. Eugène E, Hoffmann I, Pujol C, Couraud PO, Bourdoulous S, Nassif X. 2002. Microvilli-like structures are associated with the internalization of virulent capsulated *Neisseria meningitidis* into vascular endothelial cells. *J Cell Sci* **115**:1231–1241.

80. Soyer M, Charles-Orszag A, Lagache T, Machata S, Imhaus AF, Dumont A, Millien C, Olivo-Marin JC, Duménil G. 2014. Early sequence of events triggered by the interaction of *Neisseria meningitidis* with endothelial cells. *Cell Microbiol* **16**:878–895.

81. Mikaty G, Soyer M, Mairey E, Henry N, Dyer D, Forest KT, Morand P, Guadagnini S, Prévost MC, Nassif X, Duménil G. 2009. Extracellular bacterial pathogen induces host cell surface reorganization to resist shear stress. *PLoS Pathog* **5**:e1000314.

82. Merz AJ, So M. 1997. Attachment of piliated, Opa- and Opc- gonococci and meningococci to epithelial cells elicits cortical actin rearrangements and clustering of tyrosine-phosphorylated proteins. *Infect Immun* **65**:4341–4349.

83. Charles-Orszag A, Tsai FC, Bonazzi D, Manriquez V, Sachse M, Mallet A, Salles A, Melican K, Staneva R, Bertin A, Millien C, Goussard S, Lafaye P, Shorte S, Piel M, Krijnse-Locker J, Brochard-Wyart F, Bassereau P, Dumenil G. 2018. Adhesion to nanofibers drives cell membrane remodeling through one-dimensional wetting. *Nat Commun* **9**:4450.

84. Hoen B, Duval X. 2013. Infective endocarditis. *N Engl J Med* **369**:785.

85. Cahill TJ, Prendergast BD. 2016. Infective endocarditis. *Lancet* **387**:882–893.

86. Vilcant V, Hai O. 2018. *Endocarditis, Bacterial*. Stat Pearls, Treasure Island, FL.

87. McDonald JR, Olaison L, Anderson DJ, Hoen B, Miro JM, Eykyn S, Abrutyn E, Fowler VG Jr, Habib G, Selton-Suty C, Pappas PA, Cabell CH, Corey GR, Marco F, Sexton DJ. 2005. Enterococcal endocarditis: 107 cases from the international collaboration on endocarditis merged database. *Am J Med* 118:759–766.

88. Yew HS, Murdoch DR. 2012. Global trends in infective endocarditis epidemiology. *Curr Infect Dis Rep* 14: 367–372.

89. Widmer E, Que YA, Entenza JM, Moreillon P. 2006. New concepts in the pathophysiology of infective endocarditis. *Curr Infect Dis Rep* 8:271–279.

90. Hemler ME, Elices MJ, Parker C, Takada Y. 1990. Structure of the integrin VLA-4 and its cell-cell and cell-matrix adhesion functions. *Immunol Rev* 114:45–65.

91. Foster TJ, Höök M. 1998. Surface protein adhesins of *Staphylococcus aureus*. *Trends Microbiol* 6:484–488.

92. Chavakis T, Wiechmann K, Preissner KT, Herrmann M. 2005. *Staphylococcus aureus* interactions with the endothelium: the role of bacterial "secretable expanded repertoire adhesive molecules" (SERAM) in disturbing host defense systems. *Thromb Haemost* 94:278–285.

93. Moreillon P, Que YA, Bayer AS. 2002. Pathogenesis of streptococcal and staphylococcal endocarditis. *Infect Dis Clin North Am* 16:297–318.

94. Werdan K, Dietz S, Löffler B, Niemann S, Bushnaq H, Silber RE, Peters G, Müller-Werdan U. 2014. Mechanisms of infective endocarditis: pathogen-host interaction and risk states. *Nat Rev Cardiol* 11:35–50.

95. Haslinger-Löffler B, Kahl BC, Grundmeier M, Strangfeld K, Wagner B, Fischer U, Cheung AL, Peters G, Schulze-Osthoff K, Sinha B. 2005. Multiple virulence factors are required for *Staphylococcus aureus*-induced apoptosis in endothelial cells. *Cell Microbiol* 7:1087–1097.

96. Brouqui P, Raoult D. 2001. Endocarditis due to rare and fastidious bacteria. *Clin Microbiol Rev* 14:177–207.

97. Fournier PE, Lelievre H, Eykyn SJ, Mainardi JL, Marrie TJ, Bruneel F, Roure C, Nash J, Clave D, James E, Benoit-Lemercier C, Deforges L, Tissot-Dupont H, Raoult D. 2001. Epidemiologic and clinical characteristics of *Bartonella quintana* and *Bartonella henselae* endocarditis: a study of 48 patients. *Medicine (Baltimore)* 80:245–251.

98. Raoult D, Fournier PE, Vandenesch F, Mainardi JL, Eykyn SJ, Nash J, James E, Benoit-Lemercier C, Marrie TJ. 2003. Outcome and treatment of *Bartonella* endocarditis. *Arch Intern Med* 163:226–230.

99. Raoult D, Fournier PE, Drancourt M, Marrie TJ, Etienne J, Cosserat J, Cacoub P, Poinsignon Y, Leclercq P, Sefton AM. 1996. Diagnosis of 22 new cases of *Bartonella* endocarditis. *Ann Intern Med* 125:646–652.

100. Dehio C. 2004. Molecular and cellular basis of bartonella pathogenesis. *Annu Rev Microbiol* 58:365–390.

101. Breitschwerdt EB, Kordick DL. 2000. *Bartonella* infection in animals: carriership, reservoir potential, pathogenicity, and zoonotic potential for human infection. *Clin Microbiol Rev* 13:428–438.

102. Chomel BB. 2000. Cat-scratch disease. *Rev Sci Tech* 19:136–150.

103. Koehler JE, Tappero JW. 1993. Bacillary angiomatosis and bacillary peliosis in patients infected with human immunodeficiency virus. *Clin Infect Dis* 17:612–624.

104. Regnery RL, Childs JE, Koehler JE. 1995. Infections associated with *Bartonella* species in persons infected with human immunodeficiency virus. *Clin Infect Dis* 21(Suppl 1): S94–S98.

105. Kostianovsky M, Greco MA. 1994. Angiogenic process in bacillary angiomatosis. *Ultrastruct Pathol* 18:349–355.

106. Manders SM. 1996. Bacillary angiomatosis. *Clin Dermatol* 14:295–299.

107. Dehio C, Meyer M, Berger J, Schwarz H, Lanz C. 1997. Interaction of *Bartonella henselae* with endothelial cells results in bacterial aggregation on the cell surface and the subsequent engulfment and internalisation of the bacterial aggregate by a unique structure, the invasome. *J Cell Sci* 110:2141–2154.

108. Verma A, Davis GE, Ihler GM. 2000. Infection of human endothelial cells with *Bartonella bacilliformis* is dependent on Rho and results in activation of Rho. *Infect Immun* 68:5960–5969.

109. Dramsi S, Cossart P. 1998. Intracellular pathogens and the actin cytoskeleton. *Annu Rev Cell Dev Biol* 14: 137–166.

110. Kirby JE, Nekorchuk DM. 2002. Bartonella-associated endothelial proliferation depends on inhibition of apoptosis. *Proc Natl Acad Sci USA* 99:4656–4661.

111. Schulein R, Dehio C. 2002. The VirB/VirD4 type IV secretion system of *Bartonella* is essential for establishing intraerythrocytic infection. *Mol Microbiol* 46:1053–1067.

112. Seubert A, Hiestand R, de la Cruz F, Dehio C. 2003. A bacterial conjugation machinery recruited for pathogenesis. *Mol Microbiol* 49:1253–1266.

113. Torisu H, Ono M, Kiryu H, Furue M, Ohmoto Y, Nakayama J, Nishioka Y, Sone S, Kuwano M. 2000. Macrophage infiltration correlates with tumor stage and angiogenesis in human malignant melanoma: possible involvement of TNFα and IL-1α. *Int J Cancer* 85:182–188.

114. Musso T, Badolato R, Ravarino D, Stornello S, Panzanelli P, Merlino C, Savoia D, Cavallo R, Ponzi AN, Zucca M. 2001. Interaction of *Bartonella henselae* with the murine macrophage cell line J774: infection and proinflammatory response. *Infect Immun* 69:5974–5980.

115. Kempf VA, Volkmann B, Schaller M, Sander CA, Alitalo K, Riess T, Autenrieth IB. 2001. Evidence of a leading role for VEGF in *Bartonella henselae*-induced endothelial cell proliferations. *Cell Microbiol* 3:623–632.

116. Resto-Ruiz SI, Schmiederer M, Sweger D, Newton C, Klein TW, Friedman H, Anderson BE. 2002. Induction of a potential paracrine angiogenic loop between human THP-1 macrophages and human microvascular endothelial cells during *Bartonella henselae* infection. *Infect Immun* 70:4564–4570.

117. Minasyan H. 2016. Mechanisms and pathways for the clearance of bacteria from blood circulation in health and disease. *Pathophysiology* 23:61–66.

118. Khakpour S, Wilhelmsen K, Hellman J. 2015. Vascular endothelial cell Toll-like receptor pathways in sepsis. *Innate Immun* 21:827–846.

119. **Gupta SK, Lysko PG, Pillarisetti K, Ohlstein E, Stadel JM.** 1998. Chemokine receptors in human endothelial cells. Functional expression of CXCR4 and its transcriptional regulation by inflammatory cytokines. *J Biol Chem* **273:**4282–4287.

120. **Murdoch C, Monk PN, Finn A.** 1999. Cxc chemokine receptor expression on human endothelial cells. *Cytokine* **11:**704–712.

121. **Mitchell JA, Ryffel B, Quesniaux VF, Cartwright N, Paul-Clark M.** 2007. Role of pattern-recognition receptors in cardiovascular health and disease. *Biochem Soc Trans* **35:**1449–1452.

122. **Opitz B, Eitel J, Meixenberger K, Suttorp N.** 2009. Role of Toll-like receptors, NOD-like receptors and RIG-I-like receptors in endothelial cells and systemic infections. *Thromb Haemost* **102:**1103–1109.

123. **Marceau F, Grassi J, Frobert Y, Bergeron C, Poubelle PE.** 1992. Effects of experimental conditions on the production of interleukin-1 alpha and -1 beta by human endothelial cells cultured in vitro. *Int J Immunopharmacol* **14:**525–534.

124. **Opitz B, Püschel A, Beermann W, Hocke AC, Förster S, Schmeck B, van Laak V, Chakraborty T, Suttorp N, Hippenstiel S.** 2006. *Listeria monocytogenes* activated p38 MAPK and induced IL-8 secretion in a nucleotide-binding oligomerization domain 1-dependent manner in endothelial cells. *J Immunol* **176:**484–490.

125. **Anand AR, Cucchiarini M, Terwilliger EF, Ganju RK.** 2008. The tyrosine kinase Pyk2 mediates lipopolysaccharide-induced IL-8 expression in human endothelial cells. *J Immunol* **180:**5636–5644.

126. **Faure E, Thomas L, Xu H, Medvedev A, Equils O, Arditi M.** 2001. Bacterial lipopolysaccharide and IFN-γ induce Toll-like receptor 2 and Toll-like receptor 4 expression in human endothelial cells: role of NF-κB activation. *J Immunol* **166:**2018–2024.

127. **Danese S, Dejana E, Fiocchi C.** 2007. Immune regulation by microvascular endothelial cells: directing innate and adaptive immunity, coagulation, and inflammation. *J Immunol* **178:**6017–6022.

128. **Neefjes J, Jongsma ML, Paul P, Bakke O.** 2011. Towards a systems understanding of MHC class I and MHC class II antigen presentation. *Nat Rev Immunol* **11:**823–836.

129. **Rose ML, Coles MI, Griffin RJ, Pomerance A, Yacoub MH.** 1986. Expression of class I and class II major histocompatibility antigens in normal and transplanted human heart. *Transplantation* **41:**776–780.

130. **Leeuwenberg JF, Van Damme J, Meager T, Jeunhomme TM, Buurman WA.** 1988. Effects of tumor necrosis factor on the interferon-gamma-induced major histocompatibility complex class II antigen expression by human endothelial cells. *Eur J Immunol* **18:**1469–1472.

131. **Mai J, Virtue A, Shen J, Wang H, Yang XF.** 2013. An evolving new paradigm: endothelial cells–conditional innate immune cells. *J Hematol Oncol* **6:**61.

132. **van der Poll T, van de Veerdonk FL, Scicluna BP, Netea MG.** 2017. The immunopathology of sepsis and potential therapeutic targets. *Nat Rev Immunol* **17:**407–420.

133. **Wiersinga WJ, Leopold SJ, Cranendonk DR, van der Poll T.** 2014. Host innate immune responses to sepsis. *Virulence* **5:**36–44.

134. **Levy MM, Fink MP, Marshall JC, Abraham E, Angus D, Cook D, Cohen J, Opal SM, Vincent JL, Ramsay G, SCCM/ESICM/ACCP/ATS/SIS.** 2003. 2001 SCCM/ESICM/ACCP/ATS/SIS International Sepsis Definitions Conference. *Crit Care Med* **31:**1250–1256.

135. **Rittirsch D, Flierl MA, Ward PA.** 2008. Harmful molecular mechanisms in sepsis. *Nat Rev Immunol* **8:**776–787.

136. **Hotchkiss RS, Moldawer LL, Opal SM, Reinhart K, Turnbull IR, Vincent JL.** 2016. Sepsis and septic shock. *Nat Rev Dis Primers* **2:**16045.

137. **Hotchkiss RS, Tinsley KW, Swanson PE, Grayson MH, Osborne DF, Wagner TH, Cobb JP, Coopersmith C, Karl IE.** 2002. Depletion of dendritic cells, but not macrophages, in patients with sepsis. *J Immunol* **168:**2493–2500.

138. **Hotchkiss RS, Monneret G, Payen D.** 2013. Sepsis-induced immunosuppression: from cellular dysfunctions to immunotherapy. *Nat Rev Immunol* **13:**862–874.

139. **Scumpia PO, Delano MJ, Kelly-Scumpia KM, Weinstein JS, Wynn JL, Winfield RD, Xia C, Chung CS, Ayala A, Atkinson MA, Reeves WH, Clare-Salzler MJ, Moldawer LL.** 2007. Treatment with GITR agonistic antibody corrects adaptive immune dysfunction in sepsis. *Blood* **110:**3673–3681.

140. **Boomer JS, To K, Chang KC, Takasu O, Osborne DF, Walton AH, Bricker TL, Jarman SD II, Kreisel D, Krupnick AS, Srivastava A, Swanson PE, Green JM, Hotchkiss RS.** 2011. Immunosuppression in patients who die of sepsis and multiple organ failure. *JAMA* **306:**2594–2605.

141. **Huang X, Venet F, Wang YL, Lepape A, Yuan Z, Chen Y, Swan R, Kherouf H, Monneret G, Chung CS, Ayala A.** 2009. PD-1 expression by macrophages plays a pathologic role in altering microbial clearance and the innate inflammatory response to sepsis. *Proc Natl Acad Sci USA* **106:**6303–6308.

142. **Levi M, Ten Cate H.** 1999. Disseminated intravascular coagulation. *N Engl J Med* **341:**586–592.

143. **Davis RP, Miller-Dorey S, Jenne CN.** 2016. Platelets and coagulation in infection. *Clin Transl Immunology* **5:**e89.

144. **Pernerstorfer T, Stohlawetz P, Hollenstein U, Dzirlo L, Eichler HG, Kapiotis S, Jilma B, Speiser W.** 1999. Endotoxin-induced activation of the coagulation cascade in humans: effect of acetylsalicylic acid and acetaminophen. *Arterioscler Thromb Vasc Biol* **19:**2517–2523.

145. **Østerud B, Bjørklid E.** 2001. The tissue factor pathway in disseminated intravascular coagulation. *Semin Thromb Hemost* **27:**605–618.

146. **Abraham E.** 2000. Coagulation abnormalities in acute lung injury and sepsis. *Am J Respir Cell Mol Biol* **22:**401–404.

147. **Ince C.** 2005. The microcirculation is the motor of sepsis. *Crit Care* **9**(Suppl 4):S13–S19.

Bacteria and Intracellularity
Edited by Pascale Cossart, Craig R. Roy, and Philippe Sansonetti
© 2019 American Society for Microbiology, Washington, DC
doi:10.1128/microbiolspec.BAI-0014-2019

Reaching the End of the Line: Urinary Tract Infections

6

Kevin O. Tamadonfar,[1] Natalie S. Omattage,[1] Caitlin N. Spaulding,[1,2] and Scott J. Hultgren[1,3]

INTRODUCTION

Urinary tract infections (UTIs) refer to bacterial colonization of the urinary tract and are one of the most common bacterial infections, infecting an estimated 150 million people worldwide annually. In the United States alone, nearly 11 million cases are reported each year, resulting in approximately $5 billion in indirect and direct costs annually (1, 2). More than 50% of women will experience at least one UTI in their lifetime, and, despite antibiotic intervention, 20 to 30% of women with an initial UTI will experience a recurrent UTI (rUTI) within 3 to 4 months of the initial infection (2, 3). Such infections therefore represent a great health care burden and, as such, demand further research to advance treatment options and improve patient care. This chapter outlines what is currently known about the determinants and features of *Escherichia coli* pathogenesis in UTIs and highlights how such knowledge is now being translated into tools for alleviating that burden clinically.

UROGENITAL TRACT

The principal function of the urinary tract is to collect, transport, store, and eliminate urine, which is composed of excreted metabolic products and waste generated in the kidneys (4, 5). From its proximal to distal end, the urinary tract is composed of the kidneys, ureters, bladder, and urethra, and each of these organs plays a critical role in maintaining the homeostasis of this system. The upper urinary tract consists of the kidneys, which filter blood to produce urine, and the ureters, bilateral fibromuscular tubes that carry urine from the kidneys to the bladder. The bladder is a hollow, distensible organ composed of smooth muscle, col-

lagen, and elastin (6). When devoid of urine, it adopts a tetrahedral shape; upon being filled, it becomes ovoid (7). Finally, the urethra connects to the neck of the bladder, begins at the distal end of the urethral sphincter, and serves as a duct by which urine is eliminated out of the body from the bladder (7).

In both males and females, the luminal surface of the urinary tract is lined with specialized epithelial tissue broadly known as the urothelium. The urothelium serves as a distensible and effective permeability barrier to accommodate urine flow and volume while preventing the unregulated exchange of metabolic products between the blood and urine (8). The superficial urothelium comprises a single layer of large polyhedral, multinucleated, highly differentiated umbrella cells, also termed superficial facet cells (8). Umbrella cells are decorated with a crystalline array of uroplakin proteins that form urothelial plaques. Importantly, uroplakins play a critical role in the maintenance of the superficial urothelium's permeability barrier (9–13). The intermediate and basal layers of the urothelium are significantly smaller and less differentiated, and they are believed to contain urothelial stem cells required for umbrella cell regeneration (7, 14–16).

The urinary tract is thought to be relatively sterile (17), although recently, evidence for a urinary microbiota was presented (18). As is discussed in the following sections, upon accessing the urinary tract, bacteria can exploit tissue-specific receptors to establish infection.

INFECTION OF THE URINARY TRACT

The majority of uncomplicated UTIs manifest as infections of the lower urinary tract: infection and inflamma-

[1]Department of Molecular Microbiology, Washington University School of Medicine, St. Louis, MO 63110; [2]Harvard University School of Public Health, Boston, MA 02115; [3]Center for Women's Infectious Disease Research, Washington University, School of Medicine, St. Louis, MO 63110.

tion of the urethra (urethritis) or urinary bladder (cystitis) (2). If bacteria ascend the ureters to the upper urinary tract, this results in pyelonephritis (2). This is particularly concerning, as bacteria in the kidneys may enter the bloodstream, causing sepsis (2). Asymptomatic bacteriuria (ASB) is marked by positive urine cultures in the laboratory without urinary symptoms (2). Cystitis is typically diagnosed based on symptomology, such as frequency and urgency of urination, burning pain and sensation during urination, abdominal discomfort, and/or turbid, odorous urine paired with high levels of bacteria in the urine (bacteriuria) (2). Pyelonephritis typically presents with bacteriuria, pyuria (white blood cells in the urine), flank pain, or fever and may or may not present with symptoms associated with cystitis (2). The majority (85%) of uncomplicated, community-acquired UTIs are caused by uropathogenic *E. coli* (UPEC), and the remaining 15% are caused by other Gram-negative bacilli like *Klebsiella* or Gram-positive cocci such as *Enterococcus* or *Staphylococcus* (19). Risk factors for uncomplicated UTI include sexual activity, history of UTI, contraception, and host genetics and immune responses (2, 20). *E. coli* can also exist in the urinary tract asymptomatically in a condition known as ASB (21).

In the health care setting, catheterization increases the risk of complicated UTIs (22). Catheter-associated UTIs (CAUTI) account for 30 to 40% of all health care-associated infections in the United States (23). The majority of CAUTI are asymptomatic, but these infections can present with fever, chills, malaise, and/or generalizable discomfort or as cystitis or pyelonephritis once the catheter is removed (2). The two major causative agents of CAUTI are UPEC (65%) and *Enterococcus* spp. (11%) (24). CAUTI are particularly threatening, as they have the potential to disseminate in the health care setting.

Due to their prevalence and the high rate of recurrence, UTIs are a significant cause of morbidity in women throughout their lifetime. It is estimated that one in three women will be prescribed antibiotics to treat a UTI before the age of 24 (2). In the outpatient setting, 15% of antibiotic prescriptions have been reported to be for UTI treatment (25, 26). Frequent antibiotic usage coupled with antibiotic resistance among uropathogens (27) highlights the urgent need to develop new and improved treatment and prevention options.

UTI PATHOGENESIS

Uropathogenic *Escherichia coli*

UPEC (Fig. 1) lacks a "genetic signature" (28) that distinguishes it from non-UPEC. This is likely due to the broad definition of UPEC as any strain that is recovered from the urine of a patient with a symptomatic UTI. Recently, a high-resolution, comparative genomic study performed on *E. coli* isolates from women with recurrent UTIs revealed that the isolates were diverse and represented five major *E. coli* clades: A, B1, B2, D, and E (28). Two-thirds of these strains belonged to the clade B2, which comprises the majority of UPEC strains isolated in the United States and Europe (28). Interestingly, the strain's phylogenetic background and carriage of virulence factors are not entirely predictive of its urovirulence (28). Instead, the expression of certain genes, such as those involved in motility and transport of sugars, is a better predictor of the virulence of a given strain in mice. Lending support to this is the fact that in some women suffering from recurrent UTIs with a strain different from that which caused the previous event, the new strain can actually encode fewer putative urovirulence factors than the strain that was replaced. Thus, work in multiple mouse models of UTIs has defined a "lock-and-key" mechanism of UTI pathogenesis in which the disease outcome is not completely fixed based on the pathogen or the host but, rather, is determined in part by how the fitness level of the introduced pathogen is matched against the resistance or susceptibility level of the host, which is influenced by history of infection and the presence of foreign bodies (28–30).

The type 1 pilus is an important mediator of bladder colonization (31, 32). The adhesive tip protein or adhesin (33) of the type 1 pilus FimH binds to mannose (31, 34). This ligand is present on uroplakin 1a and on $\beta 1$ and $\alpha 3$ integrin molecules on the surface of bladder urothelial cells (31, 35, 36). Changes in host cell cytoskeletal elements, thought to be mediated through Rho GTPases, allow type 1 facilitated invasion into urothelial cells (31, 37, 38). During infection, pathogen-associated molecular patterns (PAMPs) can stimulate the pattern recognition receptor Toll-like receptor 4 to activate host responses. One example of a PAMP is bacterial lipopolysaccharide (39). Cytokine production (39), the influx of inflammatory monocytes and neutrophils (40), bacterial eviction from host cells (39, 41), and the exfoliation of urothelial cells (39, 42) are all innate host responses encountered by UPEC (39) (Fig. 1C). Further, work has demonstrated that the role of urothelial exfoliation is to eliminate infected bladder cells from the body, thus reducing the UPEC burden in the bladder (43, 146). UPEC-induced exfoliation results in dead or dying shed epithelial cells, rather than the predominantly living host cells shed by chemical exfoliation (43). This exfoliation may occur by multiple pathways, including interleukin 1β (IL-1β) signaling and the NLRP3 inflammasome (42).

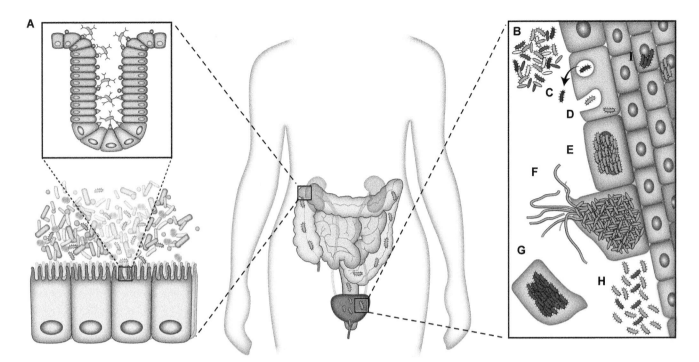

Figure 1 UPEC pathogenesis. (A) UPEC is housed in a reservoir in the gastrointestinal system. The bacteria are able to colonize the urinary tract from this reservoir. (B) Bacteria are able to adhere to and invade the bladder epithelial cells. (C) Bacterial cells can be evicted from the host cell in response. Bacterial cells can also enter the cytoplasm (D) and initiate IBC formation (E). (F) UPEC can, upon fluxing out of the host cells, filament and reinfect other urothelial cells. (G) To counteract intracellular pathogens, the host can initiate a program of host cell exfoliation. (H) Chronic cystitis in mice can occur with persistent high titers of bacteriuria. (I) QIRs can be established, in mice with resolved infections, in layers below superficial urothelial cells. Image and caption are adapted from reference 31.

Exfoliation can be a double-edged sword, as it leads to the exposure of the underlying transitional epithelium, where bacteria can invade and persist in small quiescent intracellular reservoirs (QIRs) even after resolution of bacteriuria. The bacteria localized in QIRs can subsequently reactivate to seed recurrent UTI (44). Evidence suggests that chymase, from mast cells, activates procaspase to initiate this cytolysis (43). Interestingly, mast cells have been shown to induce an anti-inflammatory response in the bladder as well. In C57BL/6 mice infected with a UPEC isolate, IL-10 expression spikes at 6 hours postinfection in the bladder and remains elevated for at least 72 hours. Mast cells, which have been shown to increase in numbers in the bladder upon UPEC infection, can secrete IL-10, which also functions to reduce the number of mature dendritic cells and possibly other immune cells (45).

In humans, UPEC infections have numerous outcomes, including ASB, acute and self-resolving UTIs, chronic UTIs, and/or recurrent UTIs (20) (Fig. 1H and I). Murine models of cystitis have been developed

that are capable of mimicking these clinical outcomes. For example, C3H/HeN mouse models have recapitulated two disease courses. Mice experience (i) acute infection followed by spontaneous resolution within 1 to 4 weeks of infection, or (ii) acute infection that then progresses to a long-lasting persistent infection termed chronic cystitis (39).

The fate of infection is determined in part by whether a host-pathogen checkpoint is activated. Activation of the checkpoint leads to elevated levels of COX2 expression (see below), which licenses the transmigration of neutrophils across the bladder epithelium, leading to the associated mucosal damage that ensues (40). Thus, activation of the host-pathogen checkpoint leads to persistent high-titer bacteriuria, which is accompanied by severe immunopathology and ablation of the terminally differentiated superficial umbrella cells in a condition we have termed chronic cystitis. Chronic and recurrent cystitis can be predicted 24 hours postinfection by increased levels of the serum biomarkers IL-5, IL-6, neutrophil cytokine CXCL1, and granulocyte colony-stimulating factor (29, 40). Similarly, in the sera of young women with acute UTI, UTI recurrence was predicted by increased levels of soluble biomarkers involved in myeloid cell development and chemotaxis (40).

While type 1 pili are important for the progression of acute and chronic cystitis, another pilus type, Fim-like (Fml) or F9, is also important for UPEC persistence in the inflamed bladder. Bladder inflammation leads to the exposure of the galactose β1-3 N-acetylgalactosamine receptor recognized by the Fml adhesin FmlH which facilitates binding to the inflamed tissue and enables persistent bacteriuria and high bladder bacterial burdens throughout chronic cystitis (46).

Furthermore, clinically, a history of cystitis is one of the key risk factors for the development of recurrent infections (rUTIs), specifically, an incidence of UTI at a young age or two or more previous incidences of UTIs (29). Mechanistically, a possible explanation for this phenomenon was recently proposed. The remodeling of the urothelium during chronic infection permanently alters its architecture, even after antibiotic therapy and convalescence from infection, resulting in hundreds of differentially expressed genes and proteins in the remodeled bladder compared to an age-matched naïve bladder (29). Thus, mice with a history of chronic infection are left with a molecular imprint on the bladder defined by a defect in terminal differentiation of the bladder epithelium, resulting in significantly smaller luminal cells and an altered transcriptome (29). Importantly, bladder remodeling changes host-pathogen interactions during acute pathogenesis by conferring resistance to early colonization events. However, mice with a history of chronic infection succumb to severe bladder infection, a process that is COX-2 dependent and leads to the transmigration of neutrophils across the bladder epithelium, mucosal wounding, and unchecked bacterial replication (29). In support of this, treatment with a COX-2 inhibitor leads to a significant reduction in both chronic and recurrent cystitis (29, 40). Thus, bladder mucosal remodeling can occur as a consequence of persistent infection, and this reprogramming of the bladder predisposes the host to more severe rUTI upon subsequent bacterial exposure, even with less pathogenic strains.

UPEC in the gastrointestinal tract

The major source of UPEC is thought to be the gastrointestinal tract, where UPEC can reside transiently or as a commensal member of the gut microbiota (3, 47–49). UPEC is then shed in the feces, inoculating the periurethral area or vagina, and subsequently introduced into the urinary tract during periods of physical manipulation, such as during sexual activity or catheterization (20). Several recent studies identified chaperone usher pathway (CUP) pilus types that promote the establishment and/or maintenance of the UPEC intestinal reservoir. Interestingly, a role for type 1 pili in UPEC intestinal colonization in mice has been reported by several groups (47, 50, 51). Additionally, a previously uncharacterized pilus, the F17-like pilus, has also been implicated in UPEC intestinal colonization in mice (47). Purified lectin domains of the type 1 and F17-like adhesins (FimH and UclD, respectively) were shown to bind within the colonic crypt, suggesting that type 1 and F17-like pili facilitate colonization within that niche (Fig. 1A). However, further studies examining the localization of whole bacteria expressing type 1 or F17-like pili within the mouse gut are required to determine if UPEC binds within the crypts during intestinal colonization in vivo. Phylogenomic and structural analyses suggest that UPEC acquired F17-like pili from intestinal pathogens, and B2 UPEC strains causing same-strain recurrences were found to be significantly enriched for the carriage of the F17-like pilus gene cluster (47). These analyses reveal that F17-like pili might have evolved to enable maintenance of a UPEC intestinal reservoir by promoting UPEC persistence in women with rUTIs. Thus, the identification of UPEC genes involved in gastrointestinal colonization provides the framework for future studies elucidating the mechanisms that underlie UPEC persistence in the gut.

Intracellular bacterial communities

Intracellular bacterial communities (IBCs) are clonal collections of bacterial cells housed within the cytoplasm of superficial facet cells of the bladder (52, 53). IBCs are encased within a biofilm-like matrix (31, 52) and are replicative, metabolically active communities (52, 54). IBCs provide a mechanism for UPEC replication in the bladder while being protected from immune responses and possible antibiotic treatment (31, 52). Studies have found that the IBCs, although studied extensively in mice (39, 55, 56), are a feature of human infection (31, 57, 58). IBC formation has also been documented in a number of bacterial species in the family Enterobacteriaceae (52). IBC formation occurs during acute infection and is restricted to the superficial umbrella cells. Exfoliation of these cells is part of an innate defense, and the ablation of the luminal epithelium restricts further IBC formation during chronic infection (39, 52).

A number of factors have been found to be critical in IBC formation. FimH, the type 1 pilus adhesin known to mediate binding to and invasion of bladder urothelium (53, 59), also plays a role in bacterial association within the IBC biomass (60). The K1 capsule also allows clumping of cells within the host cell (52). LacZ and GalK, factors involved in metabolism, have been found to be important for the establishment of IBCs. In a murine model, strains with individual deletions of the genes encoding these proteins were found to lack fitness in competitive infections against the wild type (54). YeaR, a recently described protein involved in the oxidative stress response, is critical to IBC formation in a type 1-dependent manner (54). Iron uptake systems, including siderophore biosynthetic genes, are highly upregulated in IBCs, as are reciprocal iron responses in neighboring host cells. Thus, a competition for iron occurs at the interface between the IBC and neighboring epithelial cells (61). For example, ChuA, a hemin receptor, is highly upregulated in IBCs, and neighboring epithelial cells respond by upregulating the transferrin receptor, an iron-scavenging factor (52, 61). Developmentally, bacterial cells within IBCs progress from a coccoid shape to a rod shape. Bacteria then generally take a filamentous form, mediated by SulA, a cell division regulator, as they exit host cells to the extracellular environment (52). This development and exit are of note, as they provide a mechanism of infection of neighboring cells, allowing the infection to spread in the bladder (52). It is clear that the formation of IBCs is a hallmark of UPEC pathogenesis (52) and represents a critical topic for future study.

Quiescent intracellular reservoirs

QIRs are small communities of bacterial cells contained within Lamp1⁺ vesicles in host cells (44, 52). These communities contain 4 to 10 bacterial cells, oriented in a rosette-like fashion (44), and are nonreplicating (52), in contrast to IBCs (52). QIRs can be present in both superficial epithelial and transitional bladder cells (44) and can persist for 12 weeks (44). Beyond being protected from antibiotics (62), such reservoirs are thought to be able to initiate a recurrent infection (52), as work has demonstrated that in mice possessing bladder QIRs, exfoliation of the superficial bladder epithelial cells can result in an activation of the bacteria within the QIR to cause pyuria, bacteriuria, and increased bacterial bladder titers (44). Interestingly, there may exist an interplay between the vaginal microbiome and rUTI, as it has been shown that in bladders containing QIRs, exposure to *Gardnerella vaginalis* can result in activation of the reservoir, leading to rUTI (63). Additional work has examined the contribution of host cytoskeletal elements to QIR behavior. Interrupting the host actin network causes QIRs to replicate and then

exit the vesicle into the cytosolic space (64). Considering the substantial burden of recurrent UTI, QIRs represent a rich area of study to understand the mechanisms of recurrence.

Virulence and Bacterial Colonization

The determinants by which UPEC causes UTIs (Fig. 2) have been extensively studied. To facilitate survival within human urine, an environment rich in amino acids and peptides, UPEC relies on amino acid biosynthesis and amino acid and carbohydrate metabolism (65, 66). As described above, to fulfill nutritional metal requirements to survive within host cells, UPEC utilizes iron acquisition molecules called siderophores to chelate iron from the host environment. Iron-siderophore complexes are then recognized by cognate outer membrane (OM) receptors on the bacterium for their reuptake into the bacterial cell. In particular, enterobactin, yersiniabactin, and salmochelin are important siderophores in the context of UTIs (67). UPEC also utilizes certain toxins that play important roles in pathogenesis (68, 69). Finally, surface-localized structures, such as flagella, pili, capsule, and OM adhesins, and the regulation of these factors are important for the motility, colonization, and biofilm formation of UPEC during infection (Fig. 2) (70).

CUP pilus assembly

Pili and adhesins are particularly important, as they are critical for all stages of the UPEC pathogenic cascade, except for growth in urine (71, 72). To facilitate adhesion to host- and tissue-specific niches, UPEC encodes CUP pili. *E. coli* carries genes for at least 38 CUP pili in its pangenome, and UPEC utilizes CUP pili, such as type 1 and P pili, to mediate adherence critical in cystitis and pyelonephritis, respectively (Fig. 3) (19, 73–76). Gram-negative bacteria assemble CUP pili to mediate adhesion to host and environmental surfaces, facilitate invasion into host tissues, and promote formation of intra- and extracellular biofilm communities (77). Further, as discussed above, recent work suggests that the type 1 and F17-like pilus types promote UPEC colonization within the mouse colon (47, 50, 51). Expression of type 1 pili is under the control of an invertible promoter, *fimS*, that oscillates between ON and OFF (72). Interestingly, there exist factors in the urine that promote *fimS*, in planktonic UPEC in the urine, to adopt a phase OFF orientation; however, bacteria bound to bladder cells shed into the urine remain in phase ON (72). Microarray and RNA-Seq studies of bacteria isolated from the urine of UTI patients have revealed patients with different patterns (both high and low)

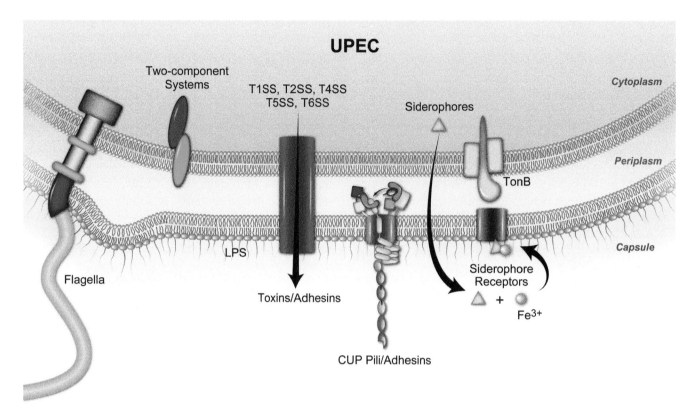

Figure 2 Overview of UPEC fitness and virulence factors. Surface-associated structures that play a role in UTI pathogenesis include lipopolysaccharide, polysaccharide capsule, flagella, pili, toxins, secretion systems (SS), and siderophore receptors. Image and caption are adapted from reference 68.

of *fim* expression (71, 78). Based on these and other human studies and from work in a murine model, one hypothesis is that planktonic bacteria in urine are (or become) nonpiliated, while bacteria colonizing the bladder tissue or bound to shed epithelial cells express type 1 pili (71, 79–81). Additionally, it has been postulated that exponential growth in human urine suppresses type 1 pilus expression (82). Taken together, these results indicate that type 1 pili are temporally and spatially regulated and are required for colonization of host tissues.

CUP pili are assembled by dedicated chaperone-usher machinery, which is encoded by operons that contain the genetic determinants required to assemble a mature pilus: a periplasmic chaperone protein, an OM usher protein, major and minor pilus subunits, and, in most cases, a tip adhesin protein (77). Adhesins are two-domain proteins, with an N-terminal lectin domain that binds to receptors with stereochemical specificity, while the C-terminal pilin domain joins the adhesin to the pilus rod (59). In CUP pilus assembly, individual pilus subunits or pilins are first exported across the in-

ner membrane to the periplasm, where they are guided to the OM usher via the chaperone (59) (Fig. 3A). Each pilin comprises a single domain having an immuno-globulin (Ig)-like structure (59) that is incomplete because it lacks a seventh C-terminal β-strand.

In a process termed donor-strand complementation, the chaperone, a boomerang-shaped protein composed of two complete Ig-like domains, provides in *trans* its G1 β-strand to transiently complete the pilin's Ig-like fold, thus catalyzing folding directly on the chaperone template (59) (Fig. 3B, C, G, and H). Chaperone-pilin complexes are then targeted to the OM usher, a β-barrel channel that catalyzes subunit-subunit interactions through a reaction called donor-strand exchange, wherein every pilin subunit has an N-terminal extension that completes the Ig fold of its neighboring subunit (59) (Fig. 3D and E). The OM usher is composed of five functional domains: a 24-stranded integral β-barrel translocation domain (TD), a β-sandwich plug domain that gates the pore of the TD, a periplasmic amino-terminal domain (NTD), and two carboxy-terminal domains (CTD1 and CTD2) (83, 84). The

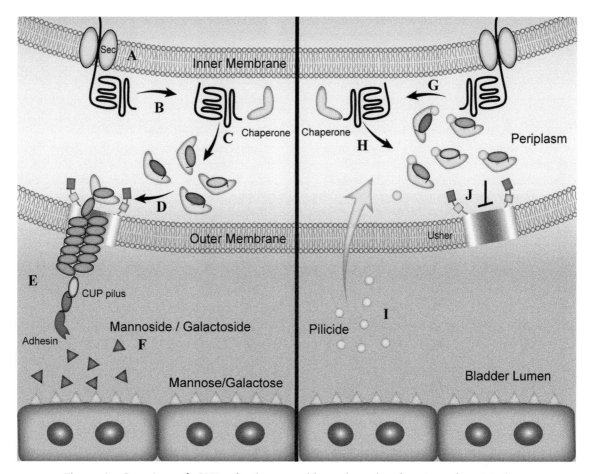

Figure 3 Overview of CUP of pilus assembly and mode of action of antivirulence compounds. (A) Sec transports unfolded subunits of the pilus structure into the periplasmic space. (B, C, G, H) Pilus subunits interact with the pilus type-specific chaperone and fold. (D) Chaperone-subunit complexes interact with the N terminus of the pilus usher. (E) Secreted subunits, bound together through donor strand exchange, form the pilus. (F) Small-molecule inhibitors, mannosides and galactosides, antagonize interactions between the adhesive tip of the pilus and its ligand. Pilicides bind to the chaperone (I) and interrupt the interaction between chaperone and the N terminus of the usher (J). Image and caption are adapted from reference 31.

concerted coordination of the usher's domains ensures that the subunits interact productively during fiber polymerization. The molecular mechanisms that drive this cooperative coordination of the different domains of the usher have been studied, and the studies have demonstrated that conformational flexibility and allostery drive this bacterial nanomachine in the absence of cellular energy at the OM (83–91). In particular, it has been shown that upon initiation of CUP pilus assembly, the TD and PD undergo marked rearrangements to accommodate transit of the growing fiber, while the periplasmic NTD and CTDs participate in substrate recruitment, catalysis of donor strand exchange, and translocation through the TD pore (83, 84).

While the OM usher serves as the assembly platform for the growing pilus fiber and anchors it to the OM, the majority of the pilus is composed of homopolymers of the major rod subunit (59). Once the pilus rod extrudes into the extracellular milieu, it coils into a right-handed helical fiber that has the ability to unwind into a linear structure (59). Recent structural studies on the type 1 and P pilus rods have identified the molecular determinants for the formation of the helical rod (92–94). Disruption of critical subunit-subunit interactions within the rod resulted in pili that were more prone to helical unwinding in the presence of shear force and displayed attenuation in murine models of cystitis and intestinal colonization by UPEC (92–94). Taken together, these studies suggest that the dynamics of rod coiling and uncoiling play a critical role in UPEC pathogenesis.

Beyond its own role in pathogenesis, the pilus rod also serves as a scaffold to present the pilus tip adhesin at the host-pathogen interface. In addition to the OM usher and pilus rod displaying conformational flexibility, recent work has shown that the two-domain adhesin protein, FimH, exists in equilibrium between conformational states as well (95). One study focusing on the type 1 pilus adhesin FimH demonstrated that it adopts two-state conformational ensembles (95). Remarkably, it appears that positively selected residues within the protein modulate the equilibrium between these two states, and this equilibrium is crucial to bacterial persistence within the bladder during the progression of UTI (95). In summary, conformational dynamics play a significant role at every level of pilus assembly.

Virulence factors

A variety of virulence factors have been the subject of study in UPEC pathogenesis. Work has revealed that surface-associated structures such as capsules are also critical for immune evasion and for the successful development of IBCs during infection (96–99) (Fig. 2). Among such virulence factors is antigen 43 (Ag43), an autotransporter protein of the AIDA-I type, which functions in the formation of biofilms and aggregation (100, 101). Ag43 is thought to be important to bladder colonization, as evidence suggests that deletion of one Ag43, Ag43a, in CFT073 causes attenuation of bladder colonization 5 days postinfection (101). Structurally, Ag43 exhibits a functionally significant L-shaped secondary structure. Along an interface of this structure, Ag43a autoaggregates in an interaction mediated by hydrogen and electrostatic bonding. As such, a "Velcro-like" mechanism has been proposed for cellular adhesion mediated by Ag43 (100). Additionally, curli, secreted amyloids which contribute to the formation of biofilm extracellular matrix (102), have been found to improve bacterial adherence to kidney epithelial cells. Curli also improve relative growth of bacteria when exposed to human antimicrobial peptide LL-37 and mouse antimicrobial peptide mCRAMP (103). A number of other characterized virulence factors are briefly described in Table 1.

Gender and UPEC UTIs

Women are more likely to experience uncomplicated, community-acquired UTIs than men. This is thought to be due to higher rates of bacterial colonization of the urethral and periurethral body sites (2). This, paired with shorter urethral lengths in women, makes it more likely for bacteria to ascend the urethra and access the bladder for colonization and to establish an infection in this population (2). However, there is a significant male patient population that experiences complicated UTIs due to risk factors that include spinal cord injuries, anatomical and physiological abnormalities in the urinary system (such as vesicoureteral reflux), diabetes, and urethral instrumentation (3).

Demographic data suggest that beyond simple anatomical differences between the male and female urinary tracts, hormones could play a role in pathogenesis (104). Cell culture work has found that estrogen aids the host defense against UTIs, increasing the expression of genes for antimicrobial peptides and proteins involved in forming cellular junctions while reducing intracellular bacterial titers *in vivo* (105). On the other hand, while community-acquired UTIs are more common among females, the rate of mortality from complicated UTI and pyelonephritis is higher in males (106). In order to study how sex influences UTI pathogenesis, surgical and nonsurgical male models for studying UTIs have been developed (106, 107). The surgical model of infection using the C3H/HeN strain of mice found that male C3H/HeN mouse bladders are colonized with UTI89 at higher levels at 6 hours postinfection than female bladders and that males were more likely to develop chronic cystitis (106). Furthermore, male C57BL/6 and C3H/HeN mice exhibited higher kidney titers with UTI89 than their female counterparts, and all of the UTI89-infected C3H/HeN mice developed renal abscesses, while less than 10% of their female counterparts developed them (106). Beyond developing a male model of UTI, the same study demonstrated that testosterone plays a role in the observed higher kidney and bladder colonization in C3H/HeN male mice (106). Discrepancies in the characteristics of UTIs between males and females represent an opportunity to further probe the features which define the natural history of UTI.

Catheter-associated UTIs caused by UPEC

Catheterization is a common phenomenon in inpatient settings, where 20 to 50% of patients can be catheterized (108). Catheterization is responsible for a substantial majority, 70 to 80%, of complicated UTIs (24), and about one-half of all CAUTI are caused by UPEC (109). Catheter-associated infections can also be caused by a number of other microorganisms, including *Enterococcus*, *Staphylococcus*, and *Proteus* (108, 110, 111). The use of urinary catheters has been shown to have an effect on the pathobiology of UPEC UTIs (30). Catheterization induces bladder inflammation and edema (30), and UPEC thus enters and colonizes a dif-

TABLE 1 Virulence factors in UPEC pathogenesis

Virulence factor(s)	Type of factor	Role in pathogenesis[a]	Reference(s)
QseBC, Cpx, and PhoPQ	Two-component regulatory systems	Regulation of virulence factor expression	130–135
SAT (secreted autotransporter toxin)	Toxin	Induction of vacuolation within the bladder and kidney cells *in vitro*; UPEC proliferation	69
CNF-1	Toxin	Activates Rho GTPases; enhances UPEC invasion of urothelial cells *in vitro*	136
HlyA (alpha-hemolysin)	Toxin	Exfoliation of urothelium; partially regulated by Cof phosphatase	42, 137, 138
YefM-YeoB	Toxin-antitoxin system	Bladder colonization in competitive infection	139
YbaJ-Hha	Toxin-antitoxin system	Bladder colonization in competitive infection	139
PasT-PasI	Toxin-antitoxin system	Kidney colonization in both competitive and noncompetitive infections; PasT promotes formation of persister cells	139
RqiL	Component of toxin-antitoxin system	GIT colonization	140
GlpG	Protease	Deficient growth in mucus medium (recapitulating the GIT mucus)	141
UpaB	Autotransporter	Bladder colonization 1 dpi	142
TosA	RTX factor	Upper urinary tract, liver, and spleen adherence	143
UpaH	Autotransporter	Bladder infection (from competitive studies); biofilm formation (CFT073)	144
neaT	Acyltransferase gene	Bacteremia	145

[a]GIT, gastrointestinal tract; dpi, day postinfection.

ferent environment than it would normally (30). For example, it has been shown that timing of infection postcatheterization can affect initial UPEC colonization (109). Furthermore, work has shown that implanted bladders exhibit lower IBC burdens than nonimplanted bladders while remaining morphologically similar. Nonetheless, implanted bladders exhibit greater exfoliation than the nonimplanted bladders, suggesting that the reduction of IBC burden results from this exfoliation phenomenon. Additionally, the mere presence of an implant activates bacteria in QIRs of previously infected mice, resulting in recurrence of infection.

This study also identified FimH as a virulence factor in CAUTI (30). Deletion of FimH reduced infectious burden in implanted mouse bladders and correspondingly affected biofilm formation *in vitro* and bacterial colonization of the implant itself. However, this study suggests that factors other than FimH could play a role in this pathogenesis (30).

TREATMENT STRATEGIES FOR UROGENITAL INFECTIONS

Antibiotic Resistance
Antibiotic resistance of UTI-causing bacteria has increased in recent years. UTIs became more difficult to treat from 1999 to 2010 according to the Drug Resis-

tance Index, which evaluates the degree of difficulty in the treatment of infections, with this trend being attributed to increasing antibiotic resistance (112). In the United Kingdom, resistance to trimethoprim specifically has become prevalent in uropathogens (27). One example of a general antibiotic resistance phenotype is ST131. ST131 represents a group of strains of extraintestinal *E. coli* exhibiting multidrug resistance (51, 113, 114). These strains exhibit resistance to beta-lactams and fluoroquinolones and, indeed, seem to be driving antibiotic resistance globally (113). Such strains have become pandemic, with isolates being identified across the globe (51, 113–115), causing, among other infections, UTIs and bacteremia (115).

Novel Lines of Treatment

Vaccines
With the substantial health care burden UTIs cause, vaccine development has become an important pillar in the effort to reduce and prevent the disease burden. Such work has leveraged current understandings of virulence factors. One group of factors targeted in vaccine development is bacterial adhesins, including FimH, FmlH, pilus, PapG, and EbpA. IgG antibodies to FimH, generated in response to vaccination with FimCH in mice and cynomolgus monkeys, were shown to protect against UTI (116, 117). It has been postulated that the

antibodies' effect is based on its ability to prevent bacterial colonization by FimH-tipped type 1 pili (116). Additionally, a FimCH experimental vaccine recently completed a phase 1a/1b trial. Vaccination of two different cohorts, whose members had a 24-month history of rUTI upon enrollment, resulted in 74% and 70% reductions in total UTI once FimH immunity was achieved. For UTIs caused specifically by *E. coli* and *Klebsiella*, 70% and 87% reductions, respectively, were observed (Gary Eldridge, personal communication). Based on these promising results, the FDA has allowed compassionate use of the vaccine for patients suffering from infections caused by multidrug-resistant UPEC strains.

Vaccination of mice with FmlH^{AD} (the lectin domain of the two-domain FmlH adhesin protein) prior to infection with CFT073 significantly decreased bladder and kidney bacterial burden 2 and 3 days after infection in mice (46). P pili, tipped with the PapG adhesin, have been shown to play a critical role in pyelonephritis in cynomolgus monkeys (75). IgG antibodies are produced when cynomolgus monkeys are vaccinated with PapDG (118). No difference in bacteriuria between vaccinated and nonvaccinated monkeys was observed, but histologically, with the exception of mononuclear cells, vaccinated monkeys exhibited none of the other recorded signs of kidney pathology, with a subset of these categories proving statistically significant, while each of these signs of pathology was found in a proportion of nonvaccinated control monkeys (118).

Enterococci express Ebp pili that are tipped with EbpA, which is a fibrinogen-binding adhesin. Urinary catheterization results in the release of fibrinogen, which subsequently coats the catheter. *Enterococcus* uses EbpA to bind to and form biofilms on the fibrinogen-coated catheter. Recent evidence has shown that antibodies to the N-terminal domain of EbpA can prevent and treat *Enterococcus*-mediated CAUTI (108). However, in a mouse model, a history of *Enterococcus* infection is not sufficient to reduce future *Enterococcal* infection (108). Beyond harnessing structural components of adhesion for vaccine development, siderophores have been found to be a promising lead. Yersiniabactin and aerobactin conjugated to bovine serum albumin and administered together to immunize mice exhibited reduced kidney colonization and pathology 48 hours postinfection compared to a nonconjugated bovine serum albumin mock vaccination, while bladder colonization and pathology remained similar (119). Vaccination and subsequent boosting with factors involved in the iron uptake are able to reduce murine bladder (LutA and IreA) and kidney (FyuA) colonization 48 hours

postinfection, and further thought has been given to generating multivalent vaccines from these iron uptake proteins (120).

Small-molecule inhibitors

The critical nature of host-pathogen interactions during the course of UPEC pathogenesis has warranted the development of ligand mimetics designed to inhibit adhesion to host tissues or block the biogenesis of CUP pili. The ultimate goal of these compounds is to create novel antibiotic-sparing therapies that selectively deplete UPEC from their various habitats in the host.

Mannosides

Mannosides are compounds developed to be ligand mimetics to the FimH adhesin that tips the type 1 pilus, which is important for establishing bladder infections (34, 121, 122). Built on a biphenyl scaffold linked to a mannose moiety, early iterations of mannosides with various substituent groups were developed and evaluated for the ability to inhibit type 1-mediated biofilm formation (122). Early iterations of mannosides demonstrated greatly improved inhibitory activity relative to methyl-α-mannose, with an increase in potency of hemagglutination inhibition on the order of approximately 10^5- to 10^7-fold (31, 34). An initially optimized compound showed, in a murine model, the ability to (i) reduce bacterial titers in bladders, both luminally and intracellularly, when administered prophylactically; (ii) efficaciously treat UTIs after oral delivery; and (iii) improve the ability of trimethoprim-sulfamethoxazole (TMP-SMX), an antibiotic, to reduce bladder bacterial load (122). Mannoside ZFH-04269 was able to render a TMP-SMX-resistant ST131 strain, EC958, sensitive to TMP-SMX treatment by preventing invasion of UPEC into the bladder epithelium, thus exposing the luminal UPEC to concentrations of TMP-SMX above the MIC (123).

Structural data and inhibitory assays suggest that interactions with the tyrosine gate associated with the binding pocket on the FimH lectin domain, composed of Tyr48 and Tyr137 and a hydrophobic region, Ile13, would generate more potent inhibitory compounds (121, 124). Continued optimization has looked to improve the stability of originally O-linked mannosides, by replacing the O linkage located between the biphenyl scaffold and alpha-D-mannose moiety with a C linkage (121). Iterations of C-linked mannosides showed improved ability to prevent and treat infections in mice (121). Moreover, in mice, oral mannoside treatment reduces intestinal colonization of genetically diverse UPEC isolates, while simultaneously treating UTI, without significantly disrupting the structural configuration of the gut microbiota. By selectively depleting the intestinal UPEC reservoir, mannosides could significantly reduce the rate of UTI and rUTI by eradicating the reservoir (47). Recently, a small-molecule compound, which is orally available, has been identified for the prevention and treatment of UTIs (125).

Galactosides

In line with this mannoside work, recent structure-based drug design efforts have resulted in the development of glycomimetic inhibitors of the FmlH adhesin from the Fml/F9 pilus involved in UPEC persistence during bladder inflammation (Fig. 3F) (33, 46). These high-affinity aryl galactosides are able to competitively block binding of the FmlH to its endogenous ligand *in vitro*, in *in vivo* murine models of UTI, and in *ex vivo* binding assays using healthy human kidney tissues (33). This study provides further evidence for the utility of the development of ligand mimetics for efficacious antivirulence strategies.

Pilicides

Pilicides are compounds capable of disrupting pilus biogenesis (126). A pipeline of pilicide development on a bicyclic 2-pyridone base structure has been established, and pilicides have been shown to reduce type 1, P, S, and Dr pilus biogenesis (126–128). Mechanistically, structural studies demonstrate that the pilicide interrupts pilus biogenesis by blocking the targeting of chaperone-subunit complexes to the usher's N terminus (126, 129). Characterization of the effect of pilicides, specifically ec240, found altered gene expression of non-CUP pilus genes, including those involved in motility and iron homeostasis, suggesting a broader antivirulence effect beyond simply pilus biogenesis (127). Such compounds could work in concert with ligand mimetics like mannosides or galactosides and prove efficacious by targeting the formation of the pilus (126) as a whole while also targeting the specific function of the pilus type.

CONCLUSION

UTIs, encompassing a variety of infectious etiologies, represent a significant threat to human health, and work in the field has broadened our understanding of the multifactorial set of determinants that contribute to colonization, pathogenesis, and morbidity. Of great significance to human health is the burden of antibiotic resistance in urinary tract-colonizing microorganisms, which dictates that the field place an increased emphasis on the development of antivirulence strategies. This has led to the targeting of the bacterial machinery necessary for establishing colonization and infection and competitive inhibition of bacterial adhesins critical in host-pathogen interactions. Such work has harnessed the field's knowledge of UTI pathogenesis and promises to deliver relief to those affected.

Acknowledgments. We thank Tom Hannan, Karen Dodson, and Gary Eldridge for their critical feedback on this work, and Roger Klein for his contribution.

Citation. Tamadonfar KO, Omattage NS, Spaulding CN, Hultgren SJ. 2019. Reaching the end of the line: urinary tract infections. Microbiol Spectr 7(3):BAI-0014-2019.

References

1. **Griebling TL.** 2005. Urologic diseases in America project: trends in resource use for urinary tract infections in women. *J Urol* **173:**1281–1287.

2. **Foxman B.** 2014. Urinary tract infection syndromes: occurrence, recurrence, bacteriology, risk factors, and disease burden. *Infect Dis Clin North Am* **28:**1–13.

3. **Foxman B.** 2002. Epidemiology of urinary tract infections: incidence, morbidity, and economic costs. *Am J Med* **113**(Suppl 1A):5–13.

4. **Fowler CJ, Griffiths D, de Groat WC.** 2008. The neural control of micturition. *Nat Rev Neurosci* **9:**453–466.

5. **Elbadawi A.** 1996. Functional anatomy of the organs of micturition. *Urol Clin North Am* **23:**177–210.

6. **Macarak EJ, Howard PS.** 1999. The role of collagen in bladder filling. *Adv Exp Med Biol* **462:**215–223, 225–233.

7. **Hickling DR, Sun TT, Wu XR.** 2015. Anatomy and physiology of the urinary tract: relation to host defense and microbial infection. *Microbiol Spectr* **3:**UTI-0016-2012.

8. **Khandelwal P, Abraham SN, Apodaca G.** 2009. Cell biology and physiology of the uroepithelium. *Am J Physiol Renal Physiol* **297:**F1477–F1501.

9. **Kachar B, Liang F, Lins U, Ding M, Wu XR, Stoffler D, Aebi U, Sun TT.** 1999. Three-dimensional analysis of the 16 nm urothelial plaque particle: luminal surface exposure, preferential head-to-head interaction, and hinge formation. *J Mol Biol* **285:**595–608.

10. **Vergara J, Longley W, Robertson JD.** 1969. A hexagonal arrangement of subunits in membrane of mouse urinary bladder. *J Mol Biol* **46:**593–596.

11. **Hicks RM, Ketterer B.** 1969. Hexagonal lattice of subunits in the thick luminal membrane of the rat urinary bladder. *Nature* **224:**1304–1305.

12. **Taylor KA, Robertson JD.** 1984. Analysis of the three-dimensional structure of the urinary bladder epithelial cell membranes. *J Ultrastruct Res* **87:**23–30.

13. **Walz T, Häner M, Wu XR, Henn C, Engel A, Sun TT, Aebi U.** 1995. Towards the molecular architecture of the asymmetric unit membrane of the mammalian urinary bladder epithelium: a closed "twisted ribbon" structure. *J Mol Biol* **248:**887–900.

14. Wu XR, Kong XP, Pellicer A, Kreibich G, Sun TT. 2009. Uroplakins in urothelial biology, function, and disease. *Kidney Int* **75**:1153–1165.

15. Ho PL, Kurtova A, Chan KS. 2012. Normal and neoplastic urothelial stem cells: getting to the root of the problem. *Nat Rev Urol* **9**:583–594.

16. Shin K, Lee J, Guo N, Kim J, Lim A, Qu L, Mysorekar IU, Beachy PA. 2011. Hedgehog/Wnt feedback supports regenerative proliferation of epithelial stem cells in bladder. *Nature* **472**:110–114.

17. O'Grady F, Cattell WR. 1966. Kinetics of urinary tract infection. II. The bladder. *Br J Urol* **38**:156–162.

18. Thomas-White K, Forster SC, Kumar N, Van Kuiken M, Putonti C, Stares MD, Hilt EE, Price TK, Wolfe AJ, Lawley TD. 2018. Culturing of female bladder bacteria reveals an interconnected urogenital microbiota. *Nat Commun* **9**:1557.

19. Ronald A. 2003. The etiology of urinary tract infection: traditional and emerging pathogens. *Dis Mon* **49**: 71–82.

20. Scholes D, Hooton TM, Roberts PL, Stapleton AE, Gupta K, Stamm WE. 2000. Risk factors for recurrent urinary tract infection in young women. *J Infect Dis* **182**:1177–1182.

21. Nicolle LE. 2015. Asymptomatic bacteriuria and bacterial interference. *Microbiol Spectr* **3**:UTI-0001-2012.

22. Sedor J, Mulholland SG. 1999. Hospital-acquired urinary tract infections associated with the indwelling catheter. *Urol Clin North Am* **26**:821–828.

23. Edwards JR, Peterson KD, Mu Y, Banerjee S, Allen-Bridson K, Morrell G, Dudeck MA, Pollock DA, Horan TC. 2009. National Healthcare Safety Network (NHSN) report: data summary for 2006 through 2008, issued December 2009. *Am J Infect Control* **37**:783–805.

24. Flores-Mireles AL, Walker JN, Caparon M, Hultgren SJ. 2015. Urinary tract infections: epidemiology, mechanisms of infection and treatment options. *Nat Rev Microbiol* **13**:269–284.

25. Kang CI, Kim J, Park DW, Kim BN, Ha US, Lee SJ, Yeo JK, Min SK, Lee H, Wie SH. 2018. Clinical practice guidelines for the antibiotic treatment of community-acquired urinary tract infections. *Infect Chemother* **50**:67–100.

26. Mazzulli T. 2002. Resistance trends in urinary tract pathogens and impact on management. *J Urol* **168**: 1720–1722.

27. Public Health England. 2017. *English Surveillance Programme for Antimicrobial Utilisation and Resistance (ESPAUR): Report 2017.* Public Health England, London, United Kingdom.

28. Schreiber HL IV, Conover MS, Chou WC, Hibbing ME, Manson AL, Dodson KW, Hannan TJ, Roberts PL, Stapleton AE, Hooton TM, Livny J, Earl AM, Hultgren SJ. 2017. Bacterial virulence phenotypes of *Escherichia coli* and host susceptibility determine risk for urinary tract infections. *Sci Transl Med* **9**:eaaf1283.

29. O'Brien VP, Hannan TJ, Yu L, Livny J, Roberson ED, Schwartz DJ, Souza S, Mendelsohn CL, Colonna M, Lewis AL, Hultgren SJ. 2016. A mucosal imprint left by prior *Escherichia coli* bladder infection sensitizes to recurrent disease. *Nat Microbiol* **2**:16196.

30. Guiton PS, Cusumano CK, Kline KA, Dodson KW, Han Z, Janetka JW, Henderson JP, Caparon MG, Hultgren SJ. 2012. Combinatorial small-molecule therapy prevents uropathogenic *Escherichia coli* catheter-associated urinary tract infections in mice. *Antimicrob Agents Chemother* **56**:4738–4745.

31. Spaulding CN, Hultgren SJ. 2016. Adhesive pili in UTI pathogenesis and drug development. *Pathogens* **5**:30.

32. Schwartz DJ, Kalas V, Pinkner JS, Chen SL, Spaulding CN, Dodson KW, Hultgren SJ. 2013. Positively selected FimH residues enhance virulence during urinary tract infection by altering FimH conformation. *Proc Natl Acad Sci USA* **110**:15530–15537.

33. Kalas V, Hibbing ME, Maddirala AR, Chugani R, Pinkner JS, Mydock-McGrane LK, Conover MS, Janetka JW, Hultgren SJ. 2018. Structure-based discovery of glycomimetic FmlH ligands as inhibitors of bacterial adhesion during urinary tract infection. *Proc Natl Acad Sci USA* **115**:E2819–E2828.

34. Han Z, Pinkner JS, Ford B, Obermann R, Nolan W, Wildman SA, Hobbs D, Ellenberger T, Cusumano CK, Hultgren SJ, Janetka JW. 2010. Structure-based drug design and optimization of mannoside bacterial FimH antagonists. *J Med Chem* **53**:4779–4792.

35. Eto DS, Jones TA, Sundsbak JL, Mulvey MA. 2007. Integrin-mediated host cell invasion by type 1-piliated uropathogenic *Escherichia coli*. *PLoS Pathog* **3**:e100.

36. Zhou G, Mo WJ, Sebbel P, Min G, Neubert TA, Glockshuber R, Wu XR, Sun TT, Kong XP. 2001. Uroplakin Ia is the urothelial receptor for uropathogenic *Escherichia coli*: evidence from in vitro FimH binding. *J Cell Sci* **114**:4095–4103.

37. Martinez JJ, Mulvey MA, Schilling JD, Pinkner JS, Hultgren SJ. 2000. Type 1 pilus-mediated bacterial invasion of bladder epithelial cells. *EMBO J* **19**: 2803–2812.

38. Martinez JJ, Hultgren SJ. 2002. Requirement of Rho-family GTPases in the invasion of type 1-piliated uropathogenic *Escherichia coli*. *Cell Microbiol* **4**:19–28.

39. Hannan TJ, Mysorekar IU, Hung CS, Isaacson-Schmid ML, Hultgren SJ. 2010. Early severe inflammatory responses to uropathogenic *E. coli* predispose to chronic and recurrent urinary tract infection. *PLoS Pathog* **6**: e1001042.

40. Hannan TJ, Roberts PL, Riehl TE, van der Post S, Binkley JM, Schwartz DJ, Miyoshi H, Mack M, Schwendener RA, Hooton TM, Stappenbeck TS, Hansson GC, Stenson WF, Colonna M, Stapleton AE, Hultgren SJ. 2014. Inhibition of cyclooxygenase-2 prevents chronic and recurrent cystitis. *EBioMedicine* **1**: 46–57.

41. Song J, Bishop BL, Li G, Grady R, Stapleton A, Abraham SN. 2009. TLR4-mediated expulsion of bacteria from infected bladder epithelial cells. *Proc Natl Acad Sci USA* **106**:14966–14971.

42. Nagamatsu K, Hannan TJ, Guest RL, Kostakioti M, Hadjifrangiskou M, Binkley J, Dodson K, Raivio TL,

Hultgren SJ. 2015. Dysregulation of *Escherichia coli* α-hemolysin expression alters the course of acute and persistent urinary tract infection. *Proc Natl Acad Sci USA* 112:E871–E880.

43. Choi HW, Bowen SE, Miao Y, Chan CY, Miao EA, Abrink M, Moeser AJ, Abraham SN. 2016. Loss of bladder epithelium induced by cytolytic mast cell granules. *Immunity* 45:1258–1269.

44. Mysorekar IU, Hultgren SJ. 2006. Mechanisms of uropathogenic *Escherichia coli* persistence and eradication from the urinary tract. *Proc Natl Acad Sci USA* 103:14170–14175.

45. Chan CY, St John AL, Abraham SN. 2013. Mast cell interleukin-10 drives localized tolerance in chronic bladder infection. *Immunity* 38:349–359.

46. Conover MS, Ruer S, Taganna J, Kalas V, De Greve H, Pinkner JS, Dodson KW, Remaut H, Hultgren SJ. 2016. Inflammation-induced adhesin-receptor interaction provides a fitness advantage to uropathogenic *E. coli* during chronic infection. *Cell Host Microbe* 20:482–492.

47. Spaulding CN, Klein RD, Ruer S, Kau AL, Schreiber HL, Cusumano ZT, Dodson KW, Pinkner JS, Fremont DH, Janetka JW, Remaut H, Gordon JI, Hultgren SJ. 2017. Selective depletion of uropathogenic *E. coli* from the gut by a FimH antagonist. *Nature* 546:528–532.

48. Moreno E, Andreu A, Pigrau C, Kuskowski MA, Johnson JR, Prats G. 2008. Relationship between *Escherichia coli* strains causing acute cystitis in women and the fecal *E. coli* population of the host. *J Clin Microbiol* 46:2529–2534.

49. Chen SL, Wu M, Henderson JP, Hooton TM, Hibbing ME, Hultgren SJ, Gordon JI. 2013. Genomic diversity and fitness of *E. coli* strains recovered from the intestinal and urinary tracts of women with recurrent urinary tract infection. *Sci Transl Med* 5:184ra60.

50. Russell CW, Fleming BA, Jost CA, Tran A, Stenquist AT, Wambaugh MA, Bronner MP, Mulvey MA. 2018. Context-dependent requirements for FimH and other canonical virulence factors in gut colonization by extra-intestinal pathogenic *Escherichia coli*. *Infect Immun* 86:e00746-17.

51. Sarkar S, Hutton ML, Vagenas D, Ruter R, Schüller S, Lyras D, Schembri MA, Totsika M. 2018. Intestinal colonization traits of pandemic multidrug-resistant *Escherichia coli* ST131. *J Infect Dis* 218:979–990.

52. Hannan TJ, Totsika M, Mansfield KJ, Moore KH, Schembri MA, Hultgren SJ. 2012. Host-pathogen checkpoints and population bottlenecks in persistent and intracellular uropathogenic *Escherichia coli* bladder infection. *FEMS Microbiol Rev* 36:616–648.

53. Chen SL, Hung CS, Pinkner JS, Walker JN, Cusumano CK, Li Z, Bouckaert J, Gordon JI, Hultgren SJ. 2009. Positive selection identifies an in vivo role for FimH during urinary tract infection in addition to mannose binding. *Proc Natl Acad Sci USA* 106:22439–22444.

54. Conover MS, Hadjifrangiskou M, Palermo JJ, Hibbing ME, Dodson KW, Hultgren SJ. 2016. Metabolic requirements of *Escherichia coli* in intracellular bacterial

communities during urinary tract infection pathogenesis. *mBio* 7:e00104-16.

55. Schwartz DJ, Chen SL, Hultgren SJ, Seed PC. 2011. Population dynamics and niche distribution of uropathogenic *Escherichia coli* during acute and chronic urinary tract infection. *Infect Immun* 79:4250–4259.

56. Duraiswamy S, Chee JLY, Chen S, Yang E, Lees K, Chen SL. 2018. Purification of intracellular bacterial communities during experimental urinary tract infection reveals an abundant and viable bacterial reservoir. *Infect Immun* 86:e00740-17.

57. Robino L, Scavone P, Araujo L, Algorta G, Zunino P, Vignoli R. 2013. Detection of intracellular bacterial communities in a child with *Escherichia coli* recurrent urinary tract infections. *Pathog Dis* 68:78–81.

58. Rosen DA, Hooton TM, Stamm WE, Humphrey PA, Hultgren SJ. 2007. Detection of intracellular bacterial communities in human urinary tract infection. *PLoS Med* 4:e329.

59. Waksman G, Hultgren SJ. 2009. Structural biology of the chaperone-usher pathway of pilus biogenesis. *Nat Rev Microbiol* 7:765–774.

60. Wright KJ, Seed PC, Hultgren SJ. 2007. Development of intracellular bacterial communities of uropathogenic *Escherichia coli* depends on type 1 pili. *Cell Microbiol* 9:2230–2241.

61. Reigstad CS, Hultgren SJ, Gordon JI. 2007. Functional genomic studies of uropathogenic *Escherichia coli* and host urothelial cells when intracellular bacterial communities are assembled. *J Biol Chem* 282:21259–21267.

62. Blango MG, Ott EM, Erman A, Veranic P, Mulvey MA. 2014. Forced resurgence and targeting of intracellular uropathogenic *Escherichia coli* reservoirs. *PLoS One* 9:e93327.

63. Gilbert NM, O'Brien VP, Lewis AL. 2017. Transient microbiota exposures activate dormant *Escherichia coli* infection in the bladder and drive severe outcomes of recurrent disease. *PLoS Pathog* 13:e1006238.

64. Eto DS, Sundsbak JL, Mulvey MA. 2006. Actin-gated intracellular growth and resurgence of uropathogenic *Escherichia coli*. *Cell Microbiol* 8:704–717.

65. Alteri CJ, Smith SN, Mobley HL. 2009. Fitness of *Escherichia coli* during urinary tract infection requires gluconeogenesis and the TCA cycle. *PLoS Pathog* 5:e1000448.

66. Hull RA, Hull SI. 1997. Nutritional requirements for growth of uropathogenic *Escherichia coli* in human urine. *Infect Immun* 65:1960–1961.

67. Henderson JP, Crowley JR, Pinkner JS, Walker JN, Tsukayama P, Stamm WE, Hooton TM, Hultgren SJ. 2009. Quantitative metabolomics reveals an epigenetic blueprint for iron acquisition in uropathogenic *Escherichia coli*. *PLoS Pathog* 5:e1000305.

68. O'Brien VP, Hannan TJ, Nielsen HV, Hultgren SJ. 2016. Drug and vaccine development for the treatment and prevention of urinary tract infections. *Microbiol Spectr* 4:UTI-0013-2012.

69. Guyer DM, Radulovic S, Jones FE, Mobley HL. 2002. Sat, the secreted autotransporter toxin of uropatho-

genic *Escherichia coli*, is a vacuolating cytotoxin for bladder and kidney epithelial cells. *Infect Immun* 70: 4539–4546.

70. Lane MC, Alteri CJ, Smith SN, Mobley HL. 2007. Expression of flagella is coincident with uropathogenic *Escherichia coli* ascension to the upper urinary tract. *Proc Natl Acad Sci USA* 104:16669–16674.

71. Hagan EC, Lloyd AL, Rasko DA, Faerber GJ, Mobley HL. 2010. *Escherichia coli* global gene expression in urine from women with urinary tract infection. *PLoS Pathog* 6:e1001187.

72. Greene SE, Hibbing ME, Janetka J, Chen SL, Hultgren SJ. 2015. Human urine decreases function and expression of type 1 pili in uropathogenic *Escherichia coli*. *mBio* 6:e00820-15.

73. Ronald AR, Nicolle LE, Stamm E, Krieger J, Warren J, Schaeffer A, Naber KG, Hooton TM, Johnson J, Chambers S, Andriole V. 2001. Urinary tract infection in adults: research priorities and strategies. *Int J Antimicrob Agents* 17:343–348.

74. Melican K, Sandoval RM, Kader A, Josefsson L, Tanner GA, Molitoris BA, Richter-Dahlfors A. 2011. Uropathogenic *Escherichia coli* P and type 1 fimbriae act in synergy in a living host to facilitate renal colonization leading to nephron obstruction. *PLoS Pathog* 7: e1001298.

75. Roberts JA, Marklund BI, Ilver D, Haslam D, Kaack MB, Baskin G, Louis M, Möllby R, Winberg J, Normark S. 1994. The Gal(alpha 1-4)Gal-specific tip adhesin of *Escherichia coli* P-fimbriae is needed for pyelonephritis to occur in the normal urinary tract. *Proc Natl Acad Sci USA* 91:11889–11893.

76. Abraham SN, Sun D, Dale JB, Beachey EH. 1988. Conservation of the D-mannose-adhesion protein among type 1 fimbriated members of the family *Enterobacteriaceae*. *Nature* 336:682–684.

77. Nuccio SP, Bäumler AJ. 2007. Evolution of the chaperone/usher assembly pathway: fimbrial classification goes Greek. *Microbiol Mol Biol Rev* 71:551–575.

78. Subashchandrabose S, Hazen TH, Brumbaugh AR, Himpsl SD, Smith SN, Ernst RD, Rasko DA, Mobley HL. 2014. Host-specific induction of *Escherichia coli* fitness genes during human urinary tract infection. *Proc Natl Acad Sci USA* 111:18327–18332.

79. Lim JK, Gunther NW IV, Zhao H, Johnson DE, Keay SK, Mobley HL. 1998. In vivo phase variation of *Escherichia coli* type 1 fimbrial genes in women with urinary tract infection. *Infect Immun* 66:3303–3310.

80. Gunther NW IV, Lockatell V, Johnson DE, Mobley HL. 2001. In vivo dynamics of type 1 fimbria regulation in uropathogenic *Escherichia coli* during experimental urinary tract infection. *Infect Immun* 69:2838–2846.

81. Hultgren SJ, Porter TN, Schaeffer AJ, Duncan JL. 1985. Role of type 1 pili and effects of phase variation on lower urinary tract infections produced by *Escherichia coli*. *Infect Immun* 50:370–377.

82. Forsyth VS, Armbruster CE, Smith SN, Pirani A, Springman AC, Walters MS, Nielubowicz GR, Himpsl SD, Snitkin ES, Mobley HLT. 2018. Rapid growth of

uropathogenic *Escherichia coli* during human urinary tract infection. *mBio* 9:e00186-18.

83. Phan G, Remaut H, Wang T, Allen WJ, Pirker KF, Lebedev A, Henderson NS, Geibel S, Volkan E, Yan J, Kunze MB, Pinkner JS, Ford B, Kay CW, Li H, Hultgren SJ, Thanassi DG, Waksman G. 2011. Crystal structure of the FimD usher bound to its cognate FimC-FimH substrate. *Nature* 474:49–53.

84. Geibel S, Procko E, Hultgren SJ, Baker D, Waksman G. 2013. Structural and energetic basis of folded-protein transport by the FimD usher. *Nature* 496:243–246.

85. Farabella I, Pham T, Henderson NS, Geibel S, Phan G, Thanassi DG, Delcour AH, Waksman G, Topf M. 2014. Allosteric signalling in the outer membrane translocation domain of PapC usher. *eLife* 3:e03532.

86. Mapingire OS, Henderson NS, Duret G, Thanassi DG, Delcour AH. 2009. Modulating effects of the plug, helix, and N- and C-terminal domains on channel properties of the PapC usher. *J Biol Chem* 284:36324–36333.

87. Pham T, Henderson NS, Werneburg GT, Thanassi DG, Delcour AH. 2015. Electrostatic networks control plug stabilization in the PapC usher. *Mol Membr Biol* 32: 198–207.

88. Remaut H, Tang C, Henderson NS, Pinkner JS, Wang T, Hultgren SJ, Thanassi DG, Waksman G, Li H. 2008. Fiber formation across the bacterial outer membrane by the chaperone/usher pathway. *Cell* 133: 640–652.

89. Saulino ET, Thanassi DG, Pinkner JS, Hultgren SJ. 1998. Ramifications of kinetic partitioning on usher-mediated pilus biogenesis. *EMBO J* 17:2177–2185.

90. Volkan E, Ford BA, Pinkner JS, Dodson KW, Henderson NS, Thanassi DG, Waksman G, Hultgren SJ. 2012. Domain activities of PapC usher reveal the mechanism of action of an *Escherichia coli* molecular machine. *Proc Natl Acad Sci USA* 109:9563–9568.

91. Volkan E, Kalas V, Pinkner JS, Dodson KW, Henderson NS, Pham T, Waksman G, Delcour AH, Thanassi DG, Hultgren SJ. 2013. Molecular basis of usher pore gating in *Escherichia coli* pilus biogenesis. *Proc Natl Acad Sci USA* 110:20741–20746.

92. Spaulding CN, Schreiber HL IV, Zheng W, Dodson KW, Hazen JE, Conover MS, Wang F, Svenmarker P, Luna-Rico A, Francetic O, Andersson M, Hultgren S, Egelman EH. 2018. Functional role of the type 1 pilus rod structure in mediating host-pathogen interactions. *eLife* 7:e31662.

93. Hospenthal MK, Zyla D, Costa TRD, Redzej A, Giese C, Lillington J, Glockshuber R, Waksman G. 2017. The cryoelectron microscopy structure of the type 1 chaperone-usher pilus rod. *Structure* 25:1829–1838.e4.

94. Hospenthal MK, Redzej A, Dodson K, Ukleja M, Frenz B, Rodrigues C, Hultgren SJ, DiMaio F, Egelman EH, Waksman G. 2016. Structure of a chaperone-usher pilus reveals the molecular basis of rod uncoiling. *Cell* 164:269–278.

95. Kalas V, Pinkner JS, Hannan TJ, Hibbing ME, Dodson KW, Holehouse AS, Zhang H, Tolia NH, Gross ML, Pappu RV, Janetka J, Hultgren SJ. 2017. Evolutionary

fine-tuning of conformational ensembles in FimH during host-pathogen interactions. *Sci Adv* 3:e1601944.

96. Bahrani-Mougeot FK, Buckles EL, Lockatell CV, Hebel JR, Johnson DE, Tang CM, Donnenberg MS. 2002. Type 1 fimbriae and extracellular polysaccharides are preeminent uropathogenic *Escherichia coli* virulence determinants in the murine urinary tract. *Mol Microbiol* 45:1079–1093.

97. Buckles EL, Wang X, Lane MC, Lockatell CV, Johnson DE, Rasko DA, Mobley HL, Donnenberg MS. 2009. Role of the K2 capsule in *Escherichia coli* urinary tract infection and serum resistance. *J Infect Dis* 199:1689–1697.

98. Burns SM, Hull SI. 1999. Loss of resistance to ingestion and phagocytic killing by O$^-$ and K$^-$ mutants of a uropathogenic *Escherichia coli* O75:K5 strain. *Infect Immun* 67:3757–3762.

99. Anderson GG, Goller CC, Justice S, Hultgren SJ, Seed PC. 2010. Polysaccharide capsule and sialic acid-mediated regulation promote biofilm-like intracellular bacterial communities during cystitis. *Infect Immun* 78:963–975.

100. Heras B, Totsika M, Peters KM, Paxman JJ, Gee CL, Jarrott RJ, Perugini MA, Whitten AE, Schembri MA. 2014. The antigen 43 structure reveals a molecular Velcro-like mechanism of autotransporter-mediated bacterial clumping. *Proc Natl Acad Sci USA* 111:457–462.

101. Ulett GC, Valle J, Beloin C, Sherlock O, Ghigo JM, Schembri MA. 2007. Functional analysis of antigen 43 in uropathogenic *Escherichia coli* reveals a role in long-term persistence in the urinary tract. *Infect Immun* 75:3233–3244.

102. Klein RD, Shu Q, Cusumano ZT, Nagamatsu K, Gualberto NC, Lynch AJL, Wu C, Wang W, Jain N, Pinkner JS, Amarasinghe GK, Hultgren SJ, Frieden C, Chapman MR. 2018. Structure-function analysis of the curli accessory protein CsgE defines surfaces essential for coordinating amyloid fiber formation. *mBio* 9:e01349-18.

103. Kai-Larsen Y, Lüthje P, Chromek M, Peters V, Wang X, Holm A, Kádas L, Hedlund KO, Johansson J, Chapman MR, Jacobson SH, Römling U, Agerberth B, Brauner A. 2010. Uropathogenic *Escherichia coli* modulates immune responses and its curli fimbriae interact with the antimicrobial peptide LL-37. *PLoS Pathog* 6:e1001010.

104. Ingersoll MA. 2017. Sex differences shape the response to infectious diseases. *PLoS Pathog* 13:e1006688.

105. Lüthje P, Brauner H, Ramos NL, Ovregaard A, Gläser R, Hirschberg AL, Aspenström P, Brauner A. 2013. Estrogen supports urothelial defense mechanisms. *Sci Transl Med* 5:190ra80.

106. Olson PD, Hruska KA, Hunstad DA. 2016. Androgens enhance male urinary tract infection severity in a new model. *J Am Soc Nephrol* 27:1625–1634.

107. Zychlinsky Scharff A, Albert ML, Ingersoll MA. 2017. Urinary tract infection in a small animal model: transurethral catheterization of male and female mice. *J Vis Exp* 2017:e54432.

108. Flores-Mireles AL, Walker JN, Potretzke A, Schreiber HL IV, Pinkner JS, Bauman TM, Park AM, Desai A, Hultgren SJ, Caparon MG. 2016. Antibody-based therapy for enterococcal catheter-associated urinary tract infections. *mBio* 7:e01653-16.

109. Rousseau M, Goh HMS, Holec S, Albert ML, Williams RB, Ingersoll MA, Kline KA. 2016. Bladder catheterization increases susceptibility to infection that can be prevented by prophylactic antibiotic treatment. *JCI Insight* 1:e88178.

110. Walker JN, Flores-Mireles AL, Pinkner CL, Schreiber HL IV, Joens MS, Park AM, Potretzke AM, Bauman TM, Pinkner JS, Fitzpatrick JAJ, Desai A, Caparon MG, Hultgren SJ. 2017. Catheterization alters bladder ecology to potentiate *Staphylococcus aureus* infection of the urinary tract. *Proc Natl Acad Sci USA* 114:E8721–E8730.

111. Armbruster CE, Forsyth-DeOrnellas V, Johnson AO, Smith SN, Zhao L, Wu W, Mobley HLT. 2017. Genome-wide transposon mutagenesis of *Proteus mirabilis*: essential genes, fitness factors for catheter-associated urinary tract infection, and the impact of polymicrobial infection on fitness requirements. *PLoS Pathog* 13:e1006434.

112. Center for Disease Dynamics, Economics & Policy. 2018. *Drug Resistance Index*. https://resistancemap.cddep.org/DRI.php. Accessed 26 July 2018.

113. Riley LW. 2014. Pandemic lineages of extraintestinal pathogenic *Escherichia coli*. *Clin Microbiol Infect* 20:380–390.

114. Totsika M, Beatson SA, Sarkar S, Phan MD, Petty NK, Bachmann N, Szubert M, Sidjabat HE, Paterson DL, Upton M, Schembri MA. 2011. Insights into a multidrug resistant *Escherichia coli* pathogen of the globally disseminated ST131 lineage: genome analysis and virulence mechanisms. *PLoS One* 6:e26578.

115. Schembri MA, Zakour NL, Phan MD, Forde BM, Stanton-Cook M, Beatson SA. 2015. Molecular characterization of the multidrug resistant *Escherichia coli* ST131 clone. *Pathogens* 4:422–430.

116. Langermann S, Palaszynski S, Barnhart M, Auguste G, Pinkner JS, Burlein J, Barren P, Koenig S, Leath S, Jones CH, Hultgren SJ. 1997. Prevention of mucosal *Escherichia coli* infection by FimH-adhesin-based systemic vaccination. *Science* 276:607–611.

117. Langermann S, Möllby R, Burlein JE, Palaszynski SR, Auguste CG, DeFusco A, Strouse R, Schenerman MA, Hultgren SJ, Pinkner JS, Winberg J, Guldevall L, Söderhäll M, Ishikawa K, Normark S, Koenig S. 2000. Vaccination with FimH adhesin protects cynomolgus monkeys from colonization and infection by uropathogenic *Escherichia coli*. *J Infect Dis* 181:774–778.

118. Roberts JA, Kaack MB, Baskin G, Chapman MR, Hunstad DA, Pinkner JS, Hultgren SJ. 2004. Antibody responses and protection from pyelonephritis following vaccination with purified *Escherichia coli* PapDG protein. *J Urol* 171:1682–1685.

119. Mike LA, Smith SN, Sumner CA, Eaton KA, Mobley HL. 2016. Siderophore vaccine conjugates protect

against uropathogenic *Escherichia coli* urinary tract infection. *Proc Natl Acad Sci USA* 113:13468–13473.

120. Mobley HL, Alteri CJ. 2015. Development of a vaccine against *Escherichia coli* urinary tract infections. *Pathogens* 5:1.

121. Mydock-McGrane L, Cusumano Z, Han Z, Binkley J, Kostakioti M, Hannan T, Pinkner JS, Klein R, Kalas V, Crowley J, Rath NP, Hultgren SJ, Janetka JW. 2016. Antivirulence C-mannosides as antibiotic-sparing, oral therapeutics for urinary tract infections. *J Med Chem* 59:9390–9408.

122. Cusumano CK, Pinkner JS, Han Z, Greene SE, Ford BA, Crowley JR, Henderson JP, Janetka JW, Hultgren SJ. 2011. Treatment and prevention of urinary tract infection with orally active FimH inhibitors. *Sci Transl Med* 3:109ra115.

123. Totsika M, Kostakioti M, Hannan TJ, Upton M, Beatson SA, Janetka JW, Hultgren SJ, Schembri MA. 2013. A FimH inhibitor prevents acute bladder infection and treats chronic cystitis caused by multidrug-resistant uropathogenic *Escherichia coli* ST131. *J Infect Dis* 208:921–928.

124. Han Z, Pinkner JS, Ford B, Chorell E, Crowley JM, Cusumano CK, Campbell S, Henderson JP, Hultgren SJ, Janetka JW. 2012. Lead optimization studies on FimH antagonists: discovery of potent and orally bioavailable ortho-substituted biphenyl mannosides. *J Med Chem* 55:3945–3959.

125. Fimbrion Therapeutics, Inc. 6 December 2018. *Fimbrion and GSK identify novel, antibiotic-sparing development candidate for urinary tract infections.* PR Newswire.

126. Åberg V, Almqvist F. 2007. Pilicides-small molecules targeting bacterial virulence. *Org Biomol Chem* 5: 1827–1834.

127. Greene SE, Pinkner JS, Chorell E, Dodson KW, Shaffer CL, Conover MS, Livny J, Hadjifrangiskou M, Almqvist F, Hultgren SJ. 2014. Pilicide ec240 disrupts virulence circuits in uropathogenic *Escherichia coli*. *mBio* 5:e02038-14.

128. Piatek R, Zalewska-Piatek B, Dzierzbicka K, Makowiec S, Pilipczuk J, Szemiako K, Cyranka-Czaja A, Wojciechowski M. 2013. Pilicides inhibit the FGL chaperone/usher assisted biogenesis of the Dr fimbrial polyadhesin from uropathogenic *Escherichia coli*. *BMC Microbiol* 13:131.

129. Chorell E, Pinkner JS, Phan G, Edvinsson S, Buelens F, Remaut H, Waksman G, Hultgren SJ, Almqvist F. 2010. Design and synthesis of C-2 substituted thiazolo and dihydrothiazolo ring-fused 2-pyridones: pilicides with increased antivirulence activity. *J Med Chem* 53: 5690–5695.

130. Sperandio V, Li CC, Kaper JB. 2002. Quorum-sensing *Escherichia coli* regulator A: a regulator of the LysR family involved in the regulation of the locus of enterocyte effacement pathogenicity island in enterohemorrhagic *E. coli*. *Infect Immun* 70:3085–3093.

131. Alteri CJ, Lindner JR, Reiss DJ, Smith SN, Mobley HL. 2011. The broadly conserved regulator PhoP links pathogen virulence and membrane potential in *Escherichia coli*. *Mol Microbiol* 82:145–163.

132. Clarke MB, Hughes DT, Zhu C, Boedeker EC, Sperandio V. 2006. The QseC sensor kinase: a bacterial adrenergic receptor. *Proc Natl Acad Sci USA* 103: 10420–10425.

133. Debnath I, Norton JP, Barber AE, Ott EM, Dhakal BK, Kulesus RR, Mulvey MA. 2013. The Cpx stress response system potentiates the fitness and virulence of uropathogenic *Escherichia coli*. *Infect Immun* 81: 1450–1459.

134. Guckes KR, Kostakioti M, Breland EJ, Gu AP, Shaffer CL, Martinez CR III, Hultgren SJ, Hadjifrangiskou M. 2013. Strong cross-system interactions drive the activation of the QseB response regulator in the absence of its cognate sensor. *Proc Natl Acad Sci USA* 110: 16592–16597.

135. Kostakioti M, Hadjifrangiskou M, Cusumano CK, Hannan TJ, Janetka JW, Hultgren SJ. 2012. Distinguishing the contribution of type 1 pili from that of other QseB-misregulated factors when QseC is absent during urinary tract infection. *Infect Immun* 80:2826–2834.

136. Doye A, Mettouchi A, Bossis G, Clément R, Buisson-Touati C, Flatau G, Gagnoux L, Piechaczyk M, Boquet P, Lemichez E. 2002. CF1 exploits the ubiquitin-proteasome machinery to restrict Rho GTPase activation for bacterial host cell invasion. *Cell* 111:553–564.

137. Dhakal BK, Mulvey MA. 2012. The UPEC pore-forming toxin α-hemolysin triggers proteolysis of host proteins to disrupt cell adhesion, inflammatory, and survival pathways. *Cell Host Microbe* 11:58–69.

138. Murthy AMV, Phan MD, Peters KM, Nhu NTK, Welch RA, Ulett GC, Schembri MA, Sweet MJ. 2018. Regulation of hemolysin in uropathogenic *Escherichia coli* fine-tunes killing of human macrophages. *Virulence* 9: 967–980.

139. Norton JP, Mulvey MA. 2012. Toxin-antitoxin systems are important for niche-specific colonization and stress resistance of uropathogenic *Escherichia coli*. *PLoS Pathog* 8:e1002954.

140. Russell CW, Mulvey MA. 2015. The extraintestinal pathogenic *Escherichia coli* factor RqlI constrains the genotoxic effects of the RecQ-like helicase RqlH. *PLoS Pathog* 11:e1005317.

141. Russell CW, Richards AC, Chang AS, Mulvey MA. 2017. The rhomboid protease GlpG promotes the persistence of extraintestinal pathogenic *Escherichia coli* within the gut. *Infect Immun* 85:e00866-16.

142. Allsopp LP, Beloin C, Ulett GC, Valle J, Totsika M, Sherlock O, Ghigo JM, Schembri MA. 2012. Molecular characterization of UpaB and UpaC, two new auto-transporter proteins of uropathogenic *Escherichia coli* CFT073. *Infect Immun* 80:321–332.

143. Vigil PD, Wiles TJ, Engstrom MD, Prasov L, Mulvey MA, Mobley HL. 2012. The repeat-in-toxin family member TosA mediates adherence of uropathogenic *Escherichia coli* and survival during bacteremia. *Infect Immun* 80:493–505.

144. Allsopp LP, Totsika M, Tree JJ, Ulett GC, Mabbett AN, Wells TJ, Kobe B, Beatson SA, Schembri MA. 2010. UpaH is a newly identified autotransporter protein that

contributes to biofilm formation and bladder colonization by uropathogenic *Escherichia coli* CFT073. *Infect Immun* 78:1659–1669.

145. Wiles TJ, Norton JP, Smith SN, Lewis AJ, Mobley HL, Casjens SR, Mulvey MA. 2013. A phyletically rare gene promotes the niche-specific fitness of an *E. coli* pathogen during bacteremia. *PLoS Pathog* 9:e1003175.

146. Mulvey MA. 1998. Induction and evasion of host defenses by type 1-piliated uropathogenic *Escherichia coli*. *Science* 282:1494–1497.

Bacteria and Intracellularity
Edited by Pascale Cossart, Craig R. Roy, and Philippe Sansonetti
© 2019 American Society for Microbiology, Washington, DC
doi:10.1128/microbiolspec.BAI-0006-2019

The Intracellular Life Cycle of *Brucella* spp.

7

Jean Celli[1]

THE *BRUCELLA* INTRACELLULAR CYCLE

Brucella Pathogenesis

Bacteria of the genus *Brucella* belong to the alpha-2 subgroup of *Alphaproteobacteria*, a phylogenetic subgroup which includes a variety of bacteria that are either animal or plant pathogens or symbionts. As such, these bacteria have experienced a long-standing coevolution with eukaryotic hosts that has likely shaped their biology. The genus *Brucella* is composed of an increasing number of species that infect a wide variety of mammals as primary hosts, such as bovines (*Brucella abortus*), goats (*B. melitensis*), swine (*B. suis*), ovines (*B. ovis*), camels, elk, bison (*B. abortus*), canines (*B. canis*), rodents (*B. neotomae* and *B. microti*), and monkeys (*B. papionis*), as well as marine mammals such as seals, porpoises, dolphins, and whales (*B. pinnipedialis* and *B. ceti*) and also amphibians (*B. inopinata*) (1). Most species cause in their hosts a disease named brucellosis, which manifests as abortion, sterility, and lameness in animals and which can also be transmitted to humans via inhalation of aerosolized bacteria or via ingestion of, or contact with, contaminated tissues or derived products, classically by the most pathogenic species, *B. melitensis*, *B. suis*, and *B. abortus*, with additional cases due to *B. canis* and *B. neotomae* (2–4). Human brucellosis is characterized by nonspecific flu-like symptoms during an early acute phase, which is followed by a chronic infection with debilitating consequences, including recurrent fever, osteomyelitis, arthritis, neurological symptoms, and endocarditis, if not treated with antibiotic therapy in a timely manner (4). Animal and human brucellosis share common pathophysiological features at the cellular level, where bacteria undergo an intracellular cycle that ensures their survival, proliferation, and persistence within phagocytic cells of various tissues, including macrophages and dendritic cells (4, 5). Initially described in placental tissues of infected animals (6), the ability of *B. abortus* to extensively proliferate in mammalian cells was reproduced in a variety of tissue culture models of epithelial and phagocytic cells that have been instrumental in defining the main features of the bacterium's intracellular cycle (7–12).

A Multistage Intracellular Cycle

Upon entry into either phagocytic or nonphagocytic cells, *Brucella* bacteria are enclosed within a membrane-bound compartment that has been named the *Brucella*-containing vacuole (BCV) (8, 13) (Fig. 1), based on the concept that the original phagosome is functionally modified by the bacterium into an idiosyncratic membrane-bound vacuole. Early microscopy-based trafficking studies established that the initial BCV normally traffics along the endocytic pathway, sequentially acquiring early and then late endosomal membrane markers (7, 8), and becomes acidified, reaching a pH of 4.5 (14–16), consistent with a complete phagosomal maturation process. Based on the endosomal nature of the bacterial vacuole at this stage of the intracellular cycle (between 0 and 8 h postinfection), it was named the endosomal BCV (eBCV) (Fig. 1 and 2A) (17).

Subsequent to eBCV interactions with the endocytic compartment, the vacuole progressively loses endosomal markers (between 8 and 12 h postinfection), concomitant with sustained interactions with endoplasmic reticulum (ER) structures, and eventually acquires ER membrane-associated markers such as calreticulin, calnexin, and Sec61β (7, 8, 13), indicating a turnover of eBCV membranes and accretion of ER-derived membranes. These vacuoles also gain structural and functional features of the ER (7, 8), further indicating a conversion of the eBCV into an ER-derived organelle. These structural and

---

[1]Paul G. Allen School for Global Animal Health, Washington State University, Pullman, WA 99164.

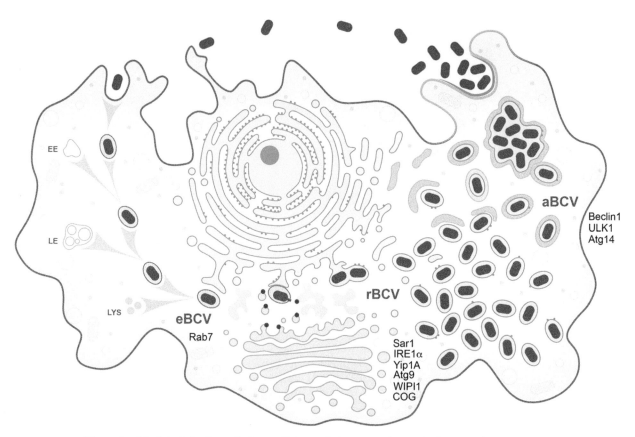

Figure 1 Model of the *Brucella* intracellular cycle in macrophages. Following phagocytic uptake by macrophages, *Brucella* spp. reside during the first 8 to 12 h postinfection within a membrane-bound vacuole that undergoes endosomal maturation via sequential interactions with early (EE) and late (LE) endosomes and lysosomes (LYS) to become an acidified eBCV. The host small GTPase Rab7 contributes to eBCV maturation, which provides physicochemical cues promoting expression of the VirB T4SS, which translocates effector proteins (red) that mediate eBCV interactions with the ER exit site and acquisition of ER and Golgi apparatus-derived membranes. These events lead to the biogenesis of replication permissive, ER-derived BCVs, called rBCVs. The host proteins Sar1, IRE1α, Yip1A, Atg9, and WIPI1 and the COG complex contribute to rBCV biogenesis. Bacteria then undergo extensive replication in rBCVs between 12 and 48 h postinfection, after which rBCVs are captured within autophagosome-like structures in a VirB T4SS-dependent manner to become aBCVs. aBCV formation requires the host autophagy proteins beclin1, ULK1, and Atg14. aBCVs harbor features of autolysosomes and are required for bacterial egress and new cycles of intracellular infections.

functional changes correlate with the onset of bacterial replication, suggesting that these organelles provide intracellular conditions that promote bacterial growth and replication. Based on these considerations, these vacuoles were named replicative BCVs (rBCVs) (Fig. 1 and 2B) (17). Original ultrastructural characterizations of rBCVs suggested that these vacuoles were individual and rarely connected with ER cisternae in either macrophage or HeLa cells (7, 8) (Fig. 2D), while other studies observed bacteria within the ER lumen of trophoblasts (6), leaving the actual organization of rBCVs uncertain. Recent electron tomography three-dimensional reconstruction of

rBCVs clearly determined that these vacuoles are intricately connected with the ER and also seem to interact with vesicular traffic between the ER and the Golgi apparatus (18), demonstrating intimate interactions with the host secretory pathway. The rBCV stage is tightly associated with bacterial proliferation (between 12 and 48 h postinfection) and causes a dramatic reorganization of the host cell ER into the rBCV network (8).

Following extensive bacterial replication, an additional stage in the *Brucella* intracellular cycle consists of the progressive capture of rBCVs by crescent-like membrane structures, leading to the formation of multi-

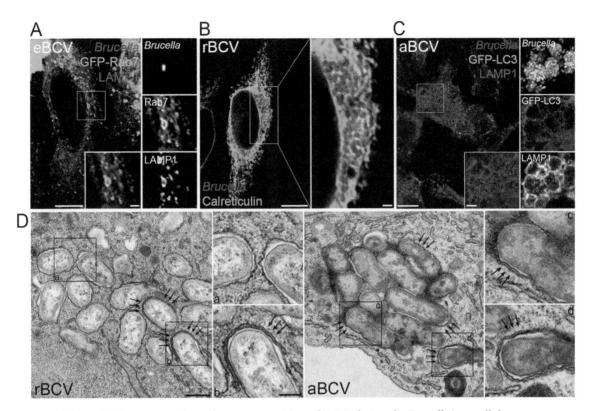

Figure 2 Structure and membrane composition of BCVs during the *Brucella* intracellular cycle. (**A**) Confocal fluorescence micrograph of HeLa cells expressing green fluorescent protein (GFP)-Rab7 and infected with DsRed$_m$-expressing *B. abortus* strain 2308 for 6 h. The inset shows an eBCV with the typical accumulation of the late endosomal/lysosomal markers Rab7 and LAMP1. Bars, 10 and 2 μm. (**B**) Confocal fluorescence micrograph of a HeLa cell infected with DsRed$_m$-expressing *B. abortus* strain 2308 for 24 h and stained for the ER marker calreticulin. The inset shows a cluster of calreticulin-positive rBCVs containing replicating bacteria and associated with the ER network. Bars, 10 and 1 μm. (**C**) Confocal fluorescence micrograph of a primary murine bone marrow-derived macrophage expressing the autophagy marker GFP-LC3 and infected with DsRed$_m$-expressing *B. abortus* strain 2308 for 72 h. The inset shows a group of aBCVs with the typical accumulation of the late endosomal/lysosomal LAMP1 but not LC3. Bars, 10 and 2 μm. (**D**) Transmission electron micrographs of bone marrow-derived macrophages infected with *B. abortus* strain 2308 for 72 h and showing the ultrastructures of rBCVs (left, single-membrane-bound vacuoles [inset a]), of forming aBCVs (inset b and arrows), and of completed double-membrane-bound aBCVs (right [insets c and d and arrows]). Bars, 500 and 200 nm. Reprinted from reference 17 with permission.

membrane vacuoles that are structurally reminiscent of autophagosomes that contain small to large groups of bacteria and acquire late endosomal/lysosomal features (17). These remodeled rBCVs, which are called autophagic BCVs (aBCVs) (Fig. 1 and 2C and D) form between 48 and 72 h postinfection and are associated with bacterial release from infected cells and new infection events, indicating that they facilitate completion of the *Brucella* intracellular cycle (17).

By their functional and spatial diversity, the sequential eBCV, rBCV, and aBCV stages of the *Brucella* intracellular cycle point towards their necessity to the bacterium's

infectious cycle. Hence, significant efforts have been made in the last 2 decades to understand the underlying mechanisms that define these stages and how the bacterium exploits the corresponding cellular pathways to complete its intracellular cycle.

The VirB Type IV Secretion System

A hallmark of *Brucella* virulence is the expression of a VirB family type IVA secretion system (T4SS), which was identified by homology to the VirB T4SS of the plant pathogen *Agrobacterium tumefaciens* and shown to be required for virulence in a murine model of chronic brucellosis and intracellular replication of *B. abortus*, *B. melitensis*, and *B. suis* in various host cell models (19–21). Indeed, deletions of various genes within the *virB* operon, or transposon insertions in different *virB* genes, rendered *Brucella* unable to convert eBCVs into rBCVs and replicate intracellularly (8, 13, 22) and unable to establish a chronic infection in mice (23, 24), emphasizing major roles of this T4SS in rBCV biogenesis and *Brucella* intracellular replication. Based on the ability of various T4SSs to deliver effector proteins or nucleoprotein complexes across biological membranes, and by analogy to those that contribute to bacterial virulence (25, 26), the VirB T4SS of *Brucella* was presumed to deliver effector proteins into host cells across the eBCV membrane to modulate specific cellular functions and mediate rBCV biogenesis. This assumption was confirmed by the discoveries of an array of *Brucella* effector proteins translocated into host cells in a T4SS-dependent manner (27–32), which opened avenues to understand at the molecular level the underlying mechanisms of the *Brucella* intracellular cycle.

THE eBCV

Early BCV Maturation

Upon uptake by phagocytes or entry into nonphagocytic cells, *Brucella* bacteria initially reside in a phagosome that rapidly acquires markers of the early endocytic compartment, including the small GTPase Rab5, which controls early endosomal maturation, and the early endosomal antigen EEA-1 (8, 13, 33). Since these markers are acquired with kinetics similar to those of classical phagosomes, it is likely that the early BCV undergoes an unaltered maturation process. Consistently, the vacuole then acquires markers of late endosomes, such as the lysosome-associated membrane proteins LAMP1 (Fig. 2A) and LAMP2, CD63, and the small GTPase Rab7 (7, 8, 13, 16), which controls fusion with late endocytic compartments and lysosomes, further indicating a normal vacuolar maturation process within the first hours postinfection. Importantly, the BCV also rapidly becomes acidified to a pH in the range of 4.5 to 5.0 (14), further supporting a maturation process into phagolysosomes. However, early attempts at detecting delivery of lysosomal luminal contents to the BCV as evidence for fusion with lysosomes failed to demonstrate accumulation of cathepsin D by immunostaining (7, 13, 34). This led to the proposal that the BCV avoids fusion with terminal degradative lysosomes, despite advanced maturation events, thus preventing bacterial killing and ensuring intracellular survival.

The eBCV: A Necessary Evil?

Several studies monitoring bacterial viability within eBCVs have revealed that a large proportion of intracellular bacteria (up to 90% in primary bone marrow-derived macrophages) are killed (8, 16), arguing for bactericidal conditions within eBCVs. Using live-cell imaging of fluorescent fluid-phase markers that were chased to terminal lysosomes, as a method that precludes any issue with detection of soluble lysosomal antigens, Starr et al. showed that eBCVs in epithelial HeLa cells undergo fusion with terminal lysosomes, although to a restricted extent (16), directly demonstrating that the eBCV matures into a compartment resembling a phagolysosome. While these findings are consistent with the loss of bacterial viability in eBCVs observed in *in vitro* models, they may appear counterintuitive with regard to *Brucella* intracellular survival. This has led to the speculation that eBCVs that undergo full lysosomal maturation are not those permissive for bacterial survival and represent dead-end paths for the bacteria, while a small fraction of BCVs that do not mature along the endocytic pathway are those that generate rBCVs and allow proliferation of the surviving bacteria. However, the following observations are inconsistent with this possibility. First, LAMP1-positive eBCVs interact with ER cisternae and acquire ER markers, arguing that they undergo conversion into rBCVs (8). Second, eBCV acidification to a pH range of terminal lysosomes is necessary for rBCV biogenesis and bacterial replication (14–16), as inhibition of lysosomal acidification prevents eBCV to rBCV conversion and bacterial replication (14–16). Third, inhibition of Rab7 activity, which controls fusion with lysosomes, also prevents eBCV conversion into rBCVs and bacterial replication (16), demonstrating that a functional late endocytic pathway and lysosomal fusion are required for *Brucella* to undergo its intracellular cycle. Fourth, eBCV acidification is essential for the induction of the *virB* operon (15, 16), which rapidly occurs postuptake in maturing eBCVs, peaking at 4 h postinfection (16, 35). Taken together, these findings rather support a model in which the eBCV stage is a necessary step in the *Brucella* intracellular cycle, which provides intravacuolar cues, including a lysosomal pH, that are necessary for the induction of the VirB T4SS and the resulting conversion of eBCVs to rBCVs.

In addition to its role in promoting *Brucella* T4SS competency, the eBCV may provide cues that initiate intracellular bacterial growth prior to completion of the replication-permissive rBCV. Deghelt et al. established using fluorescence microscopy methods that monitor chromosomal replication in intracellular *Brucella* that bacteria within LAMP1-positive eBCVs initiate chromosomal replication by 8 h postinfection, i.e., during the eBCV-to-rBCV conversion stage, while the infectious forms are in G_1-arrested phase prior to 6 h postinfection (36). Whether this cell cycle change is triggered by the endosomal conditions of the eBCV or by intravacuolar alterations during conversion to rBCV remains to be determined. However, these findings indicate that *Brucella* extensively responds to its intravacuolar environment and initiates growth at the eBCV stage, further emphasizing the importance of the endosomal stage in the *Brucella* intracellular cycle.

THE rBCV

Role of the ER in rBCV Biogenesis

Biogenesis of the rBCV is a hallmark of the *Brucella* intracellular cycle, as it consists of the conversion of the original endosomal bacterial vacuole into a specialized organelle derived from the ER that promotes bacterial proliferation. The underlying mechanisms, host functions, and bacterial effectors that mediate this process have been the subject of extensive research. The nature of the rBCV was initially discovered via its ultrastructural characterization, showing fusion with ER cisternae and studding with ribosomes, and was further confirmed by the detection of ER-associated proteins on its membrane by immunofluorescence microscopy, intravacuolar detection of glucose-6 phosphatase activity, an ER luminal enzyme, and sensitivity to the ER-vacuolating toxin aerolysin (7, 8). The first clues about how a bacterial vacuole interacting with late endocytic and lysosomal compartments could convert into an ER-derived organelle came from the demonstration that ER exit sites (ERES), an ER subcompartment where secretory transport is initiated through the formation of COPII-coated cargo vesicles (37), are functionally important for rBCV biogenesis (22). eBCVs undergo T4SS-dependent, sustained interactions with COPII coat-positive ERES structures during the eBCV-to-rBCV conversion stage (Fig. 3), and inhibition of the small GTPase Sar1, which controls COPII coat assembly and ERES formation and function, inhibits rBCV biogenesis and bacterial replication (22, 38). Consistent with these observations, *Brucella* infection upregulates production of Sar1 and the COPII components Sec23 and Sec24D by an unknown mechanism (39), suggesting that the bacterium upregulates Sar1- and COPII-mediated vesicular trafficking to promote rBCV biogenesis. Hence, *Brucella* may modulate ERES functions to promote rBCV biogenesis, by enhancing production of secretory vesicles that might fuse with the eBCV to initiate its conversion into a vacuole with ER fusogenic properties (Fig. 3), possibly creating a direct port of entry to the ER for the bacteria, while bypassing classical endosome-to-Golgi-to-ER retrograde trafficking processes.

Role of the UPR in the *Brucella* Intracellular Cycle

Another ER-mediated function associated with the *Brucella* intracellular cycle is the unfolded-protein response (UPR). Upon ER stress triggered by accumulation of misfolded proteins within the ER, signaling pathways controlled by the ER-localized UPR receptors IRE1α, PERK, and ATF6 are triggered and lead to a substantial reorganization of ER functions towards increased ER folding capacity, inhibition of protein synthesis, and activation of autophagy, all aimed at resolving ER stress (40). Although there have been disagreements about its extent, the consensus is that *Brucella* infection induces the UPR in macrophages or HeLa cells via at least the IRE1α pathway (39, 41, 42). Moreover, IRE1α is required for *Brucella* replication (43), and pharmacological compensation of protein misfolding using tauroursodeoxycholic acid impairs replication of *B. melitensis* (41), which supports the idea that the UPR is beneficial to the bacterium's intracellular cycle. However, whether and how this stress response promotes rBCV biogenesis and bacterial replication remain unclear. Taguchi et al. revealed a link between UPR induction, ERES, and rBCV biogenesis by showing that IRE1α is activated via the ERES-localized protein Yip1A, which controls formation of large vacuoles in a manner dependent on the autophagy-associated proteins Atg9 and WIPI1, and is also required for rBCV biogenesis (39). Hence, these findings support a model in which *Brucella* actively causes UPR induction via activation of the IRE1α pathway to promote an activation cascade leading to formation at ERES of vacuoles of a possible autophagic nature (43), which ultimately contributes to rBCV biogenesis (Fig. 3).

Is Autophagy Involved in rBCV Biogenesis?

Autophagy is a membrane-based process that normally captures intracellular contents, whether cytosolic contents, damaged organelles, or microorganisms, into double-membrane vesicles called autophagosomes, to deliver them for degradation to the lysosomal compartment. While it can act as an innate immune antibacterial mechanism, it can also be beneficial to some pathogens (44, 45). Based on the roles of IRE1α and Yip1A in rBCV biogenesis and *Brucella* replication, autophagosome formation at ERES may provide ER-derived membranes that may contribute to eBCV-to-rBCV conversion;

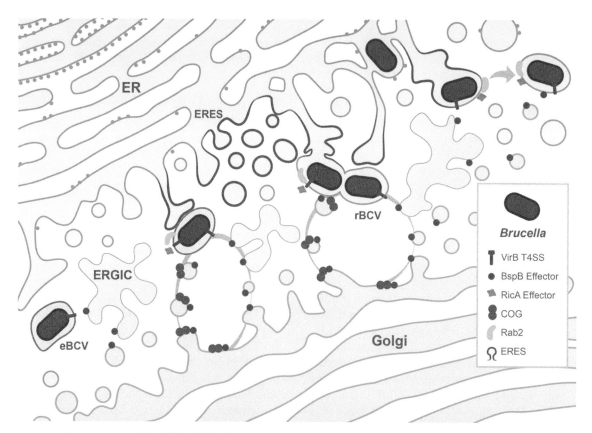

Figure 3   Model of VirB T4SS-dependent biogenesis of the rBCV. Bacteria in eBCVs induce expression of the VirB T4SS, which delivers effector proteins into the host cell. Among these, BspB traffics to Golgi membranes via the ER-to-Golgi intermediate compartment (ERGIC) and binds to the COG complex to promote redirection of Golgi apparatus-derived vesicular traffic to BCVs. RicA binds the small host secretory GTPase Rab2, which contributes to its recruitment on maturing eBCVs and role in rBCV biogenesis. Additionally, eBCV interaction with ERES is accompanied by the upregulation of COPII coat components, induction of IRE1α, and Yip1A-dependent formation of ER-derived vesicles, which are also thought to contribute to rBCV biogenesis. T4SS-dependent acquisition of ER- and Golgi apparatus-derived secretory membranes by BCVs is thought to mediate eBCV-to-rBCV conversion.

however, whether the canonical autophagic cascade is involved in rBCV biogenesis remains controversial. While a classical autophagic process was originally proposed as a mechanism for rBCV biogenesis in HeLa cells, based on the observation of multimembrane structures on BCVs and accumulation of the lysosomotropic compound monodansylcadaverine (7, 34), such structures are not seen on eBCVs in macrophages (8), nor does the autophagic marker LC3 accumulate on eBCVs, arguing against a canonical autophagic process. Furthermore, inhibition of autophagy via small-interfering-RNA (siRNA)-mediated depletion of specific autophagy components involved in the autophagosome nucleation and elongation steps, namely, ULK1, beclin1, Atg5, Atg7, ATG16L, and LC3B, does not prevent rBCV biogenesis and bacterial replication (17). Hence, there is no

substantial evidence to support a role of the canonical autophagic cascade in rBCV biogenesis. However, the demonstrated roles of the autophagosome nucleation protein WIPI1 and of the autophagy protein Atg9 in rBCV biogenesis (39) clearly invoke specific autophagy-associated machineries in this process, suggesting that rBCV biogenesis requires a subset of cellular machineries associated with autophagosome formation at ERES and Atg9-mediated delivery of membranes. Further studies are needed to clarify how these autophagy-related events actually contribute to rBCV biogenesis.

Role of the Secretory Pathway in rBCV Biogenesis

Based on the ER nature of the rBCV, the host secretory pathway certainly plays an essential role in the *Brucella* intracellular cycle. Whether secretory compartments other than the ER, such as the ER-to-Golgi intermediate compartment, the Golgi apparatus, and the *trans*-Golgi network, are important to the bacterium is a long-standing question, warranted by examples of other intracellular pathogens that exploit these compartments (46). These include *Legionella pneumophila*, which intercepts Arf1- and Rab1-dependent secretory traffic to acquire ER-derived membranes (47, 48), and *Chlamydia trachomatis*, which redirects Golgi apparatus-derived lipid trafficking pathways for acquisition of sphingolipids (49, 50). Cellular approaches based on altering specific functions along the secretory pathway using either pharmacological inhibition of host secretion, expression of dominant inactive alleles of small GTPases, or siRNA-mediated depletions have revealed that ER-Golgi secretory traffic is important for rBCV biogenesis and bacterial replication (22, 38). Inhibition of Arf1-dependent secretory traffic using brefeldin A or via siRNA treatment impairs rBCV biogenesis to levels similar to those seen with depletion of Sar1 (22, 38). Additionally, depletion of the small GTPases Rab1a and Rab2, which control anterograde and retrograde vesicular traffic between the ER and Golgi apparatus (51), negatively affects replication of *B. abortus* in macrophages (38), further indicating a complex role of vesicular traffic between these compartments in promoting *Brucella* proliferation, possibly through acquisition by the eBCV of secretory membranes during their conversion process into the rBCV. Consistent with *Brucella* exploiting these pathways, host secretory traffic is altered in *Brucella*-infected cells in a T4SS-dependent manner (30), which argues that the

bacterium actively modulates secretory functions via delivery of effectors to promote its intracellular cycle.

Bacterial Effectors of rBCV Biogenesis

The recent discoveries of several VirB T4SS effectors (27–32) and the characterization of the modes of action of some of them (Table 1) have provided opportunities to start deciphering at the molecular level the bacterial mechanisms of rBCV biogenesis and bacterial replication. VceC, identified as being coregulated with the VirB T4SS, binds the ER chaperone Grp78/BiP and induces the UPR, which triggers an inflammatory response (42), yet whether it plays a role in rBCV biogenesis has not been elucidated. TcpB/BtpA, a TIR-domain-containing effector that down-modulates proinflammatory responses (52–58), also induces the UPR and promotes bacterial proliferation once rBCVs are formed (41), suggesting that it may not contribute to rBCV biogenesis. SepA, in contrast, is possibly involved in rBCV biogenesis, as a ΔsepA mutant is retained in eBCVs (32), yet its mode of action remains unknown.

The T4SS effectors BspA, BspB, and BspF, which inhibit host protein secretion and promote bacterial replication (30, 38), support the hypothesis that *Brucella* specifically targets various host secretory functions, possibly for rBCV biogenesis purposes. While the modes of action of BspA and BspF are unknown, that of BspB has been elucidated. BspB is required for rBCV biogenesis and optimal bacterial replication in macrophages (38). This effector is delivered into host cells and traffics to the Golgi apparatus, where it interacts with the conserved oligomeric Golgi (COG) complex (38) (Fig. 3),

Table 1 *Brucella* T4SS effectors

Name	ORF in *B. abortus*	Host target	Function	Reference(s)
RicA	BAB1_1279	Rab2	Modulates rBCV biogenesis	28
VceA	BAB1_1652	Unknown	Unknown	27
VceC	BAB1_1058	Grp78/BiP	UPR activation	27, 42
BspA	BAB1_0678	Unknown	Intracellular replication	30
BspB	BAB1_0712	COG	Redirects Golgi vesicular traffic; rBCV biogenesis; intracellular replication	30, 38
BspC	BAB1_0847	Unknown	Unknown	30
BspE	BAB1_1675	Unknown	Unknown	30
BspF	BAB1_1948	Unknown	Intracellular replication	30
BtpA/TcpB	BAB1_0279	MAL	Inhibition of TLR signaling; UPR induction	52
BtpB	BAB1_0756	Unknown	Unknown	31
SepA	BAB1_1492	Unknown	eBCV trafficking	32
BPE005	BAB1_2005	Unknown	Unknown	29
BPE043	BAB1_1043	Unknown	Unknown	29
BPE275	BAB1_1275	Unknown	Unknown	29
BPE123	BAB1_0123	Unknown	Unknown	29

a CATCHR-family multisubunit tethering complex that serves as an interaction hub on Golgi membranes for secretory Rab GTPases, Golgi tethers, and SNAREs and that regulates intra-Golgi and retrograde vesicular traffic along the secretory pathway (59). COG functions are important for rBCV biogenesis and bacterial replication (38), implicating Golgi apparatus-associated functions in the *Brucella* intracellular cycle. By mechanisms that remain to be defined, BspB-COG interactions alter COG functions and lead to redirection of COG-dependent Golgi retrograde vesicular traffic to BCVs and acquisition of Golgi apparatus-derived membranes (38), demonstrating that *Brucella* likely recruits membranes from this secretory compartment during rBCV biogenesis, in addition to ER-derived membranes (Fig. 3). Interestingly, inhibition of Rab2-dependent Golgi-to-ER retrograde traffic via depletion of Rab2 suppresses the replication defect of a Δ*bspB* mutant (38), suggesting that BspB may affect retrograde secretory traffic to redirect COG-dependent Golgi vesicular traffic to the BCV. Interestingly, the T4SS effector RicA is involved in controlling rBCV biogenesis and binds the GDP-bound form of Rab2 (28) (Fig. 3). Although its mode of action is unknown, as it does not show any GEF (guanine nucleotide exchange factor) activity (28), this suggests that *Brucella* delivers several effectors that may coordinately act to modulate Rab2-dependent vesicular trafficking and promote rBCV biogenesis.

Altogether, the knowledge gained by studying VirB T4SS effectors that target the host secretory pathway has revealed yet another facet of *Brucella* interactions with this intracellular compartment and emphasizes how the identification and characterization of these effectors are key to a comprehensive understanding of how this bacterium subverts host secretory functions.

THE aBCV

While replication in ER-associated rBCVs is a key step in the pathogenesis of *Brucella*, how the bacterium completes its intracellular cycle following this proliferation stage has remained unknown for many decades. Unlike many pathogens, which cause cell death to exit the cells in which they have replicated, *Brucella* prevents cell death programs from being carried out (60, 61), thus preserving its intracellular niche. Starr et al. observed that instead, following proliferation in rBCVs, by 48 h postinfection and afterwards, the *Brucella* intracellular niche was converted from an ER-derived organelle to large vacuoles harboring features of late endosomal and lysosomal compartments, such as accumulation of LAMP1 and acidification (17). From an ultrastructural

standpoint, these vacuoles are surrounded by multiple membranes and originate from the capture of rBCVs by crescent-shaped membrane structures reminiscent of autophagosomes, despite the lack of accumulation of the canonical autophagosome marker LC3 (17) (Fig. 2). The formation of these vacuoles, named aBCVs, requires functions of the canonical autophagy nucleation but not elongation complexes, as depletion or deletion of beclin1, ULK1, and Atg14L, but not that of Atg5, Atg7, Atg4, or Atg16L, blocked their formation (17). aBCV formation therefore seems to require a subset of autophagy-associated molecular machineries, which may typify an alternate autophagic process or indicate that the bacterium actively exploits discrete functions of the canonical autophagy pathway to generate aBCVs.

Importantly, aBCV formation is tightly linked to bacterial egress, as new infection events of adjacent cells occur during the aBCV formation stage and are reduced upon inhibition of aBCV formation (17). Whether bacteria are released in a free state or contained within a membrane-bound vacuole remains to be established, but the maintenance of the originally infected cells argues that bacterial release is a nonlytic event, suggesting an exocytic process (Fig. 1). Based on the autophagic nature of the aBCV, a tempting hypothesis to explain aBCV-dependent bacterial release is that the bacterium takes advantage of the secretory functions of the autophagy pathway (62) to deliver aBCV-enclosed bacteria to the extracellular milieu.

By mediating the final step of the *Brucella* intracellular cycle, aBCV formation is likely controlled by the bacterium, potentially via the VirB T4SS. Testing this hypothesis is challenging, as the preceding step of rBCV formation is T4SS dependent, precluding the classical use of reverse genetics and VirB T4SS-deficient mutants. Transient intracellular production of the VirB11 ATPase via a tightly controlled promoter, which energizes the T4SS, allows rBCV biogenesis and bacterial replication prior to T4SS intracellular inactivation and showed a requirement for a functional VirB apparatus in aBCV formation and bacterial egress, indicating that this final step of the *Brucella* intracellular cycle is likely controlled by T4SS effectors (63). Their future identification and characterization will likely shed light on the molecular mechanisms of aBCV formation and bacterial egress.

CONCLUDING REMARKS

Bacteria of the genus *Brucella* belong to a phylogenetic group closely associated with eukaryotic hosts. In this context, *Brucella*'s long-standing coevolution with mammalian hosts has shaped its complex intracellular cycle into the sequential exploitation of intracellular compartments of the endocytic, secretory, and autophagy pathways. *Brucella* uses an array of T4SS-delivered effectors and other virulence factors to modulate discrete functions of these compartments, modifying its original phagosome into an ER-associated replication-permissive organelle that subsequently coopts autophagic functions for completion of the bacterium's intracellular cycle, thus ensuring its survival, proliferation, and egress. While a few T4SS effectors have been identified, much remains to be understood about their modes of action and contributions to *Brucella*'s intracellular cycle. Future characterization of these proteins not only will reveal unsuspected aspects of *Brucella* intracellular strategies but also will teach us a great deal about host cell functions and their roles in many aspects of bacterial pathogenesis.

Acknowledgments. We are most grateful to Andrew Rader for graphical assistance with figures. This work was supported by NIH grants AI129992 and AI127830.

Citation. Celli J. 2019. The intracellular life cycle of *Brucella* spp. Microbiol Spectrum 7(2):BAI-0006-2019.

References

1. Moreno E. 2014. Retrospective and prospective perspectives on zoonotic brucellosis. *Front Microbiol* 5:213.

2. Pappas G, Akritidis N, Bosilkovski M, Tsianos E. 2005. Brucellosis. *N Engl J Med* 352:2325–2336.

3. Pappas G, Papadimitriou P, Akritidis N, Christou L, Tsianos EV. 2006. The new global map of human brucellosis. *Lancet Infect Dis* 6:91–99.

4. Atluri VL, Xavier MN, de Jong MF, den Hartigh AB, Tsolis RM. 2011. Interactions of the human pathogenic *Brucella* species with their hosts. *Annu Rev Microbiol* 65:523–541.

5. Celli J. 2015. The changing nature of the *Brucella*-containing vacuole. *Cell Microbiol* 17:951–958.

6. Anderson TD, Cheville NF, Meador VP. 1986. Pathogenesis of placentitis in the goat inoculated with *Brucella abortus*. II. Ultrastructural studies. *Vet Pathol* 23:227–239.

7. Pizarro-Cerdá J, Méresse S, Parton RG, van der Goot G, Sola-Landa A, Lopez-Goñi I, Moreno E, Gorvel JP. 1998. *Brucella abortus* transits through the autophagic pathway and replicates in the endoplasmic reticulum of nonprofessional phagocytes. *Infect Immun* 66:5711–5724.

8. Celli J, de Chastellier C, Franchini D-M, Pizarro-Cerda J, Moreno E, Gorvel J-P. 2003. *Brucella* evades macrophage killing via VirB-dependent sustained interactions with the endoplasmic reticulum. *J Exp Med* 198:545–556.

9. Salcedo SP, Chevrier N, Lacerda TLS, Ben Amara A, Gerart S, Gorvel VA, de Chastellier C, Blasco JM, Mege J-L, Gorvel J-P. 2013. Pathogenic brucellae replicate in human trophoblasts. *J Infect Dis* 207:1075–1083.

10. Detilleux PG, Deyoe BL, Cheville NF. 1990. Entry and intracellular localization of *Brucella* spp. in Vero cells:

11. Detilleux PG, Deyoe BL, Cheville NF. 1990. Penetration and intracellular growth of *Brucella abortus* in nonphagocytic cells in vitro. *Infect Immun* 58:2320–2328.

12. Arenas GN, Staskevich AS, Aballay A, Mayorga LS. 2000. Intracellular trafficking of *Brucella abortus* in J774 macrophages. *Infect Immun* 68:4255–4263.

13. Comerci DJ, Martínez-Lorenzo MJ, Sieira R, Gorvel J-P, Ugalde RA. 2001. Essential role of the VirB machinery in the maturation of the *Brucella abortus*-containing vacuole. *Cell Microbiol* 3:159–168.

14. Porte F, Liautard JP, Köhler S. 1999. Early acidification of phagosomes containing *Brucella suis* is essential for intracellular survival in murine macrophages. *Infect Immun* 67:4041–4047.

15. Boschiroli ML, Ouahrani-Bettache S, Foulongne V, Michaux-Charachon S, Bourg G, Allardet-Servent A, Cazevieille C, Liautard JP, Ramuz M, O'Callaghan D. 2002. The *Brucella suis* virB operon is induced intracellularly in macrophages. *Proc Natl Acad Sci USA* 99:1544–1549.

16. Starr T, Ng TW, Wehrly TD, Knodler LA, Celli J. 2008. Brucella intracellular replication requires trafficking through the late endosomal/lysosomal compartment. *Traffic* 9:678–694.

17. Starr T, Child R, Wehrly TD, Hansen B, Hwang S, López-Otin C, Virgin HW, Celli J. 2012. Selective subversion of autophagy complexes facilitates completion of the Brucella intracellular cycle. *Cell Host Microbe* 11:33–45.

18. Sedzicki J, Tschon T, Low SH, Willemart K, Goldie KN, Letesson J-J, Stahlberg H, Dehio C. 2018. 3D correlative electron microscopy reveals continuity of *Brucella*-containing vacuoles with the endoplasmic reticulum. *J Cell Sci* 131:jcs210799.

19. Sieira R, Comerci DJ, Sánchez DO, Ugalde RA. 2000. A homologue of an operon required for DNA transfer in *Agrobacterium* is required in *Brucella abortus* for virulence and intracellular multiplication. *J Bacteriol* 182:4849–4855.

20. Delrue RM, Martinez-Lorenzo M, Lestrate P, Danese I, Bielarz V, Mertens P, De Bolle X, Tibor A, Gorvel JP, Letesson JJ. 2001. Identification of *Brucella* spp. genes involved in intracellular trafficking. *Cell Microbiol* 3:487–497.

21. O'Callaghan D, Cazevieille C, Allardet-Servent A, Boschiroli ML, Bourg G, Foulongne V, Frutos P, Kulakov Y, Ramuz M. 1999. A homologue of the *Agrobacterium tumefaciens* VirB and *Bordetella pertussis* Ptl type IV secretion systems is essential for intracellular survival of *Brucella suis*. *Mol Microbiol* 33:1210–1220.

22. Celli J, Salcedo SP, Gorvel J-P. 2005. *Brucella* coopts the small GTPase Sar1 for intracellular replication. *Proc Natl Acad Sci USA* 102:1673–1678.

23. Hartigh den AB, Rolán HG, de Jong MF, Tsolis RM. 2008. VirB3 to VirB6 and VirB8 to VirB11, but not VirB7, are essential for mediating persistence of *Brucella* in the reticuloendothelial system. *J Bacteriol* 190:4427–4436.

24. Lestrate P, Delrue RM, Danese I, Didembourg C, Taminiau B, Mertens P, De Bolle X, Tibor A, Tang CM, Letesson JJ.

2000. Identification and characterization of in vivo attenuated mutants of *Brucella melitensis*. *Mol Microbiol* 38: 543–551.

25. Green ER, Mecsas J. 2016. Bacterial secretion systems: an overview. *Microbiol Spectr* 4(1):VMBF-0012-2015.

26. Juhas M, Crook DW, Hood DW. 2008. Type IV secretion systems: tools of bacterial horizontal gene transfer and virulence. *Cell Microbiol* 10:2377–2386.

27. de Jong MF, Sun Y-H, den Hartigh AB, van Dijl JM, Tsolis RM. 2008. Identification of VceA and VceC, two members of the VjbR regulon that are translocated into macrophages by the *Brucella* type IV secretion system. *Mol Microbiol* 70: 1378–1396.

28. de Barsy M, Jamet A, Filopon D, Nicolas C, Laloux G, Rual J-F, Muller A, Twizere J-C, Nkengfac B, Vandenhaute J, Hill DE, Salcedo SP, Gorvel J-P, Letesson J-J, De Bolle X. 2011. Identification of a *Brucella* spp. secreted effector specifically interacting with human small GTPase Rab2. *Cell Microbiol* 13:1044–1058.

29. Marchesini MI, Herrmann CK, Salcedo SP, Gorvel J-P, Comerci DJ. 2011. In search of *Brucella abortus* type IV secretion substrates: screening and identification of four proteins translocated into host cells through VirB system. *Cell Microbiol* 13:1261–1274.

30. Myeni S, Child R, Ng TW, Kupko JJ III, Wehrly TD, Porcella SF, Knodler LA, Celli J. 2013. *Brucella* modulates secretory trafficking via multiple type IV secretion effector proteins. *PLoS Pathog* 9:e1003556.

31. Salcedo SP, Marchesini MI, Degos C, Terwagne M, Von Bargen K, Lepidi H, Herrmann CK, Santos Lacerda TL, Imbert PR, Pierre P, Alexopoulou L, Letesson JJ, Comerci DJ, Gorvel JP. 2013. BtpB, a novel *Brucella* TIR-containing effector protein with immune modulatory functions. *Front Cell Infect Microbiol* 3:28.

32. Döhmer PH, Valguarnera E, Czibener C, Ugalde JE. 2014. Identification of a type IV secretion substrate of *Brucella abortus* that participates in the early stages of intracellular survival. *Cell Microbiol* 16:396–410.

33. Chaves-Olarte E, Guzmán-Verri C, Méresse S, Desjardins M, Pizarro-Cerdá J, Badilla J, Gorvel J-P, Moreno E. 2002. Activation of Rho and Rab GTPases dissociates *Brucella abortus* internalization from intracellular trafficking. *Cell Microbiol* 4:663–676.

34. Pizarro-Cerdá J, Moreno E, Sanguedolce V, Mege JL, Gorvel JP. 1998. Virulent *Brucella abortus* prevents lysosome fusion and is distributed within autophagosome-like compartments. *Infect Immun* 66:2387–2392.

35. Sieira R, Comerci DJ, Pietrasanta LI, Ugalde RA. 2004. Integration host factor is involved in transcriptional regulation of the *Brucella abortus virB* operon. *Mol Microbiol* 54:808–822.

36. Deghelt M, Mullier C, Sternon J-F, Francis N, Laloux G, Dotreppe D, Van der Henst C, Jacobs-Wagner C, Letesson J-J, De Bolle X. 2014. G1-arrested newborn cells are the predominant infectious form of the pathogen *Brucella abortus*. *Nat Commun* 5:4366.

37. Budnik A, Stephens DJ. 2009. ER exit sites—localization and control of COPII vesicle formation. *FEBS Lett* 583: 3796–3803.

38. Miller CN, Smith EP, Cundiff JA, Knodler LA, Bailey Blackburn J, Lupashin V, Celli J. 2017. A *Brucella* type IV effector targets the COG tethering complex to remodel host secretory traffic and promote intracellular replication. *Cell Host Microbe* 22:317–329.e7.

39. Taguchi Y, Imaoka K, Kataoka M, Uda A, Nakatsu D, Horii-Okazaki S, Kunishige R, Kano F, Murata M. 2015. Yip1A, a novel host factor for the activation of the IRE1 pathway of the unfolded protein response during *Brucella* infection. *PLoS Pathog* 11:e1004747.

40. Walter P, Ron D. 2011. The unfolded protein response: from stress pathway to homeostatic regulation. *Science* 334:1081–1086.

41. Smith JA, Khan M, Magnani DD, Harms JS, Durward M, Radhakrishnan GK, Liu Y-P, Splitter GA. 2013. *Brucella* induces an unfolded protein response via TcpB that supports intracellular replication in macrophages. *PLoS Pathog* 9:e1003785.

42. de Jong MF, Starr T, Winter MG, den Hartigh AB, Child R, Knodler LA, van Dijl JM, Celli J, Tsolis RM. 2013. Sensing of bacterial type IV secretion via the unfolded protein response. *mBio* 4:e00418-12.

43. Qin Q-M, Pei J, Ancona V, Shaw BD, Ficht TA, de Figueiredo P. 2008. RNAi screen of endoplasmic reticulum-associated host factors reveals a role for IRE1α in supporting *Brucella* replication. *PLoS Pathog* 4: e1000110–e1000116.

44. Levine B, Mizushima N, Virgin HW. 2011. Autophagy in immunity and inflammation. *Nature* 469:323–335.

45. Huang J, Brumell JH. 2014. Bacteria-autophagy interplay: a battle for survival. *Nat Rev Microbiol* 12:101–114.

46. Asrat S, de Jesús DA, Hempstead AD, Ramabhadran V, Isberg RR. 2014. Bacterial pathogen manipulation of host membrane trafficking. *Annu Rev Cell Dev Biol* 30: 79–109.

47. Kagan JC, Roy CR. 2002. *Legionella* phagosomes intercept vesicular traffic from endoplasmic reticulum exit sites. *Nat Cell Biol* 4:945–954.

48. Kagan JC, Stein M-P, Pypaert M, Roy CR. 2004. *Legionella* subvert the functions of Rab1 and Sec22b to create a replicative organelle. *J Exp Med* 199:1201–1211.

49. Hackstadt T, Rockey DD, Heinzen RA, Scidmore MA. 1996. *Chlamydia trachomatis* interrupts an exocytic pathway to acquire endogenously synthesized sphingomyelin in transit from the Golgi apparatus to the plasma membrane. *EMBO J* 15:964–977.

50. Scidmore MA, Fischer ER, Hackstadt T. 1996. Sphingolipids and glycoproteins are differentially trafficked to the *Chlamydia trachomatis* inclusion. *J Cell Biol* 134: 363–374.

51. Bhuin T, Roy JK. 2014. Rab proteins: the key regulators of intracellular vesicle transport. *Exp Cell Res* 328:1–19.

52. Salcedo SP, Marchesini MI, Lelouard H, Fugier E, Jolly G, Balor S, Muller A, Lapaque N, Demaria O, Alexopoulou L, Comerci DJ, Ugalde RA, Pierre P, Gorvel J-P. 2008. Brucella control of dendritic cell maturation is dependent on the TIR-containing protein Btp1. *PLoS Pathog* 4:e21.

53. Jakka P, Namani S, Murugan S, Rai N, Radhakrishnan G. 2017. The *Brucella* effector protein TcpB induces deg-

radation of inflammatory caspases and thereby subverts non-canonical inflammasome activation in macrophages. *J Biol Chem* **292:**20613–20627.

54. Alaidarous M, Ve T, Casey LW, Valkov E, Ericsson DJ, Ullah MO, Schembri MA, Mansell A, Sweet MJ, Kobe B. 2014. Mechanism of bacterial interference with TLR4 signaling by *Brucella* Toll/interleukin-1 receptor domain-containing protein TcpB. *J Biol Chem* **289:**654–668.

55. Chaudhary A, Ganguly K, Cabantous S, Waldo GS, Micheva-Viteva SN, Nag K, Hlavacek WS, Tung C-S. 2012. The *Brucella* TIR-like protein TcpB interacts with the death domain of MyD88. *Biochem Biophys Res Commun* **417:**299–304.

56. Sengupta D, Koblansky A, Gaines J, Brown T, West AP, Zhang D, Nishikawa T, Park SG, Roop RM II, Ghosh S. 2010. Subversion of innate immune responses by *Brucella* through the targeted degradation of the TLR signaling adapter, MAL. *J Immunol* **184:**956–964.

57. Radhakrishnan GK, Yu Q, Harms JS, Splitter GA. 2009. *Brucella* TIR domain-containing protein mimics properties of the Toll-like receptor adaptor protein TIRAP. *J Biol Chem* **284:**9892–9898.

58. Cirl C, Wieser A, Yadav M, Duerr S, Schubert S, Fischer H, Stappert D, Wantia N, Rodriguez N, Wagner H, Svanborg C, Miethke T. 2008. Subversion of Toll-like receptor signaling by a unique family of bacterial Toll/interleukin-1 receptor domain-containing proteins. *Nat Med* **14:**399–406.

59. Willett R, Ungar D, Lupashin V. 2013. The Golgi puppet master: COG complex at center stage of membrane trafficking interactions. *Histochem Cell Biol* **140:**271–283.

60. Cui G, Wei P, Zhao Y, Guan Z, Yang L, Sun W, Wang S, Peng Q. 2014. *Brucella* infection inhibits macrophages apoptosis via Nedd4-dependent degradation of calpain2. *Vet Microbiol* **174:**195–205.

61. Gross A, Terraza A, Ouahrani-Bettache S, Liautard JP, Dornand J. 2000. In vitro *Brucella suis* infection prevents the programmed cell death of human monocytic cells. *Infect Immun* **68:**342–351.

62. Kimura T, Jia J, Claude-Taupin A, Kumar S, Choi SW, Gu Y, Mudd M, Dupont N, Jiang S, Peters R, Farzam F, Jain A, Lidke KA, Adams CM, Johansen T, Deretic V. 2017. Cellular and molecular mechanism for secretory autophagy. *Autophagy* **13:**1084–1085.

63. Smith EP, Miller CN, Child R, Cundiff JA, Celli J. 2016. Postreplication roles of the Brucella VirB type IV secretion system uncovered via conditional expression of the VirB11 ATPase. *mBio* **7:**e01730-16.

Bacteria and Intracellularity
Edited by Pascale Cossart, Craig R. Roy, and Philippe Sansonetti
© 2019 American Society for Microbiology, Washington, DC
doi:10.1128/microbiolspec.BAI-0024-2019

Infect and Inject: How *Mycobacterium tuberculosis* Exploits Its Major Virulence-Associated Type VII Secretion System, ESX-1

8

Sangeeta Tiwari,[1] Rosalyn Casey,[2] Celia W. Goulding,[3] Suzie Hingley-Wilson,[2] and William R. Jacobs, Jr.[1]

INTRODUCTION

Tuberculosis (TB) is a global health problem caused by the airborne pathogen *Mycobacterium tuberculosis*. Currently, one-third of the world's population is infected with *M. tuberculosis*, and this slow, tenacious bacterium kills 1.6 million people around the world each year, equating to over 4,300 deaths every day (1). Failure to eradicate this age-old disease is the result of an ineffective vaccine and extended, often insufficient, chemotherapy. To date, the only licensed vaccine available is *Mycobacterium bovis* BCG, a live attenuated strain of *M. bovis* discovered in 1919 by Albert Calmette and Camille Guérin following 230 subcultures of the original virulent isolate (2, 3). Distribution of this vaccine to various countries, and more subculturing, led to genetic variations between different BCG strains. However, all strains possess a common deletion that occurred prior to 1919. The deleted region is called region of difference 1 (RD1), and it encodes a key part of the type VII secretion system known as ESAT-6 secretion system 1 (ESX-1) (Fig. 1A); deletion(s) in this particular region are considered the major cause of BCG attenuation (4–6).

Brief History of ESX-1

ESX-1 is considered omnipresent in terms of scientific publications and functionalities, with studies showing its involvement in intercellular conjugation (7), membrane escape (8), and passage through the lung interstitium (9). ESX-1 is a complex, multifunctional type VII secretion system, producing and releasing a plethora of proteins, many of which are required for its own secretion.

Mahairas et al. first observed RD1 (*Rv3871-9*) at the genetic level in 1996 while comparing genetic differences between BCG, its parent *M. bovis,* and its cousin *M. tuberculosis* (4). Following this seminal study, comparative genomics of numerous BCG strains determined that RD1 was the first region of difference that occurred prior to attenuation in 1921 (10). ESX-1 and its four closely related homologues in *M. tuberculosis* were identified as potential secretion systems in an organism that was originally believed to have none, with additional homologues identified in other Gram-positive bacteria (11). Similar to Calmette and Guérin a century earlier, several groups saw the potential for a novel vaccine strategy, postulating that the removal of this particular attenuating region from the backbone of the strains that cause human TB, i.e., *M. tuberculosis*, would result in a vaccine that would work better than BCG. In 2003, the Jacobs, Sherman, and Cole groups were the first to create vaccine candidates based on this hypothesis, with the first two labs knocking out RD1 in *M. tuberculosis* (9, 12) and the latter taking an alternative approach by adding RD1 to BCG (13). Interestingly, RD1 knockdown strain studies in mice revealed intriguing results, wherein the bacterial count was the

[1]Department of Microbiology and Immunology, Albert Einstein College of Medicine, Bronx, NY 10461; [2]Department of Microbial Sciences, School of Biosciences and Medicine, University of Surrey, Guilford, Surrey, GU27XH, United Kingdom; [3]Department of Molecular Biology & Biochemistry and Department of Pharmaceutical Sciences, University of California Irvine, Irvine, CA 92697.

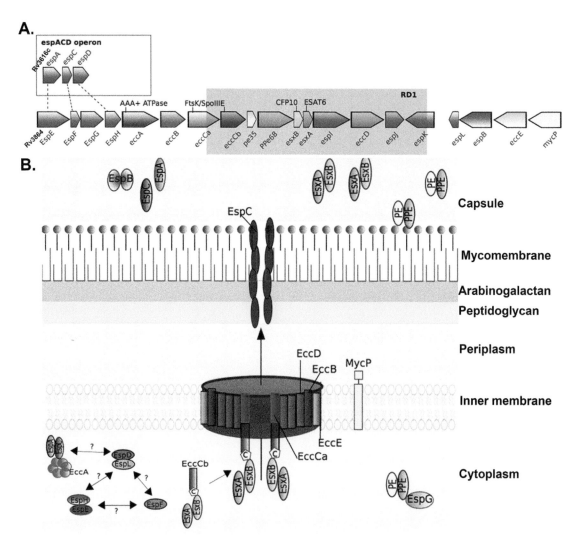

Figure 1 Schematic of the ESX-1 secretion system. (**A**) Gene map of the *esx-1* locus and the *espACD* operon in *M. tuberculosis* H37Rv. The *esx-1* locus includes *esx* genes encoding the secreted effector proteins EsxA and EsxB alongside *ecc* genes encoding ESX-conserved proteins and *esp* genes encoding ESX secretion-associated proteins (108). The *espACD* operon is at a locus distinct from the *esx-1* locus but shares sequence homology with *espE*, *espF*, and *espH* of *esx-1* (dashed lines). The spontaneous deletion (Rv3871 to Rv3878) from *esx-1* found in the vaccine strains of *M. bovis* BCG is known as region of difference 1 (RD1) and is indicated by the gray box. (**B**) Model of the ESX-1 secretion system in the mycobacterial cell envelope. In common with all ESX systems, the core structure of the ESX-1 secretion apparatus starts with the inner membrane-spanning conserved components EccB, EccC, EccD, and EccE (109). EccC is an ATP-driven translocase consisting of two subunits (a and b) that are assembled following EccB binding of target substrate, in this case, the heterodimer EsxAB, where EccCb interacts with the carboxyl-terminal signal sequence of EsxB (labeled "C") (21, 110). EsxAB secretion is codependent on the secretion of EspC/EspA, which is also dependent on interaction with the cytosolic ATPase EccA (20, 111). EspC polymerizes during secretion, indicating a role for EccA and EspA as cytosolic chaperones (18), and forms a filamentous structure thought to provide a channel for secretion of ESX-1 substrates (18). Other important ESX-1 substrates include the PE and PPE families of proteins, which form heterodimers and are recruited by the putative cytosolic chaperone EspG to initiate interaction with the core complex of proteins within the inner membrane (112–114). EspB is also secreted by ESX-1 and forms a PE-PPE-like fold, containing a C-terminal domain that is processed by the MycP$_1$ protease during secretion (26, 115). EspD to -F and EspH proteins are cytosolic and were recently shown to be stabilized by the cytosolic chaperone EspL (24–26).

same but the pathology was dramatically different (9). Protection was observed, but it never achieved the levels found with BCG vaccination in murine models of infection. However, Koch's molecular postulates were fulfilled, telling us that the removal of RD1 resulted in attenuation (14). Interestingly, a recently isolated clinical strain defective in this region has shown similar results, where there is no significant difference in bacterial count but pathology and cytokine response are remarkably different (15).

Although these studies did not lead to novel vaccine candidates, they did provide tools to study *M. tuberculosis* virulence, which may help us design better vaccines and treatment strategies. Recent advances in our understanding of TB disease and ESX-1 are discussed. However, care should be taken to differentiate between cellular functions as they pertain to different organisms; for example, there have been significant advances in *Mycobacterium marinum* studies in its zebrafish host, which have shown that ESX-1 is not virulence related in this particular species of mycobacteria (16).

Vaccine Studies That Taught Us More about Pathogenesis than Protection

No ESX-1 story is complete without the original ESX-1 knockout mutant, *M. bovis* BCG. The tale has been told many times of the 230 subcultures that Albert Calmette and Camille Guérin carried out, culminating in the attenuation of virulent *M. bovis*. The story of BCG begins at the Pasteur Institute in Lille, France, where Guérin began subculturing a virulent strain of *M. bovis* isolated from the udder of a tuberculous cow. The culture was passaged every ~3 weeks on a medium containing potato, glycerine, and ox bile. Mycobacterial cultures are notoriously clumpy, and Calmette and Guérin found that a mycobacterial stew, composed of *M. bovis* growing on potatoes that were cooked in ox bile and then dipped at one end in glycerinated ox bile, led to an emulsified culture, making it easier to standardize inoculating doses. This serendipitously resulted in attenuation of the strain, which led Calmette and Guérin to produce a vaccine utilizing this bacillus (2). By 1919, 230 subcultures had resulted in a strain that failed to produce tuberculous disease when injected into guinea pigs, rabbits, cattle, and horses (17). Following this success, preparations began for the first human clinical trials.

In the early 20th century, ethical standards were somewhat less stringent than today, and the first human "trial" of BCG was undertaken in an unlikely subject, infants. In 1921, an infant under the care of its grandmother, who had TB, was given three doses of oral BCG to prevent likely infection and possible death (3). This initial foray into attenuated TB vaccines was a success, and the child remained healthy. Following this success, a larger trial began 6 months later in which BCG was orally administered to 317 infants at birth. Ultimately, BCG proved to be safe and effective in protecting against childhood TB (3). However, vaccine safety was severely questioned in 1930 following the Lübeck disaster, in which 250 infants were vaccinated in a northern German city with a contaminated BCG strain, resulting in 73 deaths and 135 additional cases of TB. A lengthy investigation attributed the disaster to negligent vaccine preparation, leading to contamination with virulent tubercle bacilli.

Despite this early setback, BCG has subsequently proven to be one of the safest vaccines ever created and has saved the lives of countless individuals, many of them children. However, TB remains an enormous global problem, bringing attention back to BCG attenuation fundamentals, the loss of RD1, and, in turn, the absence of an ESX-1 secretion system.

THE ESX-1 SECRETION SYSTEM AND ITS PROTEINACEOUS ARMY

Many of the proteins secreted by ESX-1 are immunodominant and are at the forefront of infection and disease. The ESX type VII secretion systems are complex; the current working model of the ESX-1 secretion system is shown schematically in Fig. 1B, with the recent addition of EspC, which forms a filamentous structure spanning the bacterial cell envelope (18).

The main ESX-1 system spans the inner membrane with a channel-like structure composed of conserved ESX components (EccB to -D) that form the membrane core complex. EccB and EccC are ATPases involved in recognizing substrates and providing energy for the secretion of substrates across the mycomembrane (19–21). Interestingly, in ESX-1 and ESX-5, the *eccC* gene, encoding a FtsK/SpoIIIE-type ATPase, has split into two genes that generate the proteins EccCa and EccCb, which interact and form a functional unit for secretion through the ESX-1 system. Although the mycosin protease MycP1 is not an integral part of the central membrane complex, and its protease activity is dispensable for ESX-1-mediated protein secretion, MycP1 is a conserved membrane component associated with the membrane complex, and this association is essential for the stability of the complex (22).

In addition to membrane components, ESX-1 also has cytosolic components, including cytosolic ATPase (EccA), chaperones (EspD to -H), and secreted substrate proteins (EsxAB, PE35-PPE68, EspA to -C, and EspE) called effectors. EccA is a cytosolic AAA (ATPase associated with diverse cellular activities)-type ATPase. Most cytosolic chaperones associated with the ESX-1 system belong to ESX-1 secretion-associated proteins (Esp). EspI (Rv3876) to -L (Rv3880c) are encoded within an operon that generates ESX conserved components (Rv3868 to Rv3883c), and the EspE to -H (Rv3864 to Rv3867) genes are upstream, whereas the EspACD (3616c to 3614c) operon is at a more distant location in the genome (Fig. 1A). EspD itself is secreted by *M. tuberculosis*, although not exclusively in an ESX-1-dependent manner, but it is also required for stabilizing (EspC and EspA) and secretion (EsxA) of ESX-1 substrates (23). More recently, the EspD to -F and EspH proteins were shown to be stabilized by the chaperone EspL (24). Although some Esp proteins serve as cytosolic chaperones, some act as effectors (EspA to -C and EspE) of ESX-1 and are secreted (25, 26). EspC has been shown to form filaments in the membrane (18), whereas EspE localizes to the cell wall. Fusion of EspE with a fluorescent marker protein in *M. marinum* demonstrated that ESX-1 localizes at new poles with active peptidoglycan synthesis following cell division (27). How the Esp proteins encoded within the *esx-1* operon or distally in the genome interact with each other and with other components of the ESX-1 system and contribute to its integrity and functionality are still active areas of study.

The other major effectors secreted by the ESX-1 system are key immunogenic, highly secreted ESX proteins, including the early secreted antigenic target of 6 kDa (ESAT-6, also called EsxA) and the culture filtrate protein of 10 kDa (CFP-10 or EsxB). EsxA and EsxB are secreted as a heterodimer (EsxAB) in a codependent complex (28). Binding of the EsxAB heterodimer to the ESX-1 inner membrane core complex component EccC for secretion involves recognition of the bipartite secretion signal motif, consisting of WXG, located on EsxA, and tyrosine-X-X-X-aspartic acid/glutamic acid (YXXXD/E), located on EsxB (21, 25, 29). In contrast, secretion of the PE35-PPE68 heterodimer is dependent on direct binding to EspG (30). The ESX-1 system is highly complex, and this complexity is not restricted to the machinery and effector molecules; the regulation of ESX-1 itself also appears to be multifactorial and is indirectly regulated by PhoPR (31), WhiB6 (32), EspR (33), Lsr2 (34), and MprAB (35).

ESX-1 Lyses Membranes

The macrophage phagosome is a highly inhospitable environment; however, *M. tuberculosis* survives and replicates within this environment. It has long been debated whether *M. tuberculosis* can escape the phagosome and replicate within the cytosol, and McDonough et al. were some of the first researchers to demonstrate the controversial escape of *M. tuberculosis* from phagosomes to the cytosol using electron microscopy (36). This has since been shown to be ESX-1 mediated via ESAT-6 (37). The ESX-1 system was also found to lyse whole cells, causing macrophage and epithelial cell necrosis in *in vitro* infection experiments (4). Many researchers carried out the obvious experiments, adding ESAT-6 (EsxA) directly to cell cultures to look for membrane lysis, often in terms of measuring the release of cytoplasmic contents. However, no cell lysis was observed, until the missing link of low pH was identified (38, 39). Conrad et al. stated that contact dependence was required for ESAT-6 membrane lysis but then, in the same study, showed that low pH caused this as well (40). The Jacobs laboratory tried this experiment in 2003 before we knew of the low-pH trigger, and although our study was unsuccessful, we did demonstrate total membrane disruption in a simplified artificial membrane model with ESAT-6 or ESAT-6 and CFP-10 together, but not with CFP-10 alone (9). In addition, cryo-electron micrographs of ESAT-6 and CFP-10 proteins showed differently sized pore-like structures (Fig. 2, inset a) (8).

Phagosome Permeabilization and Its Prospective Roles

The implications of phagosomal escape have been discussed in many reviews covering mycobacterial species and other intracellular pathogens, such as *Salmonella enterica* serovar Typhimurium or *Listeria monocytogenes* (41). The reasoning includes cytoplasmic nutritional availability, antigen presentation to CD8 T cells, and dissemination. In *M. tuberculosis*, it is clear that this escape happens (37) and that it is ESX-1 mediated; however, some studies suggest that such escape is a temporal by-product of ESX-1 lysing the cell membrane to escape from the cell (42).

Nutrient-rich cytoplasm seems an attractive environment for proliferation, providing an advantage to intracellular pathogens that develop mechanisms to permeabilize, and escape from, the phagosome. Interestingly, to counter host-imposed nutrient restrictions, *M. tuberculosis* can synthesize most of the essential nutrients for its growth, but it is also capable of acquiring nutrients from the host. *M. tuberculosis* can obtain carbon, nitrogen, and some amino acids from the host (41, 43, 44), but intriguingly, it is not able to acquire arginine, methionine, or leucine from the host (45–47).

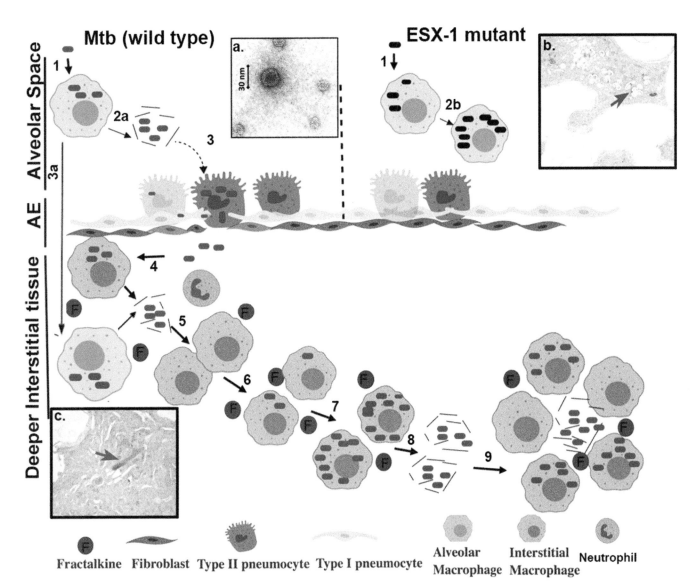

Figure 2 ESX-1-related disease progression within the lung. Steps involved in progression of disease are represented with the numbers 1 to 9. (1) Infection of alveolar macrophages with *M. tuberculosis* (wild type) or ESX-1 mutant. (2) Lysis of the phagosomal and cellular macrophage membranes is carried out by EsxA from wild-type *M. tuberculosis* (2a), while the ESX-1 mutant remains trapped in the alveolar macrophages in the alveolar space (2b). (3) Infection of type II pneumocytes in the alveolar epithelium (AE) by *M. tuberculosis*, with resulting ESAT-6-mediated lysis, allowing passage into the interstitial tissue or (3a) translocation of infected alveolar macrophage to lung interstitial tissue. (4) Translocated bacteria are ingested by and replicate within macrophages, which produce cytokines such as fractalkine. (5) Release of bacilli by necrosis of infection-dependent macrophages. (6) Recruitment of neutrophils and naive macrophages by fractalkine and infection of new macrophages and other cells by phagocytosis. (7) Intracellular replication of bacilli in recruited infected macrophages. (8) Continuation of the cycle, leading to egress of *M. tuberculosis* from the host cells into deeper interstitial tissue and dissemination within the lungs. (9) Establishment of granulomas and necrosis. (Insets) (a) Electron micrograph of EsxAB. (b) Electron micrograph of the ESX-1 mutant (blue arrow) trapped within the phagosome of an alveolar macrophage in alveolar space in a murine model. (c) Electron micrograph showing wild-type *M. tuberculosis* (red arrow) following egress to the cytoplasm and interstitial spaces in the murine lung.

In the Jacobs laboratory, we have demonstrated that arginine or methionine auxotrophy is bactericidal to *M. tuberculosis in vitro* and *in vivo*, both in macrophages and in mice (45, 46), whereas leucine auxotrophy is bacteriostatic (45–47). This finding was noteworthy, as mouse plasma has an arginine concentration of ~200 µM under normal conditions, and *M. tuberculosis* possesses arginine transporters (48, 49). *Salmonella* Typhimurium establishes an active arginine recovery system using its arginine transporter ArgT and by promoting accumulation of the host arginine transporter (mCAT1) on phagosomes (50), which does not appear to be the case with *M. tuberculosis*. This amino acid autarky is, as yet, an unexplored metabolic vulnerability. However, it does suggest that if ESX-1 is functional and provides access to the cytosol, *M. tuberculosis* amino acid auxotrophs should acquire their missing nutrient from the cytosol and proliferate and disseminate as observed with other pathogens (41, 51). However, by utilizing nutrients from the host in this manner, these pathogens also alert the host immune system. It is unclear whether *M. tuberculosis*'s ability to biosynthesize most of the amino acids and metabolic shutdown during famine of the nutrients provide an evolutionary advantage by enhancing the ability of *M. tuberculosis* to persist in the host, ultimately evading vaccine and drug treatments. Further studies are needed to better answer these questions and fully elucidate the essentiality and sufficiency of ESX-1 system to lyse phagosomal membranes and gain access to the nutrient-rich cytosol for proliferation and dissemination.

Another implication of phagosome permeabilization by *M. tuberculosis* is egress of the organism to the cytosol for dissemination and pathogenesis of disease. ESAT-6-mediated phagosome disruption activates the cytosolic inflammasome receptor NLRP3, also triggering increased necrosis (52, 53). Augenstreich et al. suggested that ESX-1, along with phthiocerol dimycocerosates, causes phagosomal rupture but leads to an alternative mode of death, specifically, apoptosis (54). Further, ESX-1-mediated phagosome permeabilization has been shown to enhance type I interferon (IFN) secretion as a pathogenic mechanism for promoting bacterial replication and manipulation of host immunity (8, 55). With so many conflicting studies, it is clear that phagosome disruption remains a much-debated topic in the TB field. Engendering further conflict in the field is the question of whether ESX-1 mediates exit from the cell by the formation of ejectosomes, membrane protrusions containing the bacilli that propel themselves by means of an actin tail. These structures have been observed in *M. marinum* (56), but whether they

occur in *M. tuberculosis*-infected human macrophages has yet to be determined, particularly as *M. tuberculosis* does not have the required active tail (57).

ESX-1 at the Site of Disease: Disease Progression via Necrosis

Orme suggested that necrosis is itself a means to progression of TB disease (58), and following intracellular replication within alveolar macrophages at the site of disease, cell death often occurs, with *M. tuberculosis* ESX-1 promoting necrosis, not apoptosis (4). Indeed, *M. tuberculosis* actively suppresses macrophage apoptosis, reducing bacterial replication (59) with ESX-1, while ESX-1-mediated necrosis enhances bacterial replication (60). *M. tuberculosis* also mediates cellular necrosis in other host cells, such as alveolar epithelial cells in the epithelial bilayer, which is needed for infection and disease progression (61–63). King believes the interaction of *M. tuberculosis* with alveolar epithelial cells is too often overlooked in TB disease, with most researchers conducting studies using macrophages and often missing these short-lived interactions, i.e., the egress across the alveolar interstitium within epithelial cells (63). Notably, studies have shown that type II pneumocytes are highly susceptible to *M. tuberculosis* infection, with the bacilli translocating into interstitial tissue through the basolateral surfaces of these cells via exocytosis or necrosis (64). In collaboration with our laboratory, King's group performed screens to find mutants of *M. tuberculosis* incapable of lysing alveolar epithelial cells, discovering that ESX-1 was required for epithelial cell lysis (9). We also observed ESX-1-mediated macrophage lysis both *in vitro* and *in vivo* (Fig. 2), with *M. tuberculosis* ESX-1 mutants remaining trapped within alveolar macrophages but wild-type bacilli escaping and egressing to the interstitial tissue (9).

Krishnan et al. predicted in 2010 that *M. tuberculosis*-infected alveolar macrophages may translocate from alveolar spaces to lung interstitium to disseminate *M. tuberculosis* (65), and recent studies support their hypothesis. Cohen et al. recently provided evidence of *M. tuberculosis*-infected alveolar macrophages being relocated to the lung interstitium due to ESX-1 and interleukin 1R (IL-1R) dependence (66). ESX-1 effector protein involved in dissemination of infected alveolar macrophages into the interstitium in mice is still undetermined (9, 66). Once *M. tuberculosis* escapes from the activated macrophage via necrosis, it needs a niche. In this instance, a growth-permissive naive macrophage serves as the perfect host where *M. tuberculosis* can survive and replicate. Therefore, to attract naive macrophages, *M. tuberculosis* has evolved a mechanism involving induction of fractalkine production by *M. tuberculosis*-infected cells.

ESX-1 and the Chemokine Fractalkine

First discovered by Bazan et al. in 1998 (67), fractalkine is a rather unusual chemokine and in a class of its own, having a strange stalk-like structure that can also tether host cells. It has been reported to attract naive macrophages to the lung, and fractalkine production from *M. tuberculosis*-infected cells has been determined to be ESX-1 regulated (68). This study also linked fractalkine levels to the influx of naive macrophages during TB infection using bronchoalveolar lavage samples taken directly from the lungs of TB patients. Other cytokines are likely involved in this influx, such as ESX-1-regulated IL-1R (66, 68, 69).

If *M. tuberculosis* ESX-1 mediates fractalkine production from the infected macrophage, what is the effector protein responsible for triggering its production? This appears to be ESAT-6, which activates the tyrosine kinase Syk (53); Syk functions in an upstream activation pathway to produce fractalkine, and its inhibition can stop *M. tuberculosis* ESX-1-mediated fractalkine production and the resulting monocytic infiltration (68). The fractalkine axis has been proposed as a treatment target via the inhibition of monocyte infiltration and thus inflammation in diseases such as Crohn's (70), and a vaccination approach has successfully been used to protect against respiratory syncytial virus infection in an animal model (71). Early establishment of infection and subsequent bacillary dissemination relies upon the availability of permissive "niche" cells. Therefore, a chemotactic signal would be a requisite for increasing the number of the cells from the approximate one macrophage per every 9 ml of lung volume (72). The question of whether other ESX-1-dependent effectors also are involved in the induction of fractalkine production by *M. tuberculosis*-infected macrophages is an open area of investigation.

DO OTHER BACTERIA HAVE ESX-1 SECRETION SYSTEMS?

Homologues of ESX-1 proteins have been detected in various members of the *Actinobacteria* (other mycobacterial species and *Streptomyces coelicolor*), *Firmicutes* (*Staphylococcus aureus*, *L. monocytogenes*, *Bacillus anthracis*, and *Bacillus subtilis*), and *Gammaproteobacteria*, such as *Helicobacter pylori* (73). These secretion systems contain at least one FtsK-SpoIII ATPase, plus one member of the WXG100 protein family (73). A type VII-like secretion system in *S. aureus* is composed of five membrane proteins (EsaA and EssA to -D), three cytosolic proteins (EsaB, -E, and -G), and five secreted virulence factors (EsxA to -D and EsaD) (74). In *S. aureus*, this specialized type VII secretion system is rapidly induced in response to interaction of the bacteria with host fluids, including blood serum, nasal secretions, and pulmonary surfactant (74). Furthermore, by generating mutants with deletions of genes homologous to the *M. tuberculosis* ESX-1 membrane core complex genes *essA*, *essB*, and *essC* in two *S. aureus* strains, Kneuper et al. demonstrated that these genes play a major role in nasal colonization and in development of pneumonia in cystic fibrosis murine infection models (75). Deletion of this secretion system in *S. aureus* leads to its attenuation via decreased bacterial growth and a subsequent decrease in the number of abscesses in host kidneys, spleen, and liver in mice (76, 77). Conversely, an ESX-1 secretion system found in *L. monocytogenes* is not required for epithelial cell invasion and intracellular multiplication in macrophages *in vitro*; indeed, in an *in vivo* murine model, the expression of the ESAT-6 homologue EsxA was detrimental to *L. monocytogenes*, resulting in decreased infection (78). Whether deletion of ESX secretion systems from these pathogens can be exploited for live-vaccine design to protect against infection remains to be investigated.

PRACTICAL IMPLICATIONS OF ESX-1

Drug Interventions and Diagnostics

Studies on ESX-1 proteins have been of continuous interest for the development of drug interventions, diagnostic markers, and vaccines. EsxA and EsxB, two of the most highly secreted proteins of *M. tuberculosis*, have formed the basis for a major breakthrough in TB diagnostics, the IFN-γ release assays (IGRAs). The addition of another ESX-1 protein, EspC, which is present in BCG but not secreted, may potentially enhance the sensitivity and specificity of these assays (79). Interestingly, lysis of *M. tuberculosis* phagosomal membranes via EsxA and EsxB is associated with NOD2-RIP2- or cGAS-STING-dependent or -independent activation of type I interferon IFN-α and IFN-β induction (80). Furthermore, Barczak et al. showed that PDIM production and export are required for coordinated secretion of ESX-1 substrates for phagosome permeabilization and induction of type I IFN response (81).

Several studies have shown that induction of type I IFNs can worsen the outcome of TB (80, 82–84). Berry et al. performed whole-blood transcript signature studies on patients with active and latent TB to identify signatures linked to the progression of active disease (85). Recently, Singhania et al. identified type I IFN as a part of the transcriptome signature that can differentiate between patients with active and latent TB (86). These studies suggest that inhibitors of *M. tuberculosis* pertaining to IFN-α and IFN-β induction are good targets for novel immunotherapeutic strategies to combat *M. tuberculosis*. In addition to the effector proteins EsxA and EsxB, potential targets include immunogenic PE (Pro-Glu) and PPE (Pro-Pro-Glu) proteins and Esp proteins. Effectors such as EspE that are localized on the *M. tuberculosis* cell surface are potential therapeutic targets for antibodies, generating antibody-dependent cell cytotoxic responses, with the aim of eliminating extracellular *M. tuberculosis*. In a recent study, IL-2 induced by stimulation of whole blood with ESX-1-secreted PE35 and PPE68, using a technique similar to that used for IGRAs, was capable of discriminating between patients latently infected with *M. tuberculosis* and those with active TB (87).

The use of ESX-1 proteins distinguishes between BCG-vaccinated and nonvaccinated humans, as BCG does not possess or secrete these proteins. Determining the difference between latent TB infection, BCG vaccination, and active TB infection could revolutionize TB treatment strategies, allowing the development of differentiating biomarkers. Better characterizations of the T-cell-stimulatory proteins secreted by ESX-1 will lead to development of improved IGRAs with enhanced prognostic value.

Why Do We Need a New Vaccine?

BCG is good at protecting a range of animals, from badgers to horses. Unfortunately, that same coverage does not translate to adult humans, resulting in a failure to eradicate TB. However, there is a silver lining with BCG, as it is able to elicit some protection against the disease in children (88). However, if we are to rid the world of TB by 2020, which is the aim of the World Health Organization, we need a better vaccine, and luckily, there are several in the clinical pipeline that are related to ESX-1 or other type VII secretion systems.

In 2012, the Tuberculosis Vaccine Initiative led the TB vaccine community to generate a blueprint for TB vaccine development (https://www.who.int/immunization/sage/3_TB_Vaccines_Strategic_Blueprint_draft_Oct2011_no-v11.pdf). TB vaccine development is difficult, as there is still no known immune correlate of protection. In 2012, there were 13 candidate TB vaccines undergoing clinical trials. In the 5 years that followed, progress of these candidates through the TB vaccine pipeline slowed or failed altogether, with very few preclinical candidates

emerging (89). This impeded progress resulted in the current pipeline of 12 TB vaccine candidates that are currently in phase 1 to 3 clinical trials (Fig. 3). This pipeline consists of a variety of delivery methods (protein/adjuvant, attenuated/killed cells or cell extract, and viral vectors), but the range of antigens and vaccine technologies is actually quite narrow; most rely on eliciting a strong T-helper 1 (Th1) and cell-mediated immune response, known to be important in anti-TB immunity, based on the attenuated *M. tuberculosis* vaccine strain (BCG).

Approaches that focus on ESX-1 and other type VII secretion systems include live, attenuated MTBVAC (90) and VPM1002 (91) and the protein subunit vaccines ID93+GLA-SE (92), H4:IC31 (93), H56:IC31 (94), and M72+AS01E (95). ID93+GLA-SE, H4:IC31, and H56:IC31 have ESAT-6 as one of the antigens secreted by ESX-1, while M72+AS01E has PPE18 secreted by ESX-5 (92–95). MTBVAC was developed from an attenuated *M. tuberculosis* clinical isolate that retained most of the discovered *M. tuberculosis* T-cell epitopes, including the immunodominant antigens EsxA and EsxB of the RD1 region deleted from BCG (Fig. 1A). MTBVAC has entered clinical trials as a preventive vaccine in newborns, adolescents, and adults. It is believed that by targeting the virulence-specific epitopes missing from the BCG vaccine, MTBVAC might afford better protection against TB in human hosts (96). VPM1002 is a recombinant BCG strain with the urease gene (*ureC*) replaced by the listeriolysin O gene *hly* from *L. monocytogenes* (91). In phase II clinical trials, VPM1002 afforded safety and immunogenicity to newborn infants as well as adults. Furthermore, the incidence of abscess formation was lower with VPM1002 than BCG (97).

However, it may be possible that *M. tuberculosis* whole-cell vaccines alone cannot confer the desired level of protection and need to be combined with novel approaches involved in enhancing host immune response, such as that taken in the development of the ID93+GLA-SE and M72+AS01E vaccine candidates. ID93+GLA-SE vaccine was rationally designed as a fusion protein of four immunogenic protein targets that are associated with either virulence (Rv3619, Rv3620, and Rv2608) or latency (Rv1813) (92, 98). Rv3619 and Rv3620 are the ESX-5 ESX protein pair (ESXM/N) paralogs called EsxV and EsxW and are uniquely expressed by *M. tuberculosis*, not *M. bovis* or BCG, while Rv2608 (PPE42) and Rv1813 are common to *M. tuberculosis*, *M. bovis*, and BCG (99–101). The immunogenicity of this vaccine candidate has been boosted by using a Toll-like receptor 4 agonist as an adjuvant, resulting in the induction of a humoral

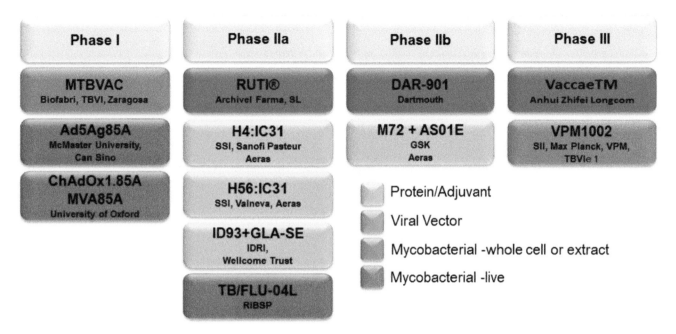

Figure 3 TB vaccines in the pipeline, undergoing phase 1 to 3 clinical trials. Current vaccine candidates in the pipeline include protein/adjuvant-based, attenuated/killed or cell extract-based, and viral vector-based vaccines.

response with a preferential increase in IgG1 and IgG3 subclasses and a Th1-type cellular response (102). Similarly, M72+AS01E includes the antigens Rv1196 (PPE18) and Rv0125, along with the adjuvant AS01E, and showed an efficacy of 54% efficacy in phase 2b trials against *M. tuberculosis* (103). Although this candidate includes an alternative agonist and is designed to promote T cell and antibody responses, we do not know if these are the only correlates that will protect.

There are also questions regarding the role of chemokines in the vaccine response. This subclass of proteins is responsible for recruiting host immune cells and has been largely neglected by TB vaccinologists. Perhaps a better chemokine-centered vaccine could be developed that could halt or contain the spread of *M. tuberculosis* upon initial infection. *M. tuberculosis* uses ESX-1 to spread into the lung interstitium from its initial encounter with the alveolar macrophage (66), in granuloma formation in a human lung tissue model (104), and to modulate the infected macrophage to produce the chemokine fractalkine, which calls in permissive macrophages that can lead to *M. tuberculosis* progression (68). Altering this chemotactic call may switch the immune response, favoring the host. It is therefore possible that ESX systems will lead the way for novel vaccine development. If so, we need to further understand how they work before we can harness their secretory host-controlling powers.

Moreover, multiple strains have been observed in the same patient (105), with mixed infections being massively underrepresented in the majority of diagnostic methods used today (106). Such incomplete diagnosis is, in itself, a huge issue with regard to curbing the spread of TB, potentially resulting in incorrect treatment regimens and enhanced TB rates, but this topic is beyond the scope of this chapter. In addition, many of the circulating strains causing TB may be other members of the *M. tuberculosis* complex (107), indicating that we may need to look for vaccines that will also protect against other members of the *M. tuberculosis* complex, including *Mycobacterium africanum*, *M. bovis*, etc.

CONCLUDING REMARKS

Without ESX-1, *M. tuberculosis* is highly attenuated. *M. tuberculosis* uses virulence-associated ESX-1 to lyse membranes, egress through cells and lung tissue, and cause tuberculous disease. We need to understand the exact role of each of the plethora of proteins that ESX-1 employs to manipulate and modulate. We urgently need novel strategies to protect against and prevent *M. tuberculosis* infections. Furthering our understanding of this proteinaceous army could enable us to target specific ESX-1 proteins involved in the hijacking of the host pathways and ultimately halt the spread of disease. Perhaps this will open new avenues leading to the development of novel immunotherapeutic strategies for TB and a variety of other bacterial diseases.

Acknowledgments. We thank Keely R. Redhage for her help with proofreading and useful comments. We thank Tsungda Hsu for useful discussions related to RD1. This work was supported by grant R01AI026170.

Citation. Tiwari S, Casey R, Goulding CW, Hingley-Wilson S, Jacobs WR Jr. 2019. Infect and Inject: how *Mycobacterium tuberculosis* exploits its major virulence-associated type VII secretion system, ESX-1. Microbiol Spectrum 7(3):BAI-0024-2019.

References

1. World Health Organization. 2018. *Global tuberculosis report 2018*. World Health Organization, Geneva, Switzerland. https://www.who.int/tb/publications/global_report/en/.

2. Calmette A. 1922. *L'infection Bacillaire et la Tuberculose chez l'Homme et chez les Animaux*, 2nd ed. Masson et Cie, Paris, France.

3. Calmette A. 1931. Preventive vaccination against tuberculosis with BCG. *Proc R Soc Med* 24:1481–1490.

4. Mahairas GG, Sabo PJ, Hickey MJ, Singh DC, Stover CK. 1996. Molecular analysis of genetic differences between *Mycobacterium bovis* BCG and virulent *M. bovis. J Bacteriol* 178:1274–1282.

5. Gröschel MI, Sayes F, Simeone R, Majlessi L, Brosch R. 2016. ESX secretion systems: mycobacterial evolution to counter host immunity. *Nat Rev Microbiol* 14:677–691.

6. van Pinxteren LA, Ravn P, Agger EM, Pollock J, Andersen P. 2000. Diagnosis of tuberculosis based on the two specific antigens ESAT-6 and CFP10. *Clin Diagn Lab Immunol* 7:155–160.

7. Gray TA, Clark RR, Boucher N, Lapierre P, Smith C, Derbyshire KM. 2016. Intercellular communication and conjugation are mediated by ESX secretion systems in mycobacteria. *Science* 354:347–350.

8. Manzanillo PS, Shiloh MU, Portnoy DA, Cox JS. 2012. *Mycobacterium tuberculosis* activates the DNA-dependent cytosolic surveillance pathway within macrophages. *Cell Host Microbe* 11:469–480.

9. Hsu T, Hingley-Wilson SM, Chen B, Chen M, Dai AZ, Morin PM, Marks CB, Padiyar J, Goulding C, Gingery M, Eisenberg D, Russell RG, Derrick SC, Collins FM, Morris SL, King CH, Jacobs WR Jr. 2003. The primary mechanism of attenuation of bacillus Calmette-Guerin is a loss of secreted lytic function required for invasion of lung interstitial tissue. *Proc Natl Acad Sci USA* 100:12420–12425.

10. Behr MA, Wilson MA, Gill WP, Salamon H, Schoolnik GK, Rane S, Small PM. 1999. Comparative genomics of BCG vaccines by whole-genome DNA microarray. *Science* 284:1520–1523.

11. Pallen MJ. 2002. The ESAT-6/WXG100 superfamily—and a new Gram-positive secretion system? *Trends Microbiol* 10:209–212.

12. Lewis KN, Liao R, Guinn KM, Hickey MJ, Smith S, Behr MA, Sherman DR. 2003. Deletion of RD1 from *Mycobacterium tuberculosis* mimics bacille Calmette-Guérin attenuation. *J Infect Dis* 187:117–123.

13. Pym AS, Brodin P, Majlessi L, Brosch R, Demangel C, Williams A, Griffiths KE, Marchal G, Leclerc C, Cole ST. 2003. Recombinant BCG exporting ESAT-6 confers enhanced protection against tuberculosis. *Nat Med* 9:533–539.

14. Falkow S. 2004. Molecular Koch's postulates applied to bacterial pathogenicity–a personal recollection 15 years later. *Nat Rev Microbiol* 2:67–72.

15. Clemmensen HS, Knudsen NPH, Rasmussen EM, Winkler J, Rosenkrands I, Ahmad A, Lillebaek T, Sherman DR, Andersen PL, Aagaard C. 2017. An attenuated *Mycobacterium tuberculosis* clinical strain with a defect in ESX-1 secretion induces minimal host immune responses and pathology. *Sci Rep* 7:46666.

16. Bosserman RE, Thompson CR, Nicholson KR, Champion PA. 2018. Esx paralogs are functionally equivalent to ESX-1 proteins but are dispensable for virulence in *Mycobacterium marinum. J Bacteriol* 200:e00726-17.

17. Sakula A. 1983. BCG: who were Calmette and Guérin? *Thorax* 38:806–812.

18. Lou Y, Rybniker J, Sala C, Cole ST. 2017. EspC forms a filamentous structure in the cell envelope of *Mycobacterium tuberculosis* and impacts ESX-1 secretion. *Mol Microbiol* 103:26–38.

19. Zhang XL, Li DF, Fleming J, Wang LW, Zhou Y, Wang DC, Zhang XE, Bi LJ. 2015. Core component EccB1 of the *Mycobacterium tuberculosis* type VII secretion system is a periplasmic ATPase. *FASEB J* 29:4804–4814.

20. Champion PA, Champion MM, Manzanillo P, Cox JS. 2009. ESX-1 secreted virulence factors are recognized by multiple cytosolic AAA ATPases in pathogenic mycobacteria. *Mol Microbiol* 73:950–962.

21. Champion PA, Stanley SA, Champion MM, Brown EJ, Cox JS. 2006. C-terminal signal sequence promotes virulence factor secretion in *Mycobacterium tuberculosis. Science* 313:1632–1636.

22. van Winden VJ, Ummels R, Piersma SR, Jiménez CR, Korotkov KV, Bitter W, Houben EN. 2016. Mycosins are required for the stabilization of the ESX-1 and ESX-5 type VII secretion membrane complexes. *mBio* 7:e01471-16.

23. Chen JM, Boy-Röttger S, Dhar N, Sweeney N, Buxton RS, Pojer F, Rosenkrands I, Cole ST. 2012. EspD is critical for the virulence-mediating ESX-1 secretion system in *Mycobacterium tuberculosis. J Bacteriol* 194:884–893.

24. Sala C, Odermatt NT, Soler-Arnedo P, Gülen MF, von Schultz S, Benjak A, Cole ST. 2018. EspL is essential for virulence and stabilizes EspE, EspF and EspH levels in *Mycobacterium tuberculosis. PLoS Pathog* 14:e1007491.

25. Fortune SM, Jaeger A, Sarracino DA, Chase MR, Sassetti CM, Sherman DR, Bloom BR, Rubin EJ. 2005. Mutually dependent secretion of proteins required for

mycobacterial virulence. *Proc Natl Acad Sci USA* **102:** 10676–10681.

26. Solomonson M, Setiaputra D, Makepeace KAT, Lameignere E, Petrotchenko EV, Conrady DG, Bergeron JR, Vuckovic M, DiMaio F, Borchers CH, Yip CK, Strynadka NCJ. 2015. Structure of EspB from the ESX-1 type VII secretion system and insights into its export mechanism. *Structure* 23:571–583.

27. Carlsson F, Joshi SA, Rangell L, Brown EJ. 2009. Polar localization of virulence-related Esx-1 secretion in mycobacteria. *PLoS Pathog* 5:e1000285.

28. Renshaw PS, Lightbody KL, Veverka V, Muskett FW, Kelly G, Frenkiel TA, Gordon SV, Hewinson RG, Burke B, Norman J, Williamson RA, Carr MD. 2005. Structure and function of the complex formed by the tuberculosis virulence factors CFP-10 and ESAT-6. *EMBO J* 24:2491–2498.

29. Daleke MH, Ummels R, Bawono P, Heringa J, Vandenbroucke-Grauls CM, Luirink J, Bitter W. 2012. General secretion signal for the mycobacterial type VII secretion pathway. *Proc Natl Acad Sci USA* 109: 11342–11347.

30. Ates LS, Houben EN, Bitter W. 2016. Type VII secretion: a highly versatile secretion system. *Microbiol Spectr* 4:VMBF-0011-2015.

31. Frigui W, Bottai D, Majlessi L, Monot M, Josselin E, Brodin P, Garnier T, Gicquel B, Martin C, Leclerc C, Cole ST, Brosch R. 2008. Control of *M. tuberculosis* ESAT-6 secretion and specific T cell recognition by PhoP. *PLoS Pathog* 4:e33.

32. Solans L, Aguiló N, Samper S, Pawlik A, Frigui W, Martín C, Brosch R, Gonzalo-Asensio J. 2014. A specific polymorphism in *Mycobacterium tuberculosis* H37Rv causes differential ESAT-6 expression and identifies WhiB6 as a novel ESX-1 component. *Infect Immun* 82:3446–3456.

33. Raghavan S, Manzanillo P, Chan K, Dovey C, Cox JS. 2008. Secreted transcription factor controls *Mycobacterium tuberculosis* virulence. *Nature* 454:717–721.

34. Gordon BR, Li Y, Wang L, Sintsova A, van Bakel H, Tian S, Navarre WW, Xia B, Liu J. 2010. Lsr2 is a nucleoid-associated protein that targets AT-rich sequences and virulence genes in *Mycobacterium tuberculosis*. *Proc Natl Acad Sci USA* 107:5154–5159.

35. Pang X, Samten B, Cao G, Wang X, Tvinnereim AR, Chen XL, Howard ST. 2013. MprAB regulates the *espA* operon in *Mycobacterium tuberculosis* and modulates ESX-1 function and host cytokine response. *J Bacteriol* 195:66–75.

36. McDonough KA, Kress Y, Bloom BR. 1993. Pathogenesis of tuberculosis: interaction of *Mycobacterium tuberculosis* with macrophages. *Infect Immun* 61:2763–2773.

37. Houben D, Demangel C, van Ingen J, Perez J, Baldeón L, Abdallah AM, Caleechurn L, Bottai D, van Zon M, de Punder K, van der Laan T, Kant A, Bossers-de Vries R, Willemsen P, Bitter W, van Soolingen D, Brosch R, van der Wel N, Peters PJ. 2012. ESX-1-mediated translocation to the cytosol controls virulence of mycobacteria. *Cell Microbiol* 14:1287–1298.

38. De Leon J, Jiang G, Ma Y, Rubin E, Fortune S, Sun J. 2012. *Mycobacterium tuberculosis* ESAT-6 exhibits a unique membrane-interacting activity that is not found in its ortholog from non-pathogenic *Mycobacterium smegmatis*. *J Biol Chem* 287:44184–44191.

39. de Jonge MI, Pehau-Arnaudet G, Fretz MM, Romain F, Bottai D, Brodin P, Honoré N, Marchal G, Jiskoot W, England P, Cole ST, Brosch R. 2007. ESAT-6 from *Mycobacterium tuberculosis* dissociates from its putative chaperone CFP-10 under acidic conditions and exhibits membrane-lysing activity. *J Bacteriol* 189:6028–6034.

40. Conrad WH, Osman MM, Shanahan JK, Chu F, Takaki KK, Cameron J, Hopkinson-Woolley D, Brosch R, Ramakrishnan L. 2017. Mycobacterial ESX-1 secretion system mediates host cell lysis through bacterium contact-dependent gross membrane disruptions. *Proc Natl Acad Sci USA* **114:**1371–1376.

41. Gouzy A, Poquet Y, Neyrolles O. 2014. Nitrogen metabolism in *Mycobacterium tuberculosis* physiology and virulence. *Nat Rev Microbiol* **12:**729–737.

42. Simeone R, Bobard A, Lippmann J, Bitter W, Majlessi L, Brosch R, Enninga J. 2012. Phagosomal rupture by *Mycobacterium tuberculosis* results in toxicity and host cell death. *PLoS Pathog* 8:e1002507.

43. Beste DJ, Nöh K, Niedenführ S, Mendum TA, Hawkins ND, Ward JL, Beale MH, Wiechert W, McFadden J. 2013. 13C-flux spectral analysis of host-pathogen metabolism reveals a mixed diet for intracellular *Mycobacterium tuberculosis*. *Chem Biol* 20:1012–1021.

44. Baughn AD, Rhee KY. 2014. Metabolomics of central carbon metabolism in *Mycobacterium tuberculosis*. *Microbiol Spectr* 2:MGM2-0026-2013.

45. Berney M, Berney-Meyer L, Wong KW, Chen B, Chen M, Kim J, Wang J, Harris D, Parkhill J, Chan J, Wang F, Jacobs WR Jr. 2015. Essential roles of methionine and S-adenosylmethionine in the autarkic lifestyle of *Mycobacterium tuberculosis*. *Proc Natl Acad Sci USA* 112:10008–10013.

46. Tiwari S, van Tonder AJ, Vilchèze C, Mendes V, Thomas SE, Malek A, Chen B, Chen M, Kim J, Blundell TL, Parkhill J, Weinrick B, Berney M, Jacobs WR Jr. 2018. Arginine-deprivation-induced oxidative damage sterilizes *Mycobacterium tuberculosis*. *Proc Natl Acad Sci USA* 115:9779–9784.

47. McAdam RA, Weisbrod TR, Martin J, Scuderi JD, Brown AM, Cirillo JD, Bloom BR, Jacobs WR Jr. 1995. In vivo growth characteristics of leucine and methionine auxotrophic mutants of *Mycobacterium bovis* BCG generated by transposon mutagenesis. *Infect Immun* 63: 1004–1012.

48. Gobert AP, Daulouede S, Lepoivre M, Boucher JL, Bouteille B, Buguet A, Cespuglio R, Veyret B, Vincendeau P. 2000. L-Arginine availability modulates local nitric oxide production and parasite killing in experimental trypanosomiasis. *Infect Immun* 68: 4653–4657.

49. Peteroy-Kelly M, Venketaraman V, Connell ND. 2001. Effects of *Mycobacterium bovis* BCG infection on regulation of L-arginine uptake and synthesis of reactive

nitrogen intermediates in J774.1 murine macrophages. *Infect Immun* **69**:5823–5831.

50. **Das P, Lahiri A, Lahiri A, Sen M, Iyer N, Kapoor N, Balaji KN, Chakravortty D.** 2010. Cationic amino acid transporters and *Salmonella* Typhimurium ArgT collectively regulate arginine availability towards intracellular *Salmonella* growth. *PLoS One* **5**:e15466.

51. **Zhang YJ, Rubin EJ.** 2013. Feast or famine: the host-pathogen battle over amino acids. *Cell Microbiol* **15**:1079–1087.

52. **Wong KW.** 2017. The role of ESX-1 in *Mycobacterium tuberculosis* pathogenesis. *Microbiol Spectr* **5**: TBTB2-0001-2015.

53. **Wong KW, Jacobs WR Jr.** 2011. Critical role for NLRP3 in necrotic death triggered by *Mycobacterium tuberculosis*. *Cell Microbiol* **13**:1371–1384.

54. **Augenstreich J, Arbues A, Simeone R, Haanappel E, Wegener A, Sayes F, Le Chevalier F, Chalut C, Malaga W, Guilhot C, Brosch R, Astarie-Dequeker C.** 2017. ESX-1 and phthiocerol dimycocerosates of *Mycobacterium tuberculosis* act in concert to cause phagosomal rupture and host cell apoptosis. *Cell Microbiol* **19**: e12726.

55. **Stanley SA, Johndrow JE, Manzanillo P, Cox JS.** 2007. The type I IFN response to infection with *Mycobacterium tuberculosis* requires ESX-1-mediated secretion and contributes to pathogenesis. *J Immunol* **178**: 3143–3152.

56. **Hagedorn M, Rohde KH, Russell DG, Soldati T.** 2009. Infection by tubercular mycobacteria is spread by nonlytic ejection from their amoeba hosts. *Science* **323**: 1729–1733.

57. **Stamm LM, Brown EJ.** 2004. *Mycobacterium marinum*: the generalization and specialization of a pathogenic mycobacterium. *Microbes Infect* **6**:1418–1428.

58. **Orme IM.** 2014. A new unifying theory of the pathogenesis of tuberculosis. *Tuberculosis (Edinb)* **94**:8–14.

59. **Sly LM, Hingley-Wilson SM, Reiner NE, McMaster WR.** 2003. Survival of *Mycobacterium tuberculosis* in host macrophages involves resistance to apoptosis dependent upon induction of antiapoptotic Bcl-2 family member Mcl-1. *J Immunol* **170**:430–437.

60. **Dallenga T, Repnik U, Corleis B, Eich J, Reimer R, Griffiths GW, Schaible UE.** 2017. *M. tuberculosis*-induced necrosis of infected neutrophils promotes bacterial growth following phagocytosis by nacrophages. *Cell Host Microbe* **22**:519–530.e3.

61. **Bermudez LE, Sangari FJ, Kolonoski P, Petrofsky M, Goodman J.** 2002. The efficiency of the translocation of *Mycobacterium tuberculosis* across a bilayer of epithelial and endothelial cells as a model of the alveolar wall is a consequence of transport within mononuclear phagocytes and invasion of alveolar epithelial cells. *Infect Immun* **70**:140–146.

62. **Sasindran SJ, Torrelles JB.** 2011. *Mycobacterium tuberculosis* infection and inflammation: what is beneficial for the host and for the bacterium? *Front Microbiol* **2**:2.

63. **Dobos KM, Spotts EA, Quinn FD, King CH.** 2000. Necrosis of lung epithelial cells during infection with *Mycobacterium tuberculosis* is preceded by cell permeation. *Infect Immun* **68**:6300–6310.

64. **Scordo JM, Knoell DL, Torrelles JB.** 2016. Alveolar epithelial cells in *Mycobacterium tuberculosis* infection: active players or innocent bystanders? *J Innate Immun* **8**:3–14.

65. **Krishnan N, Robertson BD, Thwaites G.** 2010. The mechanisms and consequences of the extra-pulmonary dissemination of *Mycobacterium tuberculosis*. *Tuberculosis (Edinb)* **90**:361–366.

66. **Cohen SB, Gern BH, Delahaye JL, Adams KN, Plumlee CR, Winkler JK, Sherman DR, Gerner MY, Urdahl KB.** 2018. Alveolar macrophages provide an early *Mycobacterium tuberculosis* niche and initiate dissemination. *Cell Host Microbe* **24**:439–446.e4.

67. **Bazan JF, Bacon KB, Hardiman G, Wang W, Soo K, Rossi D, Greaves DR, Zlotnik A, Schall TJ.** 1997. A new class of membrane-bound chemokine with a CX3C motif. *Nature* **385**:640–644.

68. **Hingley-Wilson SM, Connell D, Pollock K, Hsu T, Tchilian E, Sykes A, Grass L, Potiphar L, Bremang S, Kon OM, Jacobs WR Jr, Lalvani A.** 2014. ESX1-dependent fractalkine mediates chemotaxis and *Mycobacterium tuberculosis* infection in humans. *Tuberculosis (Edinb)* **94**:262–270.

69. **Volkman HE, Pozos TC, Zheng J, Davis JM, Rawls JF, Ramakrishnan L.** 2010. Tuberculous granuloma induction via interaction of a bacterial secreted protein with host epithelium. *Science* **327**:466–469.

70. **Brand S, Hofbauer K, Dambacher J, Schnitzler F, Staudinger T, Pfennig S, Seiderer J, Tillack C, Konrad A, Göke B, Ochsenkühn T, Lohse P.** 2006. Increased expression of the chemokine fractalkine in Crohn's disease and association of the fractalkine receptor T280M polymorphism with a fibrostenosing disease phenotype. *Am J Gastroenterol* **101**:99–106.

71. **Zhang W, Choi Y, Haynes LM, Harcourt JL, Anderson LJ, Jones LP, Tripp RA.** 2010. Vaccination to induce antibodies blocking the CX3C-CX3CR1 interaction of respiratory syncytial virus G protein reduces pulmonary inflammation and virus replication in mice. *J Virol* **84**: 1148–1157.

72. **Crapo JD, Barry BE, Gehr P, Bachofen M, Weibel ER.** 1982. Cell number and cell characteristics of the normal human lung. *Am Rev Respir Dis* **125**:740–745.

73. **Unnikrishnan M, Constantinidou C, Palmer T, Pallen MJ.** 2017. The enigmatic Esx proteins: looking beyond mycobacteria. *Trends Microbiol* **25**:192–204.

74. **Lopez MS, Tan IS, Yan D, Kang J, McCreary M, Modrusan Z, Austin CD, Xu M, Brown EJ.** 2017. Host-derived fatty acids activate type VII secretion in *Staphylococcus aureus*. *Proc Natl Acad Sci USA* **114**: 11223–11228.

75. **Kneuper H, Cao ZP, Twomey KB, Zoltner M, Jäger F, Cargill JS, Chalmers J, van der Kooi-Pol MM, van Dijl JM, Ryan RP, Hunter WN, Palmer T.** 2014. Heterogeneity in *ess* transcriptional organization and variable contribution of the Ess/Type VII protein secretion system to virulence across closely related

Staphylocccus aureus strains. *Mol Microbiol* **93**: 928–943.

76. Burts ML, Williams WA, DeBord K, Missiakas DM. 2005. EsxA and EsxB are secreted by an ESAT-6-like system that is required for the pathogenesis of *Staphylococcus aureus* infections. *Proc Natl Acad Sci USA* **102**: 1169–1174.

77. Wang Y, Hu M, Liu Q, Qin J, Dai Y, He L, Li T, Zheng B, Zhou F, Yu K, Fang J, Liu X, Otto M, Li M. 2016. Role of the ESAT-6 secretion system in virulence of the emerging community-associated *Staphylococcus aureus* lineage ST398. *Sci Rep* **6**:25163.

78. Pinheiro J, Reis O, Vieira A, Moura IM, Zanolli Moreno L, Carvalho F, Pucciarelli MG, García-Del Portillo F, Sousa S, Cabanes D. 2017. *Listeria monocytogenes* encodes a functional ESX-1 secretion system whose expression is detrimental to in vivo infection. *Virulence* **8**:993–1004.

79. Millington KA, Fortune SM, Low J, Garces A, Hingley-Wilson SM, Wickremasinghe M, Kon OM, Lalvani A. 2011. Rv3615c is a highly immunodominant RD1 (Region of Difference 1)-dependent secreted antigen specific for *Mycobacterium tuberculosis* infection. *Proc Natl Acad Sci USA* **108**:5730–5735.

80. Donovan ML, Schultz TE, Duke TJ, Blumenthal A. 2017. Type I interferons in the pathogenesis of tuberculosis: molecular drivers and immunological consequences. *Front Immunol* **8**:1633.

81. Barczak AK, Avraham R, Singh S, Luo SS, Zhang WR, Bray MA, Hinman AE, Thompson M, Nietupski RM, Golas A, Montgomery P, Fitzgerald M, Smith RS, White DW, Tischler AD, Carpenter AE, Hung DT. 2017. Systematic, multiparametric analysis of *Mycobacterium tuberculosis* intracellular infection offers insight into coordinated virulence. *PLoS Pathog* **13**:e1006363.

82. Manca C, Tsenova L, Bergtold A, Freeman S, Tovey M, Musser JM, Barry CE III, Freedman VH, Kaplan G. 2001. Virulence of a *Mycobacterium tuberculosis* clinical isolate in mice is determined by failure to induce Th1 type immunity and is associated with induction of IFN-alpha /beta. *Proc Natl Acad Sci USA* **98**: 5752–5757.

83. Antonelli LR, Gigliotti Rothfuchs A, Gonçalves R, Roffê E, Cheever AW, Bafica A, Salazar AM, Feng CG, Sher A. 2010. Intranasal poly-IC treatment exacerbates tuberculosis in mice through the pulmonary recruitment of a pathogen-permissive monocyte/macrophage population. *J Clin Invest* **120**:1674–1682.

84. Mayer-Barber KD, Andrade BB, Oland SD, Amaral EP, Barber DL, Gonzales J, Derrick SC, Shi R, Kumar NP, Wei W, Yuan X, Zhang G, Cai Y, Babu S, Catalfamo M, Salazar AM, Via LE, Barry CE III, Sher A. 2014. Host-directed therapy of tuberculosis based on interleukin-1 and type I interferon crosstalk. *Nature* **511**:99–103.

85. Berry MP, Graham CM, McNab FW, Xu Z, Bloch SA, Oni T, Wilkinson KA, Banchereau R, Skinner J, Wilkinson RJ, Quinn C, Blankenship D, Dhawan R, Cush JJ, Mejias A, Ramilo O, Kon OM, Pascual V, Banchereau J, Chaussabel D, O'Garra A. 2010. An interferon-inducible neutrophil-driven blood transcriptional signature in human tuberculosis. *Nature* **466**: 973–977.

86. Singhania A, Verma R, Graham CM, Lee J, Tran T, Richardson M, Lecine P, Leissner P, Berry MPR, Wilkinson RJ, Kaiser K, Rodrigue M, Woltmann G, Haldar P, O'Garra A. 2018. A modular transcriptional signature identifies phenotypic heterogeneity of human tuberculosis infection. *Nat Commun* **9**:2308.

87. Pourakbari B, Mamishi S, Marjani M, Rasulinejad M, Mariotti S, Mahmoudi S. 2015. Novel T-cell assays for the discrimination of active and latent tuberculosis infection: the diagnostic value of PPE family. *Mol Diagn Ther* **19**:309–316.

88. Abdallah AM, Bestebroer J, Savage ND, de Punder K, van Zon M, Wilson L, Korbee CJ, van der Sar AM, Ottenhoff TH, van der Wel NN, Bitter W, Peters PJ. 2011. Mycobacterial secretion systems ESX-1 and ESX-5 play distinct roles in host cell death and inflammasome activation. *J Immunol* **187**:4744–4753.

89. Voss G, Casimiro D, Neyrolles O, Williams A, Kaufmann SHE, McShane H, Hatherill M, Fletcher HA. 2018. Progress and challenges in TB vaccine development. *F1000 Res* **7**:199.

90. Marinova D, Gonzalo-Asensio J, Aguilo N, Martin C. 2017. MTBVAC from discovery to clinical trials in tuberculosis-endemic countries. *Expert Rev Vaccines* **16**:565–576.

91. Grode L, Ganoza CA, Brohm C, Weiner J III, Eisele B, Kaufmann SH. 2013. Safety and immunogenicity of the recombinant BCG vaccine VPM1002 in a phase 1 open-label randomized clinical trial. *Vaccine* **31**: 1340–1348.

92. Penn-Nicholson A, Tameris M, Smit E, Day TA, Musvosvi M, Jayashankar L, Vergara J, Mabwe S, Bilek N, Geldenhuys H, Luabeya AK, Ellis R, Ginsberg AM, Hanekom WA, Reed SG, Coler RN, Scriba TJ, Hatherill M, TBVPX-114 study team. 2018. Safety and immunogenicity of the novel tuberculosis vaccine ID93 + GLA-SE in BCG-vaccinated healthy adults in South Africa: a randomised, double-blind, placebo-controlled phase 1 trial. *Lancet Respir Med* **6**:287–298.

93. Nemes E, Geldenhuys H, Rozot V, Rutkowski KT, Ratangee F, Bilek N, Mabwe S, Makhethe L, Erasmus M, Toefy A, Mulenga H, Hanekom WA, Self SG, Bekker LG, Ryall R, Gurunathan S, DiazGranados CA, Andersen P, Kromann I, Evans T, Ellis RD, Landry B, Hokey DA, Hopkins R, Ginsberg AM, Scriba TJ, Hatherill M, C-040-404 Study Team. 2018. Prevention of *M. tuberculosis* infection with H4:IC31 vaccine or BCG revaccination. *N Engl J Med* **379**:138–149.

94. Suliman S, Luabeya AKK, Geldenhuys H, Tameris M, Hoff ST, Shi Z, Tait D, Kromann I, Ruhwald M, Rutkowski KT, Shepherd B, Hokey D, Ginsberg AM, Hanekom WA, Andersen P, Scriba TJ, Hatherill M, Oelofse RE, Stone L, Swarts AM, Onrust R, Jacobs G, Coetzee L, Khomba G, Diamond B, Companie A, Veldsman A, Mulenga H, Cloete Y, Steyn M, Africa H, Nkantsu L, Smit E, Botes J, Bilek N, Mabwe S, H56-035 Trial Group. 2019. Dose optimization of H56:

IC31 vaccine for tuberculosis-endemic populations. A double-blind, placebo-controlled, dose-selection trial. *Am J Respir Crit Care Med* 199:220–231.

95. Penn-Nicholson A, Geldenhuys H, Burny W, van der Most R, Day CL, Jongert E, Moris P, Hatherill M, Ofori-Anyinam O, Hanekom W, Bollaerts A, Demoitie MA, Kany Luabeya AK, De Ruymaeker E, Tameris M, Lapierre D, Scriba TJ, Vaccine Study Team. 2015. Safety and immunogenicity of candidate vaccine M72/AS01E in adolescents in a TB endemic setting.*Vaccine* 33:4025–4034.

96. Gonzalo-Asensio J, Marinova D, Martin C, Aguilo N. 2017. MTBVAC: attenuating the human pathogen of tuberculosis (TB) toward a promising vaccine against the TB epidemic. *Front Immunol* 8:1803.

97. Loxton AG, Knaul JK, Grode L, Gutschmidt A, Meller C, Eisele B, Johnstone H, van der Spuy G, Maertzdorf J, Kaufmann SHE, Hesseling AC, Walzl G, Cotton MF. 2017. Safety and immunogenicity of the recombinant *Mycobacterium bovis* BCG vaccine VPM1002 in HIV-unexposed newborn infants in South Africa. *Clin Vaccine Immunol* 24:e00439-16.

98. Bertholet S, Ireton GC, Kahn M, Guderian J, Mohamath R, Stride N, Laughlin EM, Baldwin SL, Vedvick TS, Coler RN, Reed SG. 2008. Identification of human T cell antigens for the development of vaccines against *Mycobacterium tuberculosis*. *J Immunol* 181: 7948–7957.

99. Shah S, Briken V. 2016. Modular organization of the ESX-5 secretion system in *Mycobacterium tuberculosis*. *Front Cell Infect Microbiol* 6:49.

100. Copin R, Coscollá M, Efstathiadis E, Gagneux S, Ernst JD. 2014. Impact of in vitro evolution on antigenic diversity of *Mycobacterium bovis* bacillus Calmette-Guerin (BCG). *Vaccine* 32:5998–6004.

101. Garnier T, Eiglmeier K, Camus JC, Medina N, Mansoor H, Pryor M, Duthoy S, Grondin S, Lacroix C, Monsempe C, Simon S, Harris B, Atkin R, Doggett J, Mayes R, Keating L, Wheeler PR, Parkhill J, Barrell BG, Cole ST, Gordon SV, Hewinson RG. 2003. The complete genome sequence of *Mycobacterium bovis*. *Proc Natl Acad Sci USA* 100:7877–7882.

102. Coler RN, Day TA, Ellis R, Piazza FM, Beckmann AM, Vergara J, Rolf T, Lu L, Alter G, Hokey D, Jayashankar L, Walker R, Snowden MA, Evans T, Ginsberg A, Reed SG, TBVPX-113 Study Team. 2018. The TLR-4 agonist adjuvant, GLA-SE, improves magnitude and quality of immune responses elicited by the ID93 tuberculosis vaccine: first-in-human trial. *NPJ Vaccines* 3:34.

103. Van Der Meeren O, Hatherill M, Nduba V, Wilkinson RJ, Muyoyeta M, Van Brakel E, Ayles HM, Henostroza G, Thienemann F, Scriba TJ, Diacon A, Blatner GL, Demoitié MA, Tameris M, Malahleha M, Innes JC, Hellström E, Martinson N, Singh T, Akite EJ, Khatoon Azam A, Bollaerts A, Ginsberg AM, Evans TG, Gillard P, Tait DR. 2018. Phase 2b controlled trial of M72/AS01$_E$ vaccine to prevent tuberculosis. *N Engl J Med* 379:1621–1634.

104. Parasa VR, Rahman MJ, Ngyuen Hoang AT, Svensson M, Brighenti S, Lerm M. 2014. Modeling *Mycobacterium tuberculosis* early granuloma formation in experimental human lung tissue. *Dis Model Mech* 7: 281–288.

105. Hingley-Wilson SM, Casey R, Connell D, Bremang S, Evans JT, Hawkey PM, Smith GE, Jepson A, Philip S, Kon OM, Lalvani A. 2013. Undetected multidrug-resistant tuberculosis amplified by first-line therapy in mixed infection. *Emerg Infect Dis* 19:1138–1141.

106. McIvor A, Koornhof H, Kana BD. 2017. Relapse, re-infection and mixed infections in tuberculosis disease. *Pathog Dis* 75:ftx020.

107. Yeboah-Manu D, Asare P, Asante-Poku A, Otchere ID, Osei-Wusu S, Danso E, Forson A, Koram KA, Gagneux S. 2016. Spatio-temporal distribution of *Mycobacterium tuberculosis* complex strains in Ghana. *PLoS One* 11: e0161892.

108. Bitter W, Houben EN, Bottai D, Brodin P, Brown EJ, Cox JS, Derbyshire K, Fortune SM, Gao LY, Liu J, Gey van Pittius NC, Pym AS, Rubin EJ, Sherman DR, Cole ST, Brosch R. 2009. Systematic genetic nomenclature for type VII secretion systems. *PLoS Pathog* 5: e1000507.

109. Houben EN, Bestebroer J, Ummels R, Wilson L, Piersma SR, Jiménez CR, Ottenhoff TH, Luirink J, Bitter W. 2012. Composition of the type VII secretion system membrane complex. *Mol Microbiol* 86:472–484.

110. Rosenberg OS, Dovala D, Li X, Connolly L, Bendebury A, Finer-Moore J, Holton J, Cheng Y, Stroud RM, Cox JS. 2015. Substrates control multimerization and activation of the multi-domain ATPase motor of type VII secretion. *Cell* 161:501–512.

111. Das C, Ghosh TS, Mande SS. 2011. Computational analysis of the ESX-1 region of *Mycobacterium tuberculosis*: insights into the mechanism of type VII secretion system. *PLoS One* 6:e27980.

112. Daleke MH, van der Woude AD, Parret AH, Ummels R, de Groot AM, Watson D, Piersma SR, Jiménez CR, Luirink J, Bitter W, Houben EN. 2012. Specific chaperones for the type VII protein secretion pathway. *J Biol Chem* 287:31939–31947.

113. Ekiert DC, Cox JS. 2014. Structure of a PE-PPE-EspG complex from *Mycobacterium tuberculosis* reveals molecular specificity of ESX protein secretion. *Proc Natl Acad Sci USA* 111:14758–14763.

114. Korotkova N, Freire D, Phan TH, Ummels R, Creekmore CC, Evans TJ, Wilmanns M, Bitter W, Parret AH, Houben EN, Korotkov KV. 2014. Structure of the *Mycobacterium tuberculosis* type VII secretion system chaperone EspG5 in complex with PE25-PPE41 dimer. *Mol Microbiol* 94:367–382.

115. Korotkova N, Piton J, Wagner JM, Boy-Röttger S, Japaridze A, Evans TJ, Cole ST, Pojer F, Korotkov KV. 2015. Structure of EspB, a secreted substrate of the ESX-1 secretion system of *Mycobacterium tuberculosis*. *J Struct Biol* 191:236–244.

Bacteria and Intracellularity
Edited by Pascale Cossart, Craig R. Roy, and Philippe Sansonetti
© 2019 American Society for Microbiology, Washington, DC
doi:10.1128/microbiolspec.BAI-0001-2019

Mycobacterium tuberculosis: Bacterial Fitness within the Host Macrophage

9

Lu Huang,[1] Evgeniya V. Nazarova,[1] and David G. Russell[1]

INTRODUCTION

The foundations of our understanding of intracellular parasitism by a range of eukaryote and prokaryote pathogens has been laid by using tissue culture infection models. These models, using defined cell lines or expanded primary cell cultures, have been invaluable in the generation of the knowledge base on which the field currently relies. However, the models artificially compress the heterogeneity that exists for all these pathogens in their natural *in vivo* infection cycle. It is the heterogeneity within the pathogen population that enhances a pathogen's capacity to adapt and survive under the different immune pressures and tissue environments within its host (1–3).

The past few years have seen the development of a new generation of tools that will enable us to better understand the functional consequences of heterogeneity both in the pathogen population and in the subsets of host cells present *in vivo* (4–6). *Mycobacterium tuberculosis* is a human pathogen and is the largest single cause of death by a single infectious agent. There are no effective vaccines against infection and no biomarkers for protective immunity (7–10). While there are drugs that are effective against *M. tuberculosis*, treatment requires a cocktail of three or four drugs taken continuously for 8 to 9 months. Such drug regimens are a serious strain on the resources of the health care systems in many resource-challenged nations, and drug-resistant strains emerge with disturbing frequency in many countries. Understanding the consequences of bacterial heterogeneity *in vivo* with respect to both drug action and immune containment remains a serious challenge to the field.

THE IMMUNE ENVIRONMENT AT THE SITE OF INFECTION

While not an obligate intracellular pathogen, *M. tuberculosis* does spend the greatest part of its infection cycle within host phagocytes, and the granuloma, the tissue response to *M. tuberculosis* infection, is an extremely macrophage-rich structure (11, 12). Recent data indicate that, following inhalation of infectious *M. tuberculosis*, the bacterium is phagocytosed by alveolar macrophages (AMs) patrolling the airway surface (13). Uptake of *M. tuberculosis* activates an inflammatory response through the stimulatory capacity of the multiple Toll-like receptor ligands on the bacterial cell wall. The infected AM invades the subtending tissue of the lung, and the proinflammatory response amplifies. This response leads to the generation of chemokines, such as CCL2, that are the primary drivers of the recruitment of interstitial macrophages (IMs) derived from peripheral blood monocytes in the circulatory system (14–17). This proinflammatory response persists until the development of an acquired immune response, which in the murine model system is delayed until 3 to 4 weeks postinfection because it is dependent on dendritic cells carrying *M. tuberculosis* antigen to draining lymph nodes to prime the initial T-cell response to infection (18, 19).

Upon initiation of a specific immune response against *M. tuberculosis*, the replication of the bacterium is restricted and the infection transitions into a containment state with a relatively static bacterial burden (Fig. 1A). In non-human primates and, by inference, in humans, the infection is paucibacillary, whereas in mice there is a much greater bacterial burden. This is one of the

[1]Microbiology and Immunology, College of Veterinary Medicine, Cornell University, Ithaca, NY 14853.

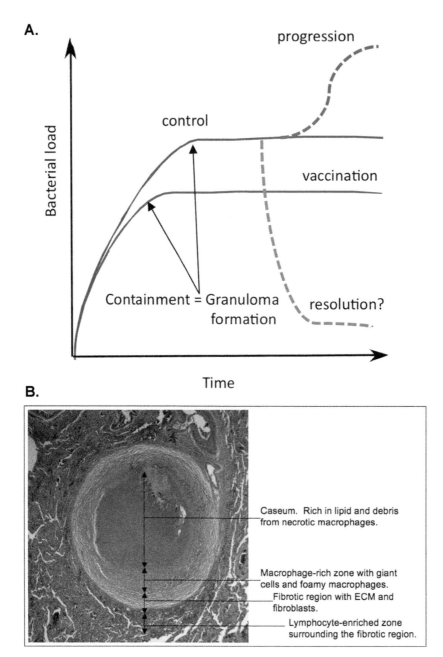

Figure 1 (**A**) Schematic illustration of the potential outcomes of infection with *M. tuberculosis*. In most hosts, *M. tuberculosis* exhibits rapid expansion of the bacterial burden during the first 3 to 4 weeks of infection. At this point, the acquired immune response has developed and controls the bacterial burden at a subclinical level but is unable to clear the infection. In vaccinated hosts, this transition to control of the bacterial burden is achieved at around 1 log fewer bacilli. While resolution of infection is theoretically possible, it is virtually impossible to demonstrate. Progression from latent disease to active disease appears to occur in the face of a robust systemic immune response that is Th1 dominant. While there are candidate indicators of early disease progression, the field lacks immunological markers to detect vaccine-induced protection. Published previously in reference 10. (**B**) The main features of the human TB granuloma. A fully formed human TB granuloma is an extremely stratified structure. The center of the granuloma is caseous and rich in lipids, thought to be derived from the lipids present in foamy macrophages. The caseum is surrounded by a macrophage-rich layer that contains foamy macrophages, multinucleated giant cells, and epithelioid macrophages. *M. tuberculosis* bacilli are observed in many of these cells. This structure is frequently encased in a fibrous capsule of collagen and other extracellular matrix proteins. Lymphocytes tend to be restricted to the periphery of the granuloma outside the fibrous outer layer. Published previously in reference 77.

features of the murine infection that raises concerns regarding its usefulness as a model for human tuberculosis (TB). During this phase of containment and cellular consolidation, new macrophage phenotypes, such as epithelioid macrophages, multinucleated giant cells, and foamy macrophages, appear within the granuloma (20). In non-human primates and humans, the granuloma is a highly stratified structure with distinct transcriptional signatures associated with the different regions (Fig. 1B). The central, caseous region of the granuloma has a proinflammatory signature, while the region surrounding the caseum shows marked enrichment for transcripts associated with anti-inflammatory programs (21, 22). Intriguingly, each granuloma functions like an independent entity, and while the systemic immune response appears to be unchanged, some granulomas may progress to active disease while others continue to control the infection, or even progress to a sterile state (23). The factors that determine the localized progression to active disease have remained elusive (24).

This phenomenon reflects one of the greatest obstacles to combating this disease. There are no reliable biomarkers for protective immunity and therefore no surrogates to inform vaccine development programs (7–9). Increasingly sensitive indicators of early disease progression have been reported (25), but these indicators require initiation of the tissue damage that accompanies actual disease, so they are not useful indicators of protective immune status. Mycobacterial growth inhibition assays are the most utilized peripheral indicator of protective immunity (26). The data look compelling because they show a functional readout linked to bacterial survival. However, recent comprehensive evaluation of extensive data sets for the application of mycobacterial growth inhibition assays to different human populations indicates that, while the data are indicative of trained innate immunity, they do not correlate with the protection status of the individual (27).

LIFE OR DEATH IN THE PHAGOCYTE

M. tuberculosis is internalized by classic phagocytosis. Inert particles phagocytosed by macrophages are delivered to the acidic, hydrolytic environment of the phagolysosome, but *M. tuberculosis* has evolved strategies to subvert the process of phagosome maturation (28). The compartment in which *M. tuberculosis* resides is slightly acidified (pH 6.4), remains interactive with the endosomal network, and shows limited acquisition of lysosomal hydrolases. Classic activation of the macrophage with interferon gamma (IFN-γ) prior to infection enables the macrophage to overcome this process and deliver the

bacterium to an acidic lysosome (29, 30). The killing of *M. tuberculosis* by activated macrophages is dependent on multiple factors, most significantly, the production of nitric oxide (NO), the low pH of the lysosome, and the delivery of antimicrobial peptides through the process of autophagy (31–33).

Several publications document the ability of *M. tuberculosis* to escape the phagosome and access the cytosol of its host cell (34–37). Escape from the phagosome appears to precipitate the necrotic death of the infected macrophage and a marked growth spurt in the intracellular bacterial population (38, 39). This transient event may have significance with respect to the pathology observed in late-stage disease but may be of less significance to long-term survival of the pathogen in its host. Data indicate that, temporally and spatially, the intravacuolar population of *M. tuberculosis* likely represents the more significant target for therapeutics (40).

UNDERLYING MECHANISMS OF IMMUNE CONTROL AND DISEASE PROGRESSION

Our understanding of immune control of TB is shaped heavily by failed immunity in the form of knockout mouse studies or catastrophic human genetic lesions (41, 42). IFN-γ is known to be important because mice deficient in IFN-γ fail to control *M. tuberculosis* infection and humans with genetic defects in the IFN-γ receptor are exquisitely susceptible to TB and to infection with *M. bovis* BCG. IFN-γ release assays have also been used, unsuccessfully, as indicators of a protective immune response or treatment efficacy (43). However, our current knowledge indicates that while a Th1-biased immune response and the production of IFN-γ are required for an effective immune response to *M. tuberculosis*, they are not sufficient to protect against either infection or disease progression. Moreover, the assumption that disease progression is the consequence of failure of Th1-dependent immune control, while widely held, is actually unsubstantiated.

A recent study used fluorescent *M. tuberculosis* fitness reporter strains to identify host phagocytes that best controlled *M. tuberculosis* growth and those that were permissive (44). The strains all expressed mCherry constitutively and expressed green fluorescent protein (GFP) either as a fusion protein with the single-strand binding protein (SSB) as a readout for replication or conditionally under regulation of the NO-responsive promoter for *hspX* (4–6) (Fig. 2). Studies in vaccinated and naïve mice demonstrated that expression of *hspX'*::GFP correlated with the development of a Th1 immune response and the expression of iNOS in the host tissue and that fluo-

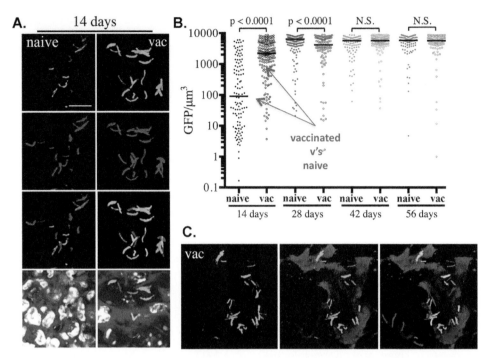

Figure 2 Usefulness of the *hspX'*::GFP reporter strain in assessing and reporting on the localized induction of inducible nitric oxide synthase at the site of infection. Phosphate-buffered saline-immunized (naïve) mice and mice vaccinated with heat-killed *M. tuberculosis* (vac) were infected with an *hspX'*::GFP *smyc'*::mCherry Erdman *M. tuberculosis* reporter strain. Fluorescence induction of the *hspX* promoter-dependent GFP is higher at 14 days in the vaccinated animals, as assessed by confocal microscopy of thick tissue sections (**A**), which were scored subsequently by Volocity (**B**). (**C**) The thick tissue sections were probed with antibodies against murine NOS2 (magenta), demonstrating the colocalization between GFP induction and NOS2 expression at the site(s) of infection. N.S., not significant. Data are from reference 5).

rescent SSB-GFP foci were less numerous in the face of a Th1 immune response (5). These data were generated with tissue sections from the murine granulomas. The phenotype of the bacterium at individual cell level was determined on cell suspensions from infected tissue (44). At 2 weeks postinfection, the bacteria were present predominantly in neutrophils, AMs, and IMs. Upon characterization of the reporter *M. tuberculosis* strains, it was found that the levels of stress induction (*hspX'*:: GFP) were higher in *M. tuberculosis* in IMs and neutrophils than in bacilli in AMs. Conversely, the SSB-GFP puncta were more frequent in *M. tuberculosis* in AMs and neutrophils than they were in *M. tuberculosis* in IMs. These data suggested that *M. tuberculosis* in AMs experienced less stress and replicated more actively than those in IMs. This result was corroborated with *M. tuberculosis* expressing a clock plasmid, pBP10, which is lost from the bacteria at a fixed rate linked to replication (45, 46).

Clodronate liposome-mediated depletion of the macrophage subsets was conducted to demonstrate the functional significance of the IM and AM host cell pop-

ulations. Delivery of clodronate liposomes to the lung airways depleted the AM population, and intravenous inoculation of clodronate liposomes depleted the blood monocytes and therefore the IM population. In the mice with depleted AMs, the bacterial burden was reduced by approximately 1 log, while in the mice with depleted IMs, the bacterial burden was increased by 1 log (Fig. 3). These data demonstrate that by altering the relative proportion of IMs and AMs available to act as host phagocytes, one can impact the bacterial load in the mice either positively or negatively, an observation consistent with previous macrophage depletion studies (14, 16, 17).

IMs AND AMs ADOPT MARKEDLY DIFFERENT METABOLIC STATES IN RESPONSE TO *M. TUBERCULOSIS* INFECTION

Analysis of the transcriptional profiles of both *M. tuberculosis*-infected and uninfected IMs and AMs showed that all four phagocyte populations had their

A. Functional consequences of depletion of Alveolar Macrophages

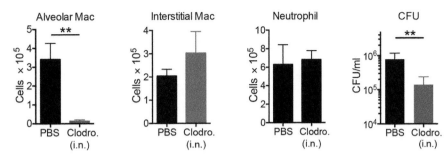

B. Functional consequences of depletion of Interstitial Macrophages

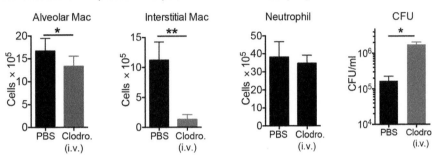

Figure 3   Selective depletion of AMs and IMs results in a decrease and an increase in bacterial burden, respectively. Mice were treated with clodronate (Clodro.) liposomes delivered either intranasally (i.n.) (**A**) or intravenously (i.v.) (**B**) to deplete the AMs or the circulating monocytes, which depleted the recruited IMs. Neither treatment impacted the neutrophil population within the infected lung tissue. Interestingly, depletion of AMs led to a reduction in bacterial burden, while depletion of IMs led to an increase in bacterial burden. The data demonstrate how modulation of the relative dimensions of the permissive (AM) and controller (IM) macrophage populations directly impacts bacterial burden. Data are from reference 44.

own discrete signatures (44). Pathway analysis of the *M. tuberculosis*-infected AMs and IMs indicated that infected AMs were enriched in transcripts associated with fatty acid metabolism and cholesterol homeostasis. In contrast, infected IMs were up-regulated in transcripts linked to inflammatory responses, glycolysis, IFN-γ signaling, and hypoxia. Treatment of infected mice with the nonhydrolyzable glucose analog 2-deoxyglucose led to a decrease in IM number without impacting the AM population. The reduction in IM number was accompanied by an increase in bacterial burden, providing an independent demonstration that the reduction in the relative proportion of IMs and AMs drives an expansion in the bacterial burden.

A functional link between host cell metabolism and bacterial growth was demonstrated through the manipulation of *M. tuberculosis*-infected bone marrow-derived macrophages with the metabolic inhibitors 2-deoxyglucose and the fatty acid oxidation inhibitor etomoxir *in vitro*. Inhibition of glycolysis in the infected bone marrow-derived macrophages enhanced bacterial growth, while inhibition of fatty acid oxidation

with etomoxir led to a reduction in bacterial growth. Neither compound had any impact on bacterial growth in rich Middlebrook 7H9 bacterial broth.

BASIS OF THE DIFFERENCE BETWEEN AMs AND IMs

Until very recently, it was thought that all macrophages in the body were differentiated from peripheral blood monocytes derived from hematopoietic precursors in the bone marrow. This is now known not to be the case; most tissue-resident macrophages, including AMs, derive from fetal yolk sac and fetal liver stem cells during embryogenesis (47, 48). These tissue-resident cells are self-maintaining and capable of replication, albeit at a low rate during homeostasis. Interestingly, recent reports suggest that *M. tuberculosis* infection arrests cell cycle in infected cells while increasing bystander macrophage replication within the infected tissue (44, 49). A similar state of monocytosis has been observed in human TB, indicating that this response is not restricted to the murine infection model (50, 51). The induction of replication within the macrophage populations in the infected lung provides another route for the selective expansion of permissive AM populations.

The larger question emerging from these studies is how the IM and AM lineages, which experience the same immune milieu generated by *M. tuberculosis* infection, adopt such divergent metabolic states. IMs and AMs are ontologically distinct macrophage lineages, suggesting that ontogeny is the dominant determinant controlling their response to infection. This interpretation is supported by recent data from an acute lung injury model where IMs and AMs exposed to lipopolysaccharide in the lung responded divergently despite experiencing the same insult (52). The accepted tissue culture model for macrophage polarization invokes the adoption of an M1 (inflammatory and antimicrobial) state in response to IFN-γ and progression to an M2 (anti-inflammatory and tissue repair) state following exposure to interleukins 4 and 13 (Fig. 4) (53–55).

While these definitions provide a useful sense of context, multiple labs report that *in vivo*, in both humans and mice, different macrophage populations coexpress numerous proteins or transcripts that *in vitro* are thought to associate exclusively with either M1 or M2 activation states (56, 57). Extensive analysis and modeling of macrophage subsets in TB infection of non-human primates have detailed different populations of macrophages that express M1 (endothelial and inducible nitric oxide synthase)- or M2 (Arg1 and Arg2)-associated markers (58). A subsequent model suggests that the ratio of M1 to M2 macrophage subsets is an accurate predictor of whether any individual granuloma is likely to progress to active disease (59). The model is consistent with data indicating that ontogenically distinct macrophage populations, the AMs and IMs, are actually preprogrammed to respond divergently when experiencing the same immunological milieu during *M. tuberculosis* infection. Analysis of peripheral blood mononucleocyte-derived macrophages and tissue-resident macrophages under homeostatic conditions suggests that the bias towards M1-like and M2-like phenotypes in these different macrophage lineages exists prior to any insult or infection (60, 61).

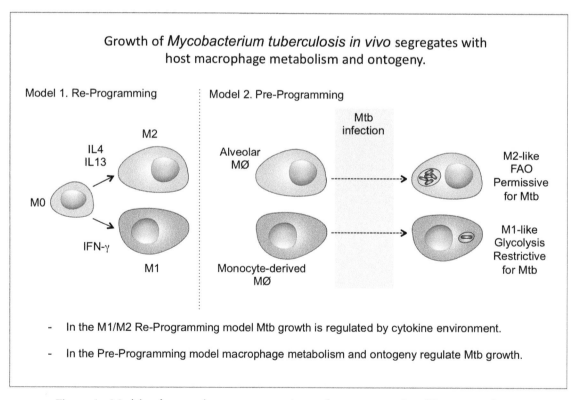

Figure 4 Models of macrophage reprogramming and preprogramming. How macrophages function in the reprogramming model (Model 1) is determined by immune signaling within the tissue niche. In the proposed preprogramming model (Model 2), the function of coexisting macrophage lineages in the lung in *M. tuberculosis* infection is determined, in large part, by the origin of the macrophage. Mtb, *M. tuberculosis*; IL, interleukin; FAO, fatty acid oxidation. Published previously in reference 44.

BACTERIAL METABOLISM IN THE HOST ENVIRONMENT

The advances in our understanding of host cell metabolism and bacterial control now connect with our appreciation of bacterial metabolism within the host cell environment. *M. tuberculosis*'s preference for lipids and fatty acids as carbon sources has been discussed since the 1950s, but the central significance of this metabolic dependence for the virulence and pathogenesis of *M. tuberculosis* has been demonstrated experimentally only recently. In 2000, McKinney and colleagues reported that mutants of *M. tuberculosis* deficient in expression of isocitrate lyase (*icl1*) could not sustain an infection in the face of immune pressure (62). Isocitrate lyase of *M. tuberculosis* is a bifunctional enzyme whose more significant activity is that of a methyl isocitrate lyase that is required for the methylcitrate cycle, which is the primary route for detoxification of propionyl coenzyme A, which accumulates upon degradation of cholesterol (63–66).

M. tuberculosis has specific transport systems dedicated to the acquisition of fatty acids and cholesterol. The Mce family of lipid transporters is conserved across the bacterial kingdom (67) and is present in *M. tuberculosis* as four distinct multigenic transporter complexes (68). Mce1 and Mce4 are the preferred uptake transporters for fatty acids and for cholesterol, respectively (69). The two transporters share some of their subunit proteins, which stabilize the transporter complexes, and most notably, all Mce transporters use a common motor, the ATPase MceG (69). The linking of fatty acid and cholesterol acquisition is not surprising given the requirement for the balanced production of downstream intermediates to feed the tricarboxylic acid cycle and provide building blocks for the synthesis of complex cell wall lipids (63, 66).

The significance of cholesterol for *M. tuberculosis* growth was also demonstrated by a large empirical screen to identify compounds active against intracellular *M. tuberculosis* (70). The screen identified several inhibitors

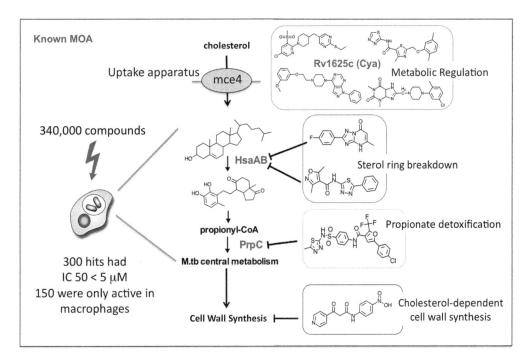

Figure 5 Major classes of cholesterol-dependent anti-*M. tuberculosis* compounds identified in a screen against intracellular *M. tuberculosis* (M.tb). The primary screen of 340,000 compounds identified 300 hits with 50% inhibitory concentrations (IC 50) less than 5 µM, 50% of which showed activity only against intracellular bacteria and had no activity against *M. tuberculosis* in rich broth. However, the majority of these compounds recovered their activity when *M. tuberculosis* was grown in medium with cholesterol or fatty acids as the limiting carbon source. Major targets or functions inhibited by the compounds are shown. Activators of an adenylate cyclase (rv1625c [Cya]) were shown to be involved in regulation of cholesterol utilization, as well as specific inhibitors of the enzymes HsaAB and PrpC, which are involved in cholesterol breakdown or propionyl coenzyme A (propionyl-CoA) detoxification. Data are from reference 70.

that blocked specific steps in bacterial cholesterol degradation or its regulation (Fig. 5). In addition, transcriptional profiling from a panel of 15 clinical strains of *M. tuberculosis* that represented the global genetic diversity of the *M. tuberculosis* complex confirmed that genes involved in the processing of cholesterol and fatty acids were up-regulated during intracellular growth as part of a common core transcriptome shared across all isolates (71).

COUPLED METABOLISM OF HOST AND PATHOGEN

While it is clear that the metabolism of *M. tuberculosis* is shifted towards heavy dependence on fatty acids and cholesterol and that the predisposition of the AM population towards fatty acid oxidation appears to provide *M. tuberculosis* with a permissive host cell population,

the modulation of host metabolism extends beyond the host cell to the surrounding tissue.

Figure 1B illustrates the caseous center of the human TB granuloma. Thin-layer chromatography and mass spectrometry analysis of the lipid species in the human granuloma demonstrated that the major lipid species were triacylglycerols, cholesterol, and cholesterol ester (21). The presence of abundant cholesterol ester in the caseum is strong evidence that these lipids came from lipid droplets present in the foamy macrophages that typically surround the caseous center of the granuloma (72, 73). When cells accumulate cholesterol, they usually esterify the sterol prior to transport from the endoplasmic reticulum and incorporation into the lipid droplet. This esterification is proposed to reduce the toxicity of the cholesterol. *M. tuberculosis* infection in culture induces a foamy macrophage phenotype in the infected cell and in uninfected bystander macrophages

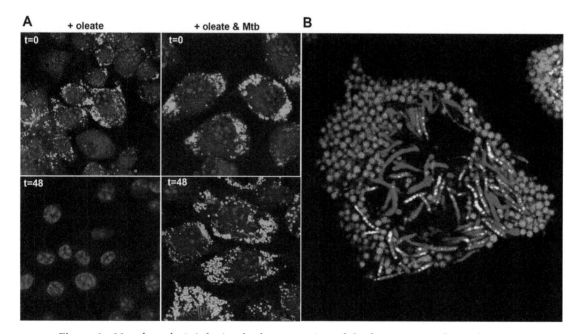

Figure 6 *M. tuberculosis* infection leads to retention of the foamy macrophage phenotype and facilitates bacterial access to host-derived lipids. (**A**) Murine bone marrow-derived macrophages were induced to form foamy cells through incubation with 400 μM oleate for 24 h. The cells were subsequently infected with *M. tuberculosis* or left uninfected. At 0 h and 48 h after infection (t=0 and t=48), cells were fixed and stained with BODIPY 493/503. *M. tuberculosis* organisms are displayed in red, BODIPY 493/503 is displayed in green, and DAPI (4′,6-diamidino-2-phenylindole)-stained nuclei are shown in blue. The absence of green stain in uninfected cells at 48 h indicates loss of oleate-induced lipid droplets. (**B**) Visualization of trafficking of host-acquired lipids into intracellular *M. tuberculosis*. Murine bone marrow-derived macrophages were infected with *M. tuberculosis* for 5 days and treated with 400 μM oleate for 24 h. The cells were incubated with the fluorescent fatty acid BODIPY FL-C16 for 60 min prior to analysis by confocal microscopy. *M. tuberculosis* organisms are displayed in red, BODIPY FL-C16 is displayed in green, and colocalization of *M. tuberculosis* with the fluorescent lipid appears in yellow. Data from reference 78.

in the same culture. The mycobacterial cell wall lipid trehalose dimycolate has been shown to induce this behavior (72). Trehalose dimycolate is recognized by the scavenger receptor MARCO and signals through both TLR2 and Mincle (74, 75). It is thought that the prolonged, chronic activation of the proinflammatory pathways in macrophages drives this transformation into foamy cells (Fig. 6), similar to the cascade invoked in atherosclerotic plaques.

CONCLUDING REMARKS

It is interesting to see how evolution appears to have driven *M. tuberculosis* to exploit the nutrient sources that it has the capacity to enhance at the site of infection, thus maximizing its chance of success. But the odds are not entirely in favor of *M. tuberculosis*. Of immune-competent individuals that acquire an *M. tuberculosis* infection, during the course of their lifetime, only 5 to 10% will progress to develop active disease. These constitute good odds for the human species. However, a problem arises with the bacterium's extraordinary efficiency of transmission, which enables a single individual with active TB to infect a large number of people. Recent estimates indicated that approximately 25% of the world's population is subclinically infected with *M. tuberculosis* (76). In areas of high HIV endemicity, such as sub-Saharan Africa, this constitutes a major challenge to human health. Not only is *M. tuberculosis* the largest single cause of death by an infectious agent, it is also the single greatest cause of death in individuals living with HIV. The challenges remain, but our increased knowledge of the physiology and metabolism of intracellular *M. tuberculosis*, and its interplay with different host macrophage populations, will likely provide new avenues to combat this pathogen.

Acknowledgments. D.G.R., E.V.N., and L.H. are supported by awards from the National Institutes of Health (AI 118582 and AI134183) and by funds from the Bill and Melinda Gates Foundation (OPP1108452 and OPP1156451).

Citation. Huang L, Nazarova EV, Russell DG. 2019. *Mycobacterium tuberculosis*: bacterial fitness within the host macrophage. Microbiol Spectrum 7(2):BAI-0001-2019.

References

1. Aldridge BB, Fernandez-Suarez M, Heller D, Ambravaneswaran V, Irimia D, Toner M, Fortune SM. 2012. Asymmetry and aging of mycobacterial cells lead to variable growth and antibiotic susceptibility. *Science* 335:100–104.

2. Manina G, Dhar N, McKinney JD. 2015. Stress and host immunity amplify *Mycobacterium tuberculosis* phenotypic heterogeneity and induce nongrowing metabolically active forms. *Cell Host Microbe* 17:32–46.

3. Rego EH, Audette RE, Rubin EJ. 2017. Deletion of a mycobacterial divisome factor collapses single-cell phenotypic heterogeneity. *Nature* 546:153–157.

4. Abramovitch RB, Rohde KH, Hsu FF, Russell DG. 2011. *aprABC*: a *Mycobacterium tuberculosis* complex-specific locus that modulates pH-driven adaptation to the macrophage phagosome. *Mol Microbiol* 80:678–694.

5. Sukumar N, Tan S, Aldridge BB, Russell DG. 2014. Exploitation of *Mycobacterium tuberculosis* reporter strains to probe the impact of vaccination at sites of infection. *PLoS Pathog* 10:e1004394.

6. Tan S, Sukumar N, Abramovitch RB, Parish T, Russell DG. 2013. *Mycobacterium tuberculosis* responds to chloride and pH as synergistic cues to the immune status of its host cell. *PLoS Pathog* 9:e1003282.

7. Bhatt K, Verma S, Ellner JJ, Salgame P. 2015. Quest for correlates of protection against tuberculosis. *Clin Vaccine Immunol* 22:258–266.

8. Cadena AM, Flynn JL, Fortune SM. 2016. The importance of first impressions: early events in *Mycobacterium tuberculosis* infection influence outcome. *mBio* 7:e00342-16.

9. Goletti D, Petruccioli E, Joosten SA, Ottenhoff TH. 2016. Tuberculosis biomarkers: from diagnosis to protection. *Infect Dis Rep* 8:6568.

10. Huang L, Russell DG. 2017. Protective immunity against tuberculosis: what does it look like and how do we find it? *Curr Opin Immunol* 48:44–50.

11. Flynn JL, Gideon HP, Mattila JT, Lin PL. 2015. Immunology studies in non-human primate models of tuberculosis. *Immunol Rev* 264:60–73.

12. Russell DG. 2007. Who puts the tubercle in tuberculosis? *Nat Rev Microbiol* 5:39–47.

13. Cohen SB, Gern BH, Delahaye JL, Adams KN, Plumlee CR, Winkler JK, Sherman DR, Gerner MY, Urdahl KB. 2018. Alveolar macrophages provide an early *Mycobacterium tuberculosis* niche and initiate dissemination. *Cell Host Microbe* 24:439–446.e4.

14. Antonelli LR, Gigliotti Rothfuchs A, Gonçalves R, Roffê E, Cheever AW, Bafica A, Salazar AM, Feng CG, Sher A. 2010. Intranasal poly-IC treatment exacerbates tuberculosis in mice through the pulmonary recruitment of a pathogen-permissive monocyte/macrophage population. *J Clin Invest* 120:1674–1682.

15. Kipnis A, Basaraba RJ, Orme IM, Cooper AM. 2003. Role of chemokine ligand 2 in the protective response to early murine pulmonary tuberculosis. *Immunology* 109:547–551.

16. Leemans JC, Juffermans NP, Florquin S, van Rooijen N, Vervoordeldonk MJ, Verbon A, van Deventer SJ, van der Poll T. 2001. Depletion of alveolar macrophages exerts protective effects in pulmonary tuberculosis in mice. *J Immunol* 166:4604–4611.

17. Samstein M, Schreiber HA, Leiner IM, Susac B, Glickman MS, Pamer EG. 2013. Essential yet limited role for CCR2+ inflammatory monocytes during *Mycobacterium tuberculosis*-specific T cell priming. *eLife* 2:e01086.

18. Wolf AJ, Desvignes L, Linas B, Banaiee N, Tamura T, Takatsu K, Ernst JD. 2008. Initiation of the adaptive immune response to *Mycobacterium tuberculosis* depends on antigen production in the local lymph node, not the lungs. *J Exp Med* 205:105–115.

19. Wolf AJ, Linas B, Trevejo-Nuñez GJ, Kincaid E, Tamura T, Takatsu K, Ernst JD. 2007. *Mycobacterium tuberculosis* infects dendritic cells with high frequency and impairs their function in vivo. *J Immunol* 179:2509–2519.

20. Flynn JL, Chan J, Lin PL. 2011. Macrophages and control of granulomatous inflammation in tuberculosis. *Mucosal Immunol* 4:271–278.

21. Kim MJ, Wainwright HC, Locketz M, Bekker LG, Walther GB, Dittrich C, Visser A, Wang W, Hsu FF, Wiehart U, Tsenova L, Kaplan G, Russell DG. 2010. Caseation of human tuberculosis granulomas correlates with elevated host lipid metabolism. *EMBO Mol Med* 2:258–274.

22. Marakalala MJ, Raju RM, Sharma K, Zhang YJ, Eugenin EA, Prideaux B, Daudelin IB, Chen PY, Booty MG, Kim JH, Eum SY, Via LE, Behar SM, Barry CE III, Mann M, Dartois V, Rubin EJ. 2016. Inflammatory signaling in human tuberculosis granulomas is spatially organized. *Nat Med* 22:531–538.

23. Lin PL, Ford CB, Coleman MT, Myers AJ, Gawande R, Ioerger T, Sacchettini J, Fortune SM, Flynn JL. 2014. Sterilization of granulomas is common in active and latent tuberculosis despite within-host variability in bacterial killing. *Nat Med* 20:75–79.

24. Cadena AM, Fortune SM, Flynn JL. 2017. Heterogeneity in tuberculosis. *Nat Rev Immunol* 17:691–702.

25. Petruccioli E, Scriba TJ, Petrone L, Hatherill M, Cirillo DM, Joosten SA, Ottenhoff TH, Denkinger CM, Goletti D. 2016. Correlates of tuberculosis risk: predictive biomarkers for progression to active tuberculosis. *Eur Respir J* 48:1751–1763.

26. Tanner R, O'Shea MK, Fletcher HA, McShane H. 2016. In vitro mycobacterial growth inhibition assays: a tool for the assessment of protective immunity and evaluation of tuberculosis vaccine efficacy. *Vaccine* 34:4656–4665.

27. Joosten SA, van Meijgaarden KE, Arend SM, Prins C, Oftung F, Korsvold GE, Kik SV, Arts RJ, van Crevel R, Netea MG, Ottenhoff TH. 2018. Mycobacterial growth inhibition is associated with trained innate immunity. *J Clin Invest* 128:1837–1851.

28. VanderVen BC, Huang L, Rohde KH, Russell DG. 2016. The minimal unit of infection: *Mycobacterium tuberculosis* in the macrophage. *Microbiol Spectr* 4:TBTB2-0025-2016.

29. Schaible UE, Sturgill-Koszycki S, Schlesinger PH, Russell DG. 1998. Cytokine activation leads to acidification and increases maturation of *Mycobacterium avium*-containing phagosomes in murine macrophages. *J Immunol* 160:1290–1296.

30. Via LE, Fratti RA, McFalone M, Pagan-Ramos E, Deretic D, Deretic V. 1998. Effects of cytokines on mycobacterial phagosome maturation. *J Cell Sci* 111:897–905.

31. Alonso S, Pethe K, Russell DG, Purdy GE. 2007. Lysosomal killing of *Mycobacterium* mediated by ubiquitin-derived

peptides is enhanced by autophagy. *Proc Natl Acad Sci USA* 104:6031–6036.

32. Gutierrez MG, Master SS, Singh SB, Taylor GA, Colombo MI, Deretic V. 2004. Autophagy is a defense mechanism inhibiting BCG and *Mycobacterium tuberculosis* survival in infected macrophages. *Cell* 119:753–766.

33. MacMicking JD, North RJ, LaCourse R, Mudgett JS, Shah SK, Nathan CF. 1997. Identification of nitric oxide synthase as a protective locus against tuberculosis. *Proc Natl Acad Sci USA* 94:5243–5248.

34. McDonough KA, Kress Y, Bloom BR. 1993. Pathogenesis of tuberculosis: interaction of *Mycobacterium tuberculosis* with macrophages. *Infect Immun* 61:2763–2773.

35. Myrvik QN, Leake ES, Wright MJ. 1984. Disruption of phagosomal membranes of normal alveolar macrophages by the H37Rv strain of *Mycobacterium tuberculosis*. A correlate of virulence. *Am Rev Respir Dis* 129:322–328.

36. Simeone R, Bobard A, Lippmann J, Bitter W, Majlessi L, Brosch R, Enninga J. 2012. Phagosomal rupture by *Mycobacterium tuberculosis* results in toxicity and host cell death. *PLoS Pathog* 8:e1002507.

37. van der Wel N, Hava D, Houben D, Fluitsma D, van Zon M, Pierson J, Brenner M, Peters PJ. 2007. *M. tuberculosis* and *M. leprae* translocate from the phagolysosome to the cytosol in myeloid cells. *Cell* 129:1287–1298.

38. Lerner TR, Borel S, Greenwood DJ, Repnik U, Russell MR, Herbst S, Jones ML, Collinson LM, Griffiths G, Gutierrez MG. 2017. *Mycobacterium tuberculosis* replicates within necrotic human macrophages. *J Cell Biol* 216:583–594.

39. Mahamed D, Boulle M, Ganga Y, Mc Arthur C, Skroch S, Oom L, Catinas O, Pillay K, Naicker M, Rampersad S, Mathonsi C, Hunter J, Wong EB, Suleman M, Sreejit G, Pym AS, Lustig G, Sigal A. 2017. Intracellular growth of *Mycobacterium tuberculosis* after macrophage cell death leads to serial killing of host cells. *eLife* 6:e22028.

40. Russell DG. 2016. The ins and outs of the *Mycobacterium tuberculosis*-containing vacuole. *Cell Microbiol* 18:1065–1069.

41. Boisson-Dupuis S, Bustamante J, El-Baghdadi J, Camcioglu Y, Parvaneh N, El Azbaoui S, Agader A, Hassani A, El Hafidi N, Mrani NA, Jouhadi Z, Ailal F, Najib J, Reisli I, Zamani A, Yosunkaya S, Gulle-Girit S, Yildiran A, Cipe FE, Torun SH, Metin A, Atikan BY, Hatipoglu N, Aydogmus C, Kilic SS, Dogu F, Karaca N, Aksu G, Kutukculer N, Keser-Emiroglu M, Somer A, Tanir G, Aytekin C, Adimi P, Mahdaviani SA, Mamishi S, Bousfiha A, Sanal O, Mansouri D, Casanova JL, Abel L. 2015. Inherited and acquired immunodeficiencies underlying tuberculosis in childhood. *Immunol Rev* 264:103–120.

42. North RJ, Jung YJ. 2004. Immunity to tuberculosis. *Annu Rev Immunol* 22:599–623.

43. Clifford V, He Y, Zufferey C, Connell T, Curtis N. 2015. Interferon gamma release assays for monitoring the response to treatment for tuberculosis: a systematic review. *Tuberculosis (Edinb)* 95:639–650.

44. Huang L, Nazarova EV, Tan S, Liu Y, Russell DG. 2018. Growth of *Mycobacterium tuberculosis* in vivo segre-

gates with host macrophage metabolism and ontogeny. *J Exp Med* 215:1135–1152.

45. Gill WP, Harik NS, Whiddon MR, Liao RP, Mittler JE, Sherman DR. 2009. A replication clock for *Mycobacterium tuberculosis*. *Nat Med* 15:211–214.

46. Rohde KH, Veiga DF, Caldwell S, Balázsi G, Russell DG. 2012. Linking the transcriptional profiles and the physiological states of *Mycobacterium tuberculosis* during an extended intracellular infection. *PLoS Pathog* 8:e1002769.

47. Guilliams M, De Kleer I, Henri S, Post S, Vanhoutte L, De Prijck S, Deswarte K, Malissen B, Hammad H, Lambrecht BN. 2013. Alveolar macrophages develop from fetal monocytes that differentiate into long-lived cells in the first week of life via GM-CSF. *J Exp Med* 210:1977–1992.

48. Jakubzick CV, Randolph GJ, Henson PM. 2017. Monocyte differentiation and antigen-presenting functions. *Nat Rev Immunol* 17:349–362.

49. Cumming BM, Rahman MA, Lamprecht DA, Rohde KH, Saini V, Adamson JH, Russell DG, Steyn AJC. 2017. *Mycobacterium tuberculosis* arrests host cycle at the G1/S transition to establish long term infection. *PLoS Pathog* 13: e1006389. CORRECTION *PLoS Pathog* 13:e1006490.

50. La Manna MP, Orlando V, Dieli F, Di Carlo P, Cascio A, Cuzzi G, Palmieri F, Goletti D, Caccamo N. 2017. Quantitative and qualitative profiles of circulating monocytes may help identifying tuberculosis infection and disease stages. *PLoS One* 12:e0171358.

51. Wang J, Yin Y, Wang X, Pei H, Kuai S, Gu L, Xing H, Zhang Y, Huang Q, Guan B. 2015. Ratio of monocytes to lymphocytes in peripheral blood in patients diagnosed with active tuberculosis. *Braz J Infect Dis* 19: 125–131.

52. Mould KJ, Barthel L, Mohning MP, Thomas SM, McCubbrey AL, Danhorn T, Leach SM, Fingerlin TE, O'Connor BP, Reisz JA, D'Alessandro A, Bratton DL, Jakubzick CV, Janssen WJ. 2017. Cell origin dictates programming of resident versus recruited macrophages during acute lung injury. *Am J Respir Cell Mol Biol* 57: 294–306.

53. Boscá L, González-Ramos S, Prieto P, Fernández-Velasco M, Mojena M, Martín-Sanz P, Alemany S. 2015. Metabolic signatures linked to macrophage polarization: from glucose metabolism to oxidative phosphorylation. *Biochem Soc Trans* 43:740–744.

54. Verdeguer F, Aouadi M. 2017. Macrophage heterogeneity and energy metabolism. *Exp Cell Res* 360:35–40.

55. Zhu L, Zhao Q, Yang T, Ding W, Zhao Y. 2015. Cellular metabolism and macrophage functional polarization. *Int Rev Immunol* 34:82–100.

56. Rückerl D, Campbell SM, Duncan S, Sutherland TE, Jenkins SJ, Hewitson JP, Barr TA, Jackson-Jones LH, Maizels RM, Allen JE. 2017. Macrophage origin limits functional plasticity in helminth-bacterial co-infection. *PLoS Pathog* 13:e1006233.

57. Zhu Y, Herndon JM, Sojka DK, Kim KW, Knolhoff BL, Zuo C, Cullinan DR, Luo J, Bearden AR, Lavine KJ, Yokoyama WM, Hawkins WG, Fields RC, Randolph GJ, DeNardo DG. 2017. Tissue-resident macrophages in pancreatic ductal adenocarcinoma originate from em-

bryonic hematopoiesis and promote tumor progression. *Immunity* 47:323–338.e6.

58. Mattila JT, Ojo OO, Kepka-Lenhart D, Marino S, Kim JH, Eum SY, Via LE, Barry CE III, Klein E, Kirschner DE, Morris SM Jr, Lin PL, Flynn JL. 2013. Microenvironments in tuberculous granulomas are delineated by distinct populations of macrophage subsets and expression of nitric oxide synthase and arginase isoforms. *J Immunol* 191:773–784.

59. Marino S, Cilfone NA, Mattila JT, Linderman JJ, Flynn JL, Kirschner DE. 2015. Macrophage polarization drives granuloma outcome during *Mycobacterium tuberculosis* infection. *Infect Immun* 83:324–338.

60. Gibbings SL, Goyal R, Desch AN, Leach SM, Prabagar M, Atif SM, Bratton DL, Janssen W, Jakubzick CV. 2015. Transcriptome analysis highlights the conserved difference between embryonic and postnatal-derived alveolar macrophages. *Blood* 126:1357–1366.

61. Gibbings SL, Thomas SM, Atif SM, McCubbrey AL, Desch AN, Danhorn T, Leach SM, Bratton DL, Henson PM, Janssen WJ, Jakubzick CV. 2017. Three unique interstitial macrophages in the murine lung at steady state. *Am J Respir Cell Mol Biol* 57:66–76.

62. McKinney JD, Höner zu Bentrup K, Muñoz-Elías EJ, Miczak A, Chen B, Chan WT, Swenson D, Sacchettini JC, Jacobs WR Jr, Russell DG. 2000. Persistence of *Mycobacterium tuberculosis* in macrophages and mice requires the glyoxylate shunt enzyme isocitrate lyase. *Nature* 406: 735–738.

63. Lee W, VanderVen BC, Fahey RJ, Russell DG. 2013. Intracellular *Mycobacterium tuberculosis* exploits host-derived fatty acids to limit metabolic stress. *J Biol Chem* 288: 6788–6800.

64. Muñoz-Elías EJ, McKinney JD. 2005. *Mycobacterium tuberculosis* isocitrate lyases 1 and 2 are jointly required for in vivo growth and virulence. *Nat Med* 11:638–644.

65. Muñoz-Elías EJ, Upton AM, Cherian J, McKinney JD. 2006. Role of the methylcitrate cycle in *Mycobacterium tuberculosis* metabolism, intracellular growth, and virulence. *Mol Microbiol* 60:1109–1122.

66. Savvi S, Warner DF, Kana BD, McKinney JD, Mizrahi V, Dawes SS. 2008. Functional characterization of a vitamin B12-dependent methylmalonyl pathway in *Mycobacterium tuberculosis*: implications for propionate metabolism during growth on fatty acids. *J Bacteriol* 190:3886–3895.

67. Ekiert DC, Bhabha G, Isom GL, Greenan G, Ovchinnikov S, Henderson IR, Cox JS, Vale RD. 2017. Architectures of lipid transport systems for the bacterial outer membrane. *Cell* 169:273–285.e17.

68. Zhang F, Xie JP. 2011. Mammalian cell entry gene family of *Mycobacterium tuberculosis*. *Mol Cell Biochem* 352: 1–10.

69. Nazarova EV, Montague CR, La T, Wilburn KM, Sukumar N, Lee W, Caldwell S, Russell DG, VanderVen BC. 2017. Rv3723/LucA coordinates fatty acid and cholesterol uptake in *Mycobacterium tuberculosis*. *eLife* 6:e26969.

70. VanderVen BC, Fahey RJ, Lee W, Liu Y, Abramovitch RB, Memmott C, Crowe AM, Eltis LD, Perola E, Deininger DD, Wang T, Locher CP, Russell DG. 2015. Novel inhib-

itors of cholesterol degradation in *Mycobacterium tuberculosis* reveal how the bacterium's metabolism is constrained by the intracellular environment. *PLoS Pathog* 11:e1004679.

71. Homolka S, Niemann S, Russell DG, Rohde KH. 2010. Functional genetic diversity among *Mycobacterium tuberculosis* complex clinical isolates: delineation of conserved core and lineage-specific transcriptomes during intracellular survival. *PLoS Pathog* 6:e1000988.

72. Peyron P, Vaubourgeix J, Poquet Y, Levillain F, Botanch C, Bardou F, Daffé M, Emile JF, Marchou B, Cardona PJ, de Chastellier C, Altare F. 2008. Foamy macrophages from tuberculous patients' granulomas constitute a nutrient-rich reservoir for *M. tuberculosis* persistence. *PLoS Pathog* 4:e1000204.

73. Russell DG, Cardona PJ, Kim MJ, Allain S, Altare F. 2009. Foamy macrophages and the progression of the human tuberculosis granuloma. *Nat Immunol* 10:943–948.

74. Bowdish DM, Sakamoto K, Kim MJ, Kroos M, Mukhopadhyay S, Leifer CA, Tryggvason K, Gordon S, Russell DG. 2009. MARCO, TLR2, and CD14 are required for macrophage cytokine responses to mycobacterial trehalose dimycolate and *Mycobacterium tuberculosis*. *PLoS Pathog* 5:e1000474.

75. Ishikawa E, Ishikawa T, Morita YS, Toyonaga K, Yamada H, Takeuchi O, Kinoshita T, Akira S, Yoshikai Y, Yamasaki S. 2009. Direct recognition of the mycobacterial glycolipid, trehalose dimycolate, by C-type lectin Mincle. *J Exp Med* 206:2879–2888.

76. Houben RM, Dodd PJ. 2016. The global burden of latent tuberculosis infection: a re-estimation using mathematical modelling. *PLoS Med* 13:e1002152.

77. Russell DG, VanderVen BC, Lee W, Abramovitch RB, Kim MJ, Homolka S, Niemann S, Rohde KH. 2010. *Mycobacterium tuberculosis* wears what it eats. *Cell Host Microbe* 8:68–76.

78. Podinovskaia M, Lee W, Caldwell S, Russell DG. 2013. Infection of macrophages with *Mycobacterium tuberculosis* induces global modifications to phagosomal function. *Cell Microbiol* 15:843–859.

Bacteria and Intracellularity
Edited by Pascale Cossart, Craig R. Roy, and Philippe Sansonetti
© 2019 American Society for Microbiology, Washington, DC
doi:10.1128/microbiolspec.BAI-0018-2019

The *Wolbachia* Endosymbionts

10

Frédéric Landmann[1]

INTRODUCTION

The species of the genus *Wolbachia* are Gram-negative members of the *Alphaproteobacteria* that belong to the order *Rickettsiales*. First discovered in the germ line of mosquitos almost a century ago, they have been shown to have extraordinary diversity, as well as an impressive number of host species (1). Early on, these endosymbionts received attention from ecologists for the diversity of phenotypes they induce in their terrestrial arthropod hosts. Later, cell and developmental biologists worked to decipher the mechanisms underlying *Wolbachia*-host interactions, followed by a growing number of experts in all biological disciplines, stimulated by the biomedical potential of these widespread intracellular bacteria, which are now used to control vector-borne diseases, while their symbiotic interaction with human parasites is targeted to fight filariasis, one of the most debilitating neglected tropical diseases (2). Horizontal transfers across species boundaries and the ability of these bacteria to be vertically transmitted through the egg are key elements of their successful pandemic. Involved in different types of symbiotic interactions, from parasitic to mutualistic, they influence the germ line biology of their host and the reproductive outcome through elaborate manipulations and integrate embryonic fate maps to navigate towards specific somatic targets and germ line precursors. Stably maintained in host populations, *Wolbachia* organisms also affect their hosts' evolution, physiology, immunity, and development (3). While most studies have focused on the phenotypes they induce, insights into their intracellular lifestyle are also emerging. This chapter provides an overview of the molecular data and the current understanding of the cell biology underlying the mechanisms used by *Wolbachia* endosymbionts in arthropod and nematode hosts to target and subvert the germ line and reproduction machinery in order to support their transmission. The chapter also reviews the basis of their intracellular lifestyle in parasitic and mutualistic symbiotic interactions.

GENETIC DIVERSITY AMONG *WOLBACHIA* ENDOSYMBIONTS

Since the discovery of *Wolbachia* endosymbionts in the germ line and somatic tissues of the mosquito *Culex pipiens* and other insects by Hertig and Wolbach in 1924, when they were identified as *Rickettsia*-like microorganisms (4), the number of *Wolbachia* strains and associated hosts that have been described has continued to grow. Based mainly on multilocus sequence typing (5), *Wolbachia* strains have been classified by major phylogenetic lineages named supergroups. Hence, most strain identifications derive from molecular identification rather than from formal descriptions. Although *Wolbachia* were first identified in arthropods only (supergroups A and B), other supergroups were later found to be strictly associated with filarial nematode species (C and D) (6, 7) (Fig. 1A). A count of 18 clades has currently been reached (supergroups A to R), almost exclusively in arthropods (8–10), with the interesting case of supergroup F being found in both filariae and arthropods (11, 12). More recently, another *Wolbachia* supergroup was discovered in plant-parasitic nematodes (13, 14). These phylogenetic analyses have highlighted the occurrence of horizontal transfers of *Wolbachia* on evolutionary time scales between different arthropod species sharing the same supergroup. Conversely, a given host species can harbor different *Wolbachia* strains according to its geographical distribution, or multiple strains at once.

A strong partition exists at the genomic level between the *Wolbachia* supergroups found in arthropods and those harbored by filariae, reflecting the peculiarities of the symbiotic interaction established with a given host

[1]CRBM, University of Montpellier, CNRS, Montpellier, France.

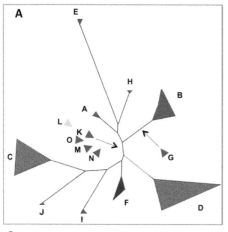

A

Supergroups

 found in arthropods only:
A, B, E, G, H, I, K, M, N, O, P,Q and R

 found in onchocercidae only: C, D and J

 found in both arthropods
and onchocercidae

△ found in plant parasite nematode
(Tylenchida) only

B

Genomic features	wBm	wMel	R. conorii	R. prowazekii
Genome size (bp)	1,080,084	1,267,782	1,268,755	1,111,523
G+C content (%)	34	35.3	32.4	29.1
Predicted protein-coding genes	806	1270	1374	835
Gene Density (functional gene/ kb)	0.75	0.94	1.37	0.75
Pseudogenes and fragmented genes	98	94	101	14
Various Repeats (% of genome)	5.4	14.2	4.9	0.3
% of coding DNA (intact proteins and RNA Genes)	67.4	81	81	76

Figure 1   Overview of *Wolbachia* diversity. (**A**) Unrooted phylogenic tree of the main *Wolbachia* supergroups. The triangle size represents the described diversity within each supergroup. (**B**) Comparison of genomic features of *Wolbachia* endosymbionts with other *Rickettsiales* pathogens. *w*Bm and *w*Mel, endosymbionts from *B. malayi* and *D. melanogaster*; *R. conorii*, *Rickettsia conorii*; *R. prowazekii*, *Rickettsia prowazekii*. Adapted from references 15 and 133.

species, from parasitic to mutualistic. These differences are noteworthy when the *Wolbachia* strain *w*Mel (supergroup A), present in the fruit fly *Drosophila melanogaster*, is compared to strain *w*Bm (supergroup D) of the filarial nematode *Brugia malayi* (Fig. 1B). These two strains have been particularly scrutinized because of the relevance of their hosts, the former being a well-known experimental model at the forefront in cell biology studies of *Wolbachia*-host interactions and the latter the sole causative agent of human filariasis that can be raised under laboratory conditions with a surrogate host.

The genomes of facultative *Wolbachia* strains found in arthropods are much larger (from 1.2 to 1.6 Mb) than those of their mutualistic counterparts found in nematodes (from 0.9 to 1.1 Mb), for reasons that may support the strategies of infection. Not only do these genomes encode more proteins, they also contain mobile genetic elements such as repeated elements, transposons, and prophages, leading to a high degree of genome plasticity, observed through the many rearrangements present in these strains (15, 16). WO prophages are present in variable numbers in the strains infecting arthropods

(17) and provide some *Wolbachia* effectors involved in the manipulation of host reproduction (18).

The genomes of *Wolbachia* supergroups associated with filarial nematodes are smaller due to the absence of prophages and fewer repeated sequences and protein-coding genes. Although this may be the result of further genetic erosion associated with mutualism (15), an alternative hypothesis comes from cophylogenetic analyses of *Wolbachia* supergroups and their filarial hosts. Their complex coevolution is marked by numerous secondary losses and horizontal transfers between clades. However, supergroup C exhibits a strong cospeciation and occupies a basal place among the *Wolbachia* groups in filariae. It has been suggested that *Wolbachia* may have first diverged within parasitic filarial species before being passed to arthropod species (8). A recent study challenged the place of supergroup C as the ancestral symbionts, nonetheless keeping the nematodes as ancestral hosts. Genomic and phylogenomic analyses of *w*Ppe, a *Wolbachia* strain derived from the root lesion nematode *Pratylenchus penetrans* (order Tylenchida), suggest instead that supergroup L is the earliest branch from which all the members of *Wolbachia* may have originated, starting with plant-parasitic nematodes as host species. Finding the ancestral *Wolbachia* may, however, remain impossible in the absence of paleontological data to position the evolutionary history of the nematodes with regard to the time scale of arthropod evolution.

All *Wolbachia* possess an evolutionary conserved type IV secretion system, clustered in two loci made of five (*virB8* to *-B11* and *virD4*) and three (*virB3*, *-B4*, and *-B6*) tandem genes (19). These two operons were found to be transcriptionally active within their nematode and arthropod hosts (16, 20–23), leaving no doubt that the secretion of effectors sustains their intracellular lifestyle and drives the manipulation of their host reproduction machineries. To date, very few *Wolbachia* effectors have been associated with a host phenotype and/or had their eukaryotic targets identified (18, 24–28); this point is developed below.

Genomic analyses have revealed disparities among supergroups in terms of number of predicted putative effectors. Although the *w*Mel genome codes for 23 ankyrin-repeat containing proteins (60 are encoded by *w*Pip from *C. pipiens*), only 5 are found in *w*Bm (15). This again echoes the differences in genome size and symbiotic relationship between these strains and their hosts. Recent bioinformatics approaches identified 163 putative effectors among the predicted 1,270 functional proteins encoded by *w*Mel (29) and 47 putative effectors in *w*Bm (30). Their expression in heterologous systems (in budding yeast or *Drosophila* S2 cells) allowed screenings (e.g., for growth defects) that proved to be very promising approaches to identify new effectors (24, 29, 30). Such experimental strategies should reveal both common and unique effectors among different *Wolbachia* strains and highlight the evolutionary history of supergroups, along with identifying the host functions they subvert in various symbioses, from those involved in the basic demands of the intracellular lifestyle to the most elegant alterations they effect in their host reproduction to favor their vertical transmission.

THE GREAT MANIPULATORS OF REPRODUCTION

The *Wolbachia* have established a wide continuum of symbiotic interactions, from being mutualistic and essential to host development, fertility, and survival (in filariae) to being facultative and parasitic, as is observed in the vast majority of *Wolbachia*-infected arthropod species. The great *Wolbachia* pandemic is in part explained by horizontal transmission events between species. They can occur through direct or indirect contacts, within a habitat, between predator and prey, or through

a shared source of food (31). In addition, *Wolbachia* organisms are endowed with extracellular survival skills for extended time periods, which can facilitate interspecies spread (32). But the key to their success, leading sometimes to 100% infected individuals in a given species (e.g., *C. pipiens*), is an extraordinary ability to manipulate the reproduction of their hosts in order to optimize their maternal transmission through the eggs. This vertical transmission selects *Wolbachia* traits favoring the infected mother, in terms of fitness, and size of the progeny. *Wolbachia* can induce a series of sex ratio distortion phenotypes in the progeny by causing parthenogenesis, feminization, or male-killing (MK), as well as a form of conditional sterility called cytoplasmic incompatibility (CI), which is the most common *Wolbachia*-induced phenotype (3, 33). Eventually, infected females are favored over their noninfected counterparts and over males if a sex ratio distortion is involved (Fig. 2).

During induction of parthenogenesis (observed in the orders Hymenoptera, Thysanoptera, and Acari), the males, which could compete for limited food resources, are no longer needed and simply disappear. In haplodiploid species, fertilized diploid eggs develop normally into females, while nonfertilized haploid eggs give rise to males. Such is the case in many parasitoid wasp and mite species. An infection by *Wolbachia* impairs the cell cycle to restore diploidy in nonfertilized eggs through various cytological mechanisms: the production of diploid gametes, an aborted anaphase during the first mitosis, or the fusion of the two first zygotic nuclei, leading to the production of infected females as almost exclusively the sole progeny (34–37). In some extreme cases, the host has totally become dependent on *Wolbachia*. When the parthenogenetic parasitoid wasp *Muscidifurax uniraptor* is artificially cured of *Wolbachia* by antibiotic treatment, males reappear in the offspring. However, these males remain sterile, and the females, reluctant to mate, possess a nonfunctional spermatheca. The thelytokous (asexual) reproduction induced by *Wolbachia* has thus evolved to become irreversible (35).

Feminization, occurring in the orders Isopoda, Lepidoptera, and Hemiptera, has been well described in the terrestrial crustacean wood louse species *Armadillidium vulgare*, where females are heterogametic and harbor ZW sexual chromosomes, while males carry a pair of ZZ chromosomes. Upon *Wolbachia* infection, the inhibition of androgenic hormone production turns genetic males into fertile phenotypic pseudofemales, developing functional ovaries by default. Since maternal transmission of *Wolbachia* is, crucially, not perfect, some males derived from noninfected eggs persist in these populations, ensuring sexual reproduction. Some wood

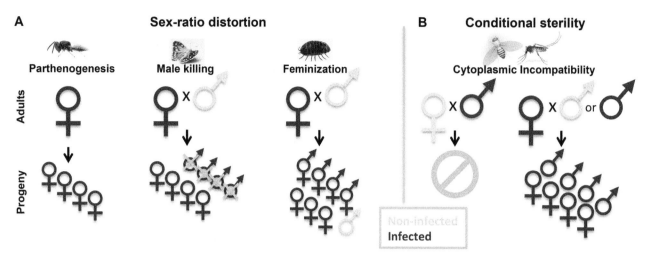

Figure 2 The four reproductive outcomes caused by *Wolbachia*, with an example of arthropod species described in the text. (**A**) Parthenogenesis, MK, and feminization cause a sex ratio distortion. (**B**) CI (left) and the rescue cross (right). Uninfected females cannot successfully mate with infected males (CI), while infected females have the selective advantage to mate with noninfected males or with males infected with a compatible strain.

louse populations were found to be devoid of true genetic females, leading to the loss of the W chromosome as an evolutionary consequence of the infection. In these instances, the *Wolbachia* infection status is the only factor ruling the phenotypic gender: pseudofemales when infected, and true males when not (38–40).

Wolbachia-induced MK, which is reported in four insect orders (Lepidoptera, Diptera, Coleoptera, and Pseudoscorpiones), leads to the embryonic death of the nontransmitting male progeny. This can provide an advantage to female siblings, because they can eat the dead eggs, thereby increasing their fitness, or because it reduces the competition for limited food supply (41, 42). A cytological description of *Wolbachia*-induced MK in *Drosophila bifasciata* suggests a defective chromatin remodeling in early male embryos (43), but the mechanisms of *Wolbachia*-induced MK remain unknown. New insights may come from the recent discovery of the Spaid toxin, produced by *Spiroplasma poulsonii*, another MK-inducing endosymbiont of *Drosophila* species (44). In *Drosophila*, the dosage compensation machinery allows transcription on the X chromosome twice more in males than in females, to achieve similar gene expression levels between both sexes. This is mediated by the male-specific lethal complex, recruited to the male X chromosome (45). Spaid is an ankyrin and OTU (ovarian tumor) deubiquitinase domain-containing toxin that recapitulates MK phenotypes when overexpressed in *D. melanogaster*, specifically in males. It has been proposed that the OTU domain promotes nuclear localization, while the ankyrin repeats mediate the interaction with the male-specific

lethal complex or its downstream targets (such as acetylation on histone H4K16). Future studies should determine to what extend *Wolbachia*-induced MK shares traits with *Spiroplasma*-associated MK.

CI is the most common *Wolbachia*-induced reproductive phenotype, observed in the orders Diptera, Coleoptera, Hemiptera, Hymenoptera, Isopoda, Lepidoptera, Orthoptera, and Acari. It describes an incompatibility occurring during fertilization between the sperm produced by a *Wolbachia*-infected male and an egg derived from either a noninfected female or a female harboring a different and incompatible *Wolbachia* strain, leading eventually to either embryonic death (in most cases) or development of haploid males in haplodiploid species (33). If the female is infected with the same (compatible) strain, compatibility is restored and the progeny is viable.

Reciprocal crosses with insects harboring different *Wolbachia* strains have revealed that CI can be uni- or bidirectional (46, 47). In case of an infection with a single *Wolbachia* strain, the infected females have the selective advantage of being able to mate with either infected or noninfected males. While the *Wolbachia* organisms are abundant during gametogenesis, they become excluded from the male gametes during the process of sperm maturation (48), suggesting that the *Wolbachia*-free sperm derived from an infected male contains *Wolbachia* secreted factors responsible for the CI phenotype.

The first cytological descriptions of CI revealed defects in paternal chromatin condensation that prevent proper chromosome segregation during the first embryonic mitosis, leading to lethal aneuploid or haploid development (33, 49). The observation of chromosomal bridges suggested the presence of incompletely replicated DNA, impeding the segregation of sister chromatids. This was confirmed by further analyses demonstrating an abnormal presence of the replicating factor PCNA specifically on the paternal chromatin during mitosis, preceded by histone deposition defects during the chromatin remodeling that shapes the sperm into a functional paternal pronucleus (50). When *Wolbachia* are present in the egg, none of these defects is induced by the *Wolbachia*-modified sperm. Hence, *Wolbachia* can modify the sperm through the potential secretion of a Mod factor(s), leading to CI, and can rescue the embryonic development when present in the egg, through the potential action of a Resc factor(s), leading to a modification-rescue model for CI. Thus, any given CI-inducing strain can be functionally defined, through combinations of host crosses, for its Mod/Resc properties. Most *Wolbachia* strains have been found to be Mod+/Resc+, but all the possible combinations have been observed (51–53).

The identification of the *Wolbachia* Mod and Resc effectors driving CI and its rescue was for decades a longstanding goal and has only been recently reached. Two studies have uncovered pairs of syntenic genes that are found in CI-inducing strains only and contained within the *Wolbachia* phage WO. The CI factors *cifA* and *cifB* of *w*Mel from *D. melanogaster*, and their orthologs *cidA* and *cidB* of *w*Pip from the mosquito *C. pipiens*, are able to recapitulate CI traits when transgenically expressed in uninfected male flies (18, 27). While these studies show subtle differences in the proposed mechanisms of action that have been recently reviewed in detail (54), they both converge on the toxic effect of the B factor, bearing a catalytically active deubiquitinase domain, which is able to recapitulate the CI-induced defects observed during the first embryonic mitosis (27). The A factor acts as an antidote, sufficient to operate the rescue (28).

The study of the genetic diversity of *w*Pip strains present in *C. pipiens* has also led to significant progress in our understanding of the CI mechanisms. All individuals of this mosquito species are naturally infected with *Wolbachia* that recently diverged into five distinct groups within *w*Pip (*w*PipI to -V), occupying different geographical areas, and resulting in a high diversity of Mod/Resc patterns when the mosquitos are crossed. Crosses are usually compatible within a *w*Pip group, while incompatibility between hosts harboring different *w*Pip groups occurs frequently. The complexity of the observed crossing types has suggested the coexistence of multiple Mod/Resc factors within a single *w*Pip strain (55). Multiple variants of CidA and CidB effectors have indeed been found to be present within single *w*Pip strains, creating a complex repertoire of effectors and matching the previously established crossing types (compatible or incompatible). This discovery also supports the hypothesis that CI and its rescue are driven by toxin-antidote interactions, whose affinity between partners determines the success of the rescue (56).

Thanks to these recent breakthrough discoveries, many questions are now waiting to be addressed. If CidA does bind to CidB *in vitro* (27), the functional relevance of this physical interaction remains to be determined. The differences in the proposed mechanisms of CI will probably be clarified with the identification of the host targets, which represents the next exciting goal. Based on the cytology, it is likely that the CI toxin perturbs the remodeling of the paternal chromatin during fertilization, and irreversible DNA damage caused by CI may explain the persistence of PCNA on the incompletely replicated paternal chromatin during the first embryonic mitosis (57). Studies on CI should also shed light on what all these mechanisms of reproduction manipulation have in common, since some *Wolbachia* strains can induce several phenotypes, depending on the host species they infect (i.e., CI or MK) (58, 59).

Beyond these elaborate manipulations of reproductive systems, a far-reaching consequence of *Wolbachia* infections is the reproductive isolation of host populations. In addition to their evolutionary impact on the mode of reproduction of their hosts, it has been proposed that *Wolbachia* could act as a factor in speciation (60–63).

ROUTES CLOSING THE CIRCLE OF VERTICAL TRANSMISSION (SOMA TO GERM LINE)

The success of *Wolbachia* resides in their ability to be efficiently passed from the host females to the offspring, by being loaded into the egg. It involves either a persistence in the germ line and its precursors throughout the embryonic, larval, and adult stages or a tropism from the soma towards the germ line, two non-mutually exclusive strategies. Aside from the germ line, *Wolbachia* are present in numerous somatic tissues, derived from infected embryonic lineages or passing from cell to cell (31). Insights into the mechanisms underlying these vertical transfers come largely from studies in the fruit fly and in *B. malayi*, an emerging experimental paradigm for the cell biology of filariae. The different routes followed by *Wolbachia* to reach the female germ line and concentrate in the eggs of insects and nematodes are reviewed below.

In insects, the female reproductive tract typically consists of a pair of ovaries, made of a series of tubes called ovarioles (Fig. 3A). Each ovariole begins with a germarium, where the germ line stem cells (GSCs) , the somatic stem cells (SSCs), and their associated niches reside. These stem cells continuously differentiate into a series of developing cysts or egg chambers, forming an ovariole. Hence, an ovariole recapitulates in the adult female the

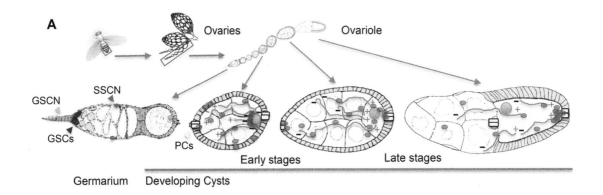

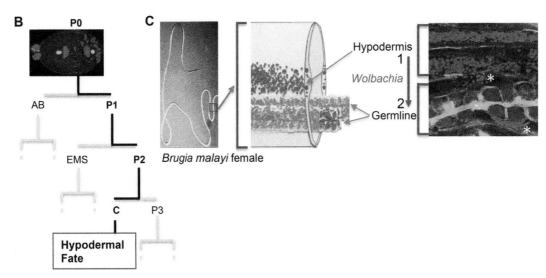

Figure 3 Germ line tropism and *Wolbachia* transmission in insect and nematode species. (**A**) Schematic representation of *D. melanogaster* oogenesis. The germ line is in white, and the surrounding somatic follicle cells are in gray. For the sake of clarity, *Wolbachia* are not represented within the germarium, where they colonize the GSCs and associated niche (GSCN) (dark and light purple, respectively), as well as the somatic stem cell niche (SSCN; pink). In developing cysts, polar cells (PCs) are yellow, the microtubule (green) polarity is indicated by plus and minus signs, and the *Wolbachia* organisms are red foci. Nuclei of developing cysts are depicted in blue. (**B**) Asymmetric segregation of *Wolbachia* during early embryogenesis in *B. malayi*. The confocal image of a fertilized egg shows the *Wolbachia* (red foci) in the posterior compartment around the centrosome (green) during the first anaphase. The route followed by *Wolbachia* to reach the hypodermis in the early lineage is highlighted in black. The P lineage represents the germ line precursor lineage, left by *Wolbachia* after the P2 division to concentrate in the hypodermal precursor C blastomere. (**C**) Schematic cross section of a *B. malayi* female, with an emphasis on the tissues infected by *Wolbachia*. The confocal image shows the tropism of some *Wolbachia* organisms from the hypodermis to the somatic gonad in a juvenile female. Asterisks indicate the entry and proliferation of *Wolbachia* in the somatic ovarian distal sheath cells.

entire process of oogenesis, from the stem cells to the mature oocytes. A cyst is composed of a syncytial cluster of nurse cells that support the growth of one oocyte, located in the posterior pole of the cyst and surrounded by various types of somatic cells. As development proceeds, the nurse cells transfer their cytoplasmic content into the growing oocyte, including crucial posterior polarity determinants (64). In *Drosophila*, *Wolbachia* are found throughout the developing cysts, in nurse cells, and in the oocyte. They are inherited from the germarium, where they are present in the GSCs.

In addition to the germ line, numerous *Wolbachia* strains have also been found to stably colonize the SSC and GSC niches in the germaria of various *Drosophila* species (65, 66). When artificially introduced through injection into the insect abdomen, the endosymbionts show a tropism towards the ovaries, and more specifically towards an SSC niche (65). Hence, targeting a niche may allow *Wolbachia* to replicate enough before they invade the fast-cycling GSCs, with the niche acting as a reservoir in long-term infections, to ensure a stable vertical transmission, and it could also represent an entry gate to the germ line when the bacteria are acquired by horizontal transfer. Although the precise mechanisms are not known, hybrid crosses between *Drosophila* species carrying different *Wolbachia* strains have revealed that the tropism for a given niche (GSC or SSC) is strain dependent and mediated by *Wolbachia*-encoded factors (66). The observation that wild-caught *Wolbachia*-infected female fruit flies can present ovarioles displaying *Wolbachia*-free early cysts (reflecting an imperfect transmission from the stem cells) and infected cysts at later stages of development suggests that soma-to-germ line transfers may have been overlooked. Such late transfers to maturing cysts in the fruit fly may originate from the polar cells, specialized somatic cells located at each pole of the cysts recently found to be targeted by *Wolbachia*, where the endosymbionts accumulate at high density (67).

Whether acquired directly from GSC divisions or indirectly from soma-to-germ line transfers, the *Wolbachia* present in the cyst must next concentrate in the oocyte. They first accumulate in the anterior of the oocyte and later concentrate in the posterior of the egg, where they incorporate the primordial germ cells during early embryonic development. In the fruit fly, the oocyte development is characterized by a dramatic reversal of microtubule orientation (Fig. 3A) (68). Genetic and cellular studies in *D. melanogaster* established that the *Wolbachia* achieve their dynamic localizations through interactions with microtubules, subverting both host dynein and kinesin motors to overcome the microtubule polarity reversal, to move first from the nurse cells to the oocyte and later to its posterior pole, where they stably associate with pole plasm components that specify primordial germ cells (69, 70).

Other genetic experiments have revealed that the actin cytoskeleton also plays a crucial role in *Wolbachia* localization and transmission (71), and biochemical studies suggest an interaction between the actin cytoskeleton and *Wolbachia* surface proteins in filariae (72). However, since the *Wolbachia* reside inside host-derived vacuoles of endoplasmic reticulum (ER) origin (73), how the bacteria directly engage in sequential associations with microtubule-associated molecular motors or with actin through surface proteins is not clear. A putative *w*Mel secreted effector able to bundle actin *in vitro* has been reported to enhance *Wolbachia* replication and/or transmission (25). It is most likely that an array of *Wolbachia* effectors able to subvert molecular motors to transport the *Wolbachia*-containing vacuole remains to be identified.

Amazingly, the *Wolbachia* have evolved to integrate embryonic fate maps, in order to reach numerous somatic target tissues and the germ line. *Wolbachia* distribution in adult tissues mostly relies on segregation patterns during oogenesis and embryonic development. In insects, although *Wolbachia* preferentially localize to the posterior of the egg to occupy the place where the primordial germ line forms in the early embryo, they also associate with the microtubules and mitotic spindles throughout the cortex of the syncytial embryo, to later persist or disappear in differentiating somatic tissues by following symmetric or asymmetric division patterns (74).

In adult filarial nematodes, the *Wolbachia* localization patterns are much simpler and almost universal among filariae, and they reflect the basic anatomy of these parasitic worms and the mutualistic relationship they have established with their host. *Wolbachia* colonize the hypodermis of both male and female individuals and the germ line exclusively of females. Transmitted by blood-feeding arthropod vector species (mosquitos, flies, or ticks), infective third larval stages develop into long threadlike adult worms in the vertebrate host. Filarial nematodes have an exceptional lifespan (more than 10 years for species infecting humans), and an adult female remains fertile long enough to deliver millions of microfilariae in the host fluids. Adults and microfilariae can cause diseases which are sometimes lethal in animals and extremely debilitating in humans (75). These nematodes live in the rich fluids of their hosts (i.e., the lymph or the blood), and most nutrients are acquired through the hypodermis rather than the digestive tract (76); *Wolbachia* are found in great abundance in this tissue, which represents a hot spot for worm metabolism. The hypodermis delivers nutrients to sustain gametogenesis and the huge demand of the embryonic development taking place entirely in the female uteri, occupying almost the entire length of the female body (77).

How do the *Wolbachia* reach the somatic hypodermis and the female germ line and avoid the male germ line during *B. malayi* development? In secernentean nematodes, such as the filarial nematode *B. malayi* and the soil-living experimental model *Caenorhabditis elegans*, the embryonic development follows an invariant cell lineage. The first asymmetric division of the egg gives rise to a posterior germ line precursor cell, and the following asymmetric divisions produce the other founder cells, a series of blastomeres producing differentiated descendants.

The similarities in cell lineage during embryonic development between *C. elegans* and *B. malayi* allowed the tracking of the endosymbionts in the filarial embryo (78). Cellular analyses of the egg-to-embryo transition in *B. malayi* revealed that the egg contains a peculiar polar microtubule organizing center of maternal origin, which is used by *Wolbachia* to concentrate in the posterior pole of the egg. Prior to the first zygotic division, this polar microtubule organizing center disappears, but the *Wolbachia* organisms remain sequestered in the posterior compartment through an interaction with the astral microtubules and the posterior cortex. This enrichment requires proper establishment of the anterior-posterior polarity in the fertilized egg and relies on dynein. Like *w*Mel in *Drosophila*, *w*Bm utilizes the host microtubule network and polarity information to navigate and asymmetrically localize in the germ line precursor lineage (79). In contrast, however, *w*Bm does not remain in the germ line precursors but concentrates preferentially in one blastomere, which gives rise to the posterior dorsal hypodermis (Fig. 3B).

How the *Wolbachia* navigate asymmetrically through several rounds of division to preferentially settle in one single blastomere out of 12 in the early embryo, and persist only within its lineage, is a mystery. Attempts to transfer *Wolbachia* into *C. elegans* have failed so far, and filariae do not offer the same genetic tools as this well-known experimental model organism to address this question. This segregation pattern is, however, conserved in several filarial species harboring either the C or D *Wolbachia* supergroup, suggesting an ancestral mode of transmission based on the colonization of the soma first (80). As a consequence, *Wolbachia* remain confined to the posterior hypodermis during embryonic development and most of the larval stage. In female larvae, the ovaries devoid of *Wolbachia* develop as tubes, whose distal tips migrate towards the posterior of the body, while the germ line proliferates (79, 80).

During the considerable growth of the larvae in the vertebrate host, *Wolbachia* colonize the entire hypodermis and eventually show a specific tropism for the very distal tips of the ovaries. The bacteria first enter the somatic gonad sheath cells and next invade the syncytial germ line (Fig. 3C). The passage of *Wolbachia* through host membranes seems to be facilitated by local depolymerization of the cortical actin fibers in filariae (80).

In summary, vertical transmission of *Wolbachia* relies on a series of asymmetric segregation events during mitotic divisions in the embryo, to reach and colonize the hypodermis. A subset of exocytosed *Wolbachia* in the pseudocoelom specifically adheres to the ovarian distal sheath cells, enters to proliferate in these somatic cells, and eventually colonizes the syncytial germ line. The basis of this germ line tropism is unknown, but it is likely to involve female-specific receptors located only on the most distal somatic gonad sheath cells, allowing *Wolbachia* to target the GSCs instead of their more proximal differentiated progeny and to stably colonize the germ line. Interestingly, the GSCs, and not their niche, act as a reservoir for *Wolbachia* in the adult filarial female.

WOLBACHIA ARE NOT PASSIVE PASSENGERS OF THE GERM LINE

Wolbachia have a unique ability to influence germ line behavior, starting with the maintenance and proliferation of GSCs. In some *Drosophila* species, *Wolbachia* induce a fecundity gain by increasing the mitotic activity of the GSCs while inhibiting the programmed cell death, leading to infected females laying four times more eggs (81). In *B. malayi*, the removal of the mutualistic *w*Bm by antibiotic treatment prevents the *in utero* embryonic development from being completed, due to a major apoptosis occurring during embryogenesis (82). Much farther upstream in the gonad, the overall GSC behavior is greatly affected in *Wolbachia*-depleted *B. malayi* females. While GSC proliferation is reduced by a third, the quiescence of a distal pool of GSCs, as well as the organization of the germ line as a monolayer of syncytial nuclei around a central rachis, is heavily perturbed, suggesting that *Wolbachia* may control GSC fate maintenance in filariae (83). In *Drosophila*, *Wolbachia* support germ line maintenance by their extraordinary ability to suppress germ line phenotypes, such as the sterility induced by mutants of *bag-of-marbles*, a gene required for GSC differentiation and germ line cyst development in females (84).

Another example is the suppression of the fertility defect induced by *Sex lethal* (*Sxl*) mutants by *w*Mel in *D. melanogaster* (85, 86). Sxl is an RNA splicing factor involved in germ line regulation and sex determination that maintains the GSCs in an undifferentiated state (87). The mechanism by which *w*Mel suppresses the *Sxl*-induced sterility phenotype was recently identified. TomO is an ankyrin repeat-containing effector that associates with *nanos* mRNA to increase its translation. Nanos, an RNA-binding protein essential to GSC self-renewal, acts by repressing an array of targets involved in differentiation (88). The elevated levels of Nanos protein induced by TomO counteract the Sxl loss by promoting the maintenance of the GSC fate (24).

The fact that the TomO ortholog from *w*Pip (the *Wolbachia* strain infecting *C. pipiens*) can rescue the *Sxl* mutation in the fruit fly suggests an evolutionary conservation of some *Wolbachia* effects on the GSCs (89). TomO has no ortholog in the *Wolbachia* strains present in filarial nematodes, and other effectors should be secreted by *w*Bm to influence the GSCs. In *B. malayi*, only the female GSCs, containing a high titer of endosymbionts, have their behavior and organization perturbed upon *Wolbachia* depletion (83). The oocytes produced by such a compromised germ line may be faulty, due to a defective developmental program to which *Wolbachia* contribute, and therefore could be unable to undergo a normal embryonic development once fertilized. Hence, the massive apoptosis undergone by the developing embryos may originate from the absence of *Wolbachia* in the germ line. The very few bacteria present within developing embryos, localized in a small subset of posterior dorsal hypodermal precursors, are unlikely to operate a nonautonomous antiapoptotic effect on the scale of the entire embryo, composed of hundreds of blastomeres (80).

Since antibiotic treatment also depletes the hypodermal *Wolbachia* population in the adult female, a somatic support for the embryonic development (i.e., a potential metabolic contribution of *Wolbachia* from the hypodermis to the uteri) cannot be excluded. Although most symbioses of *Wolbachia* with arthropods are parasitic, removal of *w*Atab3 from the parasitoid wasp *Asobara tabida* leads to female sterility. Here again, the depletion of *Wolbachia* leads to apoptosis in the germ line. However, apoptosis is restricted to a subset of maturing cysts in midoogenesis (90). It is therefore not clear yet whether *Wolbachia* directly inhibit programmed cell death, a physiological process essential to the development of fly and worm germ lines (91, 92), or whether the observed antiapoptotic effects of *Wolbachia* in filariae and parasitoid wasps are an indirect consequence due to other crucial functions carried out by *Wolbachia* in the germ line or the soma (93).

In summary, *Wolbachia* have evolved various strategies to influence host oogenesis to their advantage, such as protecting the GSCs they colonize and thus enhancing their own proliferation, while in some mutualistic associations, they prevent the maintenance of aposymbiotic germ line and/or embryonic development. Future studies focusing on effector identification and their functional analyses will teach us more about the mechanisms underlying these fascinating manipulations.

THE INFLUENCE OF *WOLBACHIA* ON HOST METABOLISM AND FITNESS, AND BIOMEDICAL APPLICATIONS

In addition to the germ line, the presence of *Wolbachia* in numerous somatic tissues observed in a plethora of arthropod species is not incidental (31). A high *Wolbachia* titer in cells and tissues can influence the host metabolism and can confer advantages in order to establish long-term, stable symbiotic associations. *Wolbachia* spp. have undergone significant gene loss, especially in metabolic pathways, and *Wolbachia* rely on their hosts to acquire amino acids and lipids. However, they have retained some biosynthetic pathways to produce, e.g., some vitamin cofactors, purines, and heme (an intact glycolysis for *w*Mel), to potentially provide metabolites to the host (15, 16). These metabolic capabilities have been proposed to sustain the mutualism with filariae by complementing biosynthetic pathways that are missing or partially missing in *B. malayi* (15). However, the genome of the closely related, *Wolbachia*-free filarial nematode *Loa loa* did not reveal additional metabolic capabilities compared to *B. malayi* (94), and a metabolomics study of nucleotide levels in *B. malayi* ovaries did not highlight differences between wild-type and *Wolbachia*-depleted germ lines (83).

Without ruling out the hypothesized metabolic complementation (95), the described mutualism is likely to rely on more subtle mechanisms. While the mutualistic symbiosis is often perceived as an array of reciprocal contributions sustaining the life of both partners, alternative scenarios can be envisaged. The *Wolbachia* metabolic demands can create new equilibriums, leading to a loss of homeostasis upon their loss. These bacteria can also participate in basic host cell or developmental functions, making them essential where they were previously not needed (96).

Nonessential *Wolbachia* can provide fitness advantages regarding fertility and/or survival, sometimes through response to various stresses (97–100). Protection against iron-induced oxidative stress has been observed in some *Wolbachia* symbioses with arthropods, through iron-buffering hemoprotein ferritins (101). In the bedbug *Cimex lectularius*, *Wolbachia* appear as nutritional mutualists, provisioning the host with B vitamins (102, 103). *Wolbachia* can affect host signaling pathways such as the insulin signaling pathway, and this may also account for their influence on host metabolism (104).

Another factor increasing host fitness is the protection conferred by *Wolbachia* against a plethora of bacterial, viral, and parasitic pathogens naturally present in arthropods (105). When artificially introduced into mosquitos, the *w*Mel strain has proved efficient in inhibiting the transmission of the most important mosquito-borne human pathogens, including arboviruses such as dengue and Zika viruses (106–112). Hence, some of the current strategies to control these diseases consist of mosquito population replacement, thanks to the CI-based spread of *Wolbachia* (2, 107, 113). Access to intracellular cholesterol appears to be a key element in *Wolbachia*-induced viral inhibition. *Wolbachia* genomes do not appear to contain any genes for lipopolysaccharide synthase, and *Wolbachia* likely incorporate cholesterol into their membranes (16, 114). This metabolite, also essential for arbovirus replication, has been shown to be esterified in the presence of *Wolbachia* in mosquito cells, and this change in cholesterol homeostasis leads to its cellular accumulation while preventing the dengue virus from accessing it (115).

While *Wolbachia* organisms are transferred from *Drosophila* to mosquitos to control the transmission of vector-borne pathogens, mutualistic *Wolbachia* organisms are conversely used as drug targets to fight filariasis (2). Not only are 120 million individuals infected with filarial nematodes, but 1.3 billion live at risk of contracting these extremely debilitating parasitic diseases, such as elephantiasis or river blindness (116). These parasites are also a burden to cattle and can be lethal in cats and dogs (117, 118). Classical anthelmintic treatments, such as ivermectin, do not kill but only sterilize adult worms, while *Wolbachia* depletion by antibiotic therapy additionally prevents larval molting and kills adult worms (75, 119–121). This reduction in life span associated with the loss of mutualistic *Wolbachia* correlates with a change in the host innate immune response (122). The presence of *Wolbachia* attracts neutrophils and protects the worm against otherwise degranulating eosinophils. Hence, the endosymbionts participate in the worm's immune escape by inducing a typical response against microbial pathogens via Toll-like receptors 2 and 4 (123, 124).

THE INTRACELLULAR LIFESTYLE OF *WOLBACHIA*

Although most efforts have focused on the comprehension of *Wolbachia*-induced host phenotypes, the use of

Drosophila and insect cell cultures has yielded novel insights into the mechanisms underlying the intracellular lifestyle of these endosymbionts. *Wolbachia* reside as individual bacteria or small clusters of bacteria inside host-derived vacuoles, suggesting a subversion of the intracellular vesicular trafficking (125, 126). Although the detailed mechanisms of membrane acquisition are not known, *Wolbachia* appear to be closely associated with the ER, and a recent study suggested that this organelle is a source of membrane for them (73, 127). Motility is achieved through transport along microtubules (74), and accordingly, genomic studies did not reveal the presence of genes related to flagellar, fimbrial, or pilus structures (15).

Although they remain mostly transmitted through mitotic divisions, *in vitro* cell culture studies revealed that *Wolbachia* organisms are likely to be secreted, and cell-to-cell infection does not require cell contact. Cell entry has been proposed to rely on phagocytosis and/or endocytosis, but precise studies are still lacking (128).

Wolbachia are pleomorphic and are present in very high titers compared to other intracellular bacteria, sometimes reaching several hundred bacteria per cell. This titer is notably influenced by dietary nutrients and is regulated in a TORC1 and insulin signaling pathway-dependent manner (129). An RNA interference screen in *Wolbachia*-infected *Drosophila* cells established that the *Wolbachia* titer relies on key players of the ER-associated protein degradation pathway (ERAD) and suggested that ERAD and ubiquitination pathways are subverted by *Wolbachia* to acquire amino acids via proteasome degradation (127). However, the proteasome activity was not found to be modulated by *Wolbachia* in other systems, such as mosquito cell lines (130), and conflicting lines of evidence emerged from different studies regarding the induction of the UPR (unfolded protein response)/ER stress by *Wolbachia*, which was found to be either down- or upregulated (115, 131), possibly because different *Wolbachia* strain-cell line associations were used, in the context of either recent or long-term infections.

The recent establishment of *Wolbachia* infections with the *w*Mel strain in distinct cellular environments (haploid female and tetraploid male *Drosophila* cell lines), leading to high titers of endosymbionts, did not perturb cell homeostasis and did not invoke the UPR and ERAD pathways, suggesting that *Wolbachia* can thrive without increasing ERAD-driven proteolysis and possesses other mechanisms of amino acid salvage (73).

Another RNA interference screen recently revealed an increased *w*Mel titer in a *Drosophila* cell line when genes coding for ribosomal or translation elongation factors were knocked down, suggesting that the host cell translation machinery is a limiting factor for *Wolbachia*. In addition, this study demonstrated that the level of host cell protein translation appears to be negatively correlated with the *Wolbachia* titer (132). This tight link between host cell translation and the number of intracellular *Wolbachia* could indicate a capacity of *Wolbachia* to modulate signaling pathways supporting translation and cell growth in order to leverage the pool of free amino acids available in the host cell. Although the mechanisms by which *Wolbachia* acquires amino acids and other nutrients remain to be explored in depth, these studies nonetheless highlight the difficulty of drawing definite conclusions with such versatile endosymbionts. Unlike in infections involving pathogenic intracellular bacteria, maintenance of cellular homeostasis is necessary to sustain long-term endosymbiont-host associations.

CONCLUSION

The most abundant endosymbionts on earth belong to the genus *Wolbachia*, which comprises a variety of strains able to exploit their hosts and induce diverse phenotypes to sustain their vertical transmission. Parasitic and mutualistic *Wolbachia* strains have similar metabolic capabilities, and cellular studies indicate that they are likely to employ the same mechanisms to survive and replicate within host cells. A better understanding of *Wolbachia*-host interactions will require large-scale identification and functional analyses of their effectors. To this end, the use of heterologous systems has proved to be a temporary alternative to the much-needed genetic manipulation of *Wolbachia*, which will eventually remove the last barriers to achieving a complete picture of their extraordinary lifestyles and symbiotic interactions.

Acknowledgments. I deeply apologize to authors whose contributions I have omitted. Some aspects of Wolbachia *biology and specific references may have been omitted due to space constraints.*

Citation. Landmann F. 2019. The *Wolbachia* endosymbionts. Microbiol Spectrum 7(2):BAI-0018-2019.

References

1. Hilgenboecker K, Hammerstein P, Schlattmann P, Telschow A, Werren JH. 2008. How many species are infected with *Wolbachia*? A statistical analysis of current data. *FEMS Microbiol Lett* 281:215–220.

2. Slatko BE, Luck AN, Dobson SL, Foster JM. 2014. *Wolbachia* endosymbionts and human disease control. *Mol Biochem Parasitol* 195:88–95.

3. Werren JH, Baldo L, Clark ME. 2008. *Wolbachia*: master manipulators of invertebrate biology. *Nat Rev Microbiol* 6:741–751.

4. Hertig M, Wolbach SB. 1924. Studies on *Rickettsia*-like micro-organisms in insects. *J Med Res* 44:329–3747.

5. Baldo L, Dunning Hotopp JC, Jolley KA, Bordenstein SR, Biber SA, Choudhury RR, Hayashi C, Maiden MCJ, Tettelin H, Werren JH. 2006. Multilocus sequence typing system for the endosymbiont *Wolbachia pipientis*. *Appl Environ Microbiol* 72:7098–7110.

6. Bandi C, Anderson TJC, Genchi C, Blaxter ML. 1998. Phylogeny of *Wolbachia* in filarial nematodes. *Proc Biol Sci* 265:2407–2413.

7. Kozek WJ. 1977. Transovarially-transmitted intracellular microorganisms in adult and larval stages of *Brugia malayi*. *J Parasitol* 63:992–1000.

8. Lefoulon E, Bain O, Makepeace BL, d'Haese C, Uni S, Martin C, Gavotte L. 2016. Breakdown of coevolution between symbiotic bacteria *Wolbachia* and their filarial hosts. *PeerJ* 4:e1840.

9. Glowska E, Dragun-Damian A, Dabert M, Gerth M. 2015. New *Wolbachia* supergroups detected in quill mites (Acari: Syringophilidae). *Infect Genet Evol* 30:140–146.

10. Wang G-H, Jia L-Y, Xiao J-H, Huang D-W. 2016. Discovery of a new *Wolbachia* supergroup in cave spider species and the lateral transfer of phage WO among distant hosts. *Infect Genet Evol* 41:1–7.

11. Casiraghi M, Anderson TJC, Bandi C, Bazzocchi C, Genchi C. 2001. A phylogenetic analysis of filarial nematodes: comparison with the phylogeny of *Wolbachia* endosymbionts. *Parasitology* 122:93–103.

12. Lo N, Casiraghi M, Salati E, Bazzocchi C, Bandi C. 2002. How many *Wolbachia* supergroups exist? *Mol Biol Evol* 19:341–346.

13. Haegeman A, Vanholme B, Jacob J, Vandekerckhove TTM, Claeys M, Borgonie G, Gheysen G. 2009. An endosymbiotic bacterium in a plant-parasitic nematode: member of a new *Wolbachia* supergroup. *Int J Parasitol* 39:1045–1054.

14. Brown AMV, Wasala SK, Howe DK, Peetz AB, Zasada IA, Denver DR. 2016. Genomic evidence for plant-parasitic nematodes as the earliest *Wolbachia* hosts. *Sci Rep* 6:34955.

15. Foster J, Ganatra M, Kamal I, Ware J, Makarova K, Ivanova N, Bhattacharyya A, Kapatral V, Kumar S, Posfai J, Vincze T, Ingram J, Moran L, Lapidus A, Omelchenko M, Kyrpides N, Ghedin E, Wang S, Goltsman E, Joukov V, Ostrovskaya O, Tsukerman K, Mazur M, Comb D, Koonin E, Slatko B. 2005. The *Wolbachia* genome of *Brugia malayi*: endosymbiont evolution within a human pathogenic nematode. *PLoS Biol* 3:e121.

16. Wu M, Sun LV, Vamathevan J, Riegler M, Deboy R, Brownlie JC, McGraw EA, Martin W, Esser C, Ahmadinejad N, Wiegand C, Madupu R, Beanan MJ, Brinkac LM, Daugherty SC, Durkin AS, Kolonay JF, Nelson WC, Mohamoud Y, Lee P, Berry K, Young MB, Utterback T, Weidman J, Nierman WC, Paulsen IT, Nelson KE, Tettelin H, O'Neill SL, Eisen JA. 2004. Phylogenomics of the reproductive parasite *Wolbachia pipientis* wMel: a streamlined genome overrun by mobile genetic elements. *PLoS Biol* 2:e69.

17. Masui S, Kamoda S, Sasaki T, Ishikawa H. 2000. Distribution and evolution of bacteriophage WO in *Wolbachia*, the endosymbiont causing sexual alterations in arthropods. *J Mol Evol* **51**:491–497.

18. LePage DP, Metcalf JA, Bordenstein SR, On J, Perlmutter JI, Shropshire JD, Layton EM, Funkhouser-Jones LJ, Beckmann JF, Bordenstein SR. 2017. Prophage WO genes recapitulate and enhance Wolbachia-nduced cytoplasmic incompatibility. *Nature* **543**:243–247.

19. Pichon S, Bouchon D, Cordaux R, Chen L, Garrett RA, Grève P. 2009. Conservation of the type IV secretion system throughout *Wolbachia* evolution. *Biochem Biophys Res Commun* **385**:557–562.

20. Li Z, Carlow CKS. 2012. Characterization of transcription factors that regulate the type IV secretion system and riboflavin biosynthesis in *Wolbachia* of *Brugia malayi*. *PLoS One* **7**:e51597.

21. Masui S, Sasaki T, Ishikawa H. 2000. Genes for the type IV secretion system in an intracellular symbiont, *Wolbachia*, a causative agent of various sexual alterations in arthropods. *J Bacteriol* **182**:6529–6531.

22. Rancès E, Voronin D, Tran-Van V, Mavingui P. 2008. Genetic and functional characterization of the type IV secretion system in *Wolbachia*. *J Bacteriol* **190**:5020–5030.

23. Félix C, Pichon S, Braquart-Varnier C, Braig H, Chen L, Garrett RA, Martin G, Grève P. 2008. Characterization and transcriptional analysis of two gene clusters for type IV secretion machinery in *Wolbachia* of *Armadillidium vulgare*. *Res Microbiol* **159**:481–485.

24. Ote M, Ueyama M, Yamamoto D. 2016. *Wolbachia* protein TomO targets *nanos* mRNA and restores germ stem cells in *Drosophila* sex-lethal mutants. *Curr Biol* **26**:2223–2232.

25. Sheehan KB, Martin M, Lesser CF, Isberg RR, Newton ILG. 2016. Identification and characterization of a candidate *Wolbachia pipientis* type IV effector that interacts with the actin cytoskeleton. *mBio* **7**:e00622-16.

26. Beckmann JF, Fallon AM. 2013. Detection of the *Wolbachia* protein WPIP0282 in mosquito spermathecae: implications for cytoplasmic incompatibility. *Insect Biochem Mol Biol* **43**:867–878.

27. Beckmann JF, Ronau JA, Hochstrasser M. 2017. A *Wolbachia* deubiquitylating enzyme induces cytoplasmic incompatibility. *Nat Microbiol* **2**:17007.

28. Shropshire JD, On J, Layton EM, Zhou H, Bordenstein SR. 2018. One prophage WO gene rescues cytoplasmic incompatibility in *Drosophila melanogaster*. *Proc Natl Acad Sci USA* **115**:4987–4991.

29. Rice DW, Sheehan KB, Newton ILG. 2017. Large-scale identification of *Wolbachia pipientis* effectors. *Genome Biol Evol* **9**:1925–1937.

30. Carpinone EM, Li Z, Mills MK, Foltz C, Brannon ER, Carlow CKS, Starai VJ. 2018. Identification of putative effectors of the type IV secretion system from the *Wolbachia* endosymbiont of *Brugia malayi*. *PLoS One* **13**:e0204736.

31. Pietri JE, DeBruhl H, Sullivan W. 2016. The rich somatic life of *Wolbachia*. *MicrobiologyOpen* **5**:923–936.

32. Rasgon JL, Gamston CE, Ren X. 2006. Survival of *Wolbachia pipientis* in cell-free medium. *Appl Environ Microbiol* **72**:6934–6937.

33. Serbus LR, Casper-Lindley C, Landmann F, Sullivan W. 2008. The genetics and cell biology of *Wolbachia*-host interactions. *Annu Rev Genet* **42**:683–707.

34. Weeks AR, Breeuwer JAJ. 2001. *Wolbachia*-induced parthenogenesis in a genus of phytophagous mites. *Proc Biol Sci* **268**:2245–2251.

35. Gottlieb Y, Zchori-Fein E. 2001. Irreversible thelytokous reproduction in *Muscidifurax uniraptor*. *Entomol Exp Appl* **100**:271–278.

36. Stouthamer R, Kazmer DJ. 1994. Cytogenetics of microbe-associated parthenogenesis and its consequences for gene flow in *Trichogramma* wasps. *Hered Edinb* **73**:317–327.

37. Adachi-Hagimori T, Miura K, Stouthamer R. 2008. A new cytogenetic mechanism for bacterial endosymbiont-induced parthenogenesis in *Hymenoptera*. *Proc Biol Sci* **275**:2667–2673.

38. Cordaux R, Bouchon D, Grève P. 2011. The impact of endosymbionts on the evolution of host sex-determination mechanisms. *Trends Genet* **27**:332–341.

39. Bouchon D, Cordaux R, Grève P. 2008. Feminizing *Wolbachia* and the evolution of sex determination in isopods, p 273–294. *In* Bourtzis K, Miller T (ed), *Insect Symbiosis*, vol 3. CRC Press, Boca Raton, FL.

40. Ferdy JB, Liu N, Sicard M. 2016. Transmission modes and the evolution of feminizing symbionts. *J Evol Biol* **29**:2395–2409.

41. Hurst GDD, Majerus MEN. 1993. Why do maternally inherited microorganisms kill males? *Hered Edinb* **71**:81–95.

42. Hurst GDD, Jiggins FM, Majerus MEN. 2003. Inherited microorganisms that selectively kill male hosts: the hidden players of insect evolution? p 177–199. *In* Bourtzis K, Miller T (ed), *Insect Symbiosis*, vol 1. CRC Press, Boca Raton, FL.

43. Riparbelli MG, Giordano R, Ueyama M, Callaini G. 2012. *Wolbachia*-mediated male killing is associated with defective chromatin remodeling. *PLoS One* **7**:e30045.

44. Harumoto T, Lemaitre B. 2018. Male-killing toxin in a bacterial symbiont of *Drosophila*. *Nature* **557**:252–255.

45. Veneti Z. 2005. A functional dosage compensation complex required for male killing in *Drosophila*. *Science* **307**:1461–1463.

46. Bordenstein SR, Werren JH. 2007. Bidirectional incompatibility among divergent *Wolbachia* and incompatibility level differences among closely related *Wolbachia* in *Nasonia*. *Hered Edinb* **99**:278–287.

47. Yen JH, Barr AR. 1971. New hypothesis of the cause of cytoplasmic incompatibility in *Culex pipiens* L. *Nature* **232**:657–658.

48. Clark ME, Veneti Z, Bourtzis K, Karr TL. 2002. The distribution and proliferation of the intracellular bacteria *Wolbachia* during spermatogenesis in *Drosophila*. *Mech Dev* **111**:3–15.

49. Callaini G, Dallai R, Riparbelli MG. 1997. *Wolbachia*-induced delay of paternal chromatin condensation does

not prevent maternal chromosomes from entering anaphase in incompatible crosses of *Drosophila simulans*. *J Cell Sci* **110**:271–280.

50. Landmann F, Orsi GA, Loppin B, Sullivan W. 2009. *Wolbachia*-mediated cytoplasmic incompatibility is associated with impaired histone deposition in the male pronucleus. *PLoS Pathog* **5**:e1000343.

51. Zabalou S, Apostolaki A, Pattas S, Veneti Z, Paraskevopoulos C, Livadaras I, Markakis G, Brissac T, Merçot H, Bourtzis K. 2008. Multiple rescue factors within a *Wolbachia* strain. *Genetics* **178**:2145–2160.

52. Atyame CM, Labbé P, Dumas E, Milesi P, Charlat S, Fort P, Weill M. 2014. *Wolbachia* divergence and the evolution of cytoplasmic incompatibility in *Culex pipiens*. *PLoS One* **9**:e87336.

53. Atyame CM, Duron O, Tortosa P, Pasteur N, Fort P, Weill M. 2011. Multiple *Wolbachia* determinants control the evolution of cytoplasmic incompatibilities in *Culex pipiens* mosquito populations. *Mol Ecol* **20**:286–298.

54. Beckmann JF, Bonneau M, Chen H, Hochstrasser M, Poinsot D, Merçot H, Weill M, Sicard M, Charlat S. 2019. The toxin-antidote model of cytoplasmic incompatibility: genetics and evolutionary implications. *Trends Genet* **35**:175–185.

55. Atyame CM, Delsuc F, Pasteur N, Weill M, Duron O. 2011. Diversification of *Wolbachia* endosymbiont in the *Culex pipiens* mosquito. *Mol Biol Evol* **28**:2761–2772.

56. Bonneau M, Atyame C, Beji M, Justy F, Cohen-Gonsaud M, Sicard M, Weill M. 2018. *Culex pipiens* crossing type diversity is governed by an amplified and polymorphic operon of *Wolbachia*. *Nat Commun* **9**:319.

57. Choe KN, Moldovan GL. 2017. Forging ahead through darkness: PCNA, still the principal conductor at the replication fork. *Mol Cell* **65**:380–392.

58. Jaenike J. 2007. Spontaneous emergence of a new *Wolbachia* phenotype. *Evolution* **61**:2244–2252.

59. Sasaki T, Massaki N, Kubo T. 2005. *Wolbachia* variant that induces two distinct reproductive phenotypes in different hosts. *Hered Edinb* **95**:389–393.

60. Moran NA, McCutcheon JP, Nakabachi A. 2008. Genomics and evolution of heritable bacterial symbionts. *Annu Rev Genet* **42**:165–190.

61. Telschow A, Flor M, Kobayashi Y, Hammerstein P, Werren JH. 2007. *Wolbachia*-induced unidirectional cytoplasmic incompatibility and speciation: mainland-island model. *PLoS One* **2**:e701.

62. Rokas A. 2000. *Wolbachia* as a speciation agent. *Trends Ecol Evol* **15**:44–45.

63. Karr TL, Ballard B. 2006. Speciation and *Wolbachia*, p 245–260. *In Encyclopedia of Life Sciences*. John Wiley & Sons, Ltd, Chichester, United Kingdom.

64. Chang C-W, Nashchekin D, Wheatley L, Irion U, Dahlgaard K, Montague TG, Hall J, St Johnston D. 2011. Anterior-posterior axis specification in *Drosophila* oocytes: identification of novel bicoid and oskar mRNA localization factors. *Genetics* **188**:883–896.

65. Frydman HM, Li JM, Robson DN, Wieschaus E. 2006. Somatic stem cell niche tropism in *Wolbachia*. *Nature* **441**:509–512.

66. Toomey ME, Panaram K, Fast EM, Beatty C, Frydman HM. 2013. Evolutionarily conserved *Wolbachia*-encoded factors control pattern of stem-cell niche tropism in *Drosophila* ovaries and favor infection. *Proc Natl Acad Sci USA* **110**:10788–10793.

67. Kamath AD, Deehan MA, Frydman HM. 2018. Polar cell fate stimulates Wolbachia intracellular growth. *Development* **145**:158097.

68. Steinhauer J, Kalderon D. 2006. Microtubule polarity and axis formation in the *Drosophila* oocyte. *Dev Dyn* **235**:1455–1468.

69. Ferree PM, Frydman HM, Li JM, Cao J, Wieschaus E, Sullivan W. 2005. *Wolbachia* utilizes host microtubules and dynein for anterior localization in the *Drosophila* oocyte. *PLoS Pathog* **1**:e14.

70. Serbus LR, Sullivan W. 2007. A cellular basis for *Wolbachia* recruitment to the host germline. *PLoS Pathog* **3**:1930–1937.

71. Newton ILG, Savytskyy O, Sheehan KB. 2015. *Wolbachia* utilize host actin for efficient maternal transmission in *Drosophila melanogaster*. *PLoS Pathog* **11**:e1004798.

72. Melnikow E, Xu S, Liu J, Bell AJ, Ghedin E, Unnasch TR, Lustigman S. 2013. A potential role for the interaction of *Wolbachia* surface proteins with the *Brugia malayi* glycolytic enzymes and cytoskeleton in maintenance of endosymbiosis. *PLoS Negl Trop Dis* **7**:e2151.

73. Fattouh N, Cazevieille C, Landmann F. Wolbachia endosymbionts subvert the endoplasmic reticulum to acquire host membranes without triggering ER stress. *PLoS Negl Trop Dis*, in press.

74. Albertson R, Casper-Lindley C, Cao J, Tram U, Sullivan W. 2009. Symmetric and asymmetric mitotic segregation patterns influence *Wolbachia* distribution in host somatic tissue. *J Cell Sci* **122**:4570–4583.

75. Foster JM, Hoerauf A, Slatko BE, Taylor MJ. 2013. The *Wolbachia* bacterial endosymbionts of filarial nematodes, p 308–336. *In* Kennedy MW, Harnett W (ed), *Parasitic Nematodes: Molecular Biology, Biochemistry and Immunology*, 2nd ed. CABI, Wallingford, United Kingdom.

76. Howells RE, Mendis AM, Bray PG. 1983. The mechanisms of amino acid uptake by *Brugia pahangi* in vitro. *Z Parasitenkd* **69**:247–253.

77. Landmann F, Foster JM, Slatko B, Sullivan W. 2010. Asymmetric *Wolbachia* segregation during early *Brugia malayi* embryogenesis determines its distribution in adult host tissues. *PLoS Negl Trop Dis* **4**:e758.

78. Lefoulon E, Gavotte L, Junker K, Barbuto M, Uni S, Landmann F, Laaksonen S, Saari S, Nikander S, de Souza Lima S, Casiraghi M, Bain O, Martin C. 2012. A new type F *Wolbachia* from Splendidofilariinae (Onchocercidae) supports the recent emergence of this supergroup. *Int J Parasitol* **42**:1025–1036.

79. Landmann F, Foster JM, Michalski ML, Slatko BE, Sullivan W. 2014. Co-evolution between an endosymbiont and its nematode host: *Wolbachia* asymmetric posterior localization and AP polarity establishment. *PLoS Negl Trop Dis* **8**:e3096.

80. Landmann F, Bain O, Martin C, Uni S, Taylor MJ, Sullivan W. 2012. Both asymmetric mitotic segregation and cell-to-cell invasion are required for stable germline transmission of *Wolbachia* in filarial nematodes. *Biol Open* 1:536–547.

81. Fast EM, Toomey ME, Panaram K, Desjardins D, Kolaczyk ED, Frydman HM. 2011. *Wolbachia* enhance *Drosophila* stem cell proliferation and target the germline stem cell niche. *Science* 334:990–992.

82. Landmann F, Voronin D, Sullivan W, Taylor MJ. 2011. Anti-filarial activity of antibiotic therapy is due to extensive apoptosis after *Wolbachia* depletion from filarial nematodes. *PLoS Pathog* 7:e1002351.

83. Foray V, Pérez-Jiménez MM, Fattouh N, Landmann F. 2018. *Wolbachia* control stem cell behavior and stimulate germline proliferation in filarial nematodes. *Dev Cell* 45:198–211.e3.

84. Flores HA, Bubnell JE, Aquadro CF, Barbash DA. 2015. The *Drosophila* bag of marbles gene interacts genetically with *Wolbachia* and shows female-specific effects of divergence. *PLoS Genet* 11:e1005453.

85. Starr DJ, Cline TW. 2002. A host parasite interaction rescues *Drosophila* oogenesis defects. *Nature* 418:76–79.

86. Sun S, Cline TW. 2009. Effects of *Wolbachia* infection and ovarian tumor mutations on sex-lethal germline functioning in *Drosophila*. *Genetics* 181:1291–1301.

87. Hashiyama K, Hayashi Y, Kobayashi S. 2011. *Drosophila* Sex lethal gene initiates female development in germline progenitors. *Science* 333:885–888.

88. Slaidina M, Lehmann R. 2014. Translational control in germline stem cell development. *J Cell Biol* 207:13–21.

89. Ote M, Yamamoto D. 2018. Enhancing Nanos expression via the bacterial TomO protein is a conserved strategy used by the symbiont *Wolbachia* to fuel germ stem cell maintenance in infected *Drosophila* females. *Arch Insect Biochem Physiol* 98:e21471.

90. Dedeine F, Vavre F, Fleury F, Loppin B, Hochberg ME, Bouletreau M. 2001. Removing symbiotic *Wolbachia* bacteria specifically inhibits oogenesis in a parasitic wasp. *Proc Natl Acad Sci USA* 98:6247–6252.

91. Peterson JS, Timmons AK, Mondragon AA, McCall K. 2015. The end of the beginning; cell death in the germline. *Curr Top Dev Biol* 114:93–119.

92. Gumienny TL, Lambie E, Hartwieg E, Horvitz HR, Hengartner MO. 1999. Genetic control of programmed cell death in the *Caenorhabditis elegans* hermaphrodite germline. *Development* 126:1011–1022.

93. Pannebakker BA, Loppin B, Elemans CPH, Humblot L, Vavre F. 2007. Parasitic inhibition of cell death facilitates symbiosis. *Proc Natl Acad Sci USA* 104:213–215.

94. Desjardins CA, Cerqueira GC, Goldberg JM, Dunning Hotopp JC, Haas BJ, Zucker J, Ribeiro JM, Saif S, Levin JZ, Fan L, Zeng Q, Russ C, Wortman JR, Fink DL, Birren BW, Nutman TB. 2013. Genomics of *Loa loa*, a *Wolbachia*-free filarial parasite of humans. *Nat Genet* 45:495–500.

95. Voronin D, Bachu S, Shlossman M, Unnasch TR, Ghedin E, Lustigman S. 2016. Glucose and glycogen metabolism in brugia malayi is associated with *Wolbachia* symbiont fitness. *PLoS One* 11:e0153812.

96. Sullivan W. 2017. *Wolbachia*, bottled water, and the dark side of symbiosis. *Mol Biol Cell* 28:2343–2346.

97. Fry AJ, Palmer MR, Rand DM. 2004. Variable fitness effects of *Wolbachia* infection in *Drosophila melanogaster*. *Hered Edinb* 93:379–389.

98. Fraser JE, De Bruyne JT, Iturbe-Ormaetxe I, Stepnell J, Burns RL, Flores HA, O'Neill SL. 2017. Novel *Wolbachia*-transinfected *Aedes aegypti* mosquitoes possess diverse fitness and vector competence phenotypes. *PLoS Pathog* 13:e1006751.

99. Maistrenko OM, Serga SV, Vaiserman AM, Kozeretska IA. 2016. Longevity-modulating effects of symbiosis: insights from *Drosophila-Wolbachia* interaction. *Biogerontology* 17:785–803.

100. Alexandrov ID, Alexandrova MV, Goryacheva II, Rochina NV, Shaikevich EV, Zakharov IA. 2007. Removing endosymbiotic *Wolbachia* specifically decreases lifespan of females and competitiveness in a laboratory strain of *Drosophila melanogaster*. *Russ J Genet* 43:1147–1152.

101. Kremer N, Voronin D, Charif D, Mavingui P, Mollereau B, Vavre F. 2009. *Wolbachia* interferes with ferritin expression and iron metabolism in insects. *PLoS Pathog* 5:e1000630.

102. Hosokawa T, Koga R, Kikuchi Y, Meng X-Y, Fukatsu T. 2010. *Wolbachia* as a bacteriocyte-associated nutritional mutualist. *Proc Natl Acad Sci USA* 107:769–774.

103. Moriyama M, Nikoh N, Hosokawa T, Fukatsu T. 2015. Riboflavin provisioning underlies *Wolbachia*'s fitness contribution to its insect host. *mBio* 6:e01732-15.

104. Ikeya T, Broughton S, Alic N, Grandison R, Partridge L. 2009. The endosymbiont *Wolbachia* increases insulin/IGF-like signalling in *Drosophila*. *Proc Biol Sci* 276:3799–3807.

105. Eleftherianos I, Atri J, Accetta J, Castillo JC. 2013. Endosymbiotic bacteria in insects: guardians of the immune system? *Front Physiol* 4:46.

106. Hoffmann AA, Iturbe-Ormaetxe I, Callahan AG, Phillips BL, Billington K, Axford JK, Montgomery B, Turley AP, O'Neill SL. 2014. Stability of the wMel *Wolbachia* infection following invasion into *Aedes aegypti* populations. *PLoS Negl Trop Dis* 8:e3115.

107. Hoffmann AA, Montgomery BL, Popovici J, Iturbe-Ormaetxe I, Johnson PH, Muzzi F, Greenfield M, Durkan M, Leong YS, Dong Y, Cook H, Axford J, Callahan AG, Kenny N, Omodei C, McGraw EA, Ryan PA, Ritchie SA, Turelli M, O'Neill SL. 2011. Successful establishment of *Wolbachia* in *Aedes* populations to suppress dengue transmission. *Nature* 476:454–457.

108. Teixeira L, Ferreira A, Ashburner M. 2008. The bacterial symbiont *Wolbachia* induces resistance to RNA viral infections in *Drosophila melanogaster*. *PLoS Biol* 6:2753–2763.

109. Moreira LA, Iturbe-Ormaetxe I, Jeffery JA, Lu G, Pyke AT, Hedges LM, Rocha BC, Hall-Mendelin S, Day A, Riegler M, Hugo LE, Johnson KN, Kay BH, McGraw EA, van den Hurk AF, Ryan PA, O'Neill SL. 2009. A

Wolbachia symbiont in *Aedes aegypti* limits infection with dengue, Chikungunya, and *Plasmodium. Cell* **139**: 1268–1278.

110. Caragata EP, Dutra HL, O'Neill SL, Moreira LA. 2016. Zika control through the bacterium *Wolbachia pipientis. Future Microbiol* **11**:1499–1502.

111. Bian G, Xu Y, Lu P, Xie Y, Xi Z. 2010. The endosymbiotic bacterium *Wolbachia* induces resistance to dengue virus in *Aedes aegypti. PLoS Pathog* **6**:e1000833.

112. Frentiu FD, Zakir T, Walker T, Popovici J, Pyke AT, van den Hurk A, McGraw EA, O'Neill SL. 2014. Limited dengue virus replication in field-collected *Aedes aegypti* mosquitoes infected with *Wolbachia. PLoS Negl Trop Dis* **8**:e2688.

113. Jiggins FM. 2017. The spread of *Wolbachia* through mosquito populations. *PLoS Biol* **15**:e2002780.

114. Lin M, Rikihisa Y. 2003. *Ehrlichia chaffeensis* and *Anaplasma phagocytophilum* lack genes for lipid A biosynthesis and incorporate cholesterol for their survival. *Infect Immun* **71**:5324–5331.

115. Geoghegan V, Stainton K, Rainey SM, Ant TH, Dowle AA, Larson T, Hester S, Charles PD, Thomas B, Sinkins SP. 2017. Perturbed cholesterol and vesicular trafficking associated with dengue blocking in *Wolbachia*-infected *Aedes aegypti* cells. *Nat Commun* **8**:526.

116. Taylor MJ, Hoerauf A, Bockarie M. 2010. Lymphatic filariasis and onchocerciasis. *Lancet* **376**:1175–1185.

117. McCall JW, Genchi C, Kramer LH, Guerrero J, Venco L. 2008. Heartworm disease in animals and humans. *Adv Parasitol* **66**:193–285.

118. Hildebrandt JC, Eisenbarth A, Renz A, Streit A. 2014. Reproductive biology of *Onchocerca ochengi*, a nodule forming filarial nematode in zebu cattle. *Vet Parasitol* **205**:318–329.

119. Taylor MJ, Makunde WH, McGarry HF, Turner JD, Mand S, Hoerauf A. 2005. Macrofilaricidal activity after doxycycline treatment of *Wuchereria bancrofti*: a double-blind, randomised placebo-controlled trial. *Lancet* **365**:2116–2121.

120. Slatko BE, Taylor MJ, Foster JM. 2010. The *Wolbachia* endosymbiont as an anti-filarial nematode target. *Symbiosis* **51**:55–65.

121. Turner JD, Sharma R, Al Jayoussi G, Tyrer HE, Gamble J, Hayward L, Priestley RS, Murphy EA, Davies J, Waterhouse D, Cook DAN, Clare RH, Cassidy A, Steven A, Johnston KL, McCall J, Ford L, Hemingway J, Ward SA, Taylor MJ. 2017. Albendazole and antibiotics synergize to deliver short-course anti-*Wolbachia* curative treatments in preclinical models of filariasis. *Proc Natl Acad Sci USA* **114**:E9712–E9721.

122. Hansen RDE, Trees AJ, Bah GS, Hetzel U, Martin C, Bain O, Tanya VN, Makepeace BL. 2011. A worm's best friend: recruitment of neutrophils by *Wolbachia* confounds eosinophil degranulation against the filarial nematode *Onchocerca ochengi. Proc Biol Sci* **278**: 2293–2302.

123. Brattig NW, Bazzocchi C, Kirschning CJ, Reiling N, Büttner DW, Ceciliani F, Geisinger F, Hochrein H, Ernst M, Wagner H, Bandi C, Hoerauf A. 2004. The major surface protein of *Wolbachia* endosymbionts in filarial nematodes elicits immune responses through TLR2 and TLR4. *J Immunol* **173**:437–445.

124. Darby AC, Armstrong SD, Bah GS, Kaur G, Hughes MA, Kay SM, Koldkjær P, Rainbow L, Radford AD, Blaxter ML, Tanya VN, Trees AJ, Cordaux R, Wastling JM, Makepeace BL. 2012. Analysis of gene expression from the *Wolbachia* genome of a filarial nematode supports both metabolic and defensive roles within the symbiosis. *Genome Res* **22**:2467–2477.

125. Chagas-Moutinho VA, Silva R, de Souza W, Motta MCM. 2015. Identification and ultrastructural characterization of the *Wolbachia* symbiont in *Litomosoides chagasfilhoi. Parasit Vectors* **8**:74.

126. Fischer K, Beatty WL, Weil GJ, Fischer PU. 2014. High pressure freezing/freeze substitution fixation improves the ultrastructural assessment of *Wolbachia* endosymbiont-filarial nematode host interaction. *PLoS One* **9**:e86383.

127. White PM, Serbus LR, Debec A, Codina A, Bray W, Guichet A, Lokey RS, Sullivan W. 2017. Reliance of *Wolbachia* on high rates of host proteolysis revealed by a genome-wide RNAi screen of *Drosophila* cells. *Genetics* **205**:1473–1488.

128. White PM, Pietri JE, Debec A, Russell S, Patel B, Sullivan W. 2017. Mechanisms of horizontal cell-to-cell transfer of *Wolbachia* spp. in *Drosophila melanogaster. Appl Environ Microbiol* **83**:e03425-16.

129. Serbus LR, White PM, Silva JP, Rabe A, Teixeira L, Albertson R, Sullivan W. 2015. The impact of host diet on *Wolbachia* titer in *Drosophila. PLoS Pathog* **11**: e1004777.

130. Fallon AM, Witthuhn BA. 2009. Proteasome activity in a naïve mosquito cell line infected with *Wolbachia pipientis* wAlbB. *In Vitro Cell Dev Biol Anim* **45**:460–466.

131. Xi Z, Gavotte L, Xie Y, Dobson SL. 2008. Genome-wide analysis of the interaction between the endosymbiotic bacterium *Wolbachia* and its *Drosophila* host. *BMC Genomics* **9**:1–12.

132. Grobler Y, Yun CY, Kahler DJ, Bergman CM, Lee H, Oliver B, Lehmann R. 2018. Whole genome screen reveals a novel relationship between *Wolbachia* levels and *Drosophila* host translation. *PLoS Pathog* **14**:e1007445.

133. Lefoulon E. 2015. *L'association tripartie Wolbachia - nématode Onchocercidae - vertébré: de l'histoire évolutive au dialogue moléculaire entre les trois partenaires.* Thesis, National museum of natural history, Paris, France.

Bacteria and Intracellularity
Edited by Pascale Cossart, Craig R. Roy, and Philippe Sansonetti
© 2019 American Society for Microbiology, Washington, DC
doi:10.1128/microbiolspec.BAI-0005-2019

Make It a Sweet Home: Responses of *Chlamydia trachomatis* to the Challenges of an Intravacuolar Lifestyle

11

Sébastien Triboulet[1] and Agathe Subtil[1]

INTRODUCTION

Unlike viruses, which can fuse with the plasma membrane to enter host cells, bacteria have only one way to penetrate a cell while preserving their integrity: engulfment through the invagination and closure of the plasma membrane. Therefore, the very first seconds of bacterial intracellular life inevitably occur within a vacuole. From there, two paths open: either to stay inside this vacuole, separated from the host cytoplasm, or to breach the membranous barrier and multiply in the cytosol. Both strategies have been adopted through evolution, and some microbes can even multiply in both environments. Remaining in a vacuole protects the bacteria from some aspects of the cytosolic innate host defense and allows them to build an environment perfectly adapted to their needs. However, this comes at a high price: the host resources are not readily accessible, as they cannot permeate the lipid bilayer that surrounds the bacteria. In addition, the area of this lipid bilayer needs to expand to accommodate bacterial multiplication. This requires building material and energy that are not directly invested in bacterial growth.

This review describes the strategies acquired by the obligate intracellular pathogen *Chlamydia trachomatis* to circumvent the difficulties raised by an intravacuolar lifestyle and turn the vacuole into a "sweet" home, not only because it is perfectly suited to sustain chlamydial proliferation but also because it is extremely rich in glycogen, which can be catabolized into sugar. In the field of *Chlamydia* research, the vacuole is termed an inclusion, and it is so designated here. Its membrane is the key to the exchanges that the bacteria establish with the host in order to access its resources. This chapter starts with an overview of the origin and composition of this membrane. Acquisition of host resources is largely, although not exclusively, mediated by interactions with membranous compartments of the eukaryotic cell, and we describe how the inclusion modifies the architecture of the cell and distribution of the neighboring compartments. Subsequently, we describe the four mechanisms characterized so far by which the bacteria acquire resources from the host: (i) transport/diffusion mechanisms across the inclusion membrane, (ii) fusion of this membrane with host compartments, (iii) direct transfer of lipids at membrane contact sites, and (iv) engulfment by the inclusion membrane of large cytoplasmic entities.

THE MAKING OF THE INCLUSION

Epithelial cells of the genital tract and those of the eye conjunctiva constitute the main sites of proliferation of *C. trachomatis*. In these cell types, over the course of 48 to 72 hours, bacteria divide several times, so that one bacterium can give rise to a progeny of several hundred. The bacteria remain confined in the inclusion, whose volume increases considerably, exceeding, for instance, that of the host cell nucleus (Fig. 1). The membrane of the inclusion, which starts as a small piece of plasma membrane engulfing the invasive pathogen, needs to expand considerably over time, and the nature and origin of its constituents have been extensively studied.

---

[1]Institut Pasteur, Cell Biology of Microbial Infection, 75015 Paris, France.

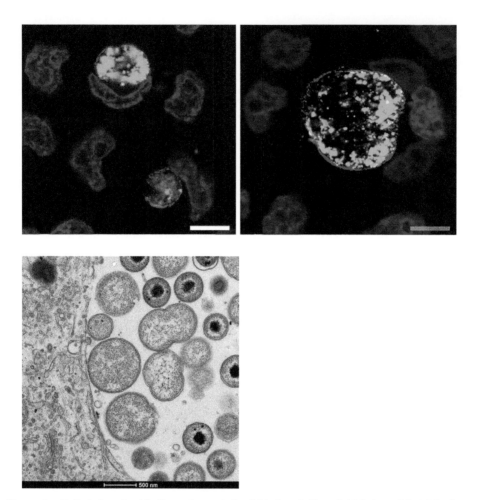

Figure 1 Cells infected with *C. trachomatis* for 24 h (top left) and 48 h (top right). The bacteria were stably transformed to express the green fluorescent protein and appear in green; the inclusion lumen was labeled in red with an antibody against one Inc protein. DNA was stained in blue. Distortion of the nucleus due to the growth of the inclusion is already visible 24 hours postinfection. Infected cells are often multinucleated, as shown in the 48-hour infection example here, due to a failure to proceed through cytokinesis. Bar, 10 μm. Chlamydiae undergo a biphasic developmental cycle. The infectious form, called the elementary body (EB), is not replicative. Once internalized, it differentiates into a reticulate body (RB). RBs multiply several times in the inclusion before differentiating into EBs. Differentiation is not synchronous, and mature inclusions contain both EBs and RBs. The electron micrograph (bottom) shows part of a mature inclusion, with bacteria in contact with the inclusion membrane. The EBs can be distinguished from the RBs by their smaller size and their condensed chromatin.

Incorporation of Lipids from the Host

The pioneering work of Ted Hackstadt demonstrated that ceramide, after transit through the Golgi apparatus, is transformed into sphingomyelin and incorporated into the bacteria (1, 2). Cholesterol appears to follow a similar Golgi-dependent pathway (3). We describe the transport mechanisms at work below, but the important point is that these elegant studies demonstrated lipid transit from the host to the inclusion membrane and from there to the bacteria. They also gave support to the claim that *Chlamydia* utilizes lipids from the host for making its own membranes, so that its lipid composition resembles that of the host rather than that of classical Gram-negative bacteria (4). This idea has recently been challenged by the Rock lab, and although the bacteria selectively scavenge host saturated fatty acids to use for *de novo* synthesis of its membrane constituents (5), it seems that the direct incorporation of host lipids into *C. trachomatis* membrane may be more marginal than previously thought (6). Still, incorporation of fluorescent lipid probes from the host into the bacteria suggests that host lipids also sustain the growth of the inclusion membrane. Whether lipids of bacterial origin are also present is not known. It has been suggested that some bacterial proteins might be delivered to the host cytoplasm packaged in outer membrane vesicles emanating from the bacteria, which could fuse with the inner leaflet of the inclusion membrane. If this is true, then bacterial lipids would also *de facto* make their way to the inclusion membrane. Purification of the inclusion membrane, in the absence of contamination by bacteria, would solve this question, since *Chlamydia*, like many bacteria, produce branched-chain fatty acids that can be resolved from host fatty acids by mass spectrometry. However, the close association between the bacteria and the inclusion membrane makes this task extremely challenging.

Domination by Proteins of Bacterial Origin?

While the contribution of the host to the lipid composition of the inclusion membrane was established early, initial attempts to detect host proteins in this compartment yielded negative results. It was soon concluded that the inclusion membrane is largely disconnected from the endocytic traffic (7–9). In fact, no particular host compartment marker appears to be highly enriched in the inclusion membrane. A recent study of the protein composition of isolated inclusions showed that several host proteins, normally associated with a variety of cellular compartments, are associated with the inclusion membrane, but no compartment clearly dominates (10). It might reflect the diversity of the pathways used by the bacteria to build this inclusion, which we discuss below, so that no cellular constituent makes a significant contribution to its composition. It probably also reflects the fact that the bacteria provide the lion's share of the protein content of the inclusion membrane. Quantitative data to determine the proportion of bacterial versus host proteins in this membrane are lacking, but it is clear that chlamydiae devote a large proportion (around 10%) of their genome to making bacterial inclusion (Inc) proteins (11). The most abundant of these proteins can easily be detected by immunofluorescence. Considering the difficulty in detecting any endogenous host membrane protein in the inclusion membrane, it is reasonable to think that bacterial proteins might dominate this landscape in terms of number. These proteins are translocated into the inclusion membrane via a secretion machinery, known as the type III secretion system (11, 12). Type III secretion apparatuses are made by several Gram-negative bacteria and allow the translocation of so-called effector proteins into the host cytoplasm (13). *C. trachomatis* secretes a number of soluble effector proteins, but Inc proteins possess a bilobal hydrophobic domain which allows the hairpin insertion of the protein into the inclusion membrane, with the rest of the protein being exposed to the cytosol. This feature has allowed the identification of putative *inc* genes, and many Inc protein candidates have been observed at the inclusion membrane by using antibodies or epitope tags (11, 14–16). Variations exist as to the kinetics of their expression (17), meaning that at different stages of the infectious cycle, the composition of the inclusion membrane varies, probably allowing subtle changes in its interactions with the host. Eukaryotic partners for many Inc proteins have been identified (Table 1); however, a majority remain orphaned. While one function of Inc proteins is clearly to recruit specific eukaryotic proteins to the inclusion periphery, some data suggest that they also have an important structural role in shaping the inclusion architecture and dynamics (18). A search for Inc-Inc interactions conducted on a subset of 21 Inc proteins indicated that a majority of these transmembrane proteins are engaged in homo- and heterodimeric interactions with other Inc proteins, suggesting that these proteins assemble to form specific multimolecular complexes (19).

The Making of the Inclusion's Niche: Remodeling of the Cell Architecture

The inclusion should be considered just another cellular compartment, fully integrated into its eukaryotic surrounding. Its presence modifies the distribution of several other intracellular compartments and the organization of the cytoskeleton.

A few hours after invasion, the inclusion migrates towards the microtubule organizing center (MTOC), in a microtubule- and dynein-dependent manner (20). This move brings the inclusion in proximity to the nucleus, and the expansion of the inclusion has a strong impact on the morphology of the nucleus, which takes a typical bean shape (Fig. 1). Deformation of the nucleus, while the inclusion remains spherical, suggests that the inclusion is more rigid. This is likely due to its ability to remodel cytoskeleton elements on its surface, building a solid, although dynamic, structure at its periphery. Indeed, the inclusion is encased in a scaffold of host cytoskeletal structures made up of a network of F-actin, septins, and intermediate filaments that act cooperatively to stabilize the pathogen-containing vacuole (21, 22). Microtubules also assemble into an interlinked scaffold at the inclusion surface (23). Microtubule cages around

Table 1 Identified Inc-host interactions

Locus name in:				
C. trachomatis D/UW-3/CX	*C. trachomatis* L2/434/Bu	Protein name	Host partner	Proposed function
CT005	CTL0260	IncV	VAP	Contacts the endoplasmic reticulum (32)
CT101	CTL0356	MrcA	ITPR3	Recruitment of ITPR3 and regulation of extrusion rate (62)
CT115	CTL0370	IncD	CERT	Ceramide import (29)
CT116	CTL0371	IncE	SNX5/6	Sequestration of retromer components (52), hijacking of retrograde pathway (10)
CT118	CTL0373	IncG	14-3-3β	Recruitment of host proteins such as BAD (63) and Raf-1 (64)
CT119	CTL0374	IncA	IncA, SNARE proteins	Homotypic fusion of inclusions (65), modulation of SNARE-controlled intracellular traffic (50)
CT147	CTL0402			EEA1 mimicry (66)
CT222	CTL0475			See CT850
CT223	CTL0476	IPAM	CEP170	Control of microtubule assembly (26)
CT228	CTL0480		MYPT1	Host cell exit by extrusion (67)
CT229	CTL0481	CpoS	Several Rab GTPases	Suppresses type I interferon responses (68), inclusion membrane stability (69)
CT232	CTL0484	IncB		See CT850
CT233	CTL0485	IncC		Inclusion membrane stability (69)
CT288	CTL0480		CCDC146	Contributes to inclusion positioning (70)
CT383	CTL0639			Inclusion membrane stability (69)
CT813	CTL0184	InaC	ARF and 14.3.3 proteins	Modulation of the cytoskeleton and Golgi redistribution (25, 52)
CT850	CTL0223		DYNLT1	Inclusion positioning at the MTOC (71), in complex with IncB, CT101, and CT222 (72); also includes IncC, CT223, CT224, and CT288 (16)

the inclusion are enriched in posttranslationally modified alpha-tubulin, particularly acetylated and detyrosinated tubulin, which stabilizes the network.

Migration of the inclusion to the MTOC also brings it in close proximity to the Golgi apparatus, which becomes fragmented late in infection. Microtubules stabilized by posttranslational modifications are necessary for positioning the Golgi stacks around the inclusion (23). The inclusion protein CT813/InaC recruits and activates host ADP-ribosylation factor 1 (ARF1) and ARF4, whose activities are required to couple posttranslationally modified microtubules and Golgi complex repositioning at the inclusion (24, 25). A second inclusion protein, CT223/IPAM, has also been proposed to play a role in the formation of the microtubule cage surrounding the inclusion by recruiting the centrosomal protein, CEP170 (26). Repositioning of the Golgi complex in proximity to the inclusion may facilitate acquisition of material. However, it is dispensable for normal *C. trachomatis* development and sphingolipid traffic to the bacteria (24, 27). Glycosylation and export to the plasma membrane of secreted proteins is not significantly changed, indi-

cating that this organelle functions normally during infection (28).

The tubular network of the endoplasmic reticulum is very often observed adjacent to the inclusion membrane (29), extending the list of membrane contact sites established between the endoplasmic reticulum and organelles, which usually contain the endoplasmic reticulum proteins VAPA (VAMP-associated protein A) and VAPB (30). Several host proteins are recruited at these sites (31), such as the Inc protein IncV, which displays FFAT motifs that contribute to the recruitment of the VAPs (32). Observations by electron tomography suggested that contact between the rough endoplasmic reticulum and the inclusion membrane occurred when bacteria were also in contact with the inner side of the inclusion membrane, indicating that bacteria had an active role in forming these close contacts (33). The same study reported the presence of transmembrane and luminal proteins of the endoplasmic reticulum in the inclusion membrane and lumen. These results need to be confirmed, as another report did not reach the same conclusions using comparable techniques (34).

The impact of the inclusion on the distribution and morphology of other cellular organelles, in particular the mitochondria and the endosomal compartment, was recently measured by quantitative image analysis. It was reported that an elongation of the mitochondria was observed early in infection by *C. trachomatis* (6 to 12 h), in agreement with the observed increase in phosphorylation of a residue of the protein Drp1, which makes it inactive at promoting fission (35). The authors noted that this situation evolved during infection, since at later times (24 to 48 h), mitochondria became fragmented. These observations contradict to some extent a previous report implicating the upregulation of host microRNAs upon infection with *C. trachomatis* in preventing mitochondrial fragmentation, even at late times of infection (36). The uptake and recycling of the endosomal marker transferrin were for the most part unchanged, except in cells with a very large inclusion (37). Altogether, while the inclusion deeply modifies the cell architecture, the bacteria manage to preserve the normal functionality of intracellular organelles. This is understandable, considering that they need to keep the host cell as healthy as possible until the end of their developmental cycle. It remains a remarkable achievement, implicating a fine tuning of host cell homeostasis at multiple levels.

TRANSPORT TO THE INCLUSION

Intravacuolar pathogens face two challenges: they need to obtain the essential molecules that they cannot synthesize themselves from the host cytoplasm, which lies beyond a lipid barrier, and they need to expand the area of this barrier. To ensure that host resources reach the inclusion lumen, the bacteria have acquired the ability to use or mimic fundamental mechanisms of transport across and between lipid bilayers, such as (i) transport/diffusion mechanisms across the inclusion membrane, through the use of pores and/or transporters; (ii) fusion of this membrane with host compartments; (iii) direct transfer of lipids at membrane contact sites; and (iv) engulfment by the inclusion membrane of large cytoplasmic entities (Fig. 2). The underlying molecular mechanisms of these processes are often unknown, but they are likely orchestrated by bacterial proteins secreted in the inclusion membrane or in the host cytoplasm.

Transport and Diffusion across the Inclusion Membrane

The use of fluorescent tracers has shown that molecules even as small as 520 Da are unable to diffuse into the inclusion lumen (38). The inclusion appears to be freely permeable to cytoplasmic H^+, Na^+, K^+, and Ca^{2+} (39). Ca^{2+} has an atomic mass of 45 Da, suggesting the existence of pores with a size between 45 and 520 Da. How these pores are made remains unknown. The ability of Inc proteins to assemble in multimolecular structures makes them attractive candidates, but translocon proteins which form the pore for type III secretion could also play that role. The *Shigella* translocon protein IpaB forms cation-selective ion channels in the membranes into which it inserts (40). This ability of translocon proteins to form persistent channels, even after detachment of the bacteria, was recently confirmed in the case of the contact between *Pseudomonas aeruginosa* and the plasma membrane (41). Similarly, by remaining anchored within the inclusion membrane, even after bacterial detachment, the translocon proteins CopB and/or CopB2 (42) could form channels permeable to ions. Alternatively, host proteins making pores in the plasma membrane or cellular compartments might be relocated to the inclusion membrane.

Little is known regarding the insertion of specific transporters in this membrane. Here again, Inc proteins might be implicated. Very few host transporters were found among the inclusion-associated host proteins, but this is likely due to technical limitations, as integral membrane proteins are difficult to solubilize and detect by mass spectrometry (10). The literature provides evidence for the inclusion relocation of three host transporters (Fig. 2). The mammalian sodium multivitamin transporter, which transports lipoic acid, biotin, and pantothenic acid into cells, has been observed by immunofluorescence at the inclusion membrane and could ensure biotin supply to the bacteria (43). The lipid transporters ABCA1 and CLA1 were also detected on the inclusion membrane of *C. trachomatis*-infected cells, where they could supply the bacteria with host lipids such as phosphatidylcholine. Interestingly, their extracellular acceptor, ApoA-I, was detected in the inclusion lumen, where it colocalized with fluorescent lipid probes (44, 45). Finally, electron microscopy observations detected the sugar transporter SLC35D2 on the inclusion membrane (46). This transporter contributes to the uptake of UDP-glucose from the host, which is used as a substrate for glycogen synthesis by bacterial enzymes present in the lumen of the inclusion.

The presence of host transporters in the inclusion membrane raises the question of their transport from their genuine cellular location to this novel compartment. As these transporters are integral membrane proteins, they can be relocated in the inclusion membrane only via vesicular traffic, described below.

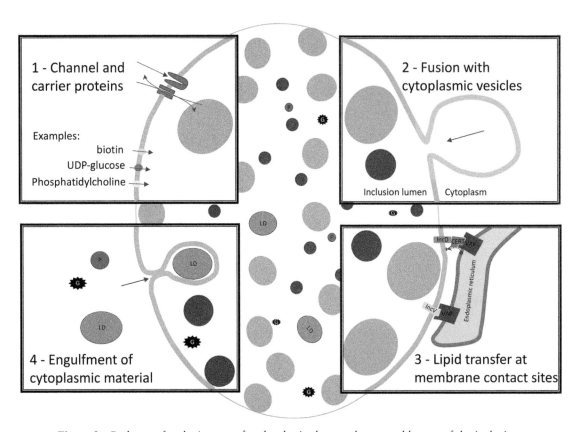

Figure 2 Pathways for the import of molecules in the membrane and lumen of the inclusion. This schematic view of an inclusion depicts reticulate bodies and elementary bodies in light and dark gray, respectively. The four boxes show enlargements of the different suspected mechanisms for material import in the inclusion, with the purple arrow pointing to the direction of transport. (1) Channel proteins have not been identified yet, but the type 3 translocon proteins CopB and -B2 are attractive candidates for cation transport. Specific transport proteins have been observed at the inclusion membrane, and some of their substrates are listed as examples. (2) Fusion with host compartments is required to import host integral membrane proteins, and several host and Inc proteins have been implicated in the regulation of this process. However, the exact nature of the donor compartment(s) which fuses with the inclusion membrane is not known. (3) The endoplasmic reticulum makes close contacts with the inclusion membrane, and by co-opting a dedicated host machinery, the bacteria induce direct transfer of ceramide to the inclusion membrane. (4) Whether the engulfment of lipid droplets (LD), peroxisomes (P), and glycogen (G) proceeds via the same pathway, with inward invagination and scission of the inclusion membrane, remains to be determined.

Vesicular Traffic to and from the Inclusion Membrane

Fusion of vesicles with the inclusion membrane appears to be advantageous, as it would simultaneously feed inclusion membrane expansion, bring transporters to the inclusion membrane, and deliver the luminal content of the vesicles into the inclusion lumen. Indeed, several observations point to the existence of vesicular flow towards the inclusion membrane.

We mention above the observation of ceramide transport from the Golgi apparatus to the inclusion. Although we point out below that this transport is probably not exclusively vesicular, its sensitivity to temperature and to a drug that targets a vesicular transport step, brefeldin A, strongly supports the idea that the inclusion intersects a vesicular transport pathway emanating from the Golgi apparatus (2, 3, 47). A number of host players have been implicated in the vesicular transport of ceramide to the inclusion (48).

Several small GTPases of the Rab family, which regulate vesicular transport between cellular compartments, have been observed at the inclusion membrane (48, 49). For several of them, protein extinction by small interfering RNA results in a reduction of bacterial progeny.

Although it is not clear whether this effect is due only to decreased vesicular traffic to the inclusion or to indirect consequences of disturbing intracellular traffic on host cell homeostasis, it speaks strongly to a high degree of interconnection between the inclusion membrane and vesicular traffic.

The second essential players in the regulation of vesicular traffic in eukaryotic cells, the SNARE (*N*-ethylmaleimide-sensitive factor activating protein receptor) proteins, also appear to contribute to the regulation of the vesicular traffic to the inclusion membrane (48). The inclusion protein IncA provided the first description of SNARE domain mimicry by a bacterial protein (50), and other Inc proteins displayed similarities with SNARE domains. Several host SNARE proteins were observed in the vicinity of the inclusion membrane, and IncA was shown to be able to interact with those proteins. As some SNARE proteins, such as Vamp8, were observed on the inclusion membrane at the ultrastructural level, it is possible that SNARE-mediated events indeed contribute to vesicular fusion with the inclusion membrane. Interaction of Inc proteins with SNARE proteins could also have inhibitory functions and could, for instance, contribute to the prevention of fusion with late endocytic compartments (50, 51).

Two independent approaches revealed that several subunits of the retromer are recruited to the inclusion membrane (10, 52). The retromer is a multiprotein complex essential for recycling of cargo receptors out of the endolysosomal pathway and for transporting them to the *trans*-Golgi network. The inclusion protein, IncE, interacts with the retromer components sortin nexins, specifically SNX5 and SNX6, explaining their relocation, together with some but not all retromer components, to the inclusion membrane. The exact significance of this observation in terms of vesicular traffic is still unclear. Silencing of retromer components enhances bacterial proliferation, suggesting that retromer activity somehow restricts bacterial growth, but how it does so remains to be determined.

Finally, the conserved oligomeric Golgi (COG) complex was also implicated in vesicular transport to the *C. trachomatis* inclusion (53). This ubiquitously expressed membrane-associated protein complex functions in retrograde intra-Golgi trafficking through associations with coiled-coil tethers, SNAREs, Rabs, and COPI (coatomer protein I). Several subunits of this complex appear to be present on the inclusion membrane, as well as the Golgi vesicular SNARE GS15. Based on this observation, and on the fact that disruption of the complex was detrimental to bacterial growth, the authors proposed that *C. trachomatis* hijacks the COG complex to redirect the population of Golgi-derived retrograde vesicles to inclusions. However, one cannot rule out the possibility that the effect of the COG disruption on bacterial growth is indirect.

So far, bacterial proteins implicated in the control of the interactions between the inclusion and host intracellular traffic all belong to the Inc family. Secreted bacterial proteins, not anchored to the inclusion membrane, could also be involved. We recently showed that secreted proteins that share a domain of unknown function called DUF582 interact with components of the ESCRT machinery (54). This machinery is involved in several cellular processes requiring membrane constriction and could constitute an interesting target for material supply to the inclusion. However, we showed that the ESCRT machinery was dispensable for inclusion growth and bacterial multiplication. Therefore, if the DUF582 proteins target ESCRT components to acquire material from the host, redundant pathways must exist to explain the normal bacterial growth in their absence.

Importantly, all these vesicular transport mechanisms were examined in the context of understanding the uptake of host material by the inclusion to sustain the multiplication of bacteria and the expansion of the inclusion membrane. The observation that only a subset of proteins, emanating from the Golgi apparatus or from other cellular compartments, are observed on the inclusion membrane suggests that sorting occurs in this compartment as in other compartments of the cells and that unwanted proteins are retrieved from the inclusion membrane. In support of this hypothesis, abundant bacterial proteins, as well as IncA, were detected at the ultrastructural level in the endoplasmic reticulum, indicating vesicular traffic exiting the inclusion (55). If this is the case, some of the molecules implicated in material uptake might actually play a role in the reverse process. How selection of proteins retained in the inclusion membrane would take place is unknown. Again, Inc proteins could be implicated by specifically retaining some host molecules in the inclusion membrane.

Direct Lipid Transfer at Membrane Contact Sites

The membrane contact sites between the endoplasmic reticulum and the inclusion described above are the sites of direct lipid transfer between the two membranes. The Inc protein IncV contributes to the tethering of the two compartments by displaying an eukaryotic FFAT motif recognized by VAP, a protein resident of the endoplasmic reticulum (32). A second Inc protein, IncD, interacts with a lipid transfer protein called CERT, which normally operates between the endoplasmic reticulum and the Golgi apparatus (29). By co-opting this mammalian lipid transfer machinery, the bacteria bring ceramide to the inclusion membrane, where it is converted to sphingomyelin by a host sphingomyelin synthase, also recruited at this site (29, 56). Sphingomyelin does not accumulate on the inclusion membrane but is rapidly taken up by the bacteria (47). Thus, this direct transfer mechanism represents an alternative to vesicular traffic for sphingomyelin acquisition by the bacteria.

Engulfment of Cytoplasmic Material

The first hint that the inclusion was able to engulf a large amount of cytoplasmic material came from the observation that lipid droplets are found in the inclusion lumen (57). It is supposed that this occurs by inward budding of the inclusion membrane, although this has not been formally demonstrated. Bacterial proteins with tropism for lipid droplets might be implicated in this process (57, 58). What use the bacteria have for luminal lipid droplets is an open question. Several human lipid-binding or modifying enzymes were detected in the inclusion lumen, suggesting that host proteins assist bacterial lipid metabolism in the inclusion (59, 60). Lipid droplets, by bringing acylglycerol, sterol esters, and peripheral phospholipids and enzymes, likely represent at least one source of substrates and enzymes for this activity. Genetic ablation of the formation of lipid droplets was reported to have negatively affected *C. trachomatis* growth in one study and to have no effect in another (58, 60). It is likely that *C. trachomatis* relies on several redundant pathways to fulfill its needs, and a difference in cell types may account for this discrepancy.

Also mysterious is the role of peroxisomes in the inclusion lumen. These organelles can occasionally be observed inside inclusions (61). Cells deficient in peroxisome biogenesis gave rise to normal infectious progeny, indicating that import of this organelle is not required for optimal bacterial growth *in vitro*. Bacteria make use of at least one enzymatic capacity of peroxisomes, i.e., their ability to make plasmalogens, since these typically eukaryotic lipids were recovered in purified bacteria (61).

The latest example of trafficking of large cytoplasmic components into the inclusion lumen came from the observation that host glycogen is imported into this compartment (46). This process contributes to the huge accumulation of luminal glycogen that *C. trachomatis* conducts throughout its developmental cycle. Here again, *C. trachomatis* has set up redundant pathways to achieve uptake of host material, since bulk uptake of host cytoplasm probably represents a minor pathway compared to *de novo* synthesis by bacterial enzymes present in the inclusion lumen. Glycogen surrounded by one or several membranes was occasionally observed in the inclusion lumen, supporting the hypothesis that engulfment proceeds through invagination of the inclusion membrane (46). However, as for lipid droplets and peroxisome import, the molecular machinery at work remains to be identified.

Other open questions are whether the three examples follow the same pathway and how selectivity operates. Selective import of cytoplasmic constituents could represent Trojan horses for certain host proteins that are detected in the inclusion lumen. For instance, association of the human acyl coenzyme A carrier hACBD6 with lipid droplets may explain their detection in the inclusion lumen (59).

CONCLUSION

In the mid-1990s, researchers were puzzled by the observation that *C. trachomatis*' inclusion appeared largely disconnected from the endosomal traffic and did not significantly retain classical markers for membrane compartments (7). Two decades of research have revealed that *C. trachomatis* exploits all the mechanisms for material exchange between or across compartments that are known to take place in a eukaryotic cell. Molecular mimicry by secreted bacterial proteins and recruitment of specific host machineries are continuously being used to hijack host material. Often, redundant pathways operate in parallel to ensure an ample supply of host resources, with the consequence that interfering with one pathway does not always affect bacterial growth.

Still, these 2 decades of research do not close the book on the solutions brought by *C. trachomatis* to the challenges of an intravacuolar lifestyle. Although we have now gathered evidence that the aforementioned four mechanisms contribute to *C. trachomatis*' supply of host material, most of the molecular details are still missing. Also, whether host protein sorting and vesicular membrane retrieval occurs at the inclusion membrane needs to be examined. Many of these questions will probably be answered by the functional study of Inc proteins, which can now be facilitated by the tools for gene disruption and overexpression. Undoubtedly, the next 2 decades should open several doors into *C. trachomatis*' sweet home.

Acknowledgments. We thank Chloé Charendoff for critical reading of the manuscript. S.T. is supported by the Agence Nationale pour la Recherche, grant Expendo.

Citation. Triboulet S, Subtil A. 2019. Make it a sweet home: responses of *Chlamydia trachomatis* to the challenges of an intravacuolar lifestyle. Microbiol Spectrum 7(2):BAI-0005-2019.

References

1. Hackstadt T, Scidmore MA, Rockey DD. 1995. Lipid metabolism in *Chlamydia trachomatis*-infected cells: directed trafficking of Golgi-derived sphingolipids to the chlamydial inclusion. *Proc Natl Acad Sci USA* **92**: 4877–4881.

2. Moore ER, Fischer ER, Mead DJ, Hackstadt T. 2008. The chlamydial inclusion preferentially intercepts basolaterally directed sphingomyelin-containing exocytic vacuoles. *Traffic* **9**:2130–2140.

3. Carabeo RA, Mead DJ, Hackstadt T. 2003. Golgi-dependent transport of cholesterol to the *Chlamydia trachomatis* inclusion. *Proc Natl Acad Sci USA* **100**:6771–6776.

4. Wylie JL, Hatch GM, McClarty G. 1997. Host cell phospholipids are trafficked to and then modified by *Chlamydia trachomatis*. *J Bacteriol* **179**:7233–7242.

5. Yao J, Dodson VJ, Frank MW, Rock CO. 2015. *Chlamydia trachomatis* scavenges host fatty acids for phospholipid synthesis via an acyl-acyl carrier protein synthetase. *J Biol Chem* **290**:22163–22173.

6. Yao J, Cherian PT, Frank MW, Rock CO. 2015. *Chlamydia trachomatis* relies on autonomous phospholipid synthesis for membrane biogenesis. *J Biol Chem* **290**:18874–18888.

7. Taraska T, Ward DM, Ajioka RS, Wyrick PB, Davis-Kaplan SR, Davis CH, Kaplan J. 1996. The late chlamydial inclusion membrane is not derived from the endocytic pathway and is relatively deficient in host proteins. *Infect Immun* **64**:3713–3727.

8. Heinzen RA, Scidmore MA, Rockey DD, Hackstadt T. 1996. Differential interaction with endocytic and exocytic pathways distinguish parasitophorous vacuoles of *Coxiella burnetii* and *Chlamydia trachomatis*. *Infect Immun* **64**:796–809.

9. Scidmore MA, Fischer ER, Hackstadt T. 2003. Restricted fusion of *Chlamydia trachomatis* vesicles with endocytic compartments during the initial stages of infection. *Infect Immun* **71**:973–984.

10. Aeberhard L, Banhart S, Fischer M, Jehmlich N, Rose L, Koch S, Laue M, Renard BY, Schmidt F, Heuer D. 2015. The proteome of the isolated *Chlamydia trachomatis* containing vacuole reveals a complex trafficking platform enriched for retromer components. *PLoS Pathog* **11**: e1004883.

11. Dehoux P, Flores R, Dauga C, Zhong G, Subtil A. 2011. Multi-genome identification and characterization of chlamydiae-specific type III secretion substrates: the Inc proteins. *BMC Genomics* **12**:109.

12. Subtil A, Parsot C, Dautry-Varsat A. 2001. Secretion of predicted Inc proteins of *Chlamydia pneumoniae* by a heterologous type III machinery. *Mol Microbiol* **39**:792–800.

13. Galán JE, Lara-Tejero M, Marlovits TC, Wagner S. 2014. Bacterial type III secretion systems: specialized nanomachines for protein delivery into target cells. *Annu Rev Microbiol* **68**:415–438.

14. Bannantine JP, Griffiths RS, Viratyosin W, Brown WJ, Rockey DD. 2000. A secondary structure motif predictive of protein localization to the chlamydial inclusion membrane. *Cell Microbiol* **2**:35–47.

15. Lutter EI, Martens C, Hackstadt T. 2012. Evolution and conservation of predicted inclusion membrane proteins in chlamydiae. *Comp Funct Genomics* **2012**:362104.

16. Weber MM, Bauler LD, Lam J, Hackstadt T. 2015. Expression and localization of predicted inclusion membrane proteins in *Chlamydia trachomatis*. *Infect Immun* **83**:4710–4718.

17. Shaw EI, Dooley CA, Fischer ER, Scidmore MA, Fields KA, Hackstadt T. 2000. Three temporal classes of gene expression during the *Chlamydia trachomatis* developmental cycle. *Mol Microbiol* **37**:913–925.

18. Mital J, Miller NJ, Dorward DW, Dooley CA, Hackstadt T. 2013. Role for chlamydial inclusion membrane proteins in inclusion membrane structure and biogenesis. *PLoS One* **8**:e63426.

19. Gauliard E, Ouellette SP, Rueden KJ, Ladant D. 2015. Characterization of interactions between inclusion membrane proteins from *Chlamydia trachomatis*. *Front Cell Infect Microbiol* **5**:13.

20. Grieshaber SS, Grieshaber NA, Hackstadt T. 2003. *Chlamydia trachomatis* uses host cell dynein to traffic to the microtubule-organizing center in a p50 dynamitin-independent process. *J Cell Sci* **116**:3793–3802.

21. Kumar Y, Valdivia RH. 2008. Actin and intermediate filaments stabilize the *Chlamydia trachomatis* vacuole by forming dynamic structural scaffolds. *Cell Host Microbe* **4**:159–169.

22. Volceanov L, Herbst K, Biniossek M, Schilling O, Haller D, Nölke T, Subbarayal P, Rudel T, Zieger B, Häcker G. 2014. Septins arrange F-actin-containing fibers on the *Chlamydia trachomatis* inclusion and are required for normal release of the inclusion by extrusion. *mBio* **5**: e01802-14.

23. Al-Zeer MA, Al-Younes HM, Kerr M, Abu-Lubad M, Gonzalez E, Brinkmann V, Meyer TF. 2014. *Chlamydia trachomatis* remodels stable microtubules to coordinate Golgi stack recruitment to the chlamydial inclusion surface. *Mol Microbiol* **94**:1285–1297.

24. Kokes M, Dunn JD, Granek JA, Nguyen BD, Barker JR, Valdivia RH, Bastidas RJ. 2015. Integrating chemical mutagenesis and whole-genome sequencing as a platform for forward and reverse genetic analysis of *Chlamydia*. *Cell Host Microbe* **17**:716–725.

25. Wesolowski J, Weber MM, Nawrotek A, Dooley CA, Calderon M, St Croix CM, Hackstadt T, Cherfils J, Paumet F. 2017. *Chlamydia* hijacks ARF GTPases to coordinate microtubule posttranslational modifications and Golgi complex positioning. *mBio* **8**:e02280-16.

26. Dumoux M, Menny A, Delacour D, Hayward RD. 2015. A *Chlamydia* effector recruits CEP170 to reprogram host microtubule organization. *J Cell Sci* **128**:3420–3434.

27. Gurumurthy RK, Chumduri C, Karlas A, Kimmig S, Gonzalez E, Machuy N, Rudel T, Meyer TF. 2014. Dynamin-mediated lipid acquisition is essential for *Chlamydia trachomatis* development. *Mol Microbiol* **94**: 186–201.

28. Scidmore MA, Fischer ER, Hackstadt T. 1996. Sphingolipids and glycoproteins are differentially trafficked to the *Chlamydia trachomatis* inclusion. *J Cell Biol* **134**:363–374.

29. Derré I, Swiss R, Agaisse H. 2011. The lipid transfer protein CERT interacts with the *Chlamydia* inclusion protein IncD and participates to ER-*Chlamydia* inclusion membrane contact sites. *PLoS Pathog* 7:e1002092.

30. Phillips MJ, Voeltz GK. 2016. Structure and function of ER membrane contact sites with other organelles. *Nat Rev Mol Cell Biol* 17:69–82.

31. Derré I. 2015. Chlamydiae interaction with the endoplasmic reticulum: contact, function and consequences. *Cell Microbiol* 17:959–966.

32. Stanhope R, Flora E, Bayne C, Derré I. 2017. IncV, a FFAT motif-containing *Chlamydia* protein, tethers the endoplasmic reticulum to the pathogen-containing vacuole. *Proc Natl Acad Sci USA* 114:12039–12044.

33. Dumoux M, Clare DK, Saibil HR, Hayward RD. 2012. Chlamydiae assemble a pathogen synapse to hijack the host endoplasmic reticulum. *Traffic* 13:1612–1627.

34. Kokes M, Valdivia RH. 2015. Differential translocation of host cellular materials into the *Chlamydia trachomatis* inclusion lumen during chemical fixation. *PLoS One* 10:e0139153.

35. Kurihara Y, Itoh R, Shimizu A, Walenna NF, Chou B, Ishii K, Soejima T, Fujikane A, Hiromatsu K. 2019. *Chlamydia trachomatis* targets mitochondrial dynamics to promote intracellular survival and proliferation. *Cell Microbiol* 21:e12962.

36. Chowdhury SR, Reimer A, Sharan M, Kozjak-Pavlovic V, Eulalio A, Prusty BK, Fraunholz M, Karunakaran K, Rudel T. 2017. *Chlamydia* preserves the mitochondrial network necessary for replication via microRNA-dependent inhibition of fission. *J Cell Biol* 216:1071–1089.

37. Larson CL, Heinzen RA. 2017. High-content imaging reveals expansion of the endosomal compartment during *Coxiella burnetii* parasitophorous vacuole maturation. *Front Cell Infect Microbiol* 7:48.

38. Heinzen RA, Hackstadt T. 1997. The *Chlamydia trachomatis* parasitophorous vacuolar membrane is not passively permeable to low-molecular-weight compounds. *Infect Immun* 65:1088–1094.

39. Grieshaber S, Swanson JA, Hackstadt T. 2002. Determination of the physical environment within the *Chlamydia trachomatis* inclusion using ion-selective ratiometric probes. *Cell Microbiol* 4:273–283.

40. Senerovic L, Tsunoda SP, Goosmann C, Brinkmann V, Zychlinsky A, Meissner F, Kolbe M. 2012. Spontaneous formation of IpaB ion channels in host cell membranes reveals how *Shigella* induces pyroptosis in macrophages. *Cell Death Dis* 3:e384.

41. Dortet L, Lombardi C, Cretin F, Dessen A, Filloux A. 2018. Pore-forming activity of the *Pseudomonas aeruginosa* type III secretion system translocon alters the host epigenome. *Nat Microbiol* 3:378–386.

42. Chellas-Géry B, Wolf K, Tisoncik J, Hackstadt T, Fields KA. 2011. Biochemical and localization analyses of putative type III secretion translocator proteins CopB and CopB2 of *Chlamydia trachomatis* reveal significant distinctions. *Infect Immun* 79:3036–3045.

43. Fisher DJ, Fernández RE, Adams NE, Maurelli AT. 2012. Uptake of biotin by *Chlamydia* spp. through the use of a bacterial transporter (BioY) and a host-cell transporter (SMVT). *PLoS One* 7:e46052.

44. Cox JV, Naher N, Abdelrahman YM, Belland RJ. 2012. Host HDL biogenesis machinery is recruited to the inclusion of *Chlamydia trachomatis*-infected cells and regulates chlamydial growth. *Cell Microbiol* 14:1497–1512.

45. Cox JV, Abdelrahman YM, Peters J, Naher N, Belland RJ. 2016. *Chlamydia trachomatis* utilizes the mammalian CLA1 lipid transporter to acquire host phosphatidylcholine essential for growth. *Cell Microbiol* 18:305–318.

46. Gehre L, Gorgette O, Perrinet S, Prevost MC, Ducatez M, Giebel AM, Nelson DE, Ball SG, Subtil A. 2016. Sequestration of host metabolism by an intracellular pathogen. *eLife* 5:e12552.

47. Hackstadt T, Rockey DD, Heinzen RA, Scidmore MA. 1996. *Chlamydia trachomatis* interrupts an exocytic pathway to acquire endogenously synthesized sphingomyelin in transit from the Golgi apparatus to the plasma membrane. *EMBO J* 15:964–977.

48. Elwell C, Mirrashidi K, Engel J. 2016. *Chlamydia* cell biology and pathogenesis. *Nat Rev Microbiol* 14:385–400.

49. Damiani MT, Gambarte Tudela J, Capmany A. 2014. Targeting eukaryotic Rab proteins: a smart strategy for chlamydial survival and replication. *Cell Microbiol* 16:1329–1338.

50. Delevoye C, Nilges M, Dehoux P, Paumet F, Perrinet S, Dautry-Varsat A, Subtil A. 2008. SNARE protein mimicry by an intracellular bacterium. *PLoS Pathog* 4:e1000022.

51. Paumet F, Wesolowski J, Garcia-Diaz A, Delevoye C, Aulner N, Shuman HA, Subtil A, Rothman JE. 2009. Intracellular bacteria encode inhibitory SNARE-like proteins. *PLoS One* 4:e7375.

52. Mirrashidi KM, Elwell CA, Verschueren E, Johnson JR, Frando A, Von Dollen J, Rosenberg O, Gulbahce N, Jang G, Johnson T, Jäger S, Gopalakrishnan AM, Sherry J, Dunn JD, Olive A, Penn B, Shales M, Cox JS, Starnbach MN, Derre I, Valdivia R, Krogan NJ, Engel J. 2015. Global mapping of the Inc-human interactome reveals that retromer restricts *Chlamydia* infection. *Cell Host Microbe* 18:109–121.

53. Pokrovskaya ID, Szwedo JW, Goodwin A, Lupashina TV, Nagarajan UM, Lupashin VV. 2012. *Chlamydia trachomatis* hijacks intra-Golgi COG complex-dependent vesicle trafficking pathway. *Cell Microbiol* 14:656–668.

54. Vromman F, Perrinet S, Gehre L, Subtil A. 2016. The DUF582 proteins of *Chlamydia trachomatis* bind to components of the ESCRT machinery, which is dispensable for bacterial growth *in vitro*. *Front Cell Infect Microbiol* 6:123.

55. Giles DK, Wyrick PB. 2008. Trafficking of chlamydial antigens to the endoplasmic reticulum of infected epithelial cells. *Microbes Infect* 10:1494–1503.

56. Elwell CA, Jiang S, Kim JH, Lee A, Wittmann T, Hanada K, Melancon P, Engel JN. 2011. *Chlamydia trachomatis* co-opts GBF1 and CERT to acquire host sphingomyelin for distinct roles during intracellular development. *PLoS Pathog* 7:e1002198 *CORRECTION PLoS Pathog* 9:10.1371/annotation/f8e7c7e3-c347-4243-9146-d-b77900cb90c.

57. Cocchiaro JL, Kumar Y, Fischer ER, Hackstadt T, Valdivia RH. 2008. Cytoplasmic lipid droplets are translocated into the lumen of the *Chlamydia trachomatis* parasitophorous vacuole. *Proc Natl Acad Sci USA* 105:9379–9384.

58. Saka HA, Thompson JW, Chen YS, Dubois LG, Haas JT, Moseley A, Valdivia RH. 2015. *Chlamydia trachomatis* infection leads to defined alterations to the lipid droplet proteome in epithelial cells. *PLoS One* 10:e0124630.

59. Soupene E, Wang D, Kuypers FA. 2015. Remodeling of host phosphatidylcholine by *Chlamydia* acyltransferase is regulated by acyl-CoA binding protein ACBD6 associated with lipid droplets. *MicrobiologyOpen* 4:235–251.

60. Recuero-Checa MA, Sharma M, Lau C, Watkins PA, Gaydos CA, Dean D. 2016. *Chlamydia trachomatis* growth and development requires the activity of host long-chain acyl-CoA synthetases (ACSLs). *Sci Rep* 6:23148.

61. Boncompain G, Müller C, Meas-Yedid V, Schmitt-Kopplin P, Lazarow PB, Subtil A. 2014. The intracellular bacteria *Chlamydia* hijack peroxisomes and utilize their enzymatic capacity to produce bacteria-specific phospholipids. *PLoS One* 9:e86196.

62. Nguyen PH, Lutter EI, Hackstadt T. 2018. *Chlamydia trachomatis* inclusion membrane protein MrcA interacts with the inositol 1,4,5-trisphosphate receptor type 3 (ITPR3) to regulate extrusion formation. *PLoS Pathog* 14:e1006911.

63. Verbeke P, Welter-Stahl L, Ying S, Hansen J, Häcker G, Darville T, Ojcius DM. 2006. Recruitment of BAD by the *Chlamydia trachomatis* vacuole correlates with host-cell survival. *PLoS Pathog* 2:e45.

64. Gurumurthy RK, Mäurer AP, Machuy N, Hess S, Pleissner KP, Schuchhardt J, Rudel T, Meyer TF. 2010. A loss-of-function screen reveals Ras- and Raf-independent MEK-ERK signaling during *Chlamydia trachomatis* infection. *Sci Signal* 3:ra21.

65. Suchland RJ, Rockey DD, Bannantine JP, Stamm WE. 2000. Isolates of *Chlamydia trachomatis* that occupy non-fusogenic inclusions lack IncA, a protein localized to the inclusion membrane. *Infect Immun* 68:360–367.

66. Belland RJ, Zhong G, Crane DD, Hogan D, Sturdevant D, Sharma J, Beatty WL, Caldwell HD. 2003. Genomic transcriptional profiling of the developmental cycle of *Chlamydia trachomatis*. *Proc Natl Acad Sci USA* 100:8478–8483.

67. Lutter EI, Barger AC, Nair V, Hackstadt T. 2013. *Chlamydia trachomatis* inclusion membrane protein CT228 recruits elements of the myosin phosphatase pathway to regulate release mechanisms. *Cell Reports* 3:1921–1931.

68. Sixt BS, Bastidas RJ, Finethy R, Baxter RM, Carpenter VK, Kroemer G, Coers J, Valdivia RH. 2016. The *Chlamydia trachomatis* inclusion membrane protein CpoS counteracts STING-mediated cellular surveillance and suicide programs. *Cell Host Microbe* 21:113–121 10.1016/j.chom.2016.12.002:1-34.

69. Weber MM, Lam JL, Dooley CA, Noriea NF, Hansen BT, Hoyt FH, Carmody AB, Sturdevant GL, Hackstadt T. 2017. Absence of specific *Chlamydia trachomatis* inclusion membrane proteins triggers premature inclusion membrane lysis and host cell death. *Cell Reports* 19:1406–1417.

70. Almeida F, Luís MP, Pereira IS, Pais SV, Mota LJ. 2018. The human centrosomal protein CCDC146 binds *Chlamydia trachomatis* inclusion membrane protein CT288 and is recruited to the periphery of the *Chlamydia*-containing vacuole. *Front Cell Infect Microbiol* 8:254.

71. Mital J, Lutter EI, Barger AC, Dooley CA, Hackstadt T. 2015. *Chlamydia trachomatis* inclusion membrane protein CT850 interacts with the dynein light chain DYNLT1 (Tctex1). *Biochem Biophys Res Commun* 462:165–170.

72. Mital J, Miller NJ, Fischer ER, Hackstadt T. 2010. Specific chlamydial inclusion membrane proteins associate with active Src family kinases in microdomains that interact with the host microtubule network. *Cell Microbiol* 12:1235–1249.

Bacteria and Intracellularity
Edited by Pascale Cossart, Craig R. Roy, and Philippe Sansonetti
© 2019 American Society for Microbiology, Washington, DC
doi:10.1128/microbiolspec.BAI-0009-2019

Salmonella Single-Cell Metabolism and Stress Responses in Complex Host Tissues

Dirk Bumann[1]

12

INTRODUCTION

Infectious diseases are the second most important cause of death worldwide (1). Public health measures are partially successful in managing infectious disease burden, but major obstacles remain. Efficacious vaccines for major pathogens are still lacking (2–4), and the dramatic decline in the development of novel antimicrobials over the last 20 years (5) together with rapidly rising antimicrobial resistance is substantially reducing treatment options (6). The emerging crisis in infectious diseases is a major threat to human health.

Infections usually start with just a few pathogen cells penetrating body surfaces. However, disease signs appear only later, when pathogens exploit host nutrients for growth to high tissue loads. The host immune system detects and attacks the infection foci, and pathogens in turn use stealth, defense, and counterattack. These coevolved combat strategies in organisms with vastly different levels of complexity represent one of the most fascinating and relevant problems in life sciences. During the past decades, infection biology research has uncovered hundreds of virulence factors in many major pathogens, as well as numerous host molecules involved in pathogen recognition, signal transduction, and deployment of microbial effector mechanisms. These mechanisms have been studied from the atomic and cellular scales up to whole-organism and epidemiology levels.

However, a principal limitation of these studies has been that they provided only bulk averages. Average data are useful to describe properties of mostly homogeneous pathogen populations, such as exponentially growing *in vitro* cultures (although even such cultures might contain small pathogen subsets with remarkable outlier behaviors [7–11]). In contrast, almost all real host-pathogen interactions occur in highly structured three-dimensional host environments that are determined by anatomy, host cell type diversity, inflammation dynamics, tissue damage, and local pathogen accumulation in infection foci (11–13). Exposure of pathogen cells to antibiotics during therapy can also differ widely in structured host tissues (14, 15).

Because of these diverse conditions, individual host-pathogen encounters involve a large variety of disparate molecular mechanisms and can have dramatically divergent outcomes. While host effector mechanisms, and/or antimicrobial chemotherapy, successfully eradicate pathogens in some areas, pathogen subpopulations with increased tolerance or rare persister subsets can survive multiple antimicrobial doses over many days, weeks, or even months (7–10, 16, 17), providing a source of subsequent relapse. A particularly well-documented example is tuberculosis, where shrinking and expanding infection foci coexist in close proximity in the same infected lung during latency, during disease, and even after clinically successful chemotherapy (17, 18). Moreover, even within individual granulomas, there are spatial gradients of inflammatory and anti-inflammatory host activities (19).

Ultimate disease outcomes—death, chronic infection, and eradication—are thus not a simple function of generally superior or inferior pathogen virulence mechanisms or host immunity. Instead, in many infectious diseases, the host is actually capable of killing many pathogen cells, even when it eventually will succumb to infection. Disease progression and eradication are thus the net result of many simultaneously occurring local encounters in which sometimes the pathogen wins and sometimes the host wins. However, we still have an only frag-

---

[1]Focal Area Infection Biology, Biozentrum, University of Basel, Basel, Switzerland.

mentary understanding of the underlying molecular and cellular mechanisms. In particular, widely used bulk-average readouts that lump together all pathogen subsets have revealed fascinating insights into host-pathogen interactions, but they cannot capture the extensive heterogeneity of host-pathogen interactions (Fig. 1).

Instead, more appropriate single-cell- and subset-based technologies are starting to offer unprecedented insights into the specific impact of, and pathogen responses to, key immunity effector molecules, such as nitric oxide (NO) and reactive oxygen species, and unravel how heterogeneous pathogen physiology modulates antimicrobial efficacy (12). Focusing on the differences between pathogen subsets can more easily identify specific pathogen responses to distinct host attacks (or antimicrobial exposure levels) (20, 21) against the complex general pathogen adaptation to infection conditions. As an example, it is possible to identify responses of pathogen cells specifically to host NO in certain tissue regions when pathogen cells with less NO exposure from the same tissue as the matched negative control are used (22, 23).

Most importantly, identifying the molecular mechanisms that distinguish successful (for the host) from failing encounters could provide a basis for entirely novel strategies in infection control, by broadening successful

host antimicrobial attacks and closing permissive niches in which pathogen subsets can thrive.

SINGLE-CELL ANALYSIS OF PATHOGENS DURING INFECTION

Heterogeneous pathogen populations consist of individual cells that differ from each other in multiple aspects of their biology. To determine mechanisms of heterogeneous host-pathogen interactions, we need to identify relevant subsets and determine their global properties and physiology.

For eukaryotic organisms, direct single-cell mRNA-seq can reveal all relevant cellular subtypes, their global gene expression profiles, and their lineages (for example, see reference 24), but such experiments are more challenging for bacterial pathogens (25). Although some methods have recently been described (26, 27), mRNA levels in bacteria are subject to large stochastic temporal variations over a few seconds due to transcriptional bursts (28), and mRNA levels may correlate poorly with protein levels, which have slower turnover (29).

In contrast, most proteins have longer lifetimes and accumulate to levels that are often higher than hundreds, or even thousands, of molecules per bacterial cell, enabling their detection at the single-cell level with anti-

a

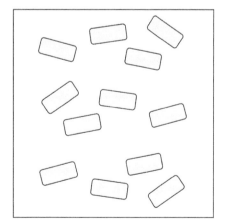

b

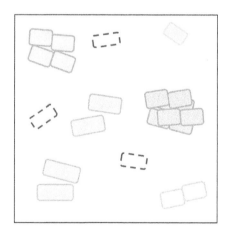

Figure 1 A paradigm shift in pathogen analysis in host tissues. (a) Common methods relied on population-level readouts that revealed average properties. This revealed many exciting insights, including identification of important vaccine antigens and antimicrobial targets. (b) Single-cell technologies reveal an additional striking heterogeneity of pathogen properties and fates that range from vigorous growth to efficient killing. All these diverse host-pathogen encounters can occur in the same host tissue at the same time. Overall disease outcome is the net result of this underlying complexity. Identifying the molecular mechanisms that distinguish successful (for the host) from failing encounters could provide a basis for entirely novel strategies in infection control, by broadening successful host antimicrobial attacks and closing permissive niches in which pathogen subsets can thrive.

bodies or as part of fusions to fluorescent proteins (29). However, such methods yield data for only a few proteins of interest per cell and are thus unsuitable for comprehensively identifying all cellular subtypes in a complex population. More global methods, such as mass spectrometry-based proteomics, still have insufficient sensitivity for single-cell analysis of bacteria (30).

Considering these current methodological limitations for bacterial single-cell analysis, an attractive strategy exploits the single-cell detection of some marker proteins to purify larger numbers of cells that belong to distinct subpopulations. Genome-scale analysis of this material can then comprehensively reveal differential gene expression patterns in the various subpopulations. As an early example of this approach for a eukaryotic pathogen, female and male *Plasmodium* gametocytes could be sorted by fluorescence-activated cell sorting (FACS) from infected blood based on gender-specific green fluorescent protein expression cassettes, followed by large-scale proteome analysis (31).

This strategy offers unique opportunities for detailed insights into pathogen heterogeneity during infection, but compared to full single-cell analysis, it has important caveats. Even if a marker reports a relevant aspect of that heterogeneity, it is likely that the detected subpopulations each contain multiple subsubsets that might differ even more among themselves than their respective parent subpopulations. It is possible to address these issues by comparing several different markers and their corresponding subpopulations, by correlating subpopulation properties and fates, and by relating subpopulations with their respective host microenvironments.

Numerous methods have been developed for single-cell analysis of microbial gene expression in axenic cultures, environmental samples, and infectious disease contexts (11–13, 32). Among these methods, fluorescent protein reporters are especially versatile for identifying and purifying pathogen subpopulations. Fluorescent proteins enable imaging from superresolution (around 50 nm) to whole-body imaging, providing host contexts for positive pathogen subpopulations. Fluorescent proteins also enable detection and sorting using flow cytometry (FACS), which combines sensitivity over several orders of magnitude with very high throughput for single cells (up to 20,000 cells per s). Fluorescent proteins come in various colors (33) and can be separated from host autofluorescence using appropriate optical filters and multicolor detection (22, 34, 35). Fluorescent-protein levels can be adjusted to nonattenuating levels by modulating translation initiation using ribosome binding site variants (36, 37). Superbright constructs are nice to observe in the microscope but may represent sick pathogen subpopula-

tions (38–41) that suffer from a stress (expression of a useless foreign protein [42]) that would be irrelevant under more physiological conditions. Three colors can be coexpressed and detected in a single pathogen cell (e.g., blue fluorescent protein–YPet [YFP for energy transfer]–mCherry or cyan fluorescent protein–green fluorescent protein–mCherry), enabling discrimination of several subpopulations in a single infection experiment (22).

Rapidly degradable variants are ideal for investigating rapid fluctuations in host microenvironments, whereas more stable variants better reflect pathogen adaptations over time scales of one or a few pathogen division cycles. Some approaches use fluorescence properties of reporter proteins themselves for identifying subpopulations. Indeed, there are many variants that show differential emission intensities depending on parameters (33) such as pH (43), concentrations of metabolites such as ATP (44), and exposure to reactive oxygen species (45).

As a caveat, conditions might change as soon as a pathogen cell is removed from its host microenvironment, and most of these signals cannot be preserved by fixation. It might thus be challenging to determine the true *in vivo* conditions and almost impossible to exploit such signals for subpopulation sorting. Retention or loss of fluorescent proteins can reflect viability of pathogen cells, in particular if microbicidal host attacks damage the pathogen cell envelope, leading to leakage of cellular contents (22, 46). However, purifying such dying and dead subsets is also challenging.

Another approach, called fluorescence dilution, loads pathogen cells with a stable fluorescent protein prior to infection and then tracks a few cell divisions based on decreasing fluorescent protein content, to monitor *in vivo* growth rates of pathogen subpopulations (47, 48). As the protein is stable, this yields a highly informative and exploitable signal for studying pathogen populations with heterogeneous growth rates with respect to their antimicrobial tolerance, metabolic activities, and interactions with host cells (49, 50). An alternative approach for monitoring pathogen growth *in vivo* utilizes the complex maturation kinetics of the fluorescent protein Timer (51, 52). The branched Timer maturation pathway yields first some green fluorescent molecules and later some additional orange fluorescent molecules (53). The green/orange ratio thus reflects the age of the molecules, and in cells with constitutive Timer expression, this is a direct function of growth rate, with rapidly growing cells emitting mostly green fluorescence, while slowly growing cells show mixed green and orange fluorescence (52). The signal can be monitored for dozens of generations, reflects the current growth rate (instead of total number of divisions, which is monitored by fluorescence dilution), is rather stable at 4°C and fixable, and can be used for purifying subpopulations for subsequent genome-scale analysis. However, oxygen tension influences fluorescence maturation, and Timer is thus best suitable for pathogens colonizing tissues with high blood flow and limited oxygen consumption, such as spleen.

Another complementary method is fluorescence recovery after photoconversion, in which pathogens expressing photoconvertible fluorescent proteins such as mKikumeGR are illuminated with a light pulse that converts all initially green fluorescent molecules to a red fluorescent form (35). The subsequent replacement of red molecules with green molecules indicates protein turnover as a proxy for metabolic activity with single-cell resolution and makes it possible to determine the impact of host effector molecules such as nitric oxide on the physiology of local *Leishmania* parasites.

Coupling fluorescent proteins with regulatory elements provides many additional opportunities for identifying and purifying pathogen subpopulations. In particular, stress-inducible promoters driving fluorescent-protein expression can highlight pathogen cells that are currently exposed to distinct stresses, such as reactive oxygen species (ROS) or reactive nitrogen species (22, 23), or grow at varying rates based on their ribosomal promoter activities (54). As an alternative to promoters, the increasing number of natural and synthetic riboswitches provides versatile biosensor constructs for a wide variety of metabolic and other conditions in the pathogen cytosol (55). Many regulatory elements respond to multiple stimuli, and it might be difficult to determine the causal stress for some highly fluorescent subpopulations unless additional information is available. On the other hand, it might not always be necessary to clarify induction specificity at an early stage, as long as the construct discriminates pathogen subpopulations with interesting differential properties. The subsequent global analysis of gene expression patterns will reveal additional information about which stimuli the corresponding subpopulation actually responded to.

For pathogen subpopulations that express fluorescent markers, flow cytometry (FACS) provides a powerful single-cell separation technique. In principle, other purification methods could offer attractive alternatives. As an example, magnetic beads coated with an antibody to an epitope that is exposed on the pathogen surface could enable rapid enrichment of pathogen cells (56).

SYSTEMIC SALMONELLOSIS AS A MODEL

Heterogeneous host-pathogen encounters *in vivo* have been investigated in only a few models (12), with a spe-

cial emphasis on *Salmonella* infections in mice (22, 50, 52, 57). Systemic *Salmonella enterica* infections are a major cause of mortality worldwide (58–62) and are becoming increasingly untreatable (63, 64). Many aspects of these systemic *Salmonella* infections can be mimicked in mouse infection models that are widely investigated (65), making murine salmonellosis one of the prime paradigms for bacterial infections. This includes the discovery of an astonishing diversity of host-*Salmonella* encounters with diverging local outcomes, which together determine disease progression (12, 13, 50, 66, 67).

The mouse typhoid fever disease model offers facile experimental accessibility, extensive literature, and a continuously increasing number of innovative approaches. This includes mechanistic studies of dozens of virulence factors, >3,000 *Salmonella* mutant virulence phenotypes, *in vivo Salmonella* proteomes, biosensors that report on *Salmonella* subpopulations in different tissue microenvironments, large-scale phenotyping of mouse mutants, extensive data on host cell infiltration and activation, immune perturbations, vaccine trials, comparisons with a recently revived human typhoid fever challenge infection model, etc. This wealth of data provides a unique basis for innovative research on heterogeneous host-pathogen encounters.

As a potential caveat, the value of mice as models for human inflammation is controversial (68, 69). However, this is less relevant for the mouse typhoid fever model, since (i) mouse models for bacterial infections have generally high predictive power for human clinical trials compared to many other medical indications (70); (ii) *Salmonella* mutant phenotypes in the mouse typhoid fever model closely correlate with those observed in experimentally infected human volunteers (71); (iii) key immune factors have comparable impact on disease progression in mouse and human typhoid fever (NADPH oxidase deficiency, interleukin 12, gamma interferon [IFN-γ], tumor necrosis factor alpha, and CD4 T cells) (72); and (iv) inflammatory responses show similarly extended time courses and participation of similar signaling networks in mouse and human typhoid fever (72).

SALMONELLA-HOST INTERACTIONS IN INFECTED SPLEEN

Several labs have used the mouse typhoid fever model to obtain intriguing initial insights into heterogeneous host-*Salmonella* interactions in mouse spleen (12, 22, 48, 52, 73–77) (Fig. 2). *Salmonella* organisms mostly reside in resident macrophages of the red pulp, which phagocytose aged erythrocytes (22, 77) (Fig. 2a, left center). Salmonellae proliferate intracellularly at rates that are

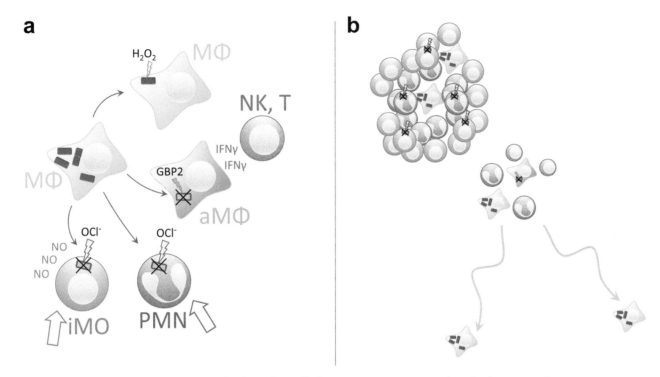

Figure 2 Working model for *Salmonella*-host interactions in an infected spleen. (a) *Salmonella* interactions with various phagocyte types. *Salmonella* proliferates in macrophages (MΦ) and spreads to other cells. When entering a macrophage, a *Salmonella* cell is exposed to a short and sublethal oxidative burst. Infiltrating NK and T cells secrete IFN-γ, which activates some macrophages, enabling them to kill intracellular salmonellae in part through guanylate-binding protein 2 (GBP2). Infection foci also attract inflammatory monocytes (iMO) and polymorphonuclear neutrophils (PMN), which kill intracellular *Salmonella* with hypochlorite (HOCl; bleach). Inflammatory monocytes generate and release large amounts of NO, which diffuses to regional salmonellae, which in turn upregulate detoxifying and damage repair enzymes. (b) Lesion formation and *Salmonella* spreading in infected tissues. Growing *Salmonella* infection foci attract inflammatory monocytes (blue) and neutrophils (magenta) that kill many *Salmonella*. However, some salmonellae escape in infected macrophages (cyan) and start new infection foci elsewhere. Early infection foci are detected by NK and T cells (green), which secrete IFN-γ and activate some of the local macrophages. Other macrophages move to yet other tissue regions, thereby spreading the infection and driving disease progression.

specific for each individual macrophage (52). Although hundreds of metabolic enzymes show differential abundance in fast-growing versus slow-growing *Salmonella*, their overall metabolic programs are qualitatively similar and reflect access to many chemically diverse nutrients, with a dominance of glycerol as the energy source, in agreement with bulk-average *in vivo* data (78). However, pathway analysis reveals a subtle shift from predominant *Salmonella* biosynthesis of several biomass components, such as nucleotides, amino acids, and carbohydrates, in the slow-growing subset to uptake of such biomass components from the host environment in the fast-growing *Salmonella* subset. Indeed, a purine-auxotrophic *Salmonella* mutant that depends completely on host purine supply splits into two distinct subsets, one with normal

growth, indicating facile access to host purines, and one with stalled growth, indicative of insufficient purine supply to meet biomass requirements. These data demonstrate that distinct microenvironments with widely varying nutrient supplies for local *Salmonella* coexist in the spleen and, at least in part, modulate the proliferation rate of local *Salmonella* subsets (52).

In contrast to their metabolic differences, rapidly and slowly growing *Salmonella* organisms show surprisingly similar levels of various stress defense proteins. These data indicate that salmonellae encounter substantial oxidative, nitrosative, and envelope stresses *in vivo* but that these stresses do not modulate *Salmonella* growth rates (52). For some stresses, such as reactive nitrogen species, *Salmonella* defense through the detoxifying enzymes NO dioxygenase (HmpA) and NO reductase (Hcp) (65), as well as YtfE, which repairs NO-damaged iron sulfur clusters, is apparently sufficient to cope with host-generated nitric oxide without compromising fitness (22), at least during acute infections (79). In contrast, *Salmonella* encounters a wide range of ROS. *Salmonella* ROS detoxification and repair are sufficient to efficiently cope with moderate hydrogen peroxide levels in macrophages (22, 80), while neutrophils and inflammatory monocytes kill *Salmonella* using highly bactericidal hypochlorite (HOCl; bleach) (22, 74). Although these bactericidal oxidative attacks are highly relevant for host control of *Salmonella* (79), methods that focus on live bacteria (such as FACS) miss these processes. Taken together, the data show that some high-intensity oxidative host attacks overwhelm *Salmonella* defense systems and kill the bacteria, while less intense oxidative attacks are insufficient to kill salmonellae or even inhibit their growth. It is possible that other attacks, such as pore formation through perforin-2 (MPEG1) (81), might have similar binary consequences (*Salmonella* death or unimpaired survival), since envelope stress responses in live *Salmonella* do not correlate with *Salmonella* growth rate (52).

Salmonella growth in spleens of genetically susceptible mice results in 10-fold daily increases in bacterial load. Surprisingly, however, most infected cells contain only one or two salmonellae at any time (75). Cells containing three or more than 20 salmonellae are rather rare, but because of their higher *Salmonella* content per cell, these cells still contain the majority of all *Salmonella* cells (82). This supports a model of stochastic transmission of intracellular *Salmonella* to new host cells which often occurs even at low intracellular *Salmonella* loads (83). Low intracellular *Salmonella* content might make detection by the host immune system more challenging. Salmonellae residing alone, or as part of large microcolonies, have comparable intracellular growth rates, arguing against an exhaustion of host supply and slowing down of expanding intracellular *Salmonella* microcolonies (52).

After being released from infected macrophages by unknown mechanisms, salmonellae enter different types of host cells. Salmonellae that enter another resident red pulp macrophage are exposed to hydrogen peroxide (H_2O_2), which causes sublethal oxidative stress (22) (see above), and proliferate again. The intrinsic motility of the host cell might facilitate *Salmonella* spreading to other tissue regions. *Salmonella* might use type III effector proteins such as SseE, SseF, or SseI/SsrfH to further manipulate this motility (84, 85). After the new infection focus has reached a certain *Salmonella* density, this is sensed by NK and T cells that secrete IFN-γ (76). This cytokine activates some, but not all, infected resident

macrophages to kill their intracellular salmonellae, with a potential contribution of the IFN-γ-inducible guanylate-binding protein 2 (73). This enables partial local restriction of expanding *Salmonella* foci.

Growing *Salmonella* infection foci attract increasing numbers of infiltrating neutrophils and inflammatory monocytes, resulting in the formation of inflammatory lesions (22, 72). Salmonellae that are released from macrophages and phagocytized by polymorphonuclear neutrophils and inflammatory monocytes are largely killed with hypochlorite (HOCl; bleach) (22, 74). Inflammatory monocytes also generate large amounts of NO, which diffuses through the tissue and triggers nonlethal stress in salmonellae residing in inflammatory monocytes or bystander cells (22). At some advanced stage, these potently bactericidal host cells reach high density and efficiently contain and eradicate all local salmonellae (Fig. 2b, upper left). However, at early stages of this process, some infected macrophages leave the area and spread to new tissue regions, where they form new foci (22, 72, 75). Overall, this spreading and formation of new foci drives the infection process more than local *Salmonella* growth in existing foci (75).

These results show that salmonellosis consists of strikingly heterogeneous and dynamic pathogen-host encounters involving diverse tissue regions, cell types, and molecular mechanisms. Importantly, these disparate encounters have divergent individual outcomes, and overall disease progression can result from failures of host control in some resting macrophages, despite successful simultaneous eradication in activated macrophages and inflammatory lesions (12).

ANTIBIOTIC ACTION *IN VIVO*

Antibiotic susceptibility depends strongly on the environment and the physiological state of the pathogen (86). Slow growth increases the tolerance of *Salmonella* to fluoroquinolone antibiotics in mouse infection models (50, 52, 57). On the other hand, many stress conditions that vary widely between different host microenvironments, such as exposure to oxidative stress and nitric oxide, might also modulate antibiotic action *in vivo*. Inhomogeneous drug penetration (14, 87) as well as human genetic diversity, lifestyle, age, and comorbidities (88, 89) might further increase variation. Even high antibiotic doses might not eradicate all bacteria, causing relapses in the absence of inherited resistance, especially in chronic infections (90–93). The *Salmonella* typhoid fever model offers diverse experimental tools that might provide unique opportunities for investigating these crucial issues in future studies.

OPEN QUESTIONS AND MAJOR CHALLENGES

Recent findings are beginning to fundamentally alter our understanding of infectious diseases and antimicrobial chemotherapy *in vivo*, but they still offer just the first glimpses into the enormous complexity of host-pathogen interactions *in vivo*. We have yet not comprehensively identified and localized even the main types of encounters, we poorly understand their cellular and molecular mechanisms, and we have few insights into their impact on overall disease outcome.

In particular, visualization of host activities that might have an impact on local pathogen cells still mostly relies on immunohistochemistry on tissue sections, providing a basically two-dimensional analysis of just a few proteins that can be detected with antibodies. Tissue sections cannot provide information about events that happen nearby but out of plane. Serial sections can be prepared and analyzed, but this is a tedious and inefficient approach for covering tissues at millimeter scales in three dimensions (3D). Exciting new 3D imaging approaches for organs have been developed in neurobiology, and some of these approaches as well as alternative methods are applicable to infected tissues (94–96). Moreover, new methods for localized mRNA sequencing in tissue sections (97) or highly multiplexed RNA fluorescent *in situ* hybridization in combination with single-cell RNA sequencing (98) might provide a much more comprehensive spatially resolved overview of host activities around infection foci.

Another challenge is how to correlate current pathogen stresses and defenses with subsequent outcomes, such as pathogen death, survival, and proliferation. Current research mostly relies on snapshots that cannot capture the crucial temporal dynamics. We know that *Salmonella* cells differentially access host nutrients, experience oxidative or nitrosative stress, etc., but what is the consequence of these encounters and what impact do they have on overall disease outcome? We detect many dead *Salmonella* cells in tissues, but which events led to their killing, and why did this not happen to the thriving *Salmonella* subsets? All these questions remain unresolved, since they require spatiotemporal measurements, which current methods cannot provide. We can detect many *Salmonella* subsets that take part in specific encounters with host cells using flow cytometry and confocal microscopy of tissue sections, but we know very little about their history, their fate, and their contribution to overall disease outcome.

Intravital microscopy offers fascinating opportunities for tracking pathogen cells in 3D over time (99–101), but data are usually limited to a few hours and areas of view that would contain only a few dozen *Salmonella* cells. This would be insufficient to answer our questions regarding systemic salmonellosis. Transparent zebrafish embryos and larvae offer whole-body infection monitoring at high spatiotemporal resolution (102), but *Salmonella* infections cause rapid lethality in this host, limiting its use for extended spatiotemporal monitoring (103).

Lineage tracing methods, in which specific cell subsets are genetically labeled using inducible recombinases and fluorescent reporters, have been highly successful for reconstructing whole-organ development and the contribution of specific cell subsets in various eukaryotic organisms (104). Some of these methods might be applicable to pathogens to track their fate and properties in host tissues over time.

Some of these approaches might help to address the fundamental issue of how heterogeneity determines ultimate disease outcome. As an example, NK and T cells secrete the cytokine IFN-γ, and this is crucial for innate (and adaptive) immunity to *Salmonella* (22, 76). However, many macrophages fail to kill *Salmonella*, and this is a primary cause of disease progression (22). Why do NK and T cells fail to activate all relevant macrophages? Can they secrete IFN-γ only after they sense a threshold density of *Salmonella* (as proposed by the working model), or are other factors more relevant? This could be the tipping point that determines overall disease outcome. Related to this issue is the question of whether fast-growing salmonellae activate their host macrophages (and hence increase the risk of being killed) or whether they suppress activation (e.g., by inhibition of NF-κB signaling [105]). Answering these questions might provide a basis for entirely novel strategies in infection control, by broadening successful host antimicrobial attacks and closing permissive niches in which pathogens can thrive.

Acknowledgments. I thank current and previous lab members for their valuable contributions. Research on pathogen heterogeneity in my laboratory is supported by Swiss National Science Foundation grants 156818 and 160702b.

Citation. Bumann D. 2019. *Salmonella* single-cell metabolism and stress responses in complex host tissues. Microbiol Spectrum 7(2):BAI-0009-2019.

References

1. Lozano R, et al. 2012. Global and regional mortality from 235 causes of death for 20 age groups in 1990 and 2010: a systematic analysis for the Global Burden of Disease Study 2010. *Lancet* 380:2095–2128. *ERRATUM Lancet* 381:628.

2. Zinkernagel RM, Hengartner H. 2004. On immunity against infections and vaccines: credo 2004. *Scand J Immunol* 60:9–13.

3. Kaufmann SH. 2007. The contribution of immunology to the rational design of novel antibacterial vaccines. *Nat Rev Microbiol* **5**:491–504.

4. Epstein JE, Giersing B, Mullen G, Moorthy V, Richie TL. 2007. Malaria vaccines: are we getting closer? *Curr Opin Mol Ther* **9**:12–24.

5. Spellberg B, Powers JH, Brass EP, Miller LG, Edwards JE Jr. 2004. Trends in antimicrobial drug development: implications for the future. *Clin Infect Dis* **38**:1279–1286.

6. Norrby SR, Nord CE, Finch R, European Society of Clinical Microbiology and Infectious Diseases. 2005. Lack of development of new antimicrobial drugs: a potential serious threat to public health. *Lancet Infect Dis* **5**:115–119.

7. Kaldalu N, Hauryliuk V, Tenson T. 2016. Persisters—as elusive as ever. *Appl Microbiol Biotechnol* **100**:6545–6553.

8. Rowe SE, Conlon BP, Keren I, Lewis K. 2016. Persisters: methods for isolation and identifying contributing factors—a review. *Methods Mol Biol* **1333**:17–28.

9. Balaban NQ, Gerdes K, Lewis K, McKinney JD. 2013. A problem of persistence: still more questions than answers? *Nat Rev Microbiol* **11**:587–591.

10. Maisonneuve E, Gerdes K. 2014. Molecular mechanisms underlying bacterial persisters. *Cell* **157**:539–548.

11. Davis KM, Isberg RR. 2016. Defining heterogeneity within bacterial populations via single cell approaches. *BioEssays* **38**:782–790.

12. Bumann D. 2015. Heterogeneous host-pathogen encounters: act locally, think globally. *Cell Host Microbe* **17**:13–19.

13. Kreibich S, Hardt WD. 2015. Experimental approaches to phenotypic diversity in infection. *Curr Opin Microbiol* **27**:25–36.

14. Prideaux B, Via LE, Zimmerman MD, Eum S, Sarathy J, O'Brien P, Chen C, Kaya F, Weiner DM, Chen PY, Song T, Lee M, Shim TS, Cho JS, Kim W, Cho SN, Olivier KN, Barry CE III, Dartois V. 2015. The association between sterilizing activity and drug distribution into tuberculosis lesions. *Nat Med* **21**:1223–1227.

15. Lehar SM, Pillow T, Xu M, Staben L, Kajihara KK, Vandlen R, DePalatis L, Raab H, Hazenbos WL, Morisaki JH, Kim J, Park S, Darwish M, Lee BC, Hernandez H, Loyet KM, Lupardus P, Fong R, Yan D, Chalouni C, Luis E, Khalfin Y, Plise E, Cheong J, Lyssikatos JP, Strandh M, Koefoed K, Andersen PS, Flygare JA, Wah Tan M, Brown EJ, Mariathasan S. 2015. Novel antibody-antibiotic conjugate eliminates intracellular *S. aureus*. *Nature* **527**:323–328.

16. Brauner A, Fridman O, Gefen O, Balaban NQ. 2016. Distinguishing between resistance, tolerance and persistence to antibiotic treatment. *Nat Rev Microbiol* **14**:320–330.

17. Malherbe ST, Shenai S, Ronacher K, Loxton AG, Dolganov G, Kriel M, Van T, Chen RY, Warwick J, Via LE, Song T, Lee M, Schoolnik G, Tromp G, Alland D, Barry CE III, Winter J, Walzl G, Lucas L, van der Spuy G, Stanley K, Thiart L, Smith B, Du Plessis N, Beltran CG, Maasdorp E, Ellmann A, Choi H, Joh J, Dodd LE,

Allwood B, Koegelenberg C, Vorster M, Griffith-Richards S, Catalysis TB–Biomarker Consortium. 2016. Persisting positron emission tomography lesion activity and *Mycobacterium tuberculosis* mRNA after tuberculosis cure. *Nat Med* **22**:1094–1100. *CORRIGENDUM Nat Med* **23**:526. *CORRIGENDUM Nat Med* **23**:1499.

18. Lenaerts A, Barry CE III, Dartois V. 2015. Heterogeneity in tuberculosis pathology, microenvironments and therapeutic responses. *Immunol Rev* **264**:288–307.

19. Marakalala MJ, Raju RM, Sharma K, Zhang YJ, Eugenin EA, Prideaux B, Daudelin IB, Chen PY, Booty MG, Kim JH, Eum SY, Via LE, Behar SM, Barry CE III, Mann M, Dartois V, Rubin EJ. 2016. Inflammatory signaling in human tuberculosis granulomas is spatially organized. *Nat Med* **22**:531–538.

20. Diard M, Garcia V, Maier L, Remus-Emsermann MN, Regoes RR, Ackermann M, Hardt WD. 2013. Stabilization of cooperative virulence by the expression of an avirulent phenotype. *Nature* **494**:353–356.

21. Ackermann M, Stecher B, Freed NE, Songhet P, Hardt WD, Doebeli M. 2008. Self-destructive cooperation mediated by phenotypic noise. *Nature* **454**:987–990.

22. Burton NA, Schürmann N, Casse O, Steeb AK, Claudi B, Zankl J, Schmidt A, Bumann D. 2014. Disparate impact of oxidative host defenses determines the fate of *Salmonella* during systemic infection in mice. *Cell Host Microbe* **15**:72–83.

23. Davis KM, Mohammadi S, Isberg RR. 2015. Community behavior and spatial regulation within a bacterial microcolony in deep tissue sites serves to protect against host attack. *Cell Host Microbe* **17**:21–31.

24. Alemany A, Florescu M, Baron CS, Peterson-Maduro J, van Oudenaarden A. 2018. Whole-organism clone tracing using single-cell sequencing. *Nature* **556**:108–112.

25. Saliba AE, Santos SC, Vogel J. 2017. New RNA-seq approaches for the study of bacterial pathogens. *Curr Opin Microbiol* **35**:78–87.

26. Kang Y, McMillan I, Norris MH, Hoang TT. 2015. Single prokaryotic cell isolation and total transcript amplification protocol for transcriptomic analysis. *Nat Protoc* **10**:974–984.

27. Avital G, Avraham R, Fan A, Hashimshony T, Hung DT, Yanai I. 2017. scDual-Seq: mapping the gene regulatory program of *Salmonella* infection by host and pathogen single-cell RNA-sequencing. *Genome Biol* **18**:200.

28. Chong S, Chen C, Ge H, Xie XS. 2014. Mechanism of transcriptional bursting in bacteria. *Cell* **158**:314–326.

29. Taniguchi Y, Choi PJ, Li GW, Chen H, Babu M, Hearn J, Emili A, Xie XS. 2010. Quantifying *E. coli* proteome and transcriptome with single-molecule sensitivity in single cells. *Science* **329**:533–538.

30. Zhang L, Vertes A. 2017. Single-cell mass spectrometry approaches to explore cellular heterogeneity. *Angew Chem Int Ed Engl* **57**:4466–4477.

31. Khan SM, Franke-Fayard B, Mair GR, Lasonder E, Janse CJ, Mann M, Waters AP. 2005. Proteome analysis of separated male and female gametocytes reveals novel sex-specific *Plasmodium* biology. *Cell* **121**:675–687.

32. Ackermann M. 2015. A functional perspective on phenotypic heterogeneity in microorganisms. *Nat Rev Microbiol* **13**:497–508.

33. Rodriguez EA, Campbell RE, Lin JY, Lin MZ, Miyawaki A, Palmer AE, Shu X, Zhang J, Tsien RY. 2017. The growing and glowing toolbox of fluorescent and photoactive proteins. *Trends Biochem Sci* **42**:111–129.

34. Bumann D. 2002. Examination of *Salmonella* gene expression in an infected mammalian host using the green fluorescent protein and two-colour flow cytometry. *Mol Microbiol* **43**:1269–1283.

35. Müller AJ, Aeschlimann S, Olekhnovitch R, Dacher M, Späth GF, Bousso P. 2013. Photoconvertible pathogen labeling reveals nitric oxide control of *Leishmania major* infection in vivo via dampening of parasite metabolism. *Cell Host Microbe* **14**:460–467.

36. Rollenhagen C, Sörensen M, Rizos K, Hurvitz R, Bumann D. 2004. Antigen selection based on expression levels during infection facilitates vaccine development for an intracellular pathogen. *Proc Natl Acad Sci USA* **101**: 8739–8744.

37. Bonde MT, Pedersen M, Klausen MS, Jensen SI, Wulff T, Harrison S, Nielsen AT, Herrgård MJ, Sommer MO. 2016. Predictable tuning of protein expression in bacteria. *Nat Methods* **13**:233.

38. Wendland M, Bumann D. 2002. Optimization of GFP levels for analyzing *Salmonella* gene expression during an infection. *FEBS Lett* **521**:105–108.

39. Rang C, Galen JE, Kaper JB, Chao L. 2003. Fitness cost of the green fluorescent protein in gastrointestinal bacteria. *Can J Microbiol* **49**:531–537.

40. Bienick MS, Young KW, Klesmith JR, Detwiler EE, Tomek KJ, Whitehead TA. 2014. The interrelationship between promoter strength, gene expression, and growth rate. *PLoS One* **9**:e109105.

41. Knodler LA, Bestor A, Ma C, Hansen-Wester I, Hensel M, Vallance BA, Steele-Mortimer O. 2005. Cloning vectors and fluorescent proteins can significantly inhibit *Salmonella enterica* virulence in both epithelial cells and macrophages: implications for bacterial pathogenesis studies. *Infect Immun* **73**:7027–7031.

42. Ceroni F, Algar R, Stan G-B, Ellis T. 2015. Quantifying cellular capacity identifies gene expression designs with reduced burden. *Nat Methods* **12**:415–418.

43. Lee EJ, Pontes MH, Groisman EA. 2013. A bacterial virulence protein promotes pathogenicity by inhibiting the bacterium's own F_1F_0 ATP synthase. *Cell* **154**: 146–156.

44. Maglica Ž, Özdemir E, McKinney JD. 2015. Single-cell tracking reveals antibiotic-induced changes in mycobacterial energy metabolism. *mBio* **6**:e02236-14.

45. van der Heijden J, Bosman ES, Reynolds LA, Finlay BB. 2015. Direct measurement of oxidative and nitrosative stress dynamics in *Salmonella* inside macrophages. *Proc Natl Acad Sci USA* **112**:560–565.

46. Barat S, Willer Y, Rizos K, Claudi B, Mazé A, Schemmer AK, Kirchhoff D, Schmidt A, Burton N, Bumann D. 2012. Immunity to intracellular *Salmonella* depends on surface-associated antigens. *PLoS Pathog* **8**:e1002966.

47. Roostalu J, Jõers A, Luidalepp H, Kaldalu N, Tenson T. 2008. Cell division in *Escherichia coli* cultures monitored at single cell resolution. *BMC Microbiol* **8**:68.

48. Helaine S, Thompson JA, Watson KG, Liu M, Boyle C, Holden DW. 2010. Dynamics of intracellular bacterial replication at the single cell level. *Proc Natl Acad Sci USA* **107**:3746–3751.

49. Saliba AE, Li L, Westermann AJ, Appenzeller S, Stapels DA, Schulte LN, Helaine S, Vogel J. 2016. Single-cell RNA-seq ties macrophage polarization to growth rate of intracellular *Salmonella*. *Nat Microbiol* **2**:16206.

50. Helaine S, Cheverton AM, Watson KG, Faure LM, Matthews SA, Holden DW. 2014. Internalization of *Salmonella* by macrophages induces formation of nonreplicating persisters. *Science* **343**:204–208.

51. Terskikh A, Fradkov A, Ermakova G, Zaraisky A, Tan P, Kajava AV, Zhao X, Lukyanov S, Matz M, Kim S, Weissman I, Siebert P. 2000. "Fluorescent timer": protein that changes color with time. *Science* **290**:1585–1588.

52. Claudi B, Spröte P, Chirkova A, Personnic N, Zankl J, Schürmann N, Schmidt A, Bumann D. 2014. Phenotypic variation of *Salmonella* in host tissues delays eradication by antimicrobial chemotherapy. *Cell* **158**:722–733.

53. Strack RL, Strongin DE, Mets L, Glick BS, Keenan RJ. 2010. Chromophore formation in DsRed occurs by a branched pathway. *J Am Chem Soc* **132**:8496–8505.

54. Manina G, Dhar N, McKinney JD. 2015. Stress and host immunity amplify *Mycobacterium tuberculosis* phenotypic heterogeneity and induce nongrowing metabolically active forms. *Cell Host Microbe* **17**:32–46.

55. Etzel M, Mörl M. 2017. Synthetic riboswitches: from plug and pray toward plug and play. *Biochemistry* **56**: 1181–1198.

56. Curkić I, Schütz M, Oberhettinger P, Diard M, Claassen M, Linke D, Hardt WD. 2016. Epitope-tagged autotransporters as single-cell reporters for gene expression by a *Salmonella* Typhimurium *wbaP* mutant. *PLoS One* **11**:e0154828.

57. Kaiser P, Regoes RR, Dolowschiak T, Wotzka SY, Lengefeld J, Slack E, Grant AJ, Ackermann M, Hardt WD. 2014. Cecum lymph node dendritic cells harbor slow-growing bacteria phenotypically tolerant to antibiotic treatment. *PLoS Biol* **12**:e1001793.

58. Ao TT, Feasey NA, Gordon MA, Keddy KH, Angulo FJ, Crump JA. 2015. Global burden of invasive nontyphoidal *Salmonella* disease, 2010. *Emerg Infect Dis* **21**: 941–949.

59. Crump JA, Luby SP, Mintz ED. 2004. The global burden of typhoid fever. *Bull World Health Organ* **82**:346–353.

60. Marks F, et al. 2017. Incidence of invasive salmonella disease in sub-Saharan Africa: a multicentre population-based surveillance study. *Lancet Glob Health* **5**:e310–e323.

61. Mogasale V, Maskery B, Ochiai RL, Lee JS, Mogasale VV, Ramani E, Kim YE, Park JK, Wierzba TF. 2014. Burden of typhoid fever in low-income and middle-income countries: a systematic, literature-based update with risk-factor adjustment. *Lancet Glob Health* **2**:e570–e580.

62. Wain J, Hendriksen RS, Mikoleit ML, Keddy KH, Ochiai RL. 2015. Typhoid fever. *Lancet* 385:1136–1145.

63. Levine MM, Simon R. 2018. The gathering storm: is untreatable typhoid fever on the way? *mBio* 9:e00482-18.

64. Kariuki S, Gordon MA, Feasey N, Parry CM. 2015. Antimicrobial resistance and management of invasive *Salmonella* disease. *Vaccine* 33(Suppl 3):C21–C29.

65. Tsolis RM, Xavier MN, Santos RL, Bäumler AJ. 2011. How to become a top model: impact of animal experimentation on human *Salmonella* disease research. *Infect Immun* 79:1806–1814.

66. Helaine S, Kugelberg E. 2014. Bacterial persisters: formation, eradication, and experimental systems. *Trends Microbiol* 22:417–424.

67. Bumann D, Cunrath O. 2017. Heterogeneity of *Salmonella*-host interactions in infected host tissues. *Curr Opin Microbiol* 39:57–63.

68. Seok J, Warren HS, Cuenca AG, Mindrinos MN, Baker HV, Xu W, Richards DR, McDonald-Smith GP, Gao H, Hennessy L, Finnerty CC, López CM, Honari S, Moore EE, Minei JP, Cuschieri J, Bankey PE, Johnson JL, Sperry J, Nathens AB, Billiar TR, West MA, Jeschke MG, Klein MB, Gamelli RL, Gibran NS, Brownstein BH, Miller-Graziano C, Calvano SE, Mason PH, Cobb JP, Rahme LG, Lowry SF, Maier RV, Moldawer LL, Herndon DN, Davis RW, Xiao W, Tompkins RG, Inflammation and Host Response to Injury, Large Scale Collaborative Research Program. 2013. Genomic responses in mouse models poorly mimic human inflammatory diseases. *Proc Natl Acad Sci USA* 110:3507–3512.

69. Takao K, Miyakawa T. 2015. Genomic responses in mouse models greatly mimic human inflammatory diseases. *Proc Natl Acad Sci USA* 112:1167–1172 CORRECTION *Proc Natl Acad Sci USA* 112:E1163–E1167.

70. Kola I, Landis J. 2004. Can the pharmaceutical industry reduce attrition rates? *Nat Rev Drug Discov* 3:711–716.

71. Bumann D, Hueck C, Aebischer T, Meyer TF. 2000. Recombinant live *Salmonella* spp. for human vaccination against heterologous pathogens. *FEMS Immunol Med Microbiol* 27:357–364.

72. Dougan G, John V, Palmer S, Mastroeni P. 2011. Immunity to salmonellosis. *Immunol Rev* 240:196–210.

73. Meunier E, Dick MS, Dreier RF, Schürmann N, Kenzelmann Broz D, Warming S, Roose-Girma M, Bumann D, Kayagaki N, Takeda K, Yamamoto M, Broz P. 2014. Caspase-11 activation requires lysis of pathogen-containing vacuoles by IFN-induced GTPases. *Nature* 509:366–370.

74. Schürmann N, Forrer P, Casse O, Li J, Felmy B, Burgener AV, Ehrenfeuchter N, Hardt WD, Recher M, Hess C, Tschan-Plessl A, Khanna N, Bumann D. 2017. Myeloperoxidase targets oxidative host attacks to *Salmonella* and prevents collateral tissue damage. *Nat Microbiol* 2:16268.

75. Sheppard M, Webb C, Heath F, Mallows V, Emilianus R, Maskell D, Mastroeni P. 2003. Dynamics of bacterial growth and distribution within the liver during *Salmonella* infection. *Cell Microbiol* 5:593–600.

76. Kupz A, Scott TA, Belz GT, Andrews DM, Greyer M, Lew AM, Brooks AG, Smyth MJ, Curtiss R III, Bedoui S, Strugnell RA. 2013. Contribution of Thy1+ NK cells to protective IFN-γ production during *Salmonella typhimurium* infections. *Proc Natl Acad Sci USA* 110:2252–2257.

77. Pilonieta MC, Moreland SM, English CN, Detweiler CS. 2014. *Salmonella enterica* infection stimulates macrophages to hemophagocytose. *mBio* 5:e02211-14.

78. Steeb B, Claudi B, Burton NA, Tienz P, Schmidt A, Farhan H, Mazé A, Bumann D. 2013. Parallel exploitation of diverse host nutrients enhances *Salmonella* virulence. *PLoS Pathog* 9:e1003301.

79. Mastroeni P, Vazquez-Torres A, Fang FC, Xu Y, Khan S, Hormaeche CE, Dougan G. 2000. Antimicrobial actions of the NADPH phagocyte oxidase and inducible nitric oxide synthase in experimental salmonellosis. II. Effects on microbial proliferation and host survival in vivo. *J Exp Med* 192:237–248.

80. Aussel L, Zhao W, Hébrard M, Guilhon AA, Viala JP, Henri S, Chasson L, Gorvel JP, Barras F, Méresse S. 2011. *Salmonella* detoxifying enzymes are sufficient to cope with the host oxidative burst. *Mol Microbiol* 80:628–640.

81. McCormack RM, de Armas LR, Shiratsuchi M, Fiorentino DG, Olsson ML, Lichtenheld MG, Morales A, Lyapichev K, Gonzalez LE, Strbo N, Sukumar N, Stojadinovic O, Plano GV, Munson GP, Tomic-Canic M, Kirsner RS, Russell DG, Podack ER. 2015. Perforin-2 is essential for intracellular defense of parenchymal cells and phagocytes against pathogenic bacteria. *eLife* 4:e06508.

82. Thöne F, Schwanhäusser B, Becker D, Ballmaier M, Bumann D. 2007. FACS-isolation of *Salmonella*-infected cells with defined bacterial load from mouse spleen. *J Microbiol Methods* 71:220–224.

83. Brown SP, Cornell SJ, Sheppard M, Grant AJ, Maskell DJ, Grenfell BT, Mastroeni P. 2006. Intracellular demography and the dynamics of *Salmonella enterica* infections. *PLoS Biol* 4:e349.

84. McLaughlin LM, Xu H, Carden SE, Fisher S, Reyes M, Heilshorn SC, Monack DM. 2014. A microfluidic-based genetic screen to identify microbial virulence factors that inhibit dendritic cell migration. *Integr Biol* 6:438–449.

85. Worley MJ, Nieman GS, Geddes K, Heffron F. 2006. *Salmonella typhimurium* disseminates within its host by manipulating the motility of infected cells. *Proc Natl Acad Sci USA* 103:17915–17920.

86. Hughes D, Andersson DI. 2017. Environmental and genetic modulation of the phenotypic expression of antibiotic resistance. *FEMS Microbiol Rev* 41:374–391.

87. Onufrak NJ, Forrest A, Gonzalez D. 2016. Pharmacokinetic and pharmacodynamic principles of anti-infective dosing. *Clin Ther* 38:1930–1947.

88. Piasecka B, Duffy D, Urrutia A, Quach H, Patin E, Posseme C, Bergstedt J, Charbit B, Rouilly V, MacPherson CR, Hasan M, Albaud B, Gentien D, Fellay J, Albert ML, Quintana-Murci L, Milieu Intérieur Consortium. 2018.

Distinctive roles of age, sex, and genetics in shaping transcriptional variation of human immune responses to microbial challenges. *Proc Natl Acad Sci USA* **115**:E488–E497.

89. **Brodin P, Davis MM.** 2017. Human immune system variation. *Nat Rev Immunol* **17**:21–29.

90. **Conlon BP.** 2014. *Staphylococcus aureus* chronic and relapsing infections: evidence of a role for persister cells. *BioEssays* **36**:991–996.

91. **World Health Organization.** 2006. *Brucellosis in Humans and Animals.* World Health Organization, Geneva, Switzerland. www.who.int/csr/resources/publications/Brucellosis.pdf.

92. **Guglietta A.** 2017. Recurrent urinary tract infections in women: risk factors, etiology, pathogenesis and prophylaxis. *Future Microbiol* **12**:239–246.

93. **Onwuezobe IA, Oshun PO, Odigwe CC.** 2012. Antimicrobials for treating symptomatic non-typhoidal *Salmonella* infection. *Cochrane Database Syst Rev* **11**:CD001167.

94. **DePas WH, Starwalt-Lee R, Van Sambeek L, Ravindra Kumar S, Gradinaru V, Newman DK.** 2016. Exposing the three-dimensional biogeography and metabolic states of pathogens in cystic fibrosis sputum via hydrogel embedding, clearing, and rRNA labeling. *mBio* **7**:e00796-16.

95. **Cronan MR, Rosenberg AF, Oehlers SH, Saelens JW, Sisk DM, Jurcic Smith KL, Lee S, Tobin DM.** 2015. CLARITY and PACT-based imaging of adult zebrafish and mouse for whole-animal analysis of infections. *Dis Model Mech* **8**:1643–1650.

96. **Arena ET, Campbell-Valois F-X, Tinevez J-Y, Nigro G, Sachse M, Moya-Nilges M, Nothelfer K, Marteyn B, Shorte SL, Sansonetti PJ.** 2015. Bioimage analysis of *Shigella* infection reveals targeting of colonic crypts. *Proc Natl Acad Sci USA* **112**:E3282–E3290.

97. **Lee JH, Daugharthy ER, Scheiman J, Kalhor R, Yang JL, Ferrante TC, Terry R, Jeanty SS, Li C, Amamoto R, Peters DT, Turczyk BM, Marblestone AH, Inverso SA, Bernard A, Mali P, Rios X, Aach J, Church GM.** 2014. Highly multiplexed subcellular RNA sequencing in situ. *Science* **343**:1360–1363.

98. **Halpern KB, Shenhav R, Matcovitch-Natan O, Tóth B, Lemze D, Golan M, Massasa EE, Baydatch S, Landen S, Moor AE, Brandis A, Giladi A, Stokar-Avihail AS, David E, Amit I, Itzkovitz S.** 2017. Single-cell spatial reconstruction reveals global division of labour in the mammalian liver. *Nature* **542**:352–356 *ERRATUM Nature* **543**:742.

99. **Müller AJ, Kaiser P, Dittmar KE, Weber TC, Haueter S, Endt K, Songhet P, Zellweger C, Kremer M, Fehling HJ, Hardt WD.** 2012. *Salmonella* gut invasion involves TTSS-2-dependent epithelial traversal, basolateral exit, and uptake by epithelium-sampling lamina propria phagocytes. *Cell Host Microbe* **11**:19–32.

100. **Egen JG, Rothfuchs AG, Feng CG, Horwitz MA, Sher A, Germain RN.** 2011. Intravital imaging reveals limited antigen presentation and T cell effector function in mycobacterial granulomas. *Immunity* **34**:807–819.

101. **Choong FX, Richter-Dahlfors A.** 2014. Intravital two-photon imaging to understand bacterial infections of the mammalian host. *Methods Mol Biol* **1197**:87–100.

102. **Ramakrishnan L.** 2013. The zebrafish guide to tuberculosis immunity and treatment. *Cold Spring Harb Symp Quant Biol* **78**:179–192.

103. **Benard EL, van AM, Ellett F, Lieschke GJ, Spaink HP, Meijer AH.** 2012. Infection of zebrafish embryos with intracellular bacterial pathogens. *J Vis Exp* **2012**(61):3781.

104. **Spanjaard B, Junker JP.** 2017. Methods for lineage tracing on the organism-wide level. *Curr Opin Cell Biol* **49**:16–21.

105. **Gunster RA, Matthews SA, Holden DW, Thurston TL.** 2017. SseK1 and SseK3 type III secretion system effectors inhibit NF-κB signaling and necroptotic cell death in *Salmonella*-infected macrophages. *Infect Immun* **85**:e00010-17.

Bacteria and Intracellularity
Edited by Pascale Cossart, Craig R. Roy, and Philippe Sansonetti
© 2019 American Society for Microbiology, Washington, DC
doi:10.1128/microbiolspec.BAI-0022-2019

Manipulation of Host Cell Organelles by Intracellular Pathogens

13

Titilayo O. Omotade[1] and Craig R. Roy[1]

INTRODUCTION

Phagocytosis is an effective countermeasure exerted primarily by host macrophages and neutrophils to internalize and degrade microbes. Following uptake, most microbes are contained in a membrane-bound compartment called a phagosome, and through a series of tightly orchestrated events, nascent phagosomes mature and eventually fuse with lysosomes. Intracellular pathogens are unique in that they have strategies to avoid lysosomal degradation. Coevolution at the host-pathogen interface has enriched for mechanisms that allow intracellular pathogens to manipulate phagosome maturation and convert the host-derived compartment into a specialized organelle that supports replication. This specialized organelle is referred to as a pathogen-containing vacuole (PCV). Conversion of the nascent phagosome into a PCV is largely achieved by pathogen-directed subversion of host membrane transport.

Organelles and vesicles in the cell have a unique molecular signature that informs the identity and function of these membrane-bound compartments. These unique signatures are largely dictated by the selective recruitment of membrane-associated small GTPases and deposition of host lipids on the membrane surface. Consequently, these key modulators of the host endomembrane system are attractive targets for vacuole-bound pathogens. To avoid degradation, intracellular pathogens are faced with two options: lyse the phagosome in which they reside or remain in the vacuole. Bacterial pathogens that remain in the vacuole face a unique set of challenges. For example, how does the pathogen prevent phagosome-lysosome fusion and degradation? How can the pathogen modify the membrane-bound organelle to fulfill the nutritional and spatial demands required to support robust replication? Finally, how does the pathogen stabilize the dynamic PCV membrane and protect the newly generated vacuole

from dedicated immune surveillance mechanisms that seek to destroy it? In other words, vacuolar pathogens must alter the phagosome from a compartment that promotes microbial degradation to a specialized organelle that supports microbial replication. Understanding how pathogens subvert cellular functions is essential for uncovering microbial infection strategies and can also reveal the inner workings of host cells, and in doing so illuminate new cell biological mechanisms.

The aim of this chapter is to highlight common mechanisms that underlie vesicular transport and organelle function through the lens of bacterial pathogens that seek to subvert these pathways to alter the fate of the phagosome. For the purpose of this chapter, vacuolar bacterial pathogens are divided into two broad groups. The first group includes pathogens that occupy vacuoles that display similarities to organelles in the canonical endocytic pathway. Members of the second group create vacuoles that rapidly diverge from the canonical endocytic route, and this bifurcation is linked to extensive remodeling and hijacking of organelles and vesicles of the secretory pathway.

MEMBRANE TRANSPORT: A BRIEF OVERVIEW

Membrane transport directs the movement of cargo between cellular organelles and the extracellular environment. Membrane transport systems support essential processes, such as signaling, nutrient acquisition/metabolism, and innate and adaptive immunity. The endomembrane system is commonly subdivided into the endocytic pathway, which directs the transport of internalized cargo, and the secretory pathway, which directs the transport of cargo delivered into the endoplasmic reticulum (ER) membrane or lumen.

---

[1]Department of Microbial Pathogenesis, Yale University, New Haven, CT.

The endocytic pathway is characterized by the internalization of extracellular macromolecules (e.g., proteins and lipids), solutes, and receptor-ligand complexes into vesicles that are subsequently delivered to specific compartments in the cell (1). Through distinct molecular mechanisms, newly formed vesicles "pinch off" from the plasma membrane and transit to early endosomes, which serve as a sorting platform. The predominant mechanism that promotes internalization is clathrin-mediated endocytosis (1). The endocytosed cargo can then be shuttled to late endosomes and lysosomes to promote degradation, be recycled back to the plasma membrane, or interact with the trans-Golgi network (TGN). The subcellular localization of endocytic vesicles is largely dictated by the differential recruitment of small GTPases and the generation of unique phospholipid signatures on the vesicular membrane (2, 3).

The secretory pathway directs the synthesis and delivery of proteins and lipids to membrane-bound organelles, the plasma membrane, and the extracellular space. Newly synthesized proteins originate from the ER and transit to the Golgi apparatus in transport vesicles. ER-derived vesicles are subjected to modifications that are introduced in specific compartments within the Golgi apparatus. The modified cargo is then sorted and distributed to the plasma membrane or subcompartments within the cell.

Rab Proteins

Rab (Ras-related proteins in brain) proteins are a large family of small GTPases that play a central role in vesicle biogenesis, transport, docking, and fusion. The differential recruitment of Rab GTPases and their associated effector proteins to target membranes directs the coordination of vesicular traffic and contributes to membrane identity and function. At the molecular level, Rab proteins cycle between two conformational states: GDP bound (inactive) and GTP bound (active). Inactivated Rab proteins associate in a tightly bound cytoplasmic complex with Rab GDP disassociation inhibitors (GDI). Guanine nucleotide exchange factors (GEFs) (4) catalyze the exchange of GDP for GTP and stimulate conversion to the active GTP-bound form, which can associate with target membranes. Activated GTPases are then deactivated by GTPase-activating proteins (GAPs), which accelerate GTP hydrolysis to remove GDP-bound Rab proteins from the membrane (5). Thus, the Rab GTPase cycle functions as a molecular switch controlled by GEFs and GAPs, which orchestrate the association and retrieval of GTP-bound Rabs from distinct membranes.

Rab5 recruitment is the earliest step in endosome maturation and is highly enriched on the surface of early endosomes (6). Following uptake, Rab5-positive phagosomes activate signaling mechanisms that promote the recruitment of Rab5 effector proteins to initiate downstream maturation events. As the phagosome matures, Rab5 is deactivated by host GAPs and extracted from these compartments. The dissociation of Rab5 is coordinated with the activation and recruitment of Rab7 to membranes; thus, Rab7 is highly enriched on the membrane of the late endosome (7). The coordinated exchange of Rab proteins on maturing vesicles is called Rab conversion. The spatial and temporal regulation of Rab conversion must be maintained in order to promote proper maturation of newly formed endosomes and direct these vesicles to the lysosome and other compartments in the cell.

Phosphoinositides

Phospholipid signatures on endosomal membranes direct endosomal maturation by contributing to the identity and fate of maturing endosomes. Phosphatidylinositol phosphate (PIP) species are generated by dedicated kinases and phosphatases that reversibly introduce a phosphate group at positions 3, 4, and 5 of the inositol ring. These reactions can generate seven distinct PIP species that are enriched on specific membranes in the cell. For example, phosphatidylinositol 4,5-bisphosphate [PI(4,5)P2] is enriched on the plasma membrane, and phosphatidylinositol 3-phosphate [PI(3)P] is an abundant marker on nascent phagosomes and early endosomes (8). Chemical alterations to the phosphoinositide pattern on the surface of host vesicles or membranes can drastically redirect the functional properties and transport of these compartments (3, 9). Proteins that modulate specific membrane transport events typically contain binding domains that recognize specific PIP signatures that mediate recruitment to vesicles to promote membrane transport and fusion (3).

The ER Regulates Protein Synthesis and Secretion

The ER is a large membranous network of tubules and flattened sacs, or cisternae, that extend from the nuclear membrane. In mammalian cells, the ER generates the majority of host proteins and lipids that comprise the endomembrane system and sustain organelle biogenesis and maintenance. Newly synthesized proteins and lipids are assembled in the ER, where molecular chaperones assist in protein folding and maturation, including posttranslational modifications (PTMs). Modified proteins are then packaged into vesicles that bud from the ER membrane and are shuttled to the Golgi apparatus. Vesicle budding and transport from the ER is mediated by a family of evolutionarily conserved proteins called coat protein complex II (COPII). COPII-coated vesicles capture proteins from ER exit sites (ERES) and deliver the cargo to the ER-Golgi intermediate compartment in a process that is regulated by the Sar1 family of GTPases (10), while retrograde transport of COPI-coated vesicles is regulated by the Arf family of GTPases (11, 12). Proteins of the membrane fusion machinery, named SNAREs (soluble *N*-ethylmaleimide-sensitive factor attachment protein receptors), drive the fusion of vesicles with target organelles. SNAREs regulate the docking and fusion of vesicles with target membranes (13). They are commonly divided into two classes: vesicle SNAREs (v-SNAREs) and target SNAREs (t-SNAREs). v-SNAREs on ER-derived vesicles pair with t-SNAREs on the *cis*-Golgi to promote fusion and subsequent delivery of the cargo into the Golgi apparatus lumen. The pairing of v-SNAREs with cognate t-SNAREs is an important event that completes the final stages of host membrane transport (14). As cargo (e.g., proteins) transits along the Golgi apparatus stacks, it is subjected to additional layers of processing before being released and delivered to the plasma membrane or specific sites in the cell. Rab GTPases are essential regulators of this process, as their association with distinct organelles or vesicles in the cell dictates the transport and fusion events in the endomembrane system. In particular, Rab1 has been implicated as being integral for ER-Golgi vesicular traffic (15). Collectively, the activities of small GTPases (Rabs, Arf, and Sar), phospholipids, and SNAREs ensure the fidelity of vesicular transport between acceptor and donor membranes in the cell.

The Golgi Apparatus Sorts and Delivers Vesicles to Subcellular Compartments

The Golgi apparatus comprises many polarized cisternae that are named relative to their position to the ER. Following protein synthesis, ER-derived vesicles interface with the *cis*-Golgi and then progress through the medial Golgi membrane network and the TGN and finally exit through the TGN in a process named cisternal progression. As proteins transit through the membranous Golgi apparatus stacks, they may be modified before they are released to their final destination (e.g., addition of sugar side chains). Cisternal progression culminates at the TGN, where proteins can be delivered to either the plasma membrane or endocytic organelles. Small GTPases, such as members of the Rab family, modulate the transport and fusion of vesicles within this dynamic compartment. For example, Rab1 is required for ER-to-Golgi vesicle transport (15), and Rab6 and Rab14 have been implicated as regulators of Golgi-to-endosome

transport (16, 17). Phosphatidylinositol 4-phosphate (PI4P) and proteins involved in P14P metabolism are very abundant on Golgi membranes (18, 19). P14P mediates distinct stages of vesicular transport, including recruitment of coat proteins that decorate secretory vesicles (20). Small GTPases and Golgi membrane-associated lipids, such as PI4P, regulate the transport of exocytic vesicles from the TGN to specific membranes in the cell.

PHAGOCYTOSIS

Phagocytosis is a form of endocytosis that refers to cellular uptake of large particles, and the organelle containing these particles is often referred to as a phagosome (8). The nascent phagosome undergoes a maturation process to convert the inner space, or lumen, into a degradative compartment. This process is marked by progressive acidification of the luminal space and the delivery of hydrolytic enzymes, which initiate the breakdown of substrates trapped in the lumen. The maturing phagosome transits along the endocytic pathway that leads to the primary degradative organelle in the cell, the lysosome. The lysosome contains hydrolytic enzymes and microbicidal compounds in a low-pH environment; this harsh environment degrades most protein substrates. Once the phagosome fuses with the lysosome and the degradation process is complete, the metabolic by-products are either recycled or repurposed to maintain cellular homeostasis. As such, phagocytosis is an indispensable component of the immune response that eliminates bacteria, viruses, or parasites that attempt to infect the cell (21).

Professional phagocytes are a class of dedicated cells that are specifically equipped to recognize and digest large substrates (e.g., dead cells and foreign material) and microorganisms. Once microorganisms are digested, professional phagocytes can use the degraded material to produce antigenic peptides that activate more complex mechanisms of the immune response (22). Phagosome maturation can be divided into three broad stages: (i) recognition and engulfment, (ii) acidification of the phagosome, and (iii) lysosomal fusion. Internalization can occur through nonspecific receptors, such as scavenger reporters, lectins, and integrins, that recognize signatures on ligands and initiate their uptake. In contrast, particles that are coated in specific proteins, or opsonized, selectively pair with cognate receptors on the cell surface in order to gain entry (e.g., complement receptors and Fcγ receptors) (21). Once internalization is initiated, the plasma membrane extends over the bacterial surface through rearrangement of the actin cytoskeleton and generates a phagosome that encompasses the bacteria. As the phagosome seals, recruitment of Rab GTPases and PI species trigger downstream signaling pathways that work in concert to convert the immature phagosome into an acidic organelle.

The hallmark of phagosome maturation is acidification. Through a series of fusion and fission events, the maturing phagosome interacts with early and late endosomes, in a process similar to endocytic maturation. The cell furnishes the newly formed phagosome with a small GTPase, Rab5, to promote localization of Rab5 effectors that extend the maturation process (6). Specifically, Rab5-positive phagosomes recruit a PI3-kinase, hVPS34, which generates a PI3P-rich compartment (23). The enrichment of PI3P on the phagosomal membrane serves as an anchor for PI3P-binding proteins, such as early endosome antigen 1 (EEA1), that regulate the fusion of early endosomes and immature phagosomes (8). Additionally, phagosomes recycle substrates to the plasma membrane, and the retrieval of these molecules may involve components of the retromer complex (e.g., sorting nexins), the coatomer, and small GTPases (24). The pH of this compartment must be lowered in order to begin the digestion process and activate resident hydrolases, which also aid in the degradation process (8). Through the activity of vacuolar ATPases, hydrogen ions are pumped across the phagosomal membrane, leading to an overall decrease in pH. This multisubunit complex is delivered to the phagosome membrane through a tightly orchestrated process (25).

The late phagosome can be characterized by Rab7 localization and the recruitment of additional effectors, such as Rab-interacting lysosomal protein (RILP), mannose-6-phosphate receptors (MPRs), and lysosome-associated membrane protein 1 (LAMP-1). RILP is a Rab7 effector that mobilizes dynein and dynactin to shuttle late phagosomes to the juxtanuclear region to promote phagosome-lysosome fusion (26, 27). MPRs deliver lysosomal enzymes to early endosomes and are enriched in late endosomes, and the proteins LAMP-1 and LAMP-2 maintain lysosomal integrity (28). The phagosome fuses with the lysosome to generate a specialized organelle called the phagolysosome. The phagolysosome completes the digestion and degradation process that was initiated in the phagocytic vacuole. This step marks the "point of no return" for pathogens that have been ingested and transited along this pathway. It is the harsh and inhospitable environment of the lysosome that makes phagocytosis an effective strategy to restrict bacterial replication and protect the cell.

The underlying mechanisms that regulate phagosome maturation are highly coordinated and complex.

Although many host factors are required for this process to run smoothly, important modulators of phagosomal maturation are Rab GTPases, phosphoinositides, and the membrane fusion machinery (e.g., SNAREs). Consequently, Rab proteins and phosphoinositides are attractive targets for bacterial pathogens that are internalized by phagocytic cells. Pathogens restricted to the phagosome have a small window to redirect the fate of the phagosome and avoid lysosomal destruction. By inhibiting, activating, or interfering with the signaling mechanisms of small GTPases and PIs, these bacterial pathogens can subvert membrane transport pathways and convert the phagosome into a nondegradative niche.

PCVs THAT RESIDE IN THE ENDOCYTIC PATHWAY

Canonical endocytic maturation involves progressive acidification of the maturing phagosome followed by lysosomal fusion. The sequential recruitment of Rab proteins and their effectors controls the acidification of maturing phagosomes and dynamic fusion with host vesicles and organelles. As phagosomes transit along the canonical route, the cell furnishes each compartment with a unique phospholipid signature that partially dictates the fate of the phagosome. Thus, the activities of activated Rab proteins and membrane-associated lipids define vesicular identity, function, and fate. Consequently, these molecules are prime targets for vacuolar pathogens that actively remodel the host-derived vacuole and alter preprogrammed delivery of the phagosome to the lysosome.

Subversion of Phosphoinositide Metabolism

Rab5 recruits hVPS34, a class III PI3-kinase that generates PI3P (8). As the nascent phagosome is converted into a functional degradative organelle, PI3P is the predominant phospholipid species that drives the maturation process and is required for phagolysosome biogenesis. Intracellular pathogens modify membrane-associated lipids, such as PI3P, to avoid lysosome-mediated degradation of the early phagosome. By modulating PI3P levels on the phagosomal surface, intracellular pathogens can directly orchestrate maturation and transport events of the early phagosome, thus avoiding lysosomal fusion and initiating early events linked to PCV biogenesis.

Mycobacterium tuberculosis causes a severe and potentially fatal infection of the lungs called tuberculosis. Local infection begins in alveolar macrophages, where phagocytosed *M. tuberculosis* bacilli remain in immature phagosomes that fail to fuse with acidified endosomes or lysosomes. *M. tuberculosis* has evolved many effector-mediated mechanisms to prevent phagosome maturation and persist in an early-endosome-like vacuole, and this activity is mediated by the ESX-1 secretion system (29). Although early endosomes are PI3P rich, the *Mycobacterium*-containing vacuole (MCV) membrane has significantly reduced levels of P13P (30). *M. tuberculosis* impairs PI3P accumulation by releasing a lipid called mannose-capped lipoarabinomannan that inserts into the phagosome membrane. This lipid interferes with Ca^{2+}-dependent signaling events that are required to activate the PI3-kinase hVPS34, which is required for PI3P production on nascent phagosomes (30, 31). When hVPS34 activity is inhibited, PI3P abundance on the MCV is severely reduced, and PI3P-binding proteins fail to accumulate on the MCV membrane (32, 33).

Pathogens that disconnect from the endocytic pathway, such as *Legionella pneumophila*, also arrest phagosomal maturation at very early stages and exploit PI3P-regulatory proteins to avoid degradation. For example, *L. pneumophila*-containing phagosomes do not recruit Rab5 or the late-endosomal markers Rab7 and LAMP-1 and -2. One mechanism that contributes to avoidance of endocytic maturation involves the effector protein VipD, which interferes with endosomal trafficking by mediating PI3P depletion by a Rab5-dependent mechanism (34). Additionally, the effector protein AnkX appears to be important for endocytic avoidance, as *ankX* mutants have a defect in preventing endocytic proteins such as LAMP-2 from being acquired on the vacuole (35, 36).

Mycobacterium also evades endocytic maturation by secreting a phosphatase called SapM that dephosphorylates PI3P (30). A recent study demonstrated that *sapM* mutants cannot resist phagosome-lysosome fusion and are readily degraded (37). Through the concerted action of proteins and lipids that target PIP species, *Mycobacterium* alters the biophysical properties of the phagosome to stall maturation and support MCV biogenesis. Conversely, *Salmonella enterica* serovar Typhimurium creates a compartment that interacts more extensively with the endocytic pathway by increasing PI3P levels to create a vacuole with properties of a late endosome. Vacuoles containing salmonellae mature significantly along the standard endocytic route and acquire late-endosome markers, such as Rab7 and LAMP-1 and -2 (38, 39). Mature *Salmonella*-containing vacuoles (SCVs) maintain high levels of PI3P on the membrane surface, and enrichment of PI3P on the SCV membrane is mediated by the *Salmonella* effector protein SopB (40, 41). Following secretion, SopB is anchored to the SCV membrane and functions as a PI phosphatase that in-

creases PI3P abundance to maintain Rab5 association and prevent lysosomal fusion. During infection, SopB phosphatase activity indirectly promotes the recruitment of the Rab5 effector hVPS34, a kinase that generates PI3P (42). SopB has also been implicated in reducing the overall negative charge of the membrane by consuming PIP2 species. Evidence suggests that manipulating the membrane charge may also prevent phagosome-lysosome fusion and SCV degradation (43–45).

Exclusion and Manipulation of Rab GTPases

Vacuolar pathogens that remain associated with the canonical endocytic pathway are trapped in phagosomes that immediately engage in this preprogrammed degradation process. To avoid lysosomal destruction, these pathogens manipulate Rab proteins to alter the "signature" on the host-derived vesicle to prevent lysosomal degradation (Fig. 1). A common theme involves effector-mediated mechanisms that selectively recruit or prevent the recruitment of specific Rab proteins to the surface of the PCV. This creates a unique Rab signature that allows these well-adapted pathogens to stall phagosomal maturation and create a nondegradative organelle. Similarly, pathogens that disconnect from the endocytic route must also possess effector-mediated mechanisms to avoid lysosomal degradation (Fig. 2). By manipulating Rab recruitment and retention, these pathogens can also direct the recruitment of Rabs that do not conventionally interact with maturing phagosomes. These pathogens exploit the conserved role of Rab GTPases to create atypical Rab signatures on the PCV membrane, which provides specialized access to vesicles, organelles, and pathways in the cell.

The differential recruitment of Rab proteins to the MCV surface locks this compartment in an immature state (46). The MCV is functionally analogous to an early endosome, because this compartment does not acidify or fuse with endosomal organelles. Consequently, late-endosome markers like Rab7 are not detected on the MCV surface, while the canonical early-endosome marker Rab5 accumulates on the MCV membrane (30, 47–49). Independent studies confirm that *M. tuberculosis* inhibits Rab5-to-Rab7 conversion on the MCV membrane, thus trapping this compartment in an undifferentiated state. Additionally, *M. tuberculosis* maintains Rab22a on the MCV membrane to inhibit Rab5-to-Rab7 conversion. In the absence of Rab22a, *M. tuberculosis* vacuoles progress along the endocytic pathway and are destroyed (49).

In contrast, *Salmonella* interferes with Rab GTPases that modulate late events in the phagocytic maturation process to create vacuoles with features of late

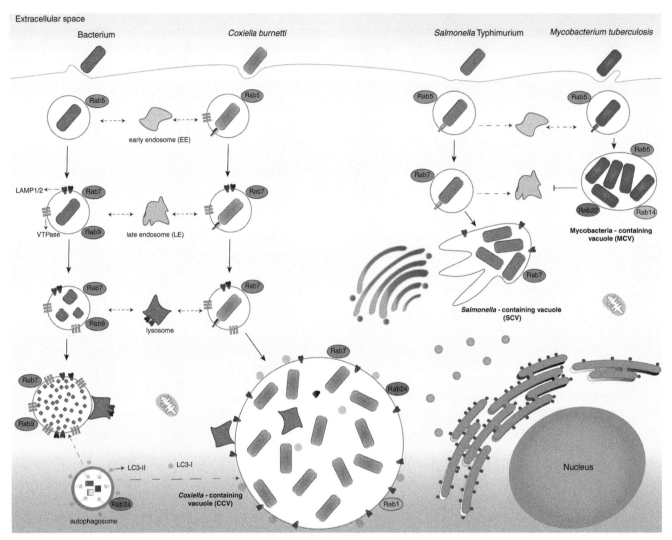

Figure 1　Rab GTPase signature of PCVs that interact with the endocytic pathway. The figure depicts canonical phagocytosis, with a subset of intracellular pathogens that manipulate endosomal traffic to avoid lysosomal degradation. When professional phagocytes recognize bacteria, local rearrangement of the actin cytoskeleton allows the plasma membrane to form protrusions that engulf bacterial cells into a host-derived membrane called the phagosome. Nascent phagosomes transiently interact with early and late endosomes to convert this compartment into an acidic and microbicidal organelle. The early-endosomal marker Rab5 associates with newly formed phagosomes, and as maturation progresses, Rab5 is displaced by the late-endosomal marker Rab7. This process culminates with lysosomal fusion, which generates a hybrid organelle called the phagolysosome that promotes complete degradation of phagocytosed bacteria. Following uptake, *M. tuberculosis* interacts with early endosomes but immediately stalls maturation to avoid acidification of the MCV. *M. tuberculosis* suspends normal transit along the endocytic route by interfering with the conversion of Rab5 to Rab7 on the MCV membrane. Consequently, by arresting the development of phagosomes during early stages of uptake, the MCV retains features of an early-endosome-like compartment and avoids delivery to the lysosome. Additionally, Rab22a and Rab14 have been detected on *M. tuberculosis* vacuoles. In contrast, the SCV transits further down the endocytic route and interacts with both early and late endosomes. The conventional (early- and late-endosome) Rab GTPases Rab5 and Rab7 localize to mature SCVs along with the late-endosome marker LAMP-1/2. Mature SCVs are dynamic compartments that closely resemble late endosomes. Unlike *Mycobacterium* and *Salmonella*, *C. burnetii* does not resist delivery to the lysosome. *C. burnetii* vacuoles progress along the standard endocytic route in a process that closely resembles canonical phagocytosis, and these compartments display many markers that associate with mature phagosomes, such as Rab5, Rab7, and LAMP-1. Delivery to the lysosome activates the T4SS machinery and triggers effector-mediated mechanisms that drastically alter properties of the lysosome and support biogenesis of the CCV. *Coxiella* repurposes the lysosome into a phenotypically distinct lysosome-derived organelle that participates in unregulated fusion events in an autophagy-dependent manner. Interestingly, additional Rab GTPases that have been linked to the autophagy pathway, Rab1 and Rab24, have been shown to contribute to *Coxiella* replication.

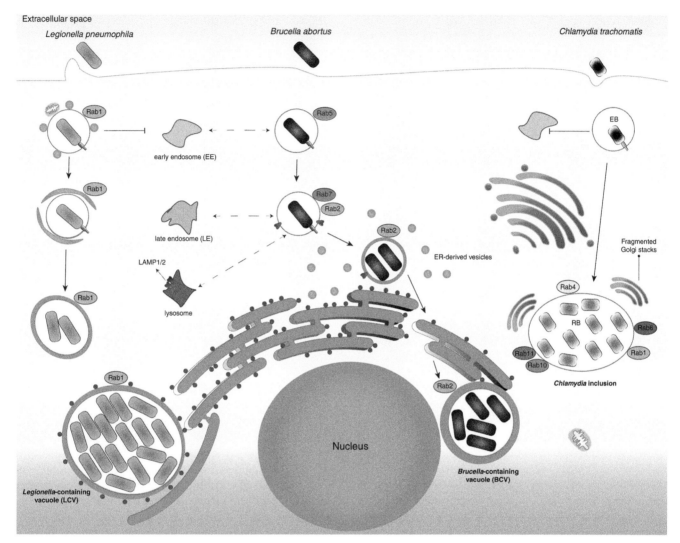

Figure 2 Rab GTPase signature of PCVs that diverge from the endocytic pathway and manipulate the pathway. The figure depicts a class of intracellular pathogens that not only avoid lysosomal degradation but also disconnect from the standard endocytic route and extensively manipulate secretory traffic. Once internalized, these pathogens manipulate Rab GTPases to create a unique molecular signature on the phagosomal membrane. Consequently, this signature rewrites the function of the original phagosome and allows each pathogen to exploit host membrane transport of secretory organelles (ER and Golgi apparatus) and their associated vesicles. As such, the atypical recruitment and association of Rab GTPases on each PCV membrane provides insight into the organelles that are hijacked and exploited for PCV biogenesis and maintenance. The *Legionella*-containing phagosome disassociates from the endocytic pathway very early after uptake, as the early-endosome marker Rab5 is not detected on this compartment. However, Rab1, an ER-associated Rab GTPase, is recruited to the *Legionella*-containing vacuole (LCV) following internalization. The localization of activated Rab1 on the LCV membrane allows this pathogen to hijack ER-derived vesicles and redirect them to the LCV surface. As the infection proceeds, the LCV matures into a ribosome-studded organelle that communicates extensively with the ER. Similar to *Legionella*, *B. abortus* remodels the phagosome into an ER-like organelle. In contrast, the BCV does not acquire Rab1 to hijack vesicles from ERES. Instead, the recruitment of Rab2 to the BCV is required to subvert ER-Golgi traffic and support BCV biogenesis. *C. trachomatis* is initially phagocytosed as an elementary body (EB), which represents the metabolically inactive and infectious form of the biphasic cycle. As the infection progresses, the EB differentiates into the metabolically active and replicative form termed the reticulate body (RB). The specialized organelle that supports *Chlamydia* replication, named the inclusion, is largely devoid of endocytic Rabs, including Rab5, Rab7, and Rab9. This indicates that *Chlamydia* divergence from the endocytic route is an early and rapid event. A wide assortment of Rab GTPases are recruited to the inclusion membrane, such as Rab1, Rab4, Rab6, Rab11, and Rab14. A hallmark of *Chlamydia* intracellular infection is the presence of fragmented Golgi stacks that surround the inclusion.

endosomes. Following uptake, the SCV colocalizes with proteins found on early endosomes (EEA1 and Rab5) and late endosomes (Rab7 and LAMP-1 and -2) (38, 39). Recruitment of late-endosome proteins also correlates with functional features associated with late endosomes, such as low pH. The mature SCV, however, is morphologically distinct from lysosomes, as hydrolytic enzymes such as the cathepsins are not delivered to this compartment (50, 51).

Given the importance of Rab GTPases in the regulation of host membrane transport, it is not surprising that vacuolar pathogens like *Salmonella* have evolved mechanisms to activate, inhibit, or redistribute these master regulators of vesicular transport. Intracellular survival relies on the expression of two type III secretion systems (T3SSs) named *Salmonella* pathogenicity islands 1 and 2 (52). Both these pathogenicity islands mediate the delivery of bacterial effectors into the host cytoplasm and contribute to SCV biogenesis and maintenance (52). One of the most striking examples of Rab manipulation is mediated by the *S.* Typhimurium effector GtgE, which is a cysteine protease that cleaves Rab29 and the closely related proteins Rab32 and Rab38 to prevent accumulation of these Rab proteins on the SCV (53, 54). Rab32 participates in the assembly of lysosome-related organelles (55) and promotes the fusion of vesicles that contain antimicrobial peptides (56). Therefore, GtgE-dependent cleavage of Rab32 protects *Salmonella* from being killed by the host cell (57).

To prevent the phagosome from maturing into a degradative compartment, *Salmonella* interferes with additional Rabs that may contribute to late-endosome maturation. During late stages of maturation, membrane tubules named *Salmonella*-induced filaments (Sifs) extend from the cytoplasmic face of mature SCVs and assemble into a dynamic tubular network (58). Sif formation is induced by the T3SS effector protein SifA, which interacts with the host protein SKIP (SifA and kinesin-interacting protein) to modulate the levels of kinesin on the SCV surface (59, 60). SifA mutants accumulate high levels of kinesin on the SCV membrane, and this enhanced enrichment compromises membrane integrity and is rapidly followed by SCV rupture (60, 61). Similar to GtgE, SifA may indirectly interfere with biogenesis of lysosome-related organelles. The SifA-SKIP complex recruits Rab9 to the SCV surface (60), and Rab9 is required for the retrograde transport of MPRs, which deliver hydrolytic enzymes to maturing lysosomes. This suggests that by forming a stable complex with Rab9, SifA indirectly antagonizes the delivery of degradative enzymes to SCVs. SifA is also required for vacuole integrity and is discussed below (see "Maintenance of the PCV").

Extensive Interactions with the Lysosome

Phagocytosis is a highly conserved innate immune response, and under the burden of selective pressure, intracellular pathogens have evolved diverse strategies with a common goal: avoiding lysosomal degradation. However, the intracellular pathogen *Coxiella burnetii* is an exception to this rule. Although most intracellular pathogens are killed if the vacuole fuses with lysosomes, *C. burnetii* requires lysosomal fusion to create the acidified vacuole in which it replicates (62, 63). After uptake, the *Coxiella*-containing vacuole (CCV) transits along the endocytic pathway and acquires the canonical endocytic markers Rab5 and Rab7 (Fig. 1) (64, 65). In fact, interfering with the function of Rab5 or Rab7 disrupts CCV biogenesis and restricts *Coxiella* intracellular replication (66, 67). This indicates that *C. burnetii* phagosomes progress along the standard endocytic route and that canonical Rab GTPases must be recruited to promote lysosome delivery (67–69). After fusion with the lysosome, the low pH within the CCV promotes bacterial metabolism and activates the Dot/Icm T4SS, which promotes the delivery of over 100 different effector proteins into the host cell that are essential for remodeling of the lysosome-derived CCV.

As *C. burnetii* replicates, the CCV expands into a spacious organelle that occupies the majority of the cytoplasmic space. CCV expansion correlates with promiscuous fusion between this organelle and most endocytic organelles in the cell. High levels of cholesterol are present on the CCV membrane, in contrast to conventional lysosomes, which typically display low levels of cholesterol (65). Although the CCV is phenotypically distinct from conventional lysosomes, it is highly enriched for lysosomal proteins such as LAMP-1, LAMP-2, LAMP-3, and vacuolar ATPases (70, 71). Effector proteins work synergistically to modulate host membrane transport and maintain the CCV in a highly fusogenic state. Interfering with *C. burnetii* protein synthesis after formation of the spacious CCV will cause the vacuole to shrink, which indicates that the bacteria must continually modulate host membrane transport to maintain this specialized organelle.

Autophagy is an evolutionarily conserved process that delivers cytoplasmic substrates to the lysosome for degradation. Under nutrient-limiting conditions, double-membrane vesicles called preautophagosomal structures are synthesized and deployed by the cell to sequester cytoplasmic cargo (72). The inner and outer membranes of mature autophagosomes are decorated with the lipidated form of the autophagy protein LC3-II (microtubule-associated light chain 3B). Conjugation of LC3 to maturing autophagosomes is required for proper autophagosome biogenesis and function (73). Once cytoplasmic cargo is captured in sealed autophagosomes, the mature autophagosome fuses with lysosomes to digest the cargo and generate a hybrid organelle called an autolysosome.

As vacuoles containing *Coxiella* mature, the protein LC3 is detected in the lumen of the CCV, which indicates that autophagosomes have fused with these pathogen-containing organelles (67, 74, 75). Early studies demonstrating the association of LC3 with the CCV suggested that autophagy was important for *Coxiella* replication (65, 74). Recent studies using host cells deficient in proteins essential for autophagy indicate that a functional autophagy system is not essential for *Coxiella* replication (67). However, autophagy does play a critical role in CCV biogenesis by promoting homotypic fusion of the this compartment with other lysosome-derived organelles in the cell (75). In the context of infection, homotypic fusion is defined as the fusion of multiple CCVs derived independently in an infected cell to create a single large acidic organelle. The *Coxiella* effector protein Cig2 is essential for this homotypic fusion process. Host cells infected with a *cig2* mutant strain of *Coxiella* display multiple tight-fitting CCVs late in the infection process rather than the single CCV displayed by cells infected with a wild-type strain. Vacuoles containing the *cig2* mutant do not accumulate the autophagy protein LC3. Thus, the ability of Cig2 to promote fusion of autophagosomes with the CCV appears to be essential for homotypic fusion of the vacuole. This strongly suggests that Cig2 locks the CCV in a state that resembles an autolysosome and that this organelle is receptive to constitutive fusion with other vesicles in the endolysosomal pathway. In addition, the protein Rab24, which has been linked to the autophagy pathway, has been implicated as being important for *Coxiella* replication, which suggests a possible role for this host factor in Cig2-mediated formation of this autolysosomal organelle (76–78).

Similar to *Coxiella*, the intracellular pathogen *Brucella* allows considerable maturation of the phagosome along the endocytic pathway and requires phagosome acidification to energize a T4SS called VirB. *Brucella abortus* is the etiological agent of brucellosis, which causes abortion and sterility in animals and severe chronic disease accompanied by fever in humans (79). Following uptake, *Brucella*-containing vacuoles (BCVs) transiently recruit early endosome proteins such as Rab5 and EEA1 (80–83). As the BCV matures, it acquires late-endosome proteins such as Rab7, LAMP-1, CD63, and the Rab7 effector RILP (80, 83–85). However, BCVs do not appear to fuse with lysosomes; rather, these pathogens exclude lysosomal-degradative enzymes through a poorly understood mechanism (80, 83). Transient interactions with acidified endosomes are required to activate VirB-mediated effector translocation and BCV biogenesis, as *virB* mutants are not able to establish infection (86). As the BCV matures, it eventually disconnects from the endocytic network, and the bacteria enter an ER-derived compartment that supports intracellular replication. Thus, in the case of *Brucella*, divergence from the endocytic continuum and direct manipulation of the secretory pathway represents another strategy employed by intracellular pathogens to convert the phagosome into a specialized organelle.

DIVERGENCE FROM THE ENDOCYTIC PATHWAY AND MANIPULATION OF THE SECRETORY PATHWAY

Following internalization, some pathogens reside in vacuoles that disconnect from the endocytic pathway and subvert host membrane transport in the secretory pathway. Although divergence from the endocytic pathway protects a pathogen from lysosomal degradation, there are challenges associated with this adaptation. PCVs that branch off from the endocytic pathway must still acquire membranes for vacuole expansion. A common strategy used by these pathogens is to modulate and manipulate the transport and fusion of vesicles in the host secretory pathway. Successful bifurcation from the endocytic pathway accompanied by extensive interactions with secretory organelles confers many advantages for a vacuolar pathogen. First, converting the nascent phagosome into a compartment that resembles an organelle in the secretory pathway can provide protection from immune surveillance systems in the cell that detect bacterial determinants in the lumens of endocytic organelles. Second, vesicles that emerge from the secretory pathway contain cargo such as proteins and lipids that can be used for bacterial replication.

Intracellular pathogens such as *L. pneumophila*, *B. abortus*, and *Chlamydia trachomatis* occupy vacuoles that diverge from the endocytic pathway, and these pathogens have the capacity to convert phagosomes into organelles that are more similar to the host ER or Golgi apparatus. How does a phagosome destined for degradation get converted into an ER-derived organelle that supports replication? Investigating how these pathogens manipulate host traffic to meet the challenges of intracellular life should reveal more about these fundamental cell biological pathways. Furthermore, by defining the biochemical function of bacterial effectors, novel cellular pathways that occur at the host-pathogen interface may be revealed.

Hijacking the ER and ER-Derived Vesicles

L. pneumophila is an intracellular pathogen commonly found in freshwater environments, where the bacteria replicate inside protozoan hosts. When *L. pneumophila* infects human macrophages, it is capable of replicating intracellularly by hijacking highly conserved and ancient pathways in the cell, which can result in a severe pneumonia called Legionnaires' disease (87). In order to establish a successful infection, *Legionella* encodes a T4SS termed Dot/Icm that translocates over 300 different effector proteins into the host cytosol (88, 89). The delivery of effector proteins is required to convert the *Legionella*-containing phagosomes into unique ER-like organelles that support intracellular replication. Within minutes of uptake, phagosome maturation is arrested and *L. pneumophila* effectors promote the rapid recruitment of ER-derived vesicles to the phagosome surface. Early studies demonstrate that canonical early (Rab5)- and late (Rab7 and LAMP)-endosomal proteins are not recruited to phagosomes harboring *Legionella* (90, 91). This demonstrates that bifurcation from the endocytic pathway is a very early event that occurs once the pathogen is internalized and that evasion of endocytic maturation prevents vacuole acidification (92). A functional Dot/Icm apparatus is required to prevent phagosome maturation and avoid lysosome-mediated death (35).

L. pneumophila subverts host membrane traffic from the secretory pathway to transform the nascent phagosome into an ER-like compartment called the *Legionella*-containing vacuole (LCV). In early morphological studies, ribosomes were detected on the cytoplasmic surface of the mature LCV (93). Independent studies have also confirmed the recruitment and localization of resident ER proteins calnexin and glucose-6-phosphatase to the LCV (94, 95). LCV biogenesis is a complex process that requires the concerted action of over 300 effector proteins that subvert host functions. Although this process is not completely understood, it is clear that extensive remodeling of the LCV is a prerequisite for intracellular replication. *Legionella* encodes dedicated effectors that mediate the retrieval of ER membranes and recruitment of ER vesicles to the LCV surface (35). Perhaps the most striking examples are *L. pneumophila*-encoded effectors that target host GTPases that regulate ER homeostasis and membrane transport in the secretory pathway.

During early stages of infection, small GTPases that regulate secretory traffic are recruited to the LCV. The host GTPase Rab1 is recruited to the vacuole membrane by the *Legionella* effector DrrA (also called SidM) (Fig. 2) (96, 97). DrrA functions as a Rab1 GEF that stimulates the GDP-to-GTP exchange to activate Rab1 (98). Activated Rab1 is capable of interacting with host tethering factors that bind ER-derived vesicles, and thus, DrrA-mediated activation of Rab1 is one mechanism by which ER vesicle recruitment to the LCV is promoted (99, 100). DrrA has a strong affinity for GDP-bound Rab1, and this is sufficient to displace Rab1-GDP from the Rab-GDI, which removes inactive Rab1 from membranes (101, 102). Thus, DrrA can directly promote Rab1 association with the LCV by coordinating the dissociation of GDI and exchange of GDP for GTP on the Rab1 protein.

Once Rab1 is recruited to the vacuole by DrrA, there are two effectors that can posttranslationally modify Rab1. The amino-terminal region of the DrrA protein has an adenylyl transferase domain that can use ATP as a substrate to add an AMP residue to the switch region of Rab1, which is a PTM known as AMPylation (103, 104). A *Legionella* effector called AnkX contains a FIC domain that can use CDP-choline as a substrate to transfer phosphorylcholine to the switch region of Rab1 (105–107). These PTMs make Rab1 resistant to deactivation by GAPs. The effector proteins SidD and Lem3 are deAMPylating and dephosphocholinating enzymes, respectively, and are responsible for removing the PTM to Rab1, which allows Rab1 to cycle off the vacuole membrane at later stages of infection (106, 108–110). Lastly, *L. pneumophila* exerts an additional layer of Rab1 modulation through the activity of LepB, which is a Rab1 GAP (111). LepB contributes to the removal of Rab1 from the LCV during the late stages of LCV biogenesis.

The small GTPase Arf1 plays a highly conserved role in vesicle transport and fusion between ER and Golgi membranes and regulates the formation of COPI-coated vesicles (12). Similar to Rab1, Arf1 is activated and recruited during early stages of LCV biogenesis. Arf-GEF proteins typically contain a conserved Sec7 domain that catalyzes the nucleotide exchange reaction (12). Similarly, the *L. pneumophila* effector RalF contains a Sec7 domain and functions as an Arf1-GEF to recruit GTP-bound Arf1 to the maturing LCV membrane (112, 113). In addition, Sar1, a small GTPase that is an essential regulator of ER vesicle budding and fusion, participates in early LCV biogenesis events. Sar1 is required for the generation of COPII-coated vesicles from ERES, and depletion of Sar1 in *L. pneumophila*-infected cells restricts replication (99, 114). Furthermore, when Sar1 function is compromised, ER-derived vesicles scavenged from the ERES fail to fuse with mature LCVs (95).

Similarly, *Brucella* spp. interact extensively with the ER and ER-derived vesicles to promote BCV biogenesis. Sar1 contributes to BCV maturation, which suggests that COPII-coated vesicles that emanate from the ERES are selectively recruited to this compartment (115). BCVs also recruit ER-associated small GTPases to drive interactions with the ER. Specifically, Rab2 is recruited to the BCV surface (116) by a process that requires the type IV effector protein RicA (117). RicA strongly interacts with GDP-bound Rab2, and *ricA* mutants display reduced recruitment of Rab2 to the BCV during infection (117). However, RicA does not possess detectable GEF activity, so the mechanisms that promote RicA-mediated recruitment of Rab2 are unclear.

A hallmark of LCV maturation is the fusion of ER-derived vesicles with the LCV membrane. The host protein Sec22b is a SNARE protein that is important for the fusion of ER-derived vesicles with the Golgi membrane (118). Sec22b associates with ER vesicles that are recruited to the LCV, and recent studies suggest that noncanonical pairing of Sec22b with plasma membrane SNAREs promotes vesicle tethering and fusion events on the LCV membrane (119, 120). However, the precise mechanisms that mediate vesicle fusion on the LCV surface have not been resolved. Through effector-mediated remodeling of early phagosome membranes, *L. pneumophila* communicates extensively with the ER to recruit ER-derived vesicles that eventually fuse to the LCV surface. ER-remodeled vacuoles transit to the ER lumen and are incorporated into this nutrient-rich organelle, thus providing an ideal environment for *Legionella* replication and vacuole expansion.

Subversion of the Golgi Apparatus and Golgi Apparatus-Derived Vesicles

C. trachomatis extensively interacts with the Golgi apparatus by co-opting host proteins to sequester TGN-derived vesicles to create a replication-permissive organelle called the inclusion. *C. trachomatis* causes a wide range of diseases in humans. The most prevalent sites of infection include colonization of the genital tract, which can lead to more serious symptoms, such as infertility (121). *Chlamydia* cycles between two morphologically distinct lifestyles characterized by the infectious elementary body and the noninfectious reticulate body. When the metabolically inactive elementary body is internalized by phagocytes, the nascent phagosome does not mature along the standard endocytic route. *C. trachomatis* delivers proteins into the host cytoplasm through a T3SS to avoid lysosomal degradation and converts the immature phagosome into the inclusion. The inclusion membrane is unique because it does not possess host receptors or proteins that are normally found on phagosomes (122), including canonical endocytic Rab GTPases (e.g., Rab5, Rab7, and Rab9) (123). Many of the effector proteins secreted by *Chlamydia* are called Inc proteins because they remain intimately associated with the inclusion membrane and are involved in remodeling of this unique compartment. During the early stages of infection, the maturing inclusion is transported to the microtubule-organizing center by an effector-mediated mechanism (122), to bring the inclusion into close contact with the Golgi apparatus.

The *Chlamydia*-occupied inclusion recruits nutrient-rich vesicles from Golgi membrane exit sites. Consequently, Rab GTPases that coordinate the sorting and delivery of cargo within the Golgi apparatus also associate with the inclusion membrane, including Rab1, Rab4, Rab6, Rab11, and Rab14 (Fig. 2) (46, 124). These Rab proteins support biogenesis and maturation of the inclusion by mediating iron and lipid acquisition and vesicle transport and fusion. Phospholipids that are enriched on Golgi membranes are also found on the *Chlamydia* inclusion and promote biogenesis of an organelle that supports intracellular replication. This process involves subversion of lipid kinases that generate PI4P, a phospholipid important for inclusion biogenesis and maintenance (125). In addition, host SNARE proteins are involved in subverting vesicle transport to maintain the inclusion. Specifically, it has been shown that the bacterial Inc proteins contain SNARE-like domains which promote homotypic fusion of individual inclusions, suggesting that these effector proteins can mimic host SNAREs (126–128). A hallmark associated with *Chlamydia* infection is fragmentation of the Golgi apparatus into small stacks that surround the mature inclusion (129). Some studies suggest that Golgi apparatus fragmentation allows for more efficient lipid transfer (130).

Interactions with the Retromer

The retromer is a multisubunit complex that mediates the retrieval of endosomal proteins (e.g., retrograde cargo receptors) and has been linked to processes associated with lysosome integrity and function (131). Accumulating evidence suggests that the retromer is often targeted by specific pathogens to enhance intracellular replication. In a genome-wide small-interfering-RNA screen, host factors that contribute to CCV biogenesis and *Coxiella* replication were identified in HeLa cells (66). This study revealed that the host retromer complex is required for *Coxiella* to generate a stable CCV and establish infection (66). In fact, depletion of retromer components impair *Coxiella* growth (66). Moreover, activated Rab7 is required for retromer recruitment to late endosomes and lysosomes (132, 133), which could be another reason that Rab7 is important for CCV biogenesis. Additionally, this suggests that the retromer subunits may remove late-endosome vesicles that would otherwise impair *Coxiella* replication.

Whereas the retromer appears to be important for *Coxiella* replication, there is evidence that retromer function is detrimental for *Legionella* replication. Specifically, it was shown that depletion of retromer subunits supported increased intracellular replication (134). The *Legionella* effector protein RidL was found to be directly involved in modulating retromer function through a direct interaction with the retromer subunit Vps29, which forms a complex with the retromer subunits Vps26 and Vps35. In the absence of RidL, the retromer complex is recruited to the LCV membrane. Importantly, ectopic expression of RidL in host cells interferes with the retrograde transport of proteins in endosomes to the Golgi apparatus, indicating that RidL interferes with retrograde vesicle transport (134). There is also evidence that *Chlamydia* interacts with components of the retrograde pathway and that interfering with retromer function enhances intracellular replication (135, 136). In addition to manipulating the retromer, the inclusion in which *Chlamydia* resides recruits the host COG complex, which is important for vesicle tethering; this, in turn, directs intra-Golgi sorting events (137). Thus, it appears that pathogens that escape the endocytic pathway have evolved mechanisms to interfere with retromer function, whereas pathogens that maintain residence in endocytic organelles require retromer function to create a vacuole that supports replication.

MAINTENANCE OF THE PCV

Most bacterial pathogens avoid lysosomal degradation by modulating endocytic maturation or diverting the phagosome from the endocytic pathway. PCVs undergo extensive remodeling that allows the pathogen to acquire nutrients and membranes from the host. However, these specialized organelles are still susceptible to cell autonomous defense mechanisms that enable cells to recognize aberrant organelles and target these compartments for destruction. Vacuole destruction results in the delivery of bacteria into the cytosol, which will trigger a number of host cell responses that are controlled by host cytosolic surveillance pathways. In particular, the host autophagy system has been identified as an ancient and evolutionarily conserved pathway used for defense against intracellular pathogens. The autophagy system has the ability to sequester damaged

organelles and cytosolic aggregates into an organelle called an autophagosome and to deliver this material to lysosomes for degradation. Autophagy can eliminate intracellular pathogens either by targeting the pathogen-occupied vacuole directly or by targeting the pathogens directly after they are delivered into the host cytosol following disruption of vacuole integrity. Thus, to evade host defenses, many vacuolar pathogens have evolved proteins that maintain vacuole integrity or block the ability of the host autophagy pathway to recognize the pathogen-occupied vacuole.

One of the first examples of a pathogen effector protein being involved in maintaining vacuole integrity was provided by studies of the *Salmonella* protein SifA. This T3SS effector was found to be essential for vacuole integrity (61). Vacuoles containing SifA-deficient *Salmonella* frequently rupture as bacteria begin to replicate intracellularly, which results in the delivery of bacteria into the cytosol (61). After vacuole disruption, the *sifA* mutants are rapidly targeted by the autophagy pathway for host destruction. Interestingly, a loss-of-function mutation in the *Salmonella* effector protein SseJ can suppress the vacuole integrity defect displayed by the *sifA* mutant (138). This implies that the activities of SseJ and SifA are tightly coordinated to maintain vacuole stability and that in the absence of SifA, the activity of SseJ creates a SCV membrane that is easily disrupted. A similar interplay of effector-mediated regulation of membrane stability was observed between the *Legionella* proteins SdhA and PlaA. Similar to *sifA* mutants, *Legionella* strains deficient in the effector protein SdhA create vacuoles with reduced stability, which results in reduced intracellular replication (139). Reduced vacuole stability displayed by the *sdhA* mutant was suppressed in a *plaA* mutant. The PlaA protein is a phospholipase, which suggests that in the absence of vacuole modifications mediated by SdhA, the phospholipase activity of PlaA weakens the LCV membrane and enhances vacuole disruption (139).

When the integrity of the PCV is compromised, the compartment is often recognized as a damaged organelle, which results in the vacuole being targeted by the host autophagy pathway (140). Carbohydrate molecules exposed on damaged membranes and on bacterial surfaces activate the autophagic response by creating a signaling platform that triggers ubiquitination and recruitment of host ubiquitin-binding proteins to these structures (141, 142). A family of ubiquitin-binding proteins serve as autophagy adaptors and bind ubiquitinated cargo through a conserved ubiquitin-binding domain (143). Autophagy adaptors also have an LC3-interacting region that promotes autophagic targeting of the ubiquitin-tagged substrates (144). At the molecular level, adaptor proteins such as p62/SQSTM1 act as molecular tethers that direct the delivery of ubiquitinated PCVs and cytosolic bacteria into autophagosomes that fuse with lysosomes to promote pathogen degradation (145, 146). Guanylate-binding proteins and galectins that are recruited to damaged phagosomes also function as autophagy-activating signals that promote adaptor-mediated targeting of pathogens by the autophagy pathway (147, 148). Thus, to enhance intracellular survival, many intracellular pathogens have evolved mechanisms to avoid autophagic targeting and destruction.

One of the most striking examples of pathogen inhibition of host autophagy was discovered by using *L. pneumophila*. Following uptake, the LCV acquires a ubiquitin coat that remains associated with this compartment throughout the infection (114); however, the ubiquitin-positive LCV avoids targeting by the autophagy pathway. It was found that one of the *Legionella* effector proteins called RavZ was both necessary and sufficient to disrupt host autophagy globally (149). One of the critical events in autophagosome biogenesis is the covalent linkage of highly conserved proteins belonging to the ATG8 family of autophagy proteins to the lipid phosphatidylethanolamine (PE) on pre-autophagosomal structures. In mammalian cells, the protein LC3 is the most common ATG8 family member that is used to identify autophagosomal structures. The effector protein RavZ was shown to be an ATG8 protease that can efficiently cleave ATG8 proteins after they are conjugated to lipids on autophagosomal structures. RavZ cleaves the penultimate peptide bond in ATG8 proteins, which results in the removal of an essential C-terminal glycine residue in the ATG8 protein that is necessary for lipid conjugation. Thus, these ATG8 proteins are irreversibly modified upon cleavage by RavZ (149, 150). Not all *Legionella* strains encode RavZ, yet most strains interfere with autophagy, suggesting that *Legionella* has additional mechanisms to evade autophagy. The effector protein LpSpl was found to be a sphingosine-1 phosphate lyase that can also suppress starvation-induced autophagy during infection (151). Thus, it is clear that *Legionella* has evolved multiple mechanisms to evade autophagy.

Unlike *Legionella*, the vacuole containing *Coxiella* subverts the host autophagy pathway to maintain the vacuole in which it resides. In a genome-wide small-interfering-RNA screen, it was found that the host protein syntaxin-17, a SNARE-like protein that promotes autophagosome-lysosome fusion, is required for homotypic fusion of the CCV (66). During infection of host cells by *Coxiella*, the pathogen has the ability to pro-

mote fusion of endocytic organelles with the CCV, including other CCVs, to create a single late-endocytic organelle in the cell. This process requires the *Coxiella* effector protein Cig2, which promotes constitutive fusion of autophagosomes with the CCV (75). Maintaining the CCV in an autolysosomal stage of maturation appears to promote robust fusion between this organelle and other endocytic compartments. Thus, the comparison between *Legionella* and *Coxiella* provides another example of how a host process can be either detrimental or beneficial to pathogen replication and survival, and this is often determined by whether the pathogen creates a modified endocytic organelle or evades endocytic interactions.

CONCLUSION

Phagosome acidification followed by lysosomal fusion is an intrinsic defense mechanism the cell uses to destroy harmful pathogens. However, pathogens that have coevolved alongside their eukaryotic hosts have evolved mechanisms to subvert this process and avoid this fate. Indeed, protracted evolution at the host-pathogen interface has enriched for unique bacterial adaptations that exploit the cell's machinery and associated organelles to ensure survival. Investigating how these pathogens manipulate host transport to build an intracellular niche provides important insights into the conserved processes in the cell.

Citation. Omotade TO, Roy CR. 2019. Manipulation of host cell organelles by intracellular pathogens. Microbiol Spectrum 7(2):BAI-0022-2019.

REFERENCES

1. Doherty GJ, McMahon HT. 2009. Mechanisms of endocytosis. *Annu Rev Biochem* 78:857–902.
2. Stenmark H. 2009. Rab GTPases as coordinators of vesicle traffic. *Nat Rev Mol Cell Biol* 10:513–525.
3. Di Paolo G, De Camilli P. 2006. Phosphoinositides in cell regulation and membrane dynamics. *Nature* 443:651–657.
4. Hutagalung AH, Novick PJ. 2011. Role of Rab GTPases in membrane traffic and cell physiology. *Physiol Rev* 91:119–149.
5. Elkin SR, Lakoduk AM, Schmid SL. 2016. Endocytic pathways and endosomal trafficking: a primer. *Wien Med Wochenschr* 166:196–204.
6. Bucci C, Parton RG, Mather IH, Stunnenberg H, Simons K, Hoflack B, Zerial M. 1992. The small GTPase rab5 functions as a regulatory factor in the early endocytic pathway. *Cell* 70:715–728.
7. Vanlandingham PA, Ceresa BP. 2009. Rab7 regulates late endocytic trafficking downstream of multivesicular

body biogenesis and cargo sequestration. *J Biol Chem* 284:12110–12124.

8. Kinchen JM, Ravichandran KS. 2008. Phagosome maturation: going through the acid test. *Nat Rev Mol Cell Biol* 9:781–795.

9. De Camilli P, Emr SD, McPherson PS, Novick P. 1996. Phosphoinositides as regulators in membrane traffic. *Science* 271:1533–1539.

10. Lee MC, Orci L, Hamamoto S, Futai E, Ravazzola M, Schekman R. 2005. Sar1p N-terminal helix initiates membrane curvature and completes the fission of a COPII vesicle. *Cell* 122:605–617.

11. Beck R, Sun Z, Adolf F, Rutz C, Bassler J, Wild K, Sinning I, Hurt E, Brügger B, Béthune J, Wieland F. 2008. Membrane curvature induced by Arf1-GTP is essential for vesicle formation. *Proc Natl Acad Sci USA* 105:11731–11736.

12. D'Souza-Schorey C, Chavrier P. 2006. ARF proteins: roles in membrane traffic and beyond. *Nat Rev Mol Cell Biol* 7:347–358.

13. Hong W. 2005. SNAREs and traffic. *Biochim Biophys Acta* 1744:493–517.

14. Chen YA, Scheller RH. 2001. SNARE-mediated membrane fusion. *Nat Rev Mol Cell Biol* 2:98–106.

15. Allan BB, Moyer BD, Balch WE. 2000. Rab1 recruitment of p115 into a cis-SNARE complex: programming budding COPII vesicles for fusion. *Science* 289:444–448.

16. Rzomp KA, Scholtes LD, Briggs BJ, Whittaker GR, Scidmore MA. 2003. Rab GTPases are recruited to chlamydial inclusions in both a species-dependent and species-independent manner. *Infect Immun* 71:5855–5870.

17. Capmany A, Damiani MT. 2010. *Chlamydia trachomatis* intercepts Golgi-derived sphingolipids through a Rab14-mediated transport required for bacterial development and replication. *PLoS One* 5:e14084.

18. Dickson EJ, Jensen JB, Hille B. 2014. Golgi and plasma membrane pools of PI(4)P contribute to plasma membrane PI(4,5)P2 and maintenance of KCNQ2/3 ion channel current. *Proc Natl Acad Sci USA* 111:E2281–E2290.

19. Clayton EL, Minogue S, Waugh MG. 2013. Mammalian phosphatidylinositol 4-kinases as modulators of membrane trafficking and lipid signaling networks. *Prog Lipid Res* 52:294–304.

20. Bishé B, Syed GH, Field SJ, Siddiqui A. 2012. Role of phosphatidylinositol 4-phosphate (PI4P) and its binding protein GOLPH3 in hepatitis C virus secretion. *J Biol Chem* 287:27637–27647.

21. Jutras I, Desjardins M. 2005. Phagocytosis: at the crossroads of innate and adaptive immunity. *Annu Rev Cell Dev Biol* 21:511–527.

22. Gruenberg J, van der Goot FG. 2006. Mechanisms of pathogen entry through the endosomal compartments. *Nat Rev Mol Cell Biol* 7:495–504.

23. Vieira OV, Botelho RJ, Rameh L, Brachmann SM, Matsuo T, Davidson HW, Schreiber A, Backer JM, Cantley LC, Grinstein S. 2001. Distinct roles of class I and class III phosphatidylinositol 3-kinases in phagosome formation and maturation. *J Cell Biol* 155:19–25.

24. Flannagan RS, Jaumouillé V, Grinstein S. 2012. The cell biology of phagocytosis. *Annu Rev Pathol* 7:61–98.

25. Xu M, Liu Y, Zhao L, Gan Q, Wang X, Yang C. 2014. The lysosomal cathepsin protease CPL-1 plays a leading role in phagosomal degradation of apoptotic cells in *Caenorhabditis elegans*. *Mol Biol Cell* 25:2071–2083.

26. Jordens I, Fernandez-Borja M, Marsman M, Dusseljee S, Janssen L, Calafat J, Janssen H, Wubbolts R, Neefjes J. 2001. The Rab7 effector protein RILP controls lysosomal transport by inducing the recruitment of dynein-dynactin motors. *Curr Biol* 11:1680–1685.

27. Harrison RE, Bucci C, Vieira OV, Schroer TA, Grinstein S. 2003. Phagosomes fuse with late endosomes and/or lysosomes by extension of membrane protrusions along microtubules: role of Rab7 and RILP. *Mol Cell Biol* 23:6494–6506.

28. Huynh KK, Eskelinen E-L, Scott CC, Malevanets A, Saftig P, Grinstein S. 2007. LAMP proteins are required for fusion of lysosomes with phagosomes. *EMBO J* 26: 313–324.

29. MacGurn JA, Cox JS. 2007. A genetic screen for *Mycobacterium tuberculosis* mutants defective for phagosome maturation arrest identifies components of the ESX-1 secretion system. *Infect Immun* 75:2668–2678.

30. Vergne I, Chua J, Lee H-H, Lucas M, Belisle J, Deretic V. 2005. Mechanism of phagolysosome biogenesis block by viable *Mycobacterium tuberculosis*. *Proc Natl Acad Sci USA* 102:4033–4038.

31. Vergne I, Chua J, Deretic V. 2003. Tuberculosis toxin blocking phagosome maturation inhibits a novel Ca2+/calmodulin-PI3K hVPS34 cascade. *J Exp Med* 198: 653–659.

32. Vieira OV, Harrison RE, Scott CC, Stenmark H, Alexander D, Liu J, Gruenberg J, Schreiber AD, Grinstein S. 2004. Acquisition of Hrs, an essential component of phagosomal maturation, is impaired by mycobacteria. *Mol Cell Biol* 24:4593–4604.

33. Fratti RA, Backer JM, Gruenberg J, Corvera S, Deretic V. 2001. Role of phosphatidylinositol 3-kinase and Rab5 effectors in phagosomal biogenesis and mycobacterial phagosome maturation arrest. *J Cell Biol* 154:631–644.

34. Gaspar AH, Machner MP. 2014. VipD is a Rab5-activated phospholipase A1 that protects *Legionella pneumophila* from endosomal fusion. *Proc Natl Acad Sci USA* 111:4560–4565.

35. Hubber A, Roy CR. 2010. Modulation of host cell function by *Legionella pneumophila* type IV effectors. *Annu Rev Cell Dev Biol* 26:261–283.

36. Campanacci V, Mukherjee S, Roy CR, Cherfils J. 2013. Structure of the *Legionella* effector AnkX reveals the mechanism of phosphocholine transfer by the FIC domain. *EMBO J* 32:1469–1477.

37. Puri RV, Reddy PV, Tyagi AK. 2013. Secreted acid phosphatase (SapM) of *Mycobacterium tuberculosis* is indispensable for arresting phagosomal maturation and growth of the pathogen in guinea pig tissues. *PLoS One* 8:e70514.

38. Méresse S, Steele-Mortimer O, Finlay BB, Gorvel JP. 1999. The rab7 GTPase controls the maturation of *Salmonella typhimurium*-containing vacuoles in HeLa cells. *EMBO J* 18:4394–4403.

39. Garcia-del Portillo F, Zwick MB, Leung KY, Finlay BB. 1993. *Salmonella* induces the formation of filamentous structures containing lysosomal membrane glycoproteins in epithelial cells. *Proc Natl Acad Sci USA* 90:10544–10548.

40. Kubori T, Galán JE. 2003. Temporal regulation of *Salmonella* virulence effector function by proteasome-dependent protein degradation. *Cell* 115:333–342.

41. Bakowski MA, Braun V, Lam GY, Yeung T, Heo WD, Meyer T, Finlay BB, Grinstein S, Brumell JH. 2010. The phosphoinositide phosphatase SopB manipulates membrane surface charge and trafficking of the *Salmonella*-containing vacuole. *Cell Host Microbe* 7:453–462.

42. Steele-Mortimer O, Knodler LA, Marcus SL, Scheid MP, Goh B, Pfeifer CG, Duronio V, Finlay BB. 2000. Activation of Akt/protein kinase B in epithelial cells by the *Salmonella typhimurium* effector sigD. *J Biol Chem* 275:37718–37724.

43. Terebiznik MR, Vieira OV, Marcus SL, Slade A, Yip CM, Trimble WS, Meyer T, Finlay BB, Grinstein S. 2002. Elimination of host cell PtdIns(4,5)P(2) by bacterial SigD promotes membrane fission during invasion by *Salmonella*. *Nat Cell Biol* 4:766–773.

44. Hernandez LD, Hueffer K, Wenk MR, Galán JE. 2004. *Salmonella* modulates vesicular traffic by altering phosphoinositide metabolism. *Science* 304:1805–1807.

45. Mallo GV, Espina M, Smith AC, Terebiznik MR, Alemán A, Finlay BB, Rameh LE, Grinstein S, Brumell JH. 2008. SopB promotes phosphatidylinositol 3-phosphate formation on *Salmonella* vacuoles by recruiting Rab5 and Vps34. *J Cell Biol* 182:741–752.

46. Sherwood RK, Roy CR. 2013. A Rab-centric perspective of bacterial pathogen-occupied vacuoles. *Cell Host Microbe* 14:256–268.

47. Via LE, Deretic D, Ulmer RJ, Hibler NS, Huber LA, Deretic V. 1997. Arrest of mycobacterial phagosome maturation is caused by a block in vesicle fusion between stages controlled by rab5 and rab7. *J Biol Chem* 272:13326–13331.

48. Perskvist N, Roberg K, Kulyté A, Stendahl O. 2002. Rab5a GTPase regulates fusion between pathogen-containing phagosomes and cytoplasmic organelles in human neutrophils. *J Cell Sci* 115:1321–1330.

49. Roberts EA, Chua J, Kyei GB, Deretic V. 2006. Higher order Rab programming in phagolysosome biogenesis. *J Cell Biol* 174:923–929.

50. Garcia-del Portillo F, Finlay BB. 1995. Targeting of *Salmonella typhimurium* to vesicles containing lysosomal membrane glycoproteins bypasses compartments with mannose 6-phosphate receptors. *J Cell Biol* 129:81–97.

51. Hashim S, Mukherjee K, Raje M, Basu SK, Mukhopadhyay A. 2000. Live *Salmonella* modulate expression of Rab proteins to persist in a specialized compartment and escape transport to lysosomes. *J Biol Chem* 275:16281–16288.

52. Galán JE. 2001. *Salmonella* interactions with host cells: type III secretion at work. *Annu Rev Cell Dev Biol* 17:53–86.

53. Spanò S, Liu X, Galán JE. 2011. Proteolytic targeting of Rab29 by an effector protein distinguishes the intracellular compartments of human-adapted and broad-host *Salmonella*. *Proc Natl Acad Sci USA* 108:18418–18423.

54. Spanò S, Galán JE. 2012. A Rab32-dependent pathway contributes to *Salmonella typhi* host restriction. *Science* 338:960–963.

55. Gerondopoulos A, Langemeyer L, Liang JR, Linford A, Barr FA. 2012. BLOC-3 mutated in Hermansky-Pudlak syndrome is a Rab32/38 guanine nucleotide exchange factor. *Curr Biol* 22:2135–2139.

56. Bultema JJ, Ambrosio AL, Burek CL, Di Pietro SM. 2012. BLOC-2, AP-3, and AP-1 proteins function in concert with Rab38 and Rab32 proteins to mediate protein trafficking to lysosome-related organelles. *J Biol Chem* 287:19550–19563.

57. Spanò S, Gao X, Hannemann S, Lara-Tejero M, Galán JE. 2016. A bacterial pathogen targets a host Rab-family GTPase defense pathway with a GAP. *Cell Host Microbe* 19:216–226.

58. Stein MA, Leung KY, Zwick M, Garcia-del Portillo F, Finlay BB. 1996. Identification of a *Salmonella* virulence gene required for formation of filamentous structures containing lysosomal membrane glycoproteins within epithelial cells. *Mol Microbiol* 20:151–164.

59. Boucrot E, Henry T, Borg JP, Gorvel JP, Méresse S. 2005. The intracellular fate of *Salmonella* depends on the recruitment of kinesin. *Science* 308:1174–1178.

60. Dumont A, Boucrot E, Drevensek S, Daire V, Gorvel JP, Poüs C, Holden DW, Méresse S. 2010. SKIP, the host target of the *Salmonella* virulence factor SifA, promotes kinesin-1-dependent vacuolar membrane exchanges. *Traffic* 11:899–911.

61. Beuzón CR, Méresse S, Unsworth KE, Ruíz-Albert J, Garvis S, Waterman SR, Ryder TA, Boucrot E, Holden DW. 2000. *Salmonella* maintains the integrity of its intracellular vacuole through the action of SifA. *EMBO J* 19:3235–3249.

62. Burton PR, Kordová N, Paretsky D. 1971. Electron microscopic studies of the rickettsia *Coxiella burnetii*: entry, lysosomal response, and fate of rickettsial DNA in L-cells. *Can J Microbiol* 17:143–150.

63. Voth DE, Heinzen RA. 2007. Lounging in a lysosome: the intracellular lifestyle of *Coxiella burnetii*. *Cell Microbiol* 9:829–840.

64. Berón W, Gutierrez MG, Rabinovitch M, Colombo MI. 2002. *Coxiella burnetii* localizes in a Rab7-labeled compartment with autophagic characteristics. *Infect Immun* 70:5816–5821.

65. Romano PS, Gutierrez MG, Berón W, Rabinovitch M, Colombo MI. 2007. The autophagic pathway is actively modulated by phase II *Coxiella burnetii* to efficiently replicate in the host cell. *Cell Microbiol* 9:891–909.

66. McDonough JA, Newton HJ, Klum S, Swiss R, Agaisse H, Roy CR. 2013. Host pathways important for

Coxiella burnetii infection revealed by genome-wide RNA interference screening. *mBio* **4**:e00606-12.

67. Newton HJ, McDonough JA, Roy CR. 2013. Effector protein translocation by the *Coxiella burnetii* Dot/Icm type IV secretion system requires endocytic maturation of the pathogen-occupied vacuole. *PLoS One* **8**:e54566.

68. Beare PA, Gilk SD, Larson CL, Hill J, Stead CM, Omsland A, Cockrell DC, Howe D, Voth DE, Heinzen RA. 2011. Dot/Icm type IVB secretion system requirements for *Coxiella burnetii* growth in human macrophages. *mBio* **2**:e00175-11.

69. Howe D, Melnicáková J, Barák I, Heinzen RA. 2003. Maturation of the *Coxiella burnetii* parasitophorous vacuole requires bacterial protein synthesis but not replication. *Cell Microbiol* **5**:469–480.

70. Heinzen RA, Scidmore MA, Rockey DD, Hackstadt T. 1996. Differential interaction with endocytic and exocytic pathways distinguish parasitophorous vacuoles of *Coxiella burnetii* and *Chlamydia trachomatis*. *Infect Immun* **64**:796–809.

71. Ghigo E, Capo C, Tung CH, Raoult D, Gorvel JP, Mege JL. 2002. *Coxiella burnetii* survival in THP-1 monocytes involves the impairment of phagosome maturation: IFN-gamma mediates its restoration and bacterial killing. *J Immunol* **169**:4488–4495.

72. He C, Klionsky DJ. 2009. Regulation mechanisms and signaling pathways of autophagy. *Annu Rev Genet* **43**:67–93.

73. Kabeya Y, Mizushima N, Ueno T, Yamamoto A, Kirisako T, Noda T, Kominami E, Ohsumi Y, Yoshimori T. 2000. LC3, a mammalian homologue of yeast Apg8p, is localized in autophagosome membranes after processing. *EMBO J* **19**:5720–5728.

74. Gutierrez MG, Vázquez CL, Munafó DB, Zoppino FC, Berón W, Rabinovitch M, Colombo MI. 2005. Autophagy induction favours the generation and maturation of the *Coxiella*-replicative vacuoles. *Cell Microbiol* **7**:981–993.

75. Kohler LJ, Reed SC, Sarraf SA, Arteaga DD, Newton HJ, Roy CR. 2016. Effector protein Cig2 decreases host tolerance of infection by directing constitutive fusion of autophagosomes with the *Coxiella*-containing vacuole. *mBio* **17**:e01127-16.

76. Munafó DB, Colombo MI. 2002. Induction of autophagy causes dramatic changes in the subcellular distribution of GFP-Rab24. *Traffic* **3**:472–482.

77. Gutierrez MG, Saka HA, Chinen I, Zoppino FC, Yoshimori T, Bocco JL, Colombo MI. 2007. Protective role of autophagy against *Vibrio cholerae* cytolysin, a pore-forming toxin from *V. cholerae*. *Proc Natl Acad Sci USA* **104**:1829–1834.

78. Campoy EM, Zoppino FC, Colombo MI. 2011. The early secretory pathway contributes to the growth of the *Coxiella*-replicative niche. *Infect Immun* **79**:402–413.

79. Pappas G, Akritidis N, Bosilkovski M, Tsianos E. 2005. Brucellosis. *N Engl J Med* **352**:2325–2336.

80. Celli J, de Chastellier C, Franchini DM, Pizarro-Cerda J, Moreno E, Gorvel JP. 2003. *Brucella* evades macrophage killing via VirB-dependent sustained interactions with the endoplasmic reticulum. *J Exp Med* **198**:545–556.

81. Comerci DJ, Martínez-Lorenzo MJ, Sieira R, Gorvel JP, Ugalde RA. 2001. Essential role of the VirB machinery in the maturation of the *Brucella abortus*-containing vacuole. *Cell Microbiol* **3**:159–168.

82. Delrue RM, Martinez-Lorenzo M, Lestrate P, Danese I, Bielarz V, Mertens P, De Bolle X, Tibor A, Gorvel JP, Letesson JJ. 2001. Identification of *Brucella* spp. genes involved in intracellular trafficking. *Cell Microbiol* **3**:487–497.

83. Pizarro-Cerdá J, Moreno E, Sanguedolce V, Mege JL, Gorvel JP. 1998. Virulent *Brucella abortus* prevents lysosome fusion and is distributed within autophagosome-like compartments. *Infect Immun* **66**:2387–2392.

84. Starr T, Ng TW, Wehrly TD, Knodler LA, Celli J. 2008. *Brucella* intracellular replication requires trafficking through the late endosomal/lysosomal compartment. *Traffic* **9**:678–694.

85. Bellaire BH, Roop RM II, Cardelli JA. 2005. Opsonized virulent *Brucella abortus* replicates within nonacidic, endoplasmic reticulum-negative, LAMP-1-positive phagosomes in human monocytes. *Infect Immun* **73**:3702–3713.

86. Boschiroli ML, Ouahrani-Bettache S, Foulongne V, Michaux-Charachon S, Bourg G, Allardet-Servent A, Cazevieille C, Liautard JP, Ramuz M, O'Callaghan D. 2002. The *Brucella suis* virB operon is induced intracellularly in macrophages. *Proc Natl Acad Sci USA* **99**:1544–1549.

87. Fraser DW, Tsai TR, Orenstein W, Parkin WE, Beecham HJ, Sharrar RG, Harris J, Mallison GF, Martin SM, McDade JE, Shepard CC, Brachman PS. 1977. Legionnaires' disease: description of an epidemic of pneumonia. *N Engl J Med* **297**:1189–1197.

88. Berger KH, Isberg RR. 1993. Two distinct defects in intracellular growth complemented by a single genetic locus in *Legionella pneumophila*. *Mol Microbiol* **7**:7–19.

89. Horwitz MA. 1987. Characterization of avirulent mutant *Legionella pneumophila* that survive but do not multiply within human monocytes. *J Exp Med* **166**:1310–1328.

90. Clemens DL, Horwitz MA. 1995. Characterization of the *Mycobacterium tuberculosis* phagosome and evidence that phagosomal maturation is inhibited. *J Exp Med* **181**:257–270.

91. Roy CR, Berger KH, Isberg RR. 1998. *Legionella pneumophila* DotA protein is required for early phagosome trafficking decisions that occur within minutes of bacterial uptake. *Mol Microbiol* **28**:663–674.

92. Horwitz MA, Maxfield FR. 1984. *Legionella pneumophila* inhibits acidification of its phagosome in human monocytes. *J Cell Biol* **99**:1936–1943.

93. Horwitz MA. 1983. Formation of a novel phagosome by the Legionnaires' disease bacterium (*Legionella pneumophila*) in human monocytes. *J Exp Med* **158**:1319–1331.

94. Ingmundson A, Roy CR. 2008. Analyzing association of the endoplasmic reticulum with the *Legionella*

pneumophila-containing vacuoles by fluorescence microscopy. *Methods Mol Biol* **445**:379–387.

95. Robinson CG, Roy CR. 2006. Attachment and fusion of endoplasmic reticulum with vacuoles containing *Legionella pneumophila*. *Cell Microbiol* **8**:793–805.

96. Kagan JC, Stein MP, Pypaert M, Roy CR. 2004. *Legionella* subvert the functions of Rab1 and Sec22b to create a replicative organelle. *J Exp Med* **199**:1201–1211.

97. Derré I, Isberg RR. 2004. *Legionella pneumophila* replication vacuole formation involves rapid recruitment of proteins of the early secretory system. *Infect Immun* **72**:3048–3053.

98. Murata T, Delprato A, Ingmundson A, Toomre DK, Lambright DG, Roy CR. 2006. The *Legionella pneumophila* effector protein DrrA is a Rab1 guanine nucleotide-exchange factor. *Nat Cell Biol* **8**:971–977.

99. Kagan JC, Roy CR. 2002. *Legionella* phagosomes intercept vesicular traffic from endoplasmic reticulum exit sites. *Nat Cell Biol* **4**:945–954.

100. Machner MP, Isberg RR. 2006. Targeting of host Rab GTPase function by the intravacuolar pathogen *Legionella pneumophila*. *Dev Cell* **11**:47–56.

101. Zhu Y, Hu L, Zhou Y, Yao Q, Liu L, Shao F. 2010. Structural mechanism of host Rab1 activation by the bifunctional *Legionella* type IV effector SidM/DrrA. *Proc Natl Acad Sci USA* **107**:4699–4704.

102. Schoebel S, Oesterlin LK, Blankenfeldt W, Goody RS, Itzen A. 2009. RabGDI displacement by DrrA from *Legionella* is a consequence of its guanine nucleotide exchange activity. *Mol Cell* **36**:1060–1072.

103. Müller MP, Peters H, Blümer J, Blankenfeldt W, Goody RS, Itzen A. 2010. The *Legionella* effector protein DrrA AMPylates the membrane traffic regulator Rab1b. *Science* **329**:946–949.

104. Hardiman CA, Roy CR. 2014. AMPylation is critical for Rab1 localization to vacuoles containing *Legionella pneumophila*. *mBio* **5**:e01035-13.

105. Pan X, Lührmann A, Satoh A, Laskowski-Arce MA, Roy CR. 2008. Ankyrin repeat proteins comprise a diverse family of bacterial type IV effectors. *Science* **320**:1651–1654.

106. Tan Y, Arnold RJ, Luo ZQ. 2011. *Legionella pneumophila* regulates the small GTPase Rab1 activity by reversible phosphorylcholination. *Proc Natl Acad Sci USA* **108**:21212–21217.

107. Mukherjee S, Liu X, Arasaki K, McDonough J, Galán JE, Roy CR. 2011. Modulation of Rab GTPase function by a protein phosphocholine transferase. *Nature* **477**:103–106.

108. Tan Y, Luo ZQ. 2011. *Legionella pneumophila* SidD is a deAMPylase that modifies Rab1. *Nature* **475**:506–509.

109. Neunuebel MR, Chen Y, Gaspar AH, Backlund PS Jr, Yergey A, Machner MP. 2011. De-AMPylation of the small GTPase Rab1 by the pathogen *Legionella pneumophila*. *Science* **333**:453–456.

110. Seto S, Tsujimura K, Koide Y. 2011. Rab GTPases regulating phagosome maturation are differentially recruited to mycobacterial phagosomes. *Traffic* **12**:407–420.

111. Ingmundson A, Delprato A, Lambright DG, Roy CR. 2007. *Legionella pneumophila* proteins that regulate Rab1 membrane cycling. *Nature* **450**:365–369.

112. Nagai H, Kagan JC, Zhu X, Kahn RA, Roy CR. 2002. A bacterial guanine nucleotide exchange factor activates ARF on *Legionella* phagosomes. *Science* **295**:679–682.

113. Amor JC, Swails J, Zhu X, Roy CR, Nagai H, Ingmundson A, Cheng X, Kahn RA. 2005. The structure of RalF, an ADP-ribosylation factor guanine nucleotide exchange factor from *Legionella pneumophila*, reveals the presence of a cap over the active site. *J Biol Chem* **280**:1392–1400.

114. Dorer MS, Kirton D, Bader JS, Isberg RR. 2006. RNA interference analysis of *Legionella* in *Drosophila* cells: exploitation of early secretory apparatus dynamics. *PLoS Pathog* **2**:e34.

115. Celli J, Salcedo SP, Gorvel J-P. 2005. *Brucella* coopts the small GTPase Sar1 for intracellular replication. *Proc Natl Acad Sci USA* **102**:1673–1678.

116. Fugier E, Salcedo SP, de Chastellier C, Pophillat M, Muller A, Arce-Gorvel V, Fourquet P, Gorvel JP. 2009. The glyceraldehyde-3-phosphate dehydrogenase and the small GTPase Rab 2 are crucial for *Brucella* replication. *PLoS Pathog* **5**:e1000487.

117. de Barsy M, Jamet A, Filopon D, Nicolas C, Laloux G, Rual JF, Muller A, Twizere JC, Nkengfac B, Vandenhaute J, Hill DE, Salcedo SP, Gorvel JP, Letesson JJ, De Bolle X. 2011. Identification of a *Brucella* spp. secreted effector specifically interacting with human small GTPase Rab2. *Cell Microbiol* **13**:1044–1058.

118. Xu D, Joglekar AP, Williams AL, Hay JC. 2000. Subunit structure of a mammalian ER/Golgi SNARE complex. *J Biol Chem* **275**:39631–39639.

119. Arasaki K, Roy CR. 2010. *Legionella pneumophila* promotes functional interactions between plasma membrane syntaxins and Sec22b. *Traffic* **11**:587–600.

120. Arasaki K, Toomre DK, Roy CR. 2012. The *Legionella pneumophila* effector DrrA is sufficient to stimulate SNARE-dependent membrane fusion. *Cell Host Microbe* **11**:46–57.

121. Menon S, Timms P, Allan JA, Alexander K, Rombauts L, Horner P, Keltz M, Hocking J, Huston WM. 2015. Human and pathogen factors associated with *Chlamydia trachomatis*-related infertility in women. *Clin Microbiol Rev* **28**:969–985.

122. Elwell C, Mirrashidi K, Engel J. 2016. Chlamydia cell biology and pathogenesis. *Nat Rev Microbiol* **14**:385–400.

123. Fields KA, Hackstadt T. 2002. The chlamydial inclusion: escape from the endocytic pathway. *Annu Rev Cell Dev Biol* **18**:221–245.

124. Rejman Lipinski A, Heymann J, Meissner C, Karlas A, Brinkmann V, Meyer TF, Heuer D. 2009. Rab6 and Rab11 regulate *Chlamydia trachomatis* development and golgin-84-dependent Golgi fragmentation. *PLoS Pathog* **5**:e1000615.

125. Moorhead AM, Jung JY, Smirnov A, Kaufer S, Scidmore MA. 2010. Multiple host proteins that function in phosphatidylinositol-4-phosphate metabolism

are recruited to the chlamydial inclusion. *Infect Immun* 78:1990–2007.

126. Ronzone E, Wesolowski J, Bauler LD, Bhardwaj A, Hackstadt T, Paumet F. 2014. An α-helical core encodes the dual functions of the chlamydial protein IncA. *J Biol Chem* 289:33469–33480.

127. Ronzone E, Paumet F. 2013. Two coiled-coil domains of *Chlamydia trachomatis* IncA affect membrane fusion events during infection. *PLoS One* 8:e69769.

128. Gauliard E, Ouellette SP, Rueden KJ, Ladant D. 2015. Characterization of interactions between inclusion membrane proteins from *Chlamydia trachomatis*. *Front Cell Infect Microbiol* 5:13.

129. Heuer D, Rejman Lipinski A, Machuy N, Karlas A, Wehrens A, Siedler F, Brinkmann V, Meyer TF. 2009. *Chlamydia* causes fragmentation of the Golgi compartment to ensure reproduction. *Nature* 457:731–735.

130. Gurumurthy RK, Chumduri C, Karlas A, Kimmig S, Gonzalez E, Machuy N, Rudel T, Meyer TF. 2014. Dynamin-mediated lipid acquisition is essential for *Chlamydia trachomatis* development. *Mol Microbiol* 94:186–201.

131. Burd C, Cullen PJ. 2014. Retromer: a master conductor of endosome sorting. *Cold Spring Harb Perspect Biol* 6:a016774.

132. Lucas M, Gershlick DC, Vidaurrazaga A, Rojas AL, Bonifacino JS, Hierro A. 2016. Structural mechanism for cargo recognition by the retromer complex. *Cell* 167:1623–1635.e1614.

133. Rojas R, Kametaka S, Haft CR, Bonifacino JS. 2007. Interchangeable but essential functions of SNX1 and SNX2 in the association of retromer with endosomes and the trafficking of mannose 6-phosphate receptors. *Mol Cell Biol* 27:1112–1124.

134. Finsel I, Ragaz C, Hoffmann C, Harrison CF, Weber S, van Rahden VA, Johannes L, Hilbi H. 2013. The *Legionella* effector RidL inhibits retrograde trafficking to promote intracellular replication. *Cell Host Microbe* 14:38–50.

135. Mirrashidi KM, Elwell CA, Verschueren E, Johnson JR, Frando A, Von Dollen J, Rosenberg O, Gulbahce N, Jang G, Johnson T, Jäger S, Gopalakrishnan AM, Sherry J, Dunn JD, Olive A, Penn B, Shales M, Cox JS, Starnbach MN, Derre I, Valdivia R, Krogan NJ, Engel J. 2015. Global mapping of the Inc-human interactome reveals that retromer restricts *Chlamydia* infection. *Cell Host Microbe* 18:109–121.

136. Aeberhard L, Banhart S, Fischer M, Jehmlich N, Rose L, Koch S, Laue M, Renard BY, Schmidt F, Heuer D. 2015. The proteome of the isolated *Chlamydia trachomatis* containing vacuole reveals a complex trafficking platform enriched for retromer components. *PLoS Pathog* 11:e1004883.

137. Smith RD, Lupashin VV. 2008. Role of the conserved oligomeric Golgi (COG) complex in protein glycosylation. *Carbohydr Res* 343:2024–2031.

138. Ruiz-Albert J, Yu XJ, Beuzón CR, Blakey AN, Galyov EE, Holden DW. 2002. Complementary activities of SseJ and SifA regulate dynamics of the *Salmonella typhimurium* vacuolar membrane. *Mol Microbiol* 44:645–661.

139. Creasey EA, Isberg RR. 2012. The protein SdhA maintains the integrity of the *Legionella*-containing vacuole. *Proc Natl Acad Sci USA* 109:3481–3486.

140. Birmingham CL, Smith AC, Bakowski MA, Yoshimori T, Brumell JH. 2006. Autophagy controls *Salmonella* infection in response to damage to the Salmonella-containing vacuole. *J Biol Chem* 281:11374–11383.

141. Noad J, von der Malsburg A, Pathe C, Michel MA, Komander D, Randow F. 2017. LUBAC-synthesized linear ubiquitin chains restrict cytosol-invading bacteria by activating autophagy and NF-κB. *Nat Microbiol* 2:17063.

142. Yoshikawa Y, Ogawa M, Hain T, Yoshida M, Fukumatsu M, Kim M, Mimuro H, Nakagawa I, Yanagawa T, Ishii T, Kakizuka A, Sztul E, Chakraborty T, Sasakawa C. 2009. *Listeria monocytogenes* ActA-mediated escape from autophagic recognition. *Nat Cell Biol* 11:1233–1240.

143. Kraft C, Peter M, Hofmann K. 2010. Selective autophagy: ubiquitin-mediated recognition and beyond. *Nat Cell Biol* 12:836–841.

144. Noda NN, Ohsumi Y, Inagaki F. 2010. Atg8-family interacting motif crucial for selective autophagy. *FEBS Lett* 584:1379–1385.

145. Bjørkøy G, Lamark T, Brech A, Outzen H, Perander M, Overvatn A, Stenmark H, Johansen T. 2005. p62/SQSTM1 forms protein aggregates degraded by autophagy and has a protective effect on huntingtin-induced cell death. *J Cell Biol* 171:603–614.

146. Bjørkøy G, Lamark T, Johansen T. 2006. p62/SQSTM1: a missing link between protein aggregates and the autophagy machinery. *Autophagy* 2:138–139.

147. Thurston TLM, Wandel MP, von Muhlinen N, Foeglein A, Randow F. 2012. Galectin 8 targets damaged vesicles for autophagy to defend cells against bacterial invasion. *Nature* 482:414–418.

148. Feeley EM, Pilla-Moffett DM, Zwack EE, Piro AS, Finethy R, Kolb JP, Martinez J, Brodsky IE, Coers J. 2017. Galectin-3 directs antimicrobial guanylate binding proteins to vacuoles furnished with bacterial secretion systems. *Proc Natl Acad Sci USA* 114:E1698–E1706.

149. Choy A, Dancourt J, Mugo B, O'Connor TJ, Isberg RR, Melia TJ, Roy CR. 2012. The *Legionella* effector RavZ inhibits host autophagy through irreversible Atg8 deconjugation. *Science* 338:1072–1076.

150. Horenkamp FA, Kauffman KJ, Kohler LJ, Sherwood RK, Krueger KP, Shteyn V, Roy CR, Melia TJ, Reinisch KM. 2015. The *Legionella* anti-autophagy effector RavZ targets the autophagosome via PI3P- and curvature-sensing motifs. *Dev Cell* 34:569–576.

151. Rolando M, Escoll P, Buchrieser C. 2016. *Legionella pneumophila* restrains autophagy by modulating the host's sphingolipid metabolism. *Autophagy* 12:1053–1054.

Subcellular Microbiology

II

Bacteria and Intracellularity
Edited by Pascale Cossart, Craig R. Roy, and Philippe Sansonetti
© 2019 American Society for Microbiology, Washington, DC
doi:10.1128/microbiolspec.BAI-0008-2019

The Role of the Type III Secretion System in the Intracellular Lifestyle of Enteric Pathogens

14

Marcela de Souza Santos[1] and Kim Orth[1,2,3]

INTRODUCTION

Many bacterial pathogens have evolved to infect host cells from the inside. In fact, some bacteria, such as *Rickettsia* spp. and *Coxiella* spp., are entirely reliant on host intracellular resources to propagate (1). The adaptation of bacteria to an intracellular life cycle is thought to confer a means to avoid the harsh extracellular milieu (low pH, physical stress, host defenses), to gain access to a nutrient-rich environment, and to facilitate the spread of the pathogen to neighboring host tissues (2, 3).

The intracellular life cycle of a bacterium initiates with its entry into a host cell. Cell entry can be a host-induced event, as in the case of bacterial uptake by phagocyte macrophages, or a bacteria-active process, as in the case of bacterial invasion of epithelial cells (4). Internalized bacteria are initially contained in a membrane-bound vacuole derived from the host cell plasma membrane (4). This vacuole is destined to traffic along the endocytic pathway, a route that defaults to vacuolar fusion with the lysosome, where vacuolar contents are degraded (i.e., bacterial killing) (5). To counteract this detrimental route, classic mechanisms used by pathogenic bacteria include avoidance of vacuole-lysosome fusion or conversion of the phagolysosomal environment into one permissive to bacterial survival (4, 5). In both instances, bacteria are referred to as vacuolar pathogens (4, 5). Alternatively, some bacteria avoid lysosomal killing by disrupting the vacuole membrane and escaping into the host cytosol; these bacteria are termed cytosolic (5). The classic vacuolar/cytosolic distinction is not always clear because, under some circumstances, some vacuolar bacteria escape into the cytosol and some cytosolic bacteria are recompartmentalized into a vacuole (5).

Crafting an intracellular lifestyle requires bacterial subversion of the host cell's machinery. One virulence factor used to subvert cellular processes is the type III secretion system (T3SS), encoded by many pathogenic Gram-negative bacteria. The T3SS is a syringe-like secretory apparatus used by the bacteria to deliver a special set of proteins, effectors, into the host cytosol (6). The apparatus is composed of 20 to 30 proteins that are relatively well conserved among different pathogens (6). The apparatus assembly initiates with formation of a basal body containing two sets of rings spanning both the inner and outer bacterial membranes (6). The basal body projects a hollow, syringe-like conduit through which the effectors travel to the eukaryotic host cell (6). At the tip of the conduit lies a protein complex that upon sensing the host cell acts as a scaffold for the formation of a translocon pore on the host cell membrane (6). The effectors, delivered through the pore, are often mimics of eukaryotic proteins; coevolution with their hosts led bacteria to usurp host protein functionalities, which were then subverted to facilitate infection (7, 8). Cellular processes commonly disrupted by T3SS effectors include the innate immune response, the cytoskeleton machinery, and cargo trafficking (7, 8).

It is expected that pathogens will distinctively employ their T3SSs to support growth inside a vacuole versus growth in the host cytosol. In this chapter we discuss how T3SSs promote the intracellular lifestyle of *Salmonella enterica* serovar Typhimurium and *Shigella flexneri*. Both bacteria are well-characterized enteric pathogens; the former is the causative agent of salmo-

---

[1]Department of Molecular Biology, [2]Department of Biochemistry, and [3]Howard Hughes Medical Institute, University of Texas Southwestern Medical Center, Dallas, TX 75390.

nellosis, one the most common foodborne illnesses, and the latter is the major causal agent of bacillary dysentery (8, 9). *S.* Typhimurium is primarily a vacuolar pathogen, while *S. flexneri* colonizes the host cytosol (8, 9). Therefore, a parallel comparison of these two pathogens' intracellular lifestyles provides a comprehensive overview of the mechanisms used by T3SSs to subvert cellular functions. Additionally, we discuss *Vibrio parahaemolyticus*, a major cause of seafoodborne enteritis (10). Recently, it was revealed that this bacterium adopts a T3SS-dependent intracellular life cycle positioning *V. parahaemolyticus* as a model for future discoveries of T3SS-mediated intracellular subversion (11, 12).

S. TYPHIMURIUM AND LIFE IN THE *SALMONELLA*-CONTAINING VACUOLE: ROLE OF THE T3SS IN VACUOLE BIOGENESIS AND MAINTENANCE

S. Typhimurium invades intestinal epithelial cells through the activity of its first T3SS, *Salmonella* pathogenicity island 1 (SPI-1) (9). Following cell entry, the bacterium is contained within a unique membranous compartment, the *Salmonella*-containing vacuole (SCV), which transiently acquires early endosomal features (9). Later, the SCV matures through selective attainment of late endosomal and lysosomal content but does not become bactericidal (9). Activation of the second T3SS, SPI-2, occurs several hours after invasion, and from that moment on, SPI-2 effectors work to adapt the SCV to a replicative niche (7).

Therefore, SPI-1 effectors are not only critical during bacterial cell invasion, but also regulate the early steps of SCV biogenesis. The SPI-1 effectors SopE and SopE2 are homologs to each other and mimics of host guanidine exchange factors (GEF), triggering the release of GDP to facilitate GTP-binding and activation of Cdc42 and Rac1 (13–15). SopE is sufficient to promote plasma membrane ruffling and *S.* Typhimurium invasion (15). While most SopE/E2 becomes degraded shortly after bacterial invasion (16), a small fraction of these effectors remain active for several hours postinvasion (17). These active pools of SopE/E2 localize to the membrane of the nascent SCV (17), where they activate the small GTPase Rab5 through their GEF activity. Rab5 promotes homotypic fusion between early-endosomal compartments and fusion events between the SCV and early endosomes (18).

The SPI-1 effector SopB (also known as SigD) is a phosphatidylinositol phosphatase that hydrolyzes a wide range of phosphoinositide substrates *in vitro* (19) with specific phosphatidylinositol 4,5-biphosphate phosphatase [PI(4,5)P$_2$] activity *in vivo* (20). Although not essential for cell invasion, SopB plays an important role in nascent SCV formation (21–23). Depletion of PI(4,5)P$_2$ by SopB promotes fusion between the SCV and vesicles containing Rab5 (23). One of the Rab5 effectors that is associated with the SCV is Vps34, a phosphatidylinositol-3 (PI-3) kinase (21, 23). Vps34 phosphorylation of local pools of phosphatidylinositol (PI) forms phosphatidylinositol 3-phosphate [PI(3)P] that recruits the early endosomal component early-endosome antigen 1 (EEA1) to the SCV membrane (21, 23). Therefore, the early biogenesis of the SCV is dependent on the activity of SopB, which promotes the acquisition of Rab5, PI(3)P, and EEA1.

The maturation of the SCV leads to the progressive loss of these early endosomal markers and acquisition of late endosomal content, such as lysosome-associated membrane protein 1 (Lamp-1) (24). Lamp-1 recruitment to the SCV is dependent on Rab7, which accumulates on the SCV early during infection (maximal level of association at 40 min postinfection) (24). Rab7 is a key regulator of late endosome trafficking to lysosomal compartments (25). During this process, Rab7 binds one of its host signaling partners, Rab-7 interacting lysosomal protein (RILP), which engages the late endosomes to the microtubule motor complex dynein-dynactin (25). This enables movement of late endosomes along microtubules toward the lysosomes located at the minus end of the microtubule-organizing center (25). Therefore, by recruiting Rab7 to the SCV, *S.* Typhimurium hijacks the endocytic pathway to promote the translocation of the SCV to the host cell perinuclear region (26, 27).

While Rab7-dependent juxtanuclear positioning of the SCV is crucial for SCV development, *Salmonella* must impede Rab7-mediated transport of the SCV to lysosomal (bactericidal) compartments. One mechanism to avoid lysosomal degradation of the SCV is to block the activity of Rab7. The SPI-2 effector SopD2 localizes to the SCV via its N-terminal domain, which also binds to Rab7 (28). SopD2 association with Rab7 precludes the interaction of the small GTPase with RILP, thereby preventing delivery of the SCV to the lysosome (28).

SopD2 further limits the interaction of the SCV with lysosomal compartments through its concerted activity with GtgE, another SPI-1 effector. GtgE is a cysteine protease that specifically cleaves the switch I region of the highly homologous Rabs 28, 29, and 32 when in their GDP-bound form, thereby disrupting interactions with downstream signaling partners (29–32). Rab32 is involved in the biogenesis of lysosome-related organelles, an intracellular membrane-bound compartment that shares many features with endosomes and lysosomes, such as Lamp-1 recruitment and acidic luminal pH (33). Because the SCV is similar to lysosome-related organelles, it can accumulate Rab32. In fact, the SCV of *S. enterica* serovar Typhi (the causal agent of typhoid fever), which lacks GtgE, accumulates Rab32, resulting in lower intracellular replicative rates than its GtgE-carrying counterpart, *S.* Typhimurium (29). Interestingly, while GtgE reduces Rab32 availability, the SCV of the *S.* Typhimurium *gtgE⁻* mutant still maintains poor association with Rab32, indicating that an additional effector(s) is involved in precluding Rab32 from this vacuole (34). The activity of SopD2 provides a striking example of cooperation between effectors. SopD2, unlike GtgE, does not affect the cellular levels of Rab32; instead, it inactivates Rab32 by accelerating hydrolysis of Rab32-GTP through its C-terminally encoded guanine-activating protein domain (34). Thereby, SopD2 enriches for Rab32-GDP, an inactive GTPase that does not interact with the SCV and the preferred form of Rab32 as the substrate for GtgE (34).

In addition to its role in early SCV biogenesis, SopB also limits SCV acquisition of late-endosomal and lysosomal content as a mechanism to avoid bacterial degradation. SopB-mediated formation of PI(3)P on the SCV allows for recruitment of sorting nexin-1, which is a component of the retromer complex involved in recycling of endosomal proteins to the trans-Golgi network (35). Sorting nexin-1 prevents accumulation of the late endosomal protein cation-independent mannose 6-phosphate receptor (MPR) on the SCV (35). Importantly, SopB-mediated hydrolysis of PI(4,5)P$_2$ at the plasma membrane generates SCVs devoid of this phosphoinositide, which is a negatively charged lipid that contributes to the net negative surface charge of the inner leaflet of the plasma membrane (36). Rab35, which promotes phagosomal-lysosomal fusion, localizes to the plasma membrane through these electrostatic interactions (36). As a result, in the absence of PI(4,5)P$_2$ the SCV membrane cannot be targeted by Rab35, and SCV-lysosome fusion is prevented (36).

While the initial nuclear apposition of the SCV is not SPI-2 dependent, the retention of the vacuole in this position is dependent on three SPI-2 effectors: SseG, SseF, and SifA (26, 37, 38). SseG and SseF share about 35% amino acid identity, bind to each other, and both interact with the Golgi network-associated protein 60/Golgi protein acyl coenzyme A binding domain-containing 3 (GCP60/ACBD3) (39, 40). The SseG, SseF, and GCP60/ACBD3 complex tethers the SCV to the Golgi

network, sustaining the SCV in its perinuclear position (40). In fact, SseG-mediated interaction with the Golgi network was shown to restrict SCV motility (26).

An additional strategy to maintain the SCV in its juxtanuclear position involves antagonizing the activity of kinesin-1, a microtubule motor protein that mediates cargo trafficking toward the cell periphery, plus-end of the microtubule-organizing center (41). PipB2, an SPI-2 effector, localizes to the SCV and directly binds kinesin light chain 1, thereby recruiting kinesin-1 to the SCV (42, 43). The accumulation of kinesin-1 directs movement of the SCV to the cell periphery and scattering of these vacuoles (44). To counteract anterograde SCV redistribution, the bacterium employs another SPI-2 effector, SifA, that interacts with the host protein SKIP (SifA and kinesin-interacting protein) and binds kinesin-1, inhibiting the centrifugal movement of the SCV (44). Therefore, *S.* Typhimurium balances the antagonizing activities of PipB2 and SifA in such a way that the inhibitory activity of SifA predominates over the activating role of PipB2 for kinesin-1 to maintain the SCV juxtanuclear position (43).

SipA is an SPI-1 effector known for its contribution during host cell invasion. This effector promotes actin polymerization and stability of actin filaments, thereby enhancing the local concentration of F-actin necessary to support membrane ruffle entry structures (45–47). Like the SPI-1 effectors discussed above, SipA remains active after *S.* Typhimurium entry into host cells (48). Following apposition to the nucleus, the SCV is stabilized by an F-actin meshwork that is less evident during *sipA⁻* mutant infections, consistent with SipA targeting of actin (48). The F-actin stabilization of the SCV in a SipA-dependent manner is important to maintain the localization of SifA on the SCV (48). In the absence of SipA, SifA exhibits poor localization to the SCV, which results in PipB2/kinesin-mediated scattering of the SCV to the cell periphery (48). Therefore, SipA cooperates to localize SifA to the SCV, thereby maintaining the nuclear positioning of the SCV.

Following apposition to the nucleus, the SCV develops tubular extensions known as *Salmonella*-induced filaments (Sifs) (49). Sif formation coincides with the onset of *S.* Typhimurium intracellular replication (50), and disruption of Sif formation correlates with attenuated virulence *in vivo* (51). Sifs elongate along microtubules in a centrifugal fashion, which implicates PipB2/kinesin-1 in this process (52, 53). In fact, SCVs formed with infection of a *pipB2⁻ S.* Typhimurium mutant result in shorter filaments compared to wild-type bacteria (42). SifA is the principal effector involved in Sif formation. SifA binds active Rab7 on Sif membranes and impedes the interaction of the small GTPase with its effector RILP (54). RILP is thereby excluded from Sifs and cannot recruit dynein, which precludes retrograde extension of the filament (54). SifA also binds the N-terminal domain RUN (RPIP8, UNC-14, and NESCA) of SKIP (53). SifA and SKIP then interact with kinesin-1 and trigger the fission of SCV-derived PipB2/kinesin-1 vesicles, whose anterograde movement contributes to Sif growth (53).

The SPI-1 effector SptP further promotes Sif formation. The N terminus of SptP contains a guanine-activating protein domain that inactivates Rac1 and Cdc42, enabling the actin cytoskeleton to recover its normal appearance after S. Typhimurium invasion (55). SptP localizes to the SCV and persists there for many hours after bacterial invasion (56). The postinvasion role of SptP relies on its C-terminally encoded phosphatase domain (56, 57). SptP directly binds to and activates, via dephosphorylation, the valosin-containing protein, a member of the AAA+ (ATPase associated with diverse cellular activities) family of ATPases. Dephosphorylated valosin-containing protein participates in vesicle fusion by binding to the t-SNARE (N-ethylmaleimide-sensitive-factor attachment protein receptor) syntaxin 5. Thereby, SptP promotes membrane fusion events that contribute to Sif formation and biogenesis of the S. Typhimurium intracellular replicative niche (56).

SifA is also involved in both inhibiting and promoting trafficking of lysosomal content to the SCV. Newly synthesized hydrolytic enzymes in the trans-Golgi network are transported to endosomes through cation-dependent and cation-independent MPRs (58). Endosomal maturation promotes activation of these hydrolases, which are then transported to lysosomes (58). One pathway that mediates recycling of MPRs from endosomes back to the trans-Golgi network involves the SNARE syntaxin 10 and its upstream effector Rab9 (58). SifA and SKIP sequester Rab9, thereby subverting the Rab9-dependent recycling of MPR, which compromises lysosomal function (58).

The fusion of lysosomes with membrane-bound compartments requires Rab7, as previously discussed, as well as the small GTPase Arl8b and the tethering factor HOPS (homotypic fusion and protein sorting) complex (59). HOPS is a hexameric complex whose subunit Vps (vacuole protein sorting) 41 is targeted to lysosomes via Arl8b. Another HOPS subunit, Vps39, interacts with SKIP (59). During S. Typhimurium infection, Arl8b localization to SCV allows recruitment of the HOPS complex (59). SKIP, localized to SCV and Sifs through binding to SifA, is also involved in recruitment of the HOPS complex (59). Tethering of the

HOPS complex to the SCV enables fusion of late endosomal and lysosomal content with the SCV, which is important for Sif formation and nutrient access that support bacterial intravacuolar replication (59).

In addition to SifA, the regulation of the SCV and Sif membrane dynamics appears to involve another SPI-2 effector, SseJ. During infection with S. Typhimurium sifA⁻ mutants, the SCV is destabilized, causing the bacterium to escape from the vacuole into the host cytosol to experience either robust replication in epithelial cells or death in macrophages (60, 61). However, during infection with the S. Typhimurium sifA⁻ sseJ⁻ double mutant, the SCV remains intact, ascribing a role for SseJ in vacuolar membrane loss (61). SseJ belongs to the GDSL motif-containing family of lipases and shares 29% amino acid identity with the glycerophospholipid-cholesterol acyltransferase (GCAT) enzyme members of this family. GCAT enzymes catalyze the transfer of fatty acid acyl groups from phospholipids to cholesterol to form cholesterol esters (62). SseJ exhibits deacylase, phospholipase A, and acyltransferase activities (62–66). Importantly, the enzymatic activity of SseJ is potentiated upon its binding to the active, GTP-bound form of RhoA (65, 66).

The esterification of cholesterol by SseJ results in the accumulation of cholesterol esters in the form of lipid droplets in infected cells, with the concurrent depletion of cholesterol from the plasma membrane and perinuclear region (63). In the absence of SseJ, cholesterol is found on the SCV and Sif membranes, whereas an excess of SseJ inhibits Sif formation. Therefore, SseJ appears to modulate membrane dynamics by regulating cholesterol levels (61, 63). The SseJ-mediated loss of SCV membrane integrity in the absence of SifA and inhibited Sif formation upon SseJ overexpression suggest an antagonist relationship between SifA and SseJ (61–63). Interestingly, SifA and SseJ were found to form a protein complex with RhoA, resulting in the formation of tubular extensions reminiscent of Sif filaments. These observations support a cooperative interaction between SseJ and SifA to fine-tune the membrane composition of SCV and Sifs (67).

One other T3SS effector involved in SCV and Sif membrane dynamics is SteA. This effector is one of a few S. Typhimurium T3SS effectors translocated by both SPI-1 and SPI-2 (68, 69). Bacterially translocated SteA localizes to the SCV and Sif membranes in a phosphatidylinositol 4-phosphate [PI(4)P]-dependent manner (70). The molecular target(s) of SteA remain uncharacterized, but deletion of this effector results in compact SCVs that contain several bacteria (as opposed to an SCV containing a single wild-type S. Typhimurium bacterium) and display a decreased number of Sifs (71). This mutant phenotype can be counteracted with pharmacological inhibition of dynein and kinesin, implicating SteA in the regulation of the activity of these microtubule protein motors (71).

Several hours (6 to 7 h) after bacterial invasion of epithelial cells, the SCV becomes surrounded by an F-actin meshwork (72). As previously discussed, the SPI-1 effector SipA participates in this process, and SipA-mediated actin accumulation around the SCV maintains Sif localization to the SCV as well as SCV perinuclear positioning (48). SPI-2 effectors also regulate actin assembly near the SCV, and this appears to contribute to maintenance of the vacuole integrity (72). The SPI-2 effector SteC is sufficient to induce F-actin accumulation around the SCV (73). At its C terminus, SteC contains a kinase domain (73) that mediates phosphorylation of MEK1, resulting in a conformational change that induces MEK-autophosphorylation and activation (74). MEK1 then stimulates a signaling cascade that includes extracellular signal-regulated kinase, myosin light chain kinase, and myosin II. The latter is responsible for the bundling of actin filaments as is observed upon ectopic expression of SteC (74).

The accumulation of F-actin around the SCV results from the *de novo* actin assembly, i.e., polymerization of actin monomers (G-actin) instead of local recruitment of preexisting filaments (72). As with many other cellular events regulated by *S*. Typhimurium, the formation of an F-actin meshwork surrounding the SCV is also the product of a bacterial fine-tuning of effectors with antagonizing activities. The SPI-2 effector SpvB, which inhibits actin polymerization by ADP-ribosylating G-actin, offsets the SteC-induced F-actin meshwork (75–77).

Altogether, these SPI effectors commandeer host vesicular trafficking and the cytoskeleton to establish a vacuolar replicative niche for *S*. Typhimurium while avoiding lysosomal degradation (Fig. 1 and Table 1).

S. FLEXNERI AND LIFE IN THE HOST CYTOSOL: ROLE FOR T3SS IN VACUOLE ESCAPE

The development of shigellosis starts with *S. flexneri* penetration of the intestinal epithelial barrier through the M cells that overlay lymphoid nodules (3, 78). Once reaching the underlying lymphoid tissue, *Shigella* is phagocytosed by resident macrophages, and shortly after, ruptures the phagosome to escape into the cytoplasm, where it initiates replication (3, 78). *Shigella*-induced death of the macrophages releases cytoplasmic

bacteria that subsequently invade the neighboring enterocytes through their basolateral surface (3, 78). Following enterocyte invasion, *S. flexneri* lyses its vacuole to replicate within and move across the host cytosol (3, 78). The encounter of a motile bacterium with the cell plasma membrane generates a protrusion that forces the bacterium into adjacent enterocytes (3, 78). Movement across two cell plasma membranes (from primary and secondary invaded host cells) causes bacterial entry into the adjacent cell through a double-membrane vacuole that is also lysed by *S. flexneri* to then initiate another round of infection (3, 78).

Therefore, the ability of *Shigella* to escape from a vacuole, be it the macrophage phagosome or the single- or double-membrane enterocyte vacuole, is paramount for this bacterium's virulence. Vacuole escape for *Shigella* is a T3SS-dependent mechanism (3). One T3SS effector involved in this process is IpgD, a $PI(4,5)P_2$ 4-phosphatase (79). Hydrolysis of $PI(4,5)P_2$ by this effector disrupts the contact between cortical actin and the plasma membrane, contributing to formation of plasma membrane ruffles at bacterial entry sites (79). Collapse of membrane ruffles and fusion with the plasma membrane leads to engulfment of the bacterium in a process similar to macropinocytosis (80). Interestingly, IpgD enhances invasion efficiency but is not required for this process (81). Internalized *Shigella* is briefly contained within a tight, uniform vacuole (*S. flexneri*-containing vacuole, *Sf*CV) that ruptures 10 min after invasion (80). Initially, the *Sf*CV is surrounded by macropinosomes formed as a result of the IpgD-ruffling activity (80). The small GTPase Rab11, known to primarily associate with recycling endosomes, is directly recruited to the *Sf*CV-surrounding macropinosomes in an IpgD-dependent manner (80, 82). Once the Rab11-macropinosomes come in contact with *Sf*CV, the bacterial vacuole ruptures by a not yet defined mechanism (80, 82). In the absence of IpgD, the availability of macropinosomes is diminished, and a delay in bacterial vacuole escape is observed (82). Additionally, the *Sf*CV of *Shigella ipgD⁻* mutants is surrounded by an actin meshwork (actin cage) that obstructs *Shigella*'s escape (82).

The overall delay effect indicates that, in addition to IpgD, other T3SS components may be playing a role in vacuole rupture. IpaB and IpaC are components of the T3SS apparatus, specifically, translocon proteins that insert into host membranes through their hydrophobic regions to form membrane pores (83, 84). The translocon-pore activity of each of these two proteins contributes to destabilizing the membrane of phagosomes, in macrophages, as well as the entry and protrusion vacuole membranes of infected epithelial cells,

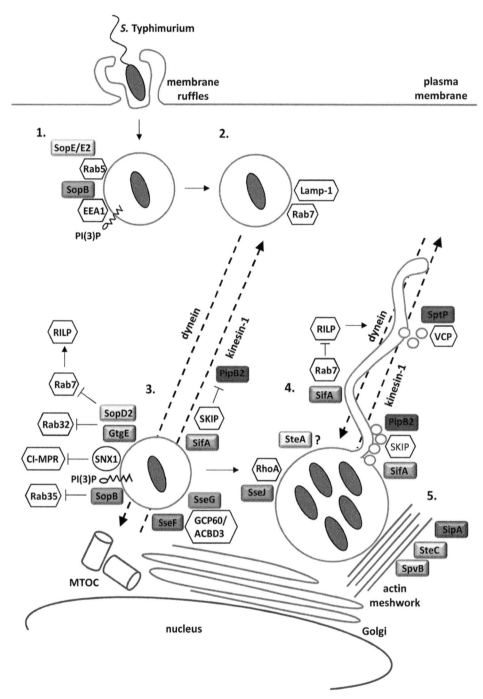

Figure 1   Schematic of the contribution of T3SS effectors to the intracellular life cycle of *S.* Typhimurium (1). Following invasion of epithelial cells, *S.* Typhimurium employs the effectors SopE/E2 and SopB to transiently recruit early endosomal markers to the *Salmonella*-containing vacuole (SCV) (2). SCV maturation and acquisition of Rab7 lead to dynein-mediated translocation of this vacuole to the host cell perinuclear region (3). Development of the SCV into a bactericidal compartment is precluded by the action of SopB, GtgE, and SopD2, which collectively, inhibit the endosomal-lysosomal fusion activities of Rab35, Rab32, and Rab7. SseF and SseG, in complex with GCP60/ACBD3, maintain the SCV juxtanuclear position. Additionally, SifA, through its eukaryotic effector SKIP, inhibits PipB2/kinesin-1-mediated centrifugal movement of the SCV (4). Next, the SCV develops Sifs, which coincides with the onset of *S.* Typhimurium intravacuolar replication. Sif formation is the product of the concerted action of SifA, PipB2, and SseJ. SifA and PipB2 coordinate the centrifugal extension of the Sifs, while SifA and SseJ regulate SCV and Sif membrane dynamics that support Sif growth. Filament growth is further promoted by SptP (5). The SCV is surrounded by an actin meshwork which contributes to maintaining SCV integrity. The effectors SipA, SpvB, and SteC modulate actin dynamics in the surroundings of the SCV.

TABLE 1   SPI-1 and SPI-2 effectors that contribute to the intracellular life cycle of *S.* Typhimurium

Effector	Secretion system	Cellular target	Biochemical activity	Biological function	References
SopE/E2	SPI-1	Cdc42 and Rac1	GEF	SCV formation	13–18
SopB	SPI-1	PI(4,5)P$_2$	Phosphatidylinositol phosphatase	SCV formation, maturation, and avoidance of lysosomal degradation	19–23, 35, 36
GtgE	SPI-1	Rab32	Cysteine protease	SCV avoidance of lysosomal degradation	29–34
SopD2	SPI-2	Rab32, Rab7	GAP	SCV avoidance of lysosomal degradation	28, 34
SseG	SPI-2	GCP60/ACBD3	Unknown	SCV perinuclear positioning	26, 37, 39, 40
SseF	SPI-2	GCP60/ACBD3	Unknown	SCV perinuclear positioning	37–40
SifA	SPI-2	SKIP	Unknown	SCV perinuclear positioning, Sif formation, SCV integrity	43, 44, 48, 49, 52–54, 58, 59
SipA	SPI-1	Actin	Actin polymerization,	SCV perinuclear positioning	45–48
PipB2	SPI-2	Kinesin-1	Unknown	Sif formation	42–44, 48, 52, 53
SptP	SPI-1	Valosin-containing protein	Phosphatase	Sif formation	55–57
SseJ	SPI-2	Cholesterol, RhoA	Glycerophospholipid: cholesterol acyltransferase	SCV and Sif membrane dynamics	60–67
SteA	SPI-1, SPI-2	Unknown	Unknown	SCV and Sif membrane dynamics	68–71
SteC	SPI-2	MEK1	Kinase	SCV-surrounding actin meshwork	73, 74
SpvB	SPI-2	G-actin	ADP-ribosylating protein	SCV-surrounding actin meshwork	75–77

allowing *S. flexneri* to escape into the host cytosol (85–88). An elegant study demonstrated that the reconstitution of *Shigella*'s T3SS apparatus into a nonpathogenic *Escherichia coli* strain was sufficient to promote bacterial escape from a vacuole (89).

Following escape into the host cytosol, *S. flexneri* employs the secreted protein IcsA (also known as VirG) to spread both across and between epithelial cells (90). IcsA is a type V secreted autotransporter that uses the Sec secretion pathway to translocate across the bacterial inner membrane (91). Despite not being a T3SS effector, IcsA plays a seminal role to the intracellular lifestyle of *S. flexneri* and, therefore, merits discussion here. IcsA is delivered to the surface of the bacterium's old pole, and this polarized distribution is sustained by outer membrane properties such as fluidity and by IcsP-mediated proteolysis of nonpolarized IcsA (92, 93). The C-terminal, transporter domain of IcsA inserts into the bacterial outer membrane, while the N-terminal, passenger domain is exposed on the bacterial surface (94). The passenger domain specifically recruits and activates neural Wiskott-Aldrich syndrome protein (N-WASP) (94–96). N-WASP possesses several domains: an N-terminal WASP homology 1, a central GTPase-binding (GDB), and a C-terminal verprolin homology/cofilin/acidic (VCA) domain. The inactive conformation of N-WASP is established through the auto-inhibitory intramolecular interaction

between the GDB and VCA domains; upon association of the Rho-GTPase Cdc42 with the GDB domain, the VCA domain is released, leading to the activation of N-WASP (97). The IcsA passenger domain directly binds both the WASP homology 1 and the GBD domain, exposing the VCA domain that subsequently binds G-actin and activates the actin filament nucleator Arp2/3 complex (94). The IcsA-mediated unidirectional actin polymerization leads to the polarized formation of an actin comet-like tail that propels the bacterium forward during intra- and intercellular motility (98).

Actin-dependent movement of *S. flexneri* enables the bacterium to protrude and enter the neighboring cell via a double-membrane vacuole (protrusion *Sf*CV) (3, 78). The T3SS effector IcsB facilitates escape from this vacuole (99–101), albeit with no role in bacterial escape from the single-membrane (entry) vacuole. IcsB binds cholesterol through its cholesterol-binding domain (102). Because there is a noted difference in plasma membrane leaflet orientation in single- and double-membrane vacuoles and membrane cholesterol content, this could account for IcsB's specific activity (101).

The protrusion *Sf*CV is targeted for autophagy through the recruitment of the autophagosome marker light chain 3 (LC3) (101). Previous works attributed a role to IcsB in autophagy evasion because higher numbers of LC3-positive vacuoles were present during infections with $icsB^{-/-}$ mutants compared to the parental strain (100, 102, 103). However, a recent study demonstrated that vacuoles containing either wild-type or $icsB^{-/-}$ bacteria equally recruit LC3, with the failure of vacuole escape in the absence of IcsB being causal for LC3 enrichment (101).

LC3 recruitment to the protrusion *Sf*CV can be modulated by the T3SS effector VirA (100, 104). VirA is a guanine-activating protein that preferentially targets the GTPase Rab1 (104). In addition to its well-established role in regulating endoplasmic reticulum-Golgi and intra-Golgi trafficking, Rab1 is also involved in autophagosome formation (105). Therefore, it has been proposed that VirA hydrolyzes Rab1 as a mechanism to control antibacterial autophagy (104).

The entry into a host cell, the escape from the vacuoles, and the movement of *Shigella* from one cell to another are mediated by a small number of effectors that use the host cell resources to facilitate invasion, replication, and virulence (Fig. 2 and Table 2).

V. PARAHAEMOLYTICUS: AN INTRACELLULAR BACTERIUM REVEALING NEW MECHANISMS FOR SURVIVAL AND REPLICATION

The diversity of T3SS-dependent mechanisms of intracellular subversion devised by *S.* Typhimurium and *S. flexneri* underscores the uniqueness of each bacterium's intracellular lifestyle and advocates for the investigation of new bacterial models as a way to uncover yet unknown mechanisms. The marine bacterium *V. parahaemolyticus* was first identified in 1950 as the causative agent of a diarrheal outbreak in Japan (106). The sequencing of the *V. parahaemolyticus* genome revealed the presence of two T3SSs: the first apparatus, T3SS1, was ancestrally acquired and is present in both environmental and clinical strains, and the second apparatus, T3SS2, was recently acquired (via horizontal transfer) and is present exclusively in clinical strains (107). T3SS2 is the virulence factor that governs acute gastroenteritis, the bacterium's principal manifestation in humans (108).

Since its discovery, this bacterium has been regarded as an exclusive extracellular bacterium, i.e., one that resides and propagates entirely outside of a host cell during infection. In fact, it was demonstrated that, *in vitro*, the potent cytotoxicity of the first T3SS masks the activity of the T3SS2 (albeit with no significant role for enterotoxicity; the T3SS1 can be activated upon culturing of the bacterium in tissue culture growth media) (109, 110). The T3SS1 effectors work in a tempo-ral manner to orchestrate the death of the host cell within about 3 hours: first, VopQ inhibits autophagic flux by disrupting the host lysosomal V-ATPase; second, VPA0450 induces plasma membrane blebbing by hydrolyzing PI(4,5)P$_2$; third, VopS contains a Fic domain that AMPylates Rho GTPases, resulting in cell rounding (111). These events, and possibly the activity of one other uncharacterized effector, VopR (112), contribute to the final lysis of the host cell.

The use of a bacterial strain lacking both the hemolysins and the T3SS1 provided insight into the pathogenesis of the T3SS2 and revealed an intracellular life cycle for *V. parahaemolyticus*. The T3SS2 effector VopC is a homolog of cytotoxic necrotizing factors that catalyzes the deamidation of Rho GTPases, specifically, Cdc42 and Rac1 (11). As a result, the deamidated Cdc42 and Rac1 adopt a constitutively active conformation resulting in dramatic rearrangements of the actin cytoskeleton (11). At sites of bacterial contact with the host epithelial cells, active Cdc42 and Rac1 reorganize the actin into membrane ruffles that promote the engulfment of *V. parahaemolyticus*, enabling bacterial invasion in nonphagocytic cells (Fig. 3) (11, 12). Upon uncovering VopC's activity, it became clear that *V. parahaemolyticus* is a facultative intracellular bacterium, i.e., one that resides and propagates both outside and inside of its host cell.

Following VopC-mediated invasion of epithelial cells, *V. parahaemolyticus* is enclosed within a vacuole that interacts with the endocytic pathway. The vacuole transiently acquires early endosomal features, such as the EEA1 protein, and subsequently matures into a late endosome-like organelle, given by the acquisition of LAMP-1 and the acidification of its lumen (12). Luminal acidification is an important cue that triggers the bacterium to break out of its vacuole and escape into the host cytosol, where prolific bacterial replication (100 to 300 bacteria/cell) takes place (Fig. 3) (12). The bacterial factors that contribute to each of these steps remain completely unknown.

A decade went by between the genome sequencing that revealed *V. parahaemolyticus*' T3SSs and the discovery of the *V. parahaemolyticus* intracellular lifestyle (11, 107). During this period, many of the bacterium's T3SS2 effectors were characterized from the realm of *V. parahaemolyticus* being an exclusively extracellular bacterium. As a result, the cellular targets and biochemical activities of these effectors were uncovered, but the relevant roles they play during invasive infection remained unknown. An example is VopL, previously identified as a potent nucleator of actin filaments that initially was thought to induce the formation of

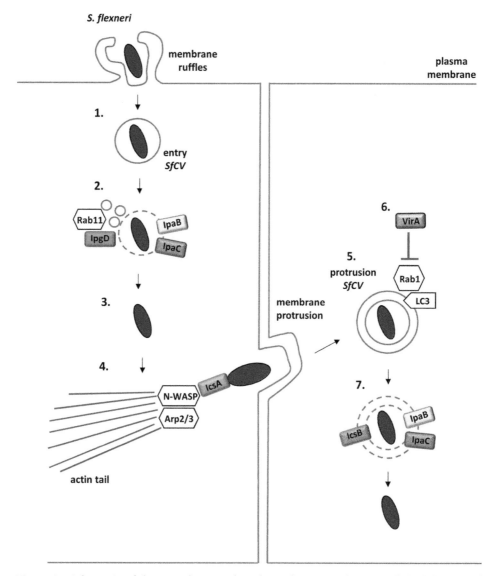

Figure 2 Schematic of the contribution of virulence factors to the intracellular life cycle of *S. flexneri* (**1**). *S. flexneri* briefly resides within its entry vacuole (*Sf*CV) (**2**). The *Sf*CV is ruptured by the pore-forming activity of the T3SS translocon proteins IpaB and IpaC. IpgD facilitates vacuolar disruption by generating Rab11-macropinosomes that fuse to *S. flexneri* (**3**). Upon rupture of the *Sf*CV, *Shigella* escapes into the host cytosol, from where the bacterium employs its IcsA to recruit actin cytoskeleton machinery, namely, N-WASP and Arp2/3 that polymerize actin filaments at one pole of the bacterium (**4**). Unidirectional actin polymerization propels the bacterium across the host cytosol, leading to protrusions that enable bacterial spread into the neighboring cell (**5**). In the secondary cell, *S. flexneri* is initially contained within a double-membrane vacuole (protrusion *Sf*CV) (**6**). Recruitment of LC3 to the protrusion vacuole is controlled by the T3SS effector VirA, which targets the Rho GTPase Rab1 (**7**). IpaB, IpaC, and the T3SS effector IcsB promote bacterial escape from the protrusion of *Sf*CV into the cytosol, enabling the bacterium to complete another infection cycle.

stress fibers but later was found to catalyze the formation of nonfunctional actin linear strings (113, 114).

Analysis of the activity of VopL demonstrated that this effector plays a critical role in a process required for *V. parahaemolyticus* intracellular survival (115). This process is the assembly and activation of the NADPH oxidase enzymatic complex. The NAPDH oxidase is a major source of bactericidal reactive oxy-

TABLE 2   Virulence factors that contribute to the intracellular life cycle of *S. flexneri*

Effector	Secretion system	Cellular target	Biochemical activity	Biological function	References
IpgD	T3SS	PI(4,5)P$_2$	4-Phosphatase	Vacuole rupture	79–82
IpaB	T3SS	Membrane lipids	Pore-forming	Vacuole rupture	83–85, 87–89
IpaC	T3SS	Membrane lipids	Pore-forming	Vacuole rupture	84, 86–89
IcsA	T5SS/T2SS	Actin	Actin filament	Cell motility	90–98
IcsB	T3SS	Unknown/cholesterol	Unknown	Vacuole rupture	99–103
VirA	T3SS	Rab1	GTPase hydrolysis	Autophagy evasion	100, 104

gen species (ROS) in host cells. In the absence of VopL, host epithelial cells produce ROS via NADPH oxidase that damage the DNA of cytosolic bacteria (115). As a result, *V. parahaemolyticus* exhibits erratic cell division with a resulting filamentous state and defective intracellular replication (115). VopL antagonizes bacterial deleterious events by inhibiting the actin-dependent movement of NADPH oxidase subunits to their site of complex assembly (host membranes), thereby precluding ROS generation (Fig. 3) (115). This was the first example of a T3SS effector that targets the actin cytoskeleton as a mechanism to suppress the ROS response.

The novel understanding of *V. parahaemolyticus* as an intracellular bacterium compares to a "rediscovery" of this bacterium, which presents itself as a model poised for future studies of T3SS-mediated disruption of intracellular processes. Like VopL, many of the already known T3SS2 effectors need to be reassessed with consideration of *V. parahaemolyticus'* intracellular life cycle to reveal their relevant biological functions. Moreover, the pathogenicity island that comprises the T3SS2 is predicted to encode additional putative effectors that likely contribute to the bacterium's intracellular lifestyle and merits investigation.

CONCLUSIONS

The coexistence of bacterial pathogens and their hosts enabled many bacteria to establish an intracellular infection as a result of convergent evolution. T3SS effectors are one of the best examples of convergent evolution, because they are often mimics of eukaryotic proteins. Mimicry of eukaryotic proteins by T3SS effectors comes in different flavors. In some instances, the mimicry is functional, as in the case of *S.* Typhimurium's SopE, which bears neither sequence nor structural homology to the Dbl family of eukaryotic GEFs of Cdc42 (116). Instead, SopE belongs to a family of bacterial WxxxE GEFs (116). Importantly, SopE and Dbl members interact with the switch I and II regions of Cdc42 in a very similar manner to facilitate nucleotide

exchange (116). In other instances, T3SS effectors are homologous to eukaryotic proteins but carry out their biochemical functions in a distinctive manner. One example of this is *S.* Typhimurium SteC, a kinase that exhibits sequence similarity to eukaryotic kinases, including its closest homolog, Raf1. These kinases target the same substrate, namely MEK, but while Raf1 phosphorylates residues within the catalytic domain of MEK, SteC phosphorylates an allosteric residue, which induces a conformational change of MEK (74).

Sometimes, different bacterial effectors possess a conserved eukaryotic domain and catalyze the same biochemical reaction but play distinct biological roles. For instance, the *S.* Typhimurium effector SopB and the *S. flexneri* effector IpgD are homologs to each other and to eukaryotic PI4,5-P$_2$ phosphatases (19, 79). PI4,5-P$_2$ hydrolysis by both SopB and IpgD results in formation of macropinosomes (22, 82). Curiously, SopB-formed macropinosomes are important as a membrane source for the formation of the spacious SCV (22). IpgD-formed macropinosomes, on the other hand, promote rupture of the *Shigella*-containing vacuole (82). Altogether, these examples underscore the extraordinary ability of bacteria to adapt protein functionalities that best suit these pathogens during infection. The study of T3SS effectors also contributes to furthering the understanding of eukaryotic cell biology. It was through the characterization of *S.* Typhimurium SifA that the protein SKIP was identified and with that, it was possible to better understand kinesin-dependent anterograde cargo trafficking (44).

The enteric pathogens *S.* Typhimurium, *S. flexneri*, and *V. parahaemolyticus* share many of the same cellular hosts but adopt distinct intracellular lifestyles to survive and propagate within these cells. *S.* Typhimurium, at large, resides within its crafted SCV, *S. flexneri* rapidly (~10 min) ruptures its vacuole to spread across the host cell, and *V. parahaemolyticus* maintains longer residence (~1 h) within its vacuole prior to its escape into the host cytosol. Adaptation into each of these distinct lifestyles is largely a result of the fact that each

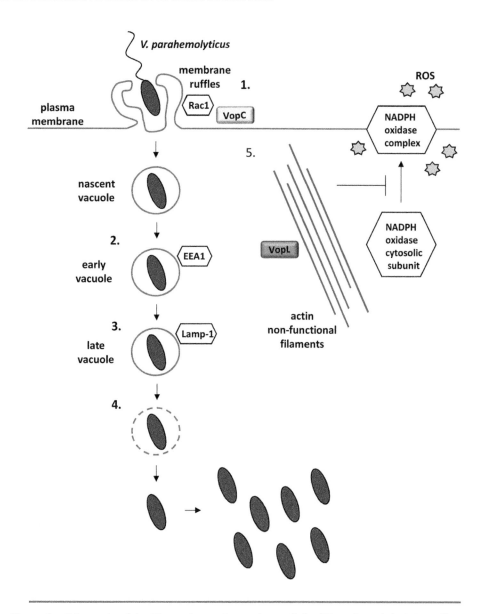

Figure 3 Schematic of the *V. parahaemolyticus* intracellular life cycle and the T3SS effectors that contribute to it (**1**). The T3SS2 effector VopC induces epithelial host cell plasma membrane ruffling that internalizes *V. parahaemolyticus* into a nascent vacuole. The nascent vacuole develops first into an early endosome-like compartment, given by its acquisition of EEA1 (**2**) and subsequently matures into a late endosome-like vacuole, given by the recruitment of Lamp-1 (**3**). (**4**) The bacterium disrupts its containing vacuole and escapes into the cytosol, where bacterial replication takes place (**5**). To evade host immune defenses, *V. parahaemolyticus* employs the T3SS2 VopL, which disrupts the actin cytoskeleton and thereby inhibits the actin-dependent assembly of the ROS-producing NADPH oxidase complex.

bacterium is equipped with a unique suite of T3SS effectors, which underlines the significance of characterizing each of these systems. *S.* Typhimurium and *S. flexneri* are established, well-studied models of intracellular infection, while *V. parahaemolyticus* provides a new model for future discoveries.

Acknowledgments. We apologize to those whose work could not be cited owing to space limitations. We thank members of the Orth lab for their helpful discussions and advice.

This work was funded by Welch Foundation grant I-1561 (K.O.) and the Once Upon a Time... Foundation (M.S., K. O.). K.O. is a Burroughs Welcome investigator in pathogenesis of infectious disease, a Beckman Young investigator, and a

W.W. Caruth, Jr. biomedical scholar and has an Earl A. Forsythe chair in biomedical science.

Citation. de Souza Santos M, Orth K. 2019. The role of the type III secretion system in the intracellular lifestyle of enteric pathogens. Microbiol Spectrum 7(3):BAI-0008-2019.

References

1. Samanta D, Mulye M, Clemente TM, Justis AV, Gilk SD. 2017. Manipulation of host cholesterol by obligate intracellular bacteria. *Front Cell Infect Microbiol* 7:165.

2. Flint A, Butcher J, Stintzi A. 2016. Stress responses, adaptation, and virulence of bacterial pathogens during host gastrointestinal colonization. *Microbiol Spectr* 4: VMBF-0007-2015.

3. Mellouk N, Enninga J. 2016. Cytosolic access of intracellular bacterial pathogens: the *Shigella* paradigm. *Front Cell Infect Microbiol* 6:35.

4. Ribet D, Cossart P. 2015. How bacterial pathogens colonize their hosts and invade deeper tissues. *Microbes Infect* 17:173–183.

5. Ray K, Marteyn B, Sansonetti PJ, Tang CM. 2009. Life on the inside: the intracellular lifestyle of cytosolic bacteria. *Nat Rev Microbiol* 7:333–340.

6. Galán JE, Waksman G. 2018. Protein-injection machines in bacteria. *Cell* 172:1306–1318.

7. Jennings E, Thurston TLM, Holden DW. 2017. Salmonella SPI-2 type III secretion system effectors: molecular mechanisms and physiological consequences. *Cell Host Microbe* 22:217–231.

8. Agaisse H. 2016. Molecular and cellular mechanisms of *Shigella flexneri* dissemination. *Front Cell Infect Microbiol* 6:29.

9. Agbor TA, McCormick BA. 2011. *Salmonella* effectors: important players modulating host cell function during infection. *Cell Microbiol* 13:1858–1869.

10. Letchumanan V, Chan KG, Lee LH. 2014. *Vibrio parahaemolyticus*: a review on the pathogenesis, prevalence, and advance molecular identification techniques. *Front Microbiol* 5:705.

11. Zhang L, Krachler AM, Broberg CA, Li Y, Mirzaei H, Gilpin CJ, Orth K. 2012. Type III effector VopC mediates invasion for *Vibrio* species. *Cell Rep* 1:453–460.

12. de Souza Santos M, Orth K. 2014. Intracellular *Vibrio parahaemolyticus* escapes the vacuole and establishes a replicative niche in the cytosol of epithelial cells. *MBio* 5:e01506-14.

13. Hardt WD, Chen LM, Schuebel KE, Bustelo XR, Galán JE. 1998. *S. typhimurium* encodes an activator of Rho GTPases that induces membrane ruffling and nuclear responses in host cells. *Cell* 93:815–826.

14. Stender S, Friebel A, Linder S, Rohde M, Mirold S, Hardt WD. 2000. Identification of SopE2 from *Salmonella typhimurium*, a conserved guanine nucleotide exchange factor for Cdc42 of the host cell. *Mol Microbiol* 36:1206–1221.

15. Humphreys D, Davidson A, Hume PJ, Koronakis V. 2012. *Salmonella* virulence effector SopE and host GEF ARNO cooperate to recruit and activate WAVE to trigger bacterial invasion. *Cell Host Microbe* 11: 129–139.

16. Kubori T, Galán JE. 2003. Temporal regulation of *Salmonella* virulence effector function by proteasome-dependent protein degradation. *Cell* 115:333–342.

17. Vonaesch P, Sellin ME, Cardini S, Singh V, Barthel M, Hardt WD. 2014. The *Salmonella* Typhimurium effector protein SopE transiently localizes to the early SCV and contributes to intracellular replication. *Cell Microbiol* 16:1723–1735.

18. Mukherjee K, Parashuraman S, Raje M, Mukhopadhyay A. 2001. SopE acts as an Rab5-specific nucleotide exchange factor and recruits non-prenylated Rab5 on *Salmonella*-containing phagosomes to promote fusion with early endosomes. *J Biol Chem* 276:23607–23615.

19. Norris FA, Wilson MP, Wallis TS, Galyov EE, Majerus PW. 1998. SopB, a protein required for virulence of *Salmonella dublin*, is an inositol phosphate phosphatase. *Proc Natl Acad Sci U S A* 95:14057–14059.

20. Terebiznik MR, Vieira OV, Marcus SL, Slade A, Yip CM, Trimble WS, Meyer T, Finlay BB, Grinstein S. 2002. Elimination of host cell PtdIns(4,5)P(2) by bacterial SigD promotes membrane fission during invasion by *Salmonella*. *Nat Cell Biol* 4:766–773.

21. Scott CC, Cuellar-Mata P, Matsuo T, Davidson HW, Grinstein S. 2002. Role of 3-phosphoinositides in the maturation of *Salmonella*-containing vacuoles within host cells. *J Biol Chem* 277:12770–12776.

22. Hernandez LD, Hueffer K, Wenk MR, Galán JE. 2004. *Salmonella* modulates vesicular traffic by altering phosphoinositide metabolism. *Science* 304:1805–1807.

23. Mallo GV, Espina M, Smith AC, Terebiznik MR, Alemán A, Finlay BB, Rameh LE, Grinstein S, Brumell JH. 2008. SopB promotes phosphatidylinositol 3-phosphate formation on *Salmonella* vacuoles by recruiting Rab5 and Vps34. *J Cell Biol* 182:741–752.

24. Méresse S, Steele-Mortimer O, Finlay BB, Gorvel JP. 1999. The rab7 GTPase controls the maturation of *Salmonella typhimurium*-containing vacuoles in HeLa cells. *EMBO J* 18:4394–4403.

25. Guerra F, Bucci C. 2016. Multiple roles of the small GTPase Rab7. *Cells* 5:E34.

26. Ramsden AE, Mota LJ, Münter S, Shorte SL, Holden DW. 2007. The SPI-2 type III secretion system restricts motility of *Salmonella*-containing vacuoles. *Cell Microbiol* 9:2517–2529.

27. Salcedo SP, Holden DW. 2003. SseG, a virulence protein that targets *Salmonella* to the Golgi network. *EMBO J* 22:5003–5014.

28. D'Costa VM, Braun V, Landekic M, Shi R, Proteau A, McDonald L, Cygler M, Grinstein S, Brumell JH. 2015. *Salmonella* disrupts host endocytic trafficking by SopD2-mediated inhibition of Rab7. *Cell Rep* 12: 1508–1518.

29. Spanò S, Galán JE. 2012. A Rab32-dependent pathway contributes to *Salmonella typhi* host restriction. *Science* 338:960–963.

30. Spanò S, Liu X, Galán JE. 2011. Proteolytic targeting of Rab29 by an effector protein distinguishes the intracellu-

lar compartments of human-adapted and broad-host *Salmonella*. *Proc Natl Acad Sci U S A* **108**:18418–18423.

31. Kohler AC, Spanò S, Galán JE, Stebbins CE. 2014. Structural and enzymatic characterization of a host-specificity determinant from *Salmonella*. *Acta Crystallogr D Biol Crystallogr* **70**:384–391.

32. Wachtel R, Bräuning B, Mader SL, Ecker F, Kaila VRI, Groll M, Itzen A. 2018. The protease GtgE from *Salmonella* exclusively targets inactive Rab GTPases. *Nat Commun* **9**:44.

33. Ohbayashi N, Fukuda M, Kanaho Y. 2017. Rab32 subfamily small GTPases: pleiotropic Rabs in endosomal trafficking. *J Biochem* **162**:65–71.

34. Spanò S, Gao X, Hannemann S, Lara-Tejero M, Galán JE. 2016. A bacterial pathogen targets a host Rab-family GTPase defense pathway with a GAP. *Cell Host Microbe* **19**:216–226.

35. Bujny MV, Ewels PA, Humphrey S, Attar N, Jepson MA, Cullen PJ. 2008. Sorting nexin-1 defines an early phase of *Salmonella*-containing vacuole-remodeling during *Salmonella* infection. *J Cell Sci* **121**:2027–2036.

36. Bakowski MA, Braun V, Lam GY, Yeung T, Heo WD, Meyer T, Finlay BB, Grinstein S, Brumell JH. 2010. The phosphoinositide phosphatase SopB manipulates membrane surface charge and trafficking of the *Salmonella*-containing vacuole. *Cell Host Microbe* **7**:453–462.

37. Kuhle V, Jäckel D, Hensel M. 2004. Effector proteins encoded by *Salmonella* pathogenicity island 2 interfere with the microtubule cytoskeleton after translocation into host cells. *Traffic* **5**:356–370.

38. Abrahams GL, Müller P, Hensel M. 2006. Functional dissection of SseF, a type III effector protein involved in positioning the *Salmonella*-containing vacuole. *Traffic* **7**:950–965.

39. Deiwick J, Salcedo SP, Boucrot E, Gilliland SM, Henry T, Petermann N, Waterman SR, Gorvel JP, Holden DW, Méresse S. 2006. The translocated *Salmonella* effector proteins SseF and SseG interact and are required to establish an intracellular replication niche. *Infect Immun* **74**:6965–6972.

40. Yu XJ, Liu M, Holden DW. 2016. *Salmonella* effectors SseF and SseG interact with mammalian protein ACBD3 (GCP60) to anchor *Salmonella*-containing vacuoles at the Golgi network. *MBio* **7**:e00474-16.

41. Mallik R, Rai AK, Barak P, Rai A, Kunwar A. 2013. Teamwork in microtubule motors. *Trends Cell Biol* **23**:575–582.

42. Knodler LA, Steele-Mortimer O. 2005. The *Salmonella* effector PipB2 affects late endosome/lysosome distribution to mediate Sif extension. *Mol Biol Cell* **16**:4108–4123.

43. Henry T, Couillault C, Rockenfeller P, Boucrot E, Dumont A, Schroeder N, Hermant A, Knodler LA, Lecine P, Steele-Mortimer O, Borg JP, Gorvel JP, Méresse S. 2006. The *Salmonella* effector protein PipB2 is a linker for kinesin-1. *Proc Natl Acad Sci U S A* **103**:13497–13502.

44. Boucrot E, Henry T, Borg JP, Gorvel JP, Méresse S. 2005. The intracellular fate of *Salmonella* depends on the recruitment of kinesin. *Science* **308**:1174–1178.

45. Zhou D, Mooseker MS, Galán JE. 1999. Role of the *S. typhimurium* actin-binding protein SipA in bacterial internalization. *Science* **283**:2092–2095.

46. Zhou D, Mooseker MS, Galán JE. 1999. An invasion-associated *Salmonella* protein modulates the actin-bundling activity of plastin. *Proc Natl Acad Sci U S A* **96**:10176–10181.

47. McGhie EJ, Hayward RD, Koronakis V. 2004. Control of actin turnover by a *Salmonella* invasion protein. *Mol Cell* **13**:497–510.

48. Brawn LC, Hayward RD, Koronakis V. 2007. *Salmonella* SPI1 effector SipA persists after entry and cooperates with a SPI2 effector to regulate phagosome maturation and intracellular replication. *Cell Host Microbe* **1**:63–75.

49. Garcia-del Portillo F, Zwick MB, Leung KY, Finlay BB. 1993. *Salmonella* induces the formation of filamentous structures containing lysosomal membrane glycoproteins in epithelial cells. *Proc Natl Acad Sci U S A* **90**:10544–10548.

50. Garcia-del Portillo F, Zwick MB, Leung KY, Finlay BB. 1993. Intracellular replication of *Salmonella* within epithelial cells is associated with filamentous structures containing lysosomal membrane glycoproteins. *Infect Agents Dis* **2**:227–231.

51. Stein MA, Leung KY, Zwick M, Garcia-del Portillo F, Finlay BB. 1996. Identification of a *Salmonella* virulence gene required for formation of filamentous structures containing lysosomal membrane glycoproteins within epithelial cells. *Mol Microbiol* **20**:151–164.

52. Brumell JH, Goosney DL, Finlay BB. 2002. SifA, a type III secreted effector of *Salmonella typhimurium*, directs *Salmonella*-induced filament (Sif) formation along microtubules. *Traffic* **3**:407–415.

53. Dumont A, Boucrot E, Drevensek S, Daire V, Gorvel JP, Poüs C, Holden DW, Méresse S. 2010. SKIP, the host target of the *Salmonella* virulence factor SifA, promotes kinesin-1-dependent vacuolar membrane exchanges. *Traffic* **11**:899–911.

54. Harrison RE, Brumell JH, Khandani A, Bucci C, Scott CC, Jiang X, Finlay BB, Grinstein S. 2004. *Salmonella* impairs RILP recruitment to Rab7 during maturation of invasion vacuoles. *Mol Biol Cell* **15**:3146–3154.

55. Fu Y, Galán JE. 1999. A *Salmonella* protein antagonizes Rac-1 and Cdc42 to mediate host-cell recovery after bacterial invasion. *Nature* **401**:293–297.

56. Humphreys D, Hume PJ, Koronakis V. 2009. The *Salmonella* effector SptP dephosphorylates host AAA+ ATPase VCP to promote development of its intracellular replicative niche. *Cell Host Microbe* **5**:225–233.

57. Kaniga K, Uralil J, Bliska JB, Galán JE. 1996. A secreted protein tyrosine phosphatase with modular effector domains in the bacterial pathogen *Salmonella* typhimurium. *Mol Microbiol* **21**:633–641.

58. McGourty K, Thurston TL, Matthews SA, Pinaud L, Mota LJ, Holden DW. 2012. *Salmonella* inhibits retrograde trafficking of mannose-6-phosphate receptors and lysosome function. *Science* **338**:963–967.

59. Sindhwani A, Arya SB, Kaur H, Jagga D, Tuli A, Sharma M. 2017. *Salmonella* exploits the host endo-lysosomal tethering factor HOPS complex to promote its intravacuolar replication. *PLoS Pathog* 13: e1006700.

60. Beuzón CR, Méresse S, Unsworth KE, Ruíz-Albert J, Garvis S, Waterman SR, Ryder TA, Boucrot E, Holden DW. 2000. *Salmonella* maintains the integrity of its intracellular vacuole through the action of SifA. *EMBO J* 19:3235–3249.

61. Ruiz-Albert J, Yu XJ, Beuzón CR, Blakey AN, Galyov EE, Holden DW. 2002. Complementary activities of SseJ and SifA regulate dynamics of the *Salmonella typhimurium* vacuolar membrane. *Mol Microbiol* 44: 645–661.

62. Ohlson MB, Fluhr K, Birmingham CL, Brumell JH, Miller SI. 2005. SseJ deacylase activity by *Salmonella enterica* serovar Typhimurium promotes virulence in mice. *Infect Immun* 73:6249–6259.

63. Nawabi P, Catron DM, Haldar K. 2008. Esterification of cholesterol by a type III secretion effector during intracellular *Salmonella* infection. *Mol Microbiol* 68: 173–185.

64. Lossi NS, Rolhion N, Magee AI, Boyle C, Holden DW. 2008. The *Salmonella* SPI-2 effector SseJ exhibits eukaryotic activator-dependent phospholipase A and glycerophospholipid : cholesterol acyltransferase activity. *Microbiology* 154:2680–2688.

65. Christen M, Coye LH, Hontz JS, LaRock DL, Pfuetzner RA, Megha, Miller SI. 2009. Activation of a bacterial virulence protein by the GTPase RhoA. *Sci Signal* 2:ra71.

66. LaRock DL, Brzovic PS, Levin I, Blanc MP, Miller SI. 2012. A *Salmonella typhimurium*-translocated glycerophospholipid:cholesterol acyltransferase promotes virulence by binding to the RhoA protein switch regions. *J Biol Chem* 287:29654–29663.

67. Ohlson MB, Huang Z, Alto NM, Blanc MP, Dixon JE, Chai J, Miller SI. 2008. Structure and function of *Salmonella* SifA indicate that its interactions with SKIP, SseJ, and RhoA family GTPases induce endosomal tubulation. *Cell Host Microbe* 4:434–446.

68. Geddes K, Worley M, Niemann G, Heffron F. 2005. Identification of new secreted effectors in *Salmonella enterica* serovar Typhimurium. *Infect Immun* 73: 6260–6271.

69. Cardenal-Muñoz E, Ramos-Morales F. 2011. Analysis of the expression, secretion and translocation of the *Salmonella enterica* type III secretion system effector SteA. *PLoS One* 6:e26930.

70. Domingues L, Ismail A, Charro N, Rodríguez-Escudero I, Holden DW, Molina M, Cid VJ, Mota LJ. 2016. The *Salmonella* effector SteA binds phosphatidylinositol 4-phosphate for subcellular targeting within host cells. *Cell Microbiol* 18:949–969.

71. Domingues L, Holden DW, Mota LJ. 2014. The *Salmonella* effector SteA contributes to the control of membrane dynamics of *Salmonella*-containing vacuoles. *Infect Immun* 82:2923–2934.

72. Méresse S, Unsworth KE, Habermann A, Griffiths G, Fang F, Martínez-Lorenzo MJ, Waterman SR, Gorvel JP, Holden DW. 2001. Remodelling of the actin cytoskeleton is essential for replication of intravacuolar *Salmonella*. *Cell Microbiol* 3:567–577.

73. Poh J, Odendall C, Spanos A, Boyle C, Liu M, Freemont P, Holden DW. 2008. SteC is a *Salmonella* kinase required for SPI-2-dependent F-actin remodelling. *Cell Microbiol* 10:20–30.

74. Odendall C, Rolhion N, Förster A, Poh J, Lamont DJ, Liu M, Freemont PS, Catling AD, Holden DW. 2012. The *Salmonella* kinase SteC targets the MAP kinase MEK to regulate the host actin cytoskeleton. *Cell Host Microbe* 12:657–668.

75. Tezcan-Merdol D, Nyman T, Lindberg U, Haag F, Koch-Nolte F, Rhen M. 2001. Actin is ADP-ribosylated by the *Salmonella enterica* virulence-associated protein SpvB. *Mol Microbiol* 39:606–619.

76. Lesnick ML, Reiner NE, Fierer J, Guiney DG. 2001. The *Salmonella* spvB virulence gene encodes an enzyme that ADP-ribosylates actin and destabilizes the cytoskeleton of eukaryotic cells. *Mol Microbiol* 39:1464–1470.

77. Miao EA, Brittnacher M, Haraga A, Jeng RL, Welch MD, Miller SI. 2003. *Salmonella* effectors translocated across the vacuolar membrane interact with the actin cytoskeleton. *Mol Microbiol* 48:401–415.

78. Mattock E, Blocker AJ. 2017. How do the virulence factors of *Shigella* work together to cause disease? *Front Cell Infect Microbiol* 7:64.

79. Niebuhr K, Giuriato S, Pedron T, Philpott DJ, Gaits F, Sable J, Sheetz MP, Parsot C, Sansonetti PJ, Payrastre B. 2002. Conversion of PtdIns(4,5)P(2) into PtdIns(5)P by the *S. flexneri* effector IpgD reorganizes host cell morphology. *EMBO J* 21:5069–5078.

80. Weiner A, Mellouk N, Lopez-Montero N, Chang YY, Souque C, Schmitt C, Enninga J. 2016. Macropinosomes are key players in early *Shigella* invasion and vacuolar escape in epithelial cells. *PLoS Pathog* 12: e1005602.

81. Allaoui A, Ménard R, Sansonetti PJ, Parsot C. 1993. Characterization of the *Shigella flexneri* ipgD and ipgF genes, which are located in the proximal part of the *mxi* locus. *Infect Immun* 61:1707–1714.

82. Mellouk N, Weiner A, Aulner N, Schmitt C, Elbaum M, Shorte SL, Danckaert A, Enninga J. 2014. *Shigella* subverts the host recycling compartment to rupture its vacuole. *Cell Host Microbe* 16:517–530.

83. De Geyter C, Wattiez R, Sansonetti P, Falmagne P, Ruysschaert JM, Parsot C, Cabiaux V. 2000. Characterization of the interaction of IpaB and IpaD, proteins required for entry of *Shigella flexneri* into epithelial cells, with a lipid membrane. *Eur J Biochem* 267: 5769–5776.

84. Veenendaal AK, Hodgkinson JL, Schwarzer L, Stabat D, Zenk SF, Blocker AJ. 2007. The type III secretion system needle tip complex mediates host cell sensing and translocon insertion. *Mol Microbiol* 63:1719–1730.

85. High N, Mounier J, Prévost MC, Sansonetti PJ. 1992. IpaB of *Shigella flexneri* causes entry into epithelial cells

and escape from the phagocytic vacuole. *EMBO J* 11: 1991–1999.

86. Bârzu S, Benjelloun-Touimi Z, Phalipon A, Sansonetti P, Parsot C. 1997. Functional analysis of the *Shigella flexneri* IpaC invasin by insertional mutagenesis. *Infect Immun* 65:1599–1605.

87. Page AL, Ohayon H, Sansonetti PJ, Parsot C. 1999. The secreted IpaB and IpaC invasins and their cytoplasmic chaperone IpgC are required for intercellular dissemination of *Shigella flexneri*. *Cell Microbiol* 1:183–193.

88. Schuch R, Sandlin RC, Maurelli AT. 1999. A system for identifying post-invasion functions of invasion genes: requirements for the Mxi-Spa type III secretion pathway of *Shigella flexneri* in intercellular dissemination. *Mol Microbiol* 34:675–689.

89. Du J, Reeves AZ, Klein JA, Twedt DJ, Knodler LA, Lesser CF. 2016. The type III secretion system apparatus determines the intracellular niche of bacterial pathogens. *Proc Natl Acad Sci U S A* 113:4794–4799.

90. Bernardini ML, Mounier J, d'Hauteville H, Coquis-Rondon M, Sansonetti PJ. 1989. Identification of *icsA*, a plasmid locus of *Shigella flexneri* that governs bacterial intra- and intercellular spread through interaction with F-actin. *Proc Natl Acad Sci U S A* 86: 3867–3871.

91. Brandon LD, Goehring N, Janakiraman A, Yan AW, Wu T, Beckwith J, Goldberg MB. 2003. IcsA, a polarly localized autotransporter with an atypical signal peptide, uses the Sec apparatus for secretion, although the Sec apparatus is circumferentially distributed. *Mol Microbiol* 50:45–60.

92. Goldberg MB, Bârzu O, Parsot C, Sansonetti PJ. 1993. Unipolar localization and ATPase activity of IcsA, a *Shigella flexneri* protein involved in intracellular movement. *J Bacteriol* 175:2189–2196.

93. Robbins JR, Monack D, McCallum SJ, Vegas A, Pham E, Goldberg MB, Theriot JA. 2001. The making of a gradient: IcsA (VirG) polarity in *Shigella flexneri*. *Mol Microbiol* 41:861–872.

94. Mauricio RP, Jeffries CM, Svergun DI, Deane JE. 2017. The *Shigella* virulence factor IcsA relieves N-WASP autoinhibition by displacing the verprolin homology/cofilin/acidic (VCA) domain. *J Biol Chem* 292:134–145.

95. Egile C, Loisel TP, Laurent V, Li R, Pantaloni D, Sansonetti PJ, Carlier MF. 1999. Activation of the CDC42 effector N-WASP by the *Shigella flexneri* IcsA protein promotes actin nucleation by Arp2/3 complex and bacterial actin-based motility. *J Cell Biol* 146: 1319–1332.

96. Suzuki T, Mimuro H, Suetsugu S, Miki H, Takenawa T, Sasakawa C. 2002. Neural Wiskott-Aldrich syndrome protein (N-WASP) is the specific ligand for *Shigella* VirG among the WASP family and determines the host cell type allowing actin-based spreading. *Cell Microbiol* 4:223–233.

97. Rohatgi R, Ma L, Miki H, Lopez M, Kirchhausen T, Takenawa T, Kirschner MW. 1999. The interaction between N-WASP and the Arp2/3 complex links Cdc42-dependent signals to actin assembly. *Cell* 97:221–231.

98. Goldberg MB, Theriot JA. 1995. *Shigella flexneri* surface protein IcsA is sufficient to direct actin-based motility. *Proc Natl Acad Sci U S A* 92:6572–6576.

99. Allaoui A, Mounier J, Prévost MC, Sansonetti PJ, Parsot C. 1992. icsB: a *Shigella flexneri* virulence gene necessary for the lysis of protrusions during intercellular spread. *Mol Microbiol* 6:1605–1616.

100. Campbell-Valois FX, Sachse M, Sansonetti PJ, Parsot C. 2015. Escape of actively secreting *Shigella flexneri* from ATG8/LC3-positive vacuoles formed during cell-to-cell spread is facilitated by IcsB and VirA. *MBio* 6:e02567-14.

101. Weddle E, Agaisse H. 2018. Spatial, temporal, and functional assessment of LC3-dependent autophagy in *Shigella flexneri* dissemination. *Infect Immun* 86: e00134-18.

102. Kayath CA, Hussey S, El hajjami N, Nagra K, Philpott D, Allaoui A. 2010. Escape of intracellular *Shigella* from autophagy requires binding to cholesterol through the type III effector, IcsB. *Microbes Infect* 12:956–966.

103. Ogawa M, Yoshimori T, Suzuki T, Sagara H, Mizushima N, Sasakawa C. 2005. Escape of intracellular *Shigella* from autophagy. *Science* 307:727–731.

104. Dong N, Zhu Y, Lu Q, Hu L, Zheng Y, Shao F. 2012. Structurally distinct bacterial TBC-like GAPs link Arf GTPase to Rab1 inactivation to counteract host defenses. *Cell* 150:1029–1041.

105. Zoppino FC, Militello RD, Slavin I, Alvarez C, Colombo MI. 2010. Autophagosome formation depends on the small GTPase Rab1 and functional ER exit sites. *Traffic* 11:1246–1261.

106. Shinoda S. 2011. Sixty years from the discovery of *Vibrio parahaemolyticus* and some recollections. *Biocontrol Sci* 16:129–137.

107. Makino K, Oshima K, Kurokawa K, Yokoyama K, Uda T, Tagomori K, Iijima Y, Najima M, Nakano M, Yamashita A, Kubota Y, Kimura S, Yasunaga T, Honda T, Shinagawa H, Hattori M, Iida T. 2003. Genome sequence of *Vibrio parahaemolyticus*: a pathogenic mechanism distinct from that of V cholerae. *Lancet* 361:743–749.

108. Ritchie JM, Rui H, Zhou X, Iida T, Kodoma T, Ito S, Davis BM, Bronson RT, Waldor MK. 2012. Inflammation and disintegration of intestinal villi in an experimental model for *Vibrio parahaemolyticus*-induced diarrhea. *PLoS Pathog* 8:e1002593.

109. Zhou X, Shah DH, Konkel ME, Call DR. 2008. Type III secretion system 1 genes in *Vibrio parahaemolyticus* are positively regulated by ExsA and negatively regulated by ExsD. *Mol Microbiol* 69:747–764.

110. Park KS, Ono T, Rokuda M, Jang MH, Okada K, Iida T, Honda T. 2004. Functional characterization of two type III secretion systems of *Vibrio parahaemolyticus*. *Infect Immun* 72:6659–6665.

111. Burdette DL, Yarbrough ML, Orvedahl A, Gilpin CJ, Orth K. 2008. *Vibrio parahaemolyticus* orchestrates a multifaceted host cell infection by induction of autophagy, cell rounding, and then cell lysis. *Proc Natl Acad Sci U S A* 105:12497–12502.

112. **Salomon D, Guo Y, Kinch LN, Grishin NV, Gardner KH, Orth K.** 2013. Effectors of animal and plant pathogens use a common domain to bind host phosphoinositides. *Nat Commun* **4:**2973.

113. **Liverman AD, Cheng HC, Trosky JE, Leung DW, Yarbrough ML, Burdette DL, Rosen MK, Orth K.** 2007. Arp2/3-independent assembly of actin by *Vibrio* type III effector VopL. *Proc Natl Acad Sci U S A* **104:** 17117–17122.

114. **Avvaru BS, Pernier J, Carlier MF.** 2015. Dimeric WH2 repeats of VopF sequester actin monomers into non-nucleating linear string conformations: an X-ray scattering study. *J Struct Biol* **190:**192–199.

115. **de Souza Santos M, Salomon D, Orth K.** 2017. T3SS effector VopL inhibits the host ROS response, promoting the intracellular survival of *Vibrio parahaemolyticus*. *PLoS Pathog* **13:**e1006438.

116. **Huang Z, Sutton SE, Wallenfang AJ, Orchard RC, Wu X, Feng Y, Chai J, Alto NM.** 2009. Structural insights into host GTPase isoform selection by a family of bacterial GEF mimics. *Nat Struct Mol Biol* **16:** 853–860.

Bacteria and Intracellularity
Edited by Pascale Cossart, Craig R. Roy, and Philippe Sansonetti
© 2019 American Society for Microbiology, Washington, DC
doi:10.1128/microbiolspec.BAI-0015-2019

Customizing Host Chromatin: A Bacterial Tale

15

Michael Connor,[1] Laurence Arbibe,[2] and Mélanie Hamon[1]

INTRODUCTION

Chromatin is located within the nuclei of eukaryotic cells and is composed of DNA wrapped around histone proteins. The highly ordered compaction of chromatin is crucial for the different functions encoded by the genetic material. These range from maintaining cell identity and genome integrity to adapting to environmental stimuli and cell replication. At the center of the chromatin language is its structural organization. This depends on the position and reversible covalent modifications to histone proteins and their cross talk with DNA and regulatory proteins. The basic unit of chromatin is the nucleosome, which is composed of an octamer of four histone proteins (H2A, H2B, H3, and H4) around which ∼147 bases of DNA are wrapped, with the linker histone (H1) outside the core structure providing structural integrity to the complex. Nucleosome remodelers are ATP-dependent enzymes that modify the chromatin structure through translocation, eviction, and introduction of histone variants (1, 2), while histone-modifying enzymes introduce reversible covalent posttranslational modifications (PTMs) to histone tails.

Nucleosome remodelers and modifying enzymes regulate chromatin dynamics by repositioning histones, winding and unwinding DNA, and adding and removing PTMs on the N-terminal histone tails that extend from the octamer complex. Each histone (H2A, H2B, H3, and H4), including the linker histone (H1) and histone variants, can be modified at multiple locations along its tail (3–7). The combined activity of remodelers and histone modifiers regulates unraveling and compaction of chromatin, leading to transcriptional regulation. Specific sets of histone marks are associated with opening of the chromatin structure, allowing transcription factors to bind, polymerase II to extend, and gene expression to occur, whereas others are associated with silent genetic regions (8–12).

Additionally, DNA itself can be methylated by DNA methyltransferases, primarily in promoter and enhancer regions preceding transcriptional start sites. DNA methylation is achieved by the covalent transfer of a methyl group to the C-5 position of the cytosine ring of DNA. Removal of this group is thought to be done indirectly through intermediate modifications, as no demethylase enzymes have been identified. DNA methylation results in silencing of the neighboring gene's expression and is important for cross regulation of histone PTMs (13).

Ultimately, through the intense remodeling of chromatin arises a histone language, which encodes additional regulatory information beyond that present in the DNA sequence (3–7). A large number of histone PTMs have been identified—acetylation, methylation, phosphorylation, ubiquitination, ADP ribosylation, deimination, and proline isomerization—highlighting the complexity of the system (13). The writers and erasers of PTMs are classified by the histone mark they deposit or erase, such as methyltransferases or demethylases, and are usually specific to a given histone residue. The combination of PTMs on a histone tail and the pattern of DNA methylation act as binding platforms onto which "reader" proteins bind and regulate cell processes. For instance, bromodomain proteins have high affinity for acetylated histones and play a role in transcriptional activation, whereas histone methylation at H3K9 will recruit silencing proteins, like heterochromatin protein 1 (HP1), and maintain a repressive genetic environment. DNA methylation is read by methyl-CpG binding proteins, which act as structural proteins to recruit histone deacetylases

[1]Institut Pasteur, G5 Chromatine et Infection, Paris, France; [2]INSERM U1151, CNRS UMR 8253, Institut Necker Enfants Malades, INEM Institute Department of Immunology, Infectiology and Hematology, Paris, France.

(HDACs) and ultimately lead to chromatin compaction and gene silencing. Histone PTMs and DNA methylation are therefore crucial in integrating environmental stimuli throughout the cell's life (13, 14).

Given the key role of chromatin in regulating host transcription, it is not surprising that bacteria have evolved to manipulate it. In this chapter, we focus on the different mechanisms by which bacteria customize host chromatin for their survival, whether it is by indirect of direct targeting of histones, DNA methylation, or even altering DNA integrity.

HISTONE MODIFICATIONS IN RESPONSE TO BACTERIAL PRODUCTS

Bacterial components are continuously sensed by host cells, and such cross talk is crucial for regulating immune responses. A balanced response must tolerate commensal bacteria in order to maintain homeostasis yet remain reactive to combat invading pathogens. How this delicate balance is achieved is not well understood; however, some evidence points to an integration of bacterial signals at the level of histone modifications to control inflammatory responses.

Proinflammatory Signaling

Sensing of bacterial components, like lipopolysaccharide (LPS), in the cellular milieu occurs in part through pattern recognition receptors, leading to activation of inflammatory responses such as the NF-κB pathway. Activation of Toll-like receptor 4 by LPS triggers NF-κB translocation into the nucleus, where it controls transcription of inflammatory mediators in sequential waves, reflecting the chromatin conformation of the genetic loci regulated (15). Indeed, immediately accessible genes are transcribed first, as they are located in regions characterized by open chromatin and are associated with high levels of H4 acetylation. In fact, all Toll-like receptor 4-responsive genes which are rapidly transcribed are maintained in a basal active state characterized by H3K9 acetylation and H3K4 trimethylation (H3K4me3) (16). Genes in this state then gain H4K5/8/12 acetylation upon activation of the signaling cascade, allowing transcriptional elongation and generation of mature full-length transcripts to occur. In contrast, late-accessibility genes require secondary signaling mediators, such as activation of mitogen-activated protein kinase (MAPK) signaling, and histone modifiers to decompact chromatin in order for NF-κB to bind (17). Therefore, regulation at the chromatin level allows transcriptional fine-tuning of genes in the same pathway. It is in this inflammatory context that pathogens and commensals need to establish their niche. Accordingly, bacteria

have developed mechanisms to tamper with host inflammatory responses for their benefit.

Anti-Inflammatory Signaling

In locations such as the gut, skin, oral cavity, and vagina, colonization by the microbiome leads to a high local level of LPS, yet in healthy individuals, strong inflammatory responses are not initiated in this environment. Some reports suggest that cells continuously exposed to LPS become unresponsive to it through mechanisms involving chromatin modifications. For instance, macrophages exposed to LPS once and those exposed multiple times display different histone marks at inflammatory gene loci (18). Upon restimulation with LPS, two classes of gene are revealed: tolerizeable (T) genes, which are transiently silenced, and nontolerizeable (NT) genes, which remain accessible. The promoters of T genes, which include inflammatory cytokines, lose the activatory H3K4me3 mark but maintain H4 acetylation levels. In contrast, the promoters of NT genes, including antimicrobial effectors such as antimicrobial defense proteins, retain H3K4me3 and are reacetylated upon restimulation with LPS. Therefore, multiple exposures to LPS lead to silencing of inflammatory genes while others remain active, and both classes of genes retain a chromatin mark reflecting their LPS encounter.

In the gut, metabolic by-products from bacterial growth are potent modulators of host responses and were recently shown to contribute to repression of LPS-inducible inflammatory responses and gut homeostasis. The short-chain fatty acid n-butyrate is produced by commensal gut bacteria and is a potent HDAC inhibitor. In the intestine, butyrate downregulates LPS-mediated inflammatory responses and modulates macrophage function (19). A related study characterized an unusual histone modification regulated by microbiota-derived short-chain fatty acids in the colon. Histone H3 crotonylation, which is an addition of a crotonyl group (C_4H_5O) to the target lysine, is regulated by class I HDACs and is induced by the microbiota (13, 20; for a review, see reference 21). Therefore, metabolic by-products of the microbiota are potent modifiers of host chromatin and may play an important role in maintaining gut homeostasis.

Similarly to the intestinal tract, the microbiota of the vaginal tract, mainly composed of *Lactobacillus* spp., is essential to maintaining a homeostatic environment. *Lactobacillus gasseri* was shown to induce the recruitment of active histone marks (H3 acetylation, H3Kme3, and the H2A.Z histone variant) to the promoter of *DEFB1* (encoding human β-defensin-1), an antimicrobial peptide (22). Intriguingly, the related species *Lactobacillus reuteri* did not. Such studies highlight the idea that maintaining homeostasis is a very delicate process which may even be species specific.

In order for pathogenic bacteria to maintain a long-term presence during chronic infection, they must also use mechanisms to limit the inflammatory response. For this, *Pseudomonas aeruginosa* generates the quorum-sensing molecule 2-aminoacetophenone, which has anti-inflammatory properties (23). Indeed, treatment with 2-aminoacetophenone prior to infection reduces the expression of proinflammatory cytokines by increased expression and activity of HDAC1 and consequent de-acetylation of histone H3 on lysine 18 at promoters of specific targets, such as tumor necrosis factor alpha (TNF-α).

BACTERIAL EFFECTORS TARGETING HISTONE MODIFICATIONS THROUGH SIGNALING EVENTS

In contrast to most colonizing bacteria, pathogens have evolved sophisticated virulence factors which subvert host defenses. Although the mechanisms are diverse, hijacking or interacting with components of host signaling cascades is common to different pathogenic bacteria (24). Targeting of such signaling cascades occurs through direct interaction of bacterial factors with host signaling components, either in the cytoplasm or in the nucleus (Fig. 1).

Cytoplasmic Effectors

Mycobacterium tuberculosis

M. tuberculosis is a facultative intracellular pathogen responsible for tuberculosis. During infection, the bacterium dampens the ability of infected macrophages to respond to gamma interferon (IFN-γ) and results in decreased expression of the transcriptional transactivator CIITA, which regulates major histocompatibility complex II (25, 26). In fact, *M. tuberculosis* blocks IFN-γ-dependent histone acetylation at the CIITA, HLA-DRα, and HLA-DRβ gene promoters. Infection was further shown to induce recruitment of a histone deacetylase complex (Sin3A), leading to histone deacetylation and gene repression. While these findings are not yet attributed to a specific effector, the *M. tuberculosis* cell wall protein LpqH has been shown to inhibit expression of CIITA, which makes it a putative candidate.

Listeria monocytogenes

L. monocytogenes is a Gram-positive foodborne pathogen that causes listeriosis (27). The internalin B (InlB) gene of *L. monocytogenes* encodes a factor that binds

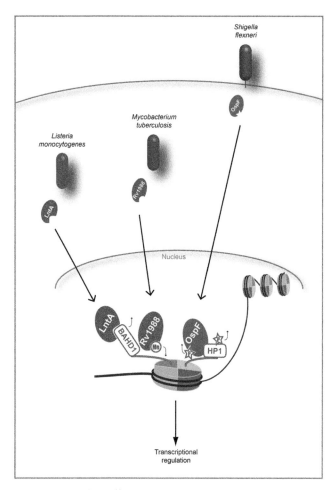

Figure 1 Nuclear effectors targeting histone marks. Secreted effectors from *L. monocytogenes*, *M. tuberculosis*, and *S. flexneri* translocate to the nucleus, where they directly act either upon the nucleosome itself (Rv1988 and OspF), bind chromatin readers to displace them (LntA), or bind chromatin readers to dephosphorylate them (OspF). Small black arrows around modifications indicate whether they are being deposited or removed.

the host receptor c-Met and activates downstream phosphatidylinositol 3-kinase/AKT signaling (28, 29). Activation of this signaling cascade during infection was shown to hijack the host deacetylase SIRT2, culminating in the translocation of SIRT2 from the cytoplasm to chromatin (30). There, SIRT2 deacetylates H3K18 at the transcriptional start sites of genes repressed during infection. The mechanism by which SIRT2 relocalization occurs was shown to depend on regulation of the phosphorylation status of SIRT2 by two phosphatases, PPM1A and PPM1B. It is this modification of SIRT2 that is crucial for chromatin association and gene regulation (31). Although the genes targeted by SIRT2 need to be further characterized, the activity of SIRT2 at the chromatin level, as well as its dephosphorylation, is essential for a productive *Listeria* infection both *in vitro* and *in vivo*.

Helicobacter pylori

H. pylori is a Gram-negative bacterium causing gastritis and stomach ulcers and is associated with gastric cancer. While the identity of the secreted effector is unknown, *H. pylori* targets H3S10 and H3T3 for dephosphorylation and H3K23 for deacetylation in a type IV secretion system (T4SS)-dependent manner. In fact, the entire *cag* pathogenicity island, which contains several virulence factors as well as the Dot/Icm T4SS, is required for chromatin modulations (32, 33). Indeed, mutants with deletions of individual virulence factors, like cytotoxin-associated gene A (*cagA*) or vacuolating cytotoxin gene A (*vacA*), fail to dephosphorylate H3S10 (34, 35). On the host side, decreases in H3S10 phosphorylation correlate with cell cycle arrest and inactivation of H3 kinases, mainly VRK1. During late stages of infection, cells reenter the cell cycle and H3S10 phosphorylation reappears (34). Such studies demonstrate that bacteria-mediated histone modifications are associated with other cell processes besides transcription, such as the cell cycle.

Pore formation

The group of toxins known as cholesterol-dependent cytolysin (CDC) are found primarily in Gram-positive bacteria and play crucial roles in virulence. These toxins are generally secreted into the extracellular milieu, where they bind to host plasma membranes in cholesterol-rich areas, oligomerize, and undergo a conformational change to form a large pore (36). The listerial toxin listeriolysin O (LLO) is one member of this family of toxins and was shown to induce H3S10 dephosphorylation and H4 deacetylation. These modifications occur independently of the cell cycle and are associated with the promoter of specific genes such as *cxcl2* and *dusp4* (37). The signaling cascades known to be induced by LLO (mainly MAPK and NF-κB) are not involved (37); rather, it is potassium efflux through toxin pores which is essential for these chromatin modifications (38).

A recent report showed that the *P. aeruginosa* T3SS translocon proteins PopB-PopD also induce H3S10 dephosphorylation in a K^+ efflux-dependent manner, similarly to LLO (39). These results suggest that the translocon acts as a pore-forming toxin and indicate that such histone modifications could represent a universal host response to a specific type of plasma membrane damage.

Nuclear Effectors

Mycobacterium tuberculosis

In addition to the modulation of cellular pathways in the cytoplasm by *M. tuberculosis*, the secreted protein Rv1988, which is found exclusively in pathogenic *Mycobacterium* species, directly targets host chromatin. This effector translocates to the nucleus, where it functions as a methyltransferase, specifically targeting H3R42me2 (40). Rv1988 is required for *M. tuberculosis* virulence, and it selectively binds to promoter regions of critical immune response genes such as *NOX1*, *NOX4*, and *NOS2* (required for host reactive-oxygen production). There, it promotes H3R42me3 and represses transcription. Interestingly, expression of Rv1988 is sufficient to confer virulence/pathogenesis *in vivo* and *in vitro* to the nonpathogenic species *Mycobacterium smegmatis*, highlighting the importance of this effector (40).

Shigella flexneri

S. flexneri is a Gram-negative pathogen and is the etiologic agent of dysentery in humans (41). Most *S. flexneri* virulence factors are secreted through the T3SS, which injects effector proteins directly into the cytoplasm of intestinal epithelial cells (41). One of these, OspF, translocates to the host nucleus upon injection, interrupts MAPK signaling, and binds to the promoter of specific genes involved in inflammatory responses. At the molecular level, OspF is a phosphothreonine lyase that blocks MAPK activation and downstream phosphorylation of histone H3S10 and the chromatin reader HP1γ (42–44). As a result, unphosphorylated HP1 accumulates at promoter sites, thereby blocking interleukin 8 (IL-8) gene transcription. Strikingly, OspF-mediated chromatin modifications and gene repression are specific and target only a subset of genes involved in inflammatory responses. *In vivo* experiments further show that OspF contributes to blocking neutrophil recruitment to the site of bacterial lesions (42).

Listeria monocytogenes

Independently of InlB and the CDC toxin LLO, *Listeria* secretes an effector, LntA, which targets the host nucleus. There, it displaces the repressive chromatin reader BAHD1 to activate gene transcription. Upon interaction with lntA, BAHD1 is displaced from chromatin, where H3K9 acetylation occurs and interferon-stimulated gene transcription is activated, leading to IFN-λ expression. In order to fine-tune host inflammatory responses, this process must be tightly regulated by the pathogen, as reflected by the observation that either constitutive expression or absence of LntA is detrimental to infection (45).

BACTERIAL FACTORS MIMICKING HOST CHROMATIN-MODIFYING ENZYMES

SET (suppressor of variegation enhancer of zeste trithorax) domain proteins are ubiquitous in eukaryotes, and this domain can be found in lysine methyltransferases, which can methylate histones in addition to other proteins. Methylated histones at specific residues are associated with different transcriptional states. Silenced genes in heterochromatin regions are marked with H3K9 methylation, whereas active transcription in euchromatin is marked with methylated H3K4 (for a review, see reference 46). To date, secreted SET domain-containing effectors have been found in obligate pathogens, such as *Chlamydia trachomatis*, *Bacillus anthracis*, and *Legionella pneumophila*. Interestingly, the SET domain of secreted bacterial effectors confers methyltransferase activity to bacteria. Due to the lack of histone substrates within bacteria, it is thought that these organisms have hijacked the SET domain to target their hosts (Fig. 2) (47–49).

Chlamydia trachomatis

While this phenomenon is not fully understood, *C. trachomatis* is able to increase global methylation of H2B, H3, and H4 through a secreted effector. This protein, NUE, translocates to the nucleus, where it automethylates and increases histone methylation (48). Since *C. trachomatis* is an obligately intracellular pathogen with a limited repertoire of protein-coding reading frames, global methylation might be essential for reprogramming the host cellular processes to support the intracellular niche of *C. trachomatis* (50).

Bacillus anthracis

The causative agent of anthrax is *B. anthracis*, a Gram-positive spore-forming bacterium (51). While anthrax toxins are among the most noted virulence factors of the organism, it also encodes several effector proteins, one of which is BaSET (47, 51). BaSET alters host gene transcription by methylating histone H1 in the promoter regions of NF-κB-controlled genes (the IL-6 gene, *c-fos*, *c-jun*, and the TNF-α gene) and counters transcriptional activation by the CREB-binding protein coactivator. Furthermore, BaSET deletion mutants fail to colonize *in vivo*, in contrast to wild-type bacteria. Therefore, it appears that downregulation of NF-κB host responses by H1 methylation plays a role in survival of the *B. anthracis* during infection (47).

Legionella pneumophila

L. pneumophila, a facultative intracellular bacterium, uses the T4SS to inject the effector RomA. Once inside

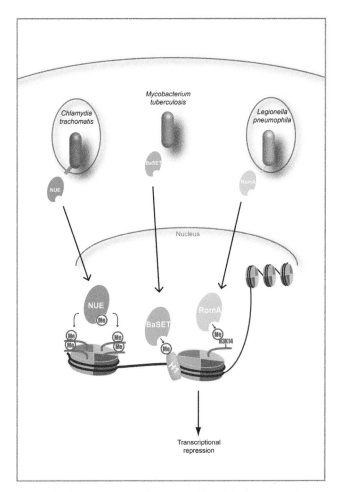

Figure 2 SET domain effectors mediate histone methylation. Effectors of *C. trachomatis*, *M. tuberculosis*, and *L. pneumophila* contain the eukaryotic SET domain. Once translocated to the nucleus, these effectors target histones for direct methylation either globally or at specific residues. For *M. tuberculosis* and *L. pneumophila*, this leads to repression of the host immune response and is thought to aid pathogen survival.

the host cell, RomA localizes to the nucleus. There, it induces histone methylation at a site not previously described, H3K14. Interestingly, methylation occurs with a simultaneous decrease in H3K14 acetylation, and thereby, an activating histone mark (acetylation) is replaced with a repressive mark (methylation). Upon infection, 4,870 gene promoter regions are targeted with the H3K14 repressive mark. Specifically, H3K14 methylation damped immunomodulatory components, such as genes coding for TNF-α, IL-6, CXCL1, CXCL2, and Nalp3 (49).

BACTERIAL TARGETING OF DNA

Aside from modifying nucleosome PTMs, bacteria can also target DNA either through methylation or by inducing genotoxicity (Fig. 3). Intriguingly, such effects on DNA are more stable than histone modifications and could have a long-lasting impact on the host.

DNA Methylation

Mycobacterium tuberculosis
Rapid hypomethylation was reported to occur upon *in vitro* infection of monocyte-derived dendritic cells with *M. tuberculosis*. Distal enhancer regions upstream of genes known to function as master regulators of the immune response were mainly targeted, with only rare detection at promoter regions (52). Such demethylation was found to correlate with an increase in activatory histone marks and the recruitment of inflammation-activated transcription factors. Although no particular phenotype or specific effector was shown to correlate with hypomethylation, this study shows that demethylation can occur and is dynamically regulated upon bacterial infection.

In contrast to the works cited above, which focused on CpG elements, another study found that a secreted effector of *M. tuberculosis*, Rv2966c, methylates DNA in regions outside CpG islands (53). This effector is a DNA methyltransferase which requires phosphorylation by either a mycobacterial or a host kinase(s) for activity. Once active, it directly methylates host DNA at CpA and CpT dinucleotides while also binding to histones 3

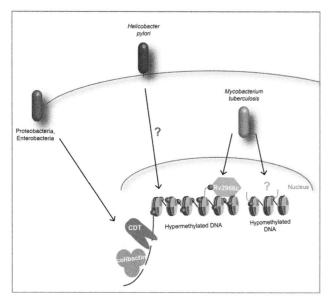

Figure 3 Targeting host DNA. Genotoxins such as CDT and colibactin induce host DNA breaks through either DNase activity (CDT) or DNA cross-linking (colibactin). *M. tuberculosis* targets host DNA directly for methylation with Rv2966c at non-CpG elements or induces hypomethylation through an unknown effector at CpG islands.

and 4. Through non-CpG methylation, Rv2966c dampens host transcription at targeted loci, such as *H2AFY2* (encoding a macrohistone 2A family member) and *GRK5* (encoding a member of the G-protein-coupled receptor kinase family) (53).

These studies clearly show that *M. tuberculosis* induces differential DNA methylation within host cells by targeting both CpG and non-CpG DNA methylation; however, whether the bacterium has more than one effector to do so remains undetermined.

Helicobacter pylori
Recent work with *H. pylori* suggests that its presence induces DNA methylation, which is strongly associated with gastric cancer (54–61). However, it is still controversial whether the elevated risk of gastric cancer is directly due to *H. pylori*-induced DNA methylation or whether it is a result of the inflammatory response to infection. Regardless, it is clear that in response to infection with *H. pylori*, transient and permanent DNA methylation changes are detected in gastric mucosa. Indeed, *H. pylori* induces specific DNA hypermethylation patterns in genomic regions termed CpG islands, mainly located in promoter regions and at transcription factor-binding motifs of tumor suppressor genes, such as *LOX* and *HAND1*, or inflammatory genes, such as *COX2* (59, 61). In addition, several of the CpG islands that undergo DNA methylation during infection remain elevated even after eradication of *H. pylori* (54). While it is accepted that *H. pylori* infection increases the risk for gastric cancer, further study is needed to directly link DNA methylation patterns with a predisposition to gastric cancer or define the role of bacterial induced inflammation in this process.

Damaging Chromatin through Bacterial Genotoxins
During infection, it is common for bacteria to induce DNA damage in their host (62–66). Such effects are often indirect, occurring through oxidative stress; however, to date, only a few *bona fide* bacterial genotoxins have been characterized.

Cytolethal distending toxin
Cytolethal distending toxin (CDT) is a family of proteins found in Gram-negative bacteria, especially in certain members of the *Proteobacteria*, such as *Escherichia coli*, *Aggregatibacter actinomycetemcomitans*, *Haemophilus ducreyi*, *Campylobacter* sp., and *Helicobacter* sp. CDT is functionally conserved in a large number of distantly related pathogenic strains, and except in *Salmonella*

enterica serovar Typhi, CDT is encoded by three genes: *cdtA*, *cdtB*, and *cdtC* (67, 68). Regardless of the microbial source of CDT, *cdtB* has been shown to be the main gene responsible for toxin activity. Although CdtB was originally described as a cyclomodulin, since intoxicated cells are arrested in their cell cycle, structural analysis of CdtB revealed homology with mammalian DNase I and potentially with inositol lipid phosphatases (67, 69–71). CdtB is an AB2-like toxin; CdtB associates with CdtA and CdtC subunits, showing ricin-like lectin folds that allow the tripartite toxin to enter host cells via endocytosis (68, 70, 72). Interestingly, CDT is the first bacterial toxin known to target the nucleus, where it exhibits DNase activity (72–74). Although other activities for CdtB have been reported, such as phosphatidylinositol phosphatase (71), cell cycle arrest is mainly attributed to its genotoxic activity. CDTs have been reported to induce apoptosis and cell senescence during infection, although the benefit to bacteria of inducing DNA breaks in the host remains mostly unclear. Interestingly, in the context of chronic exposure, the potential role of CDTs in promoting cell transformation has been raised (75–77).

Colibactin

Colibactins are synthesized by several species of *Enterobacteriaceae* and demonstrate genotoxic activity (78, 79). They are natural products of a "warhead substituted spirobicyclic" structure (80), which are biosynthesized by enzymatic machinery located in a pathogenicity island mainly conserved in virulent bacteria. Each of the 19 genes present in the *clb* genomic island is essential for the full active genotoxic effect of colibactins, and colibactin is not a unique compound but a mixture of multiple molecules (81). Contact with colibactin-expressing bacteria causes double-strand DNA breaks and eventually cell cycle arrest and death. Recently, the mechanism by which colibactin impacts chromatin integrity was shown to involve DNA interstrand cross-linking, causing replication stress and activation of DNA damage response pathways in intoxicated cells (82). Similarly to the effect of CDTs, a correlation between the presence of bacteria harboring the *clb* island and human cancers suggests that the colibactin toxin may promote inflammation-triggered colorectal cancer (83).

CONCLUSIONS AND PERSPECTIVES

Overall, many reports clearly indicate that bacteria and bacterial components reprogram the cell epigenetically. However, many questions remain unanswered regarding the role these various chromatin marks play in terms of specificity, regulation, and cellular processes.

How do bacterial effectors target specific histone residues or specific genomic regions? The effectors BaSET, NUE, and RomA all target histones for methylation; however, they each target different a histone(s) and/or residues. This suggests that the effectors are intrinsically capable of recognizing individual histones and tail residues or that their specificity occurs through synergistic interactions with unknown proteins or complexes. Similarly, bacteria target subsets of host genes for histone modifications. How this is achieved is unknown, and additional factors might be required to determine specificity. Therefore, additional work is warranted to fully understand how bacterial factors acquire specificity, whether it is to target a histone residue or a specific genomic region.

What is the impact of chromatin rearrangements on bacterial survival within the host? It is clear that bacteria are able to manipulate host chromatin, and in several cases, these modifications have been shown to affect the survival of the organism within the host (*L. monocytogenes*, *M. tuberculosis*, and *B. anthracis*). However, for other histone marks, their contribution to bacterial replication and niche establishment remains to be further defined. Indeed, the observed chromatin modifications could be a natural response of the host cell to a bacterial encounter and therefore could have no impact on bacterial growth. Thus, to gain a complete picture of chromatin-based bacterium-host interactions, the combination of the epigenetic and transcriptional responses needs to be accounted for. It is possible that future work will define modifications associated with basal responses and those associated with active bacterial manipulation. Further extending these comparisons across species, both commensal and pathogenic, will deepen our understanding of species-dependent histone marks that influence chromatin-based bacterial homeostasis or pathogenesis. Global patterns associating active chromatin remodeling, transcriptional responses, and cellular processes could then begin to be mapped systematically.

Are bacterium-induced histone marks maintained, and do they have a lasting impact on host cells? In the light of infection studies, DNA methylation is proving to be responsive to environmental stimuli; however, the lasting potential of variations in DNA methylation levels needs to be explored. Furthermore, as a clear link between DNA methylation and carcinogenesis has been established, it will be interesting to explore whether bacterium-mediated DNA methylation impacts this process. Similarly, genotoxic stress-causing toxins, depending on the time it takes the host cell to recover, could predispose the host to cancer. A lasting impact of histone modifications on transcriptional regulation of the host is another avenue of interesting studies. Recent studies put forth the idea that innate immune cells retain a memory of past encounters, which would be maintained through histone marks (84–88). Such possibilities have come to light due to the known cross-protective effects of the BCG vaccine, which is associated with H3K27 and H3K4 modifications. Whether bacteria are able to induce such memory or disrupt it remains to be explored.

As we unlock the histone code and the role this language plays in host response during bacterial disease, commensal colonization, and innate immune memory, we will discover novel mechanisms that may give rise to next-generation therapeutics, intelligently designed vaccines, and even medical advancements for microbiome dysbiosis.

Acknowledgments. We apologize to any colleagues whose work was not included in this review due to space limitations. We thank Orhan Rasid and Emmanuel Lemichez for critical reading of the manuscript. Work in the Chromatin and Infection Group is supported by the Pasteur Institute and the Agence National de la Recherche (ANR-EpiBActIn). Michael Connor is supported by the Pasteur Foundation Fellowship. Work by the genomic plasticity and infection team is supported by the Institut National de la Santé et de la Recherche Médicale (INSERM) (U1151) and by the Agence National de la Recherche (ANR- 15-CE14-0003 and ANR-16-CE15-0006-01).

Citation. Connor M, Arbibe L, Hamon M. 2019. Customizing host chromatin: a bacterial tale. Microbiol Spectrum 7(2):BAI-0015-2019.

References

1. Swygert SG, Peterson CL. 2014. Chromatin dynamics: interplay between remodeling enzymes and histone modifications. *Biochim Biophys Acta* **1839:**728–736.

2. Clapier CR, Iwasa J, Cairns BR, Peterson CL. 2017. Mechanisms of action and regulation of ATP-dependent chromatin-remodelling complexes. *Nat Rev Mol Cell Biol* **18:**407–422.

3. Strahl BD, Allis CD. 2000. The language of covalent histone modifications. *Nature* **403:**41–45.

4. Barth TK, Imhof A. 2010. Fast signals and slow marks: the dynamics of histone modifications. *Trends Biochem Sci* **35:**618–626.

5. Li B, Carey M, Workman JL. 2007. The role of chromatin during transcription. *Cell* **128:**707–719.

6. Hamon MA, Cossart P. 2008. Histone modifications and chromatin remodeling during bacterial infections. *Cell Host Microbe* **4:**100–109.

7. Saunders A, Core LJ, Lis JT. 2006. Breaking barriers to transcription elongation. *Nat Rev Mol Cell Biol* **7:**557–567.

8. Tremethick DJ. 2007. Higher-order structures of chromatin: the elusive 30 nm fiber. *Cell* **128:**651–654.

9. Kornberg RD, Lorch Y. 1999. Twenty-five years of the nucleosome, fundamental particle of the eukaryote chromosome. *Cell* **98:**285–294.

10. Kornberg RD. 1974. Chromatin structure: a repeating unit of histones and DNA. *Science* **184:**868–871.

11. Thomas JO, Kornberg RD. 1975. An octamer of histones in chromatin and free in solution. *Proc Natl Acad Sci USA* **72:**2626–2630.

12. Izzo A, Schneider R. 2016. The role of linker histone H1 modifications in the regulation of gene expression and chromatin dynamics. *Biochim Biophys Acta* **1859:**486–495.

13. Sadakierska-Chudy A, Filip M. 2015. A comprehensive view of the epigenetic landscape. Part II: histone post-translational modification, nucleosome level, and chromatin regulation by ncRNAs. *Neurotox Res* **27:**172–197.

14. Kouzarides T. 2007. Chromatin modifications and their function. *Cell* **128:**693–705.

15. Saccani S, Pantano S, Natoli G. 2001. Two waves of nuclear factor κB recruitment to target promoters. *J Exp Med* **193:**1351–1360.

16. Hargreaves DC, Horng T, Medzhitov R. 2009. Control of inducible gene expression by signal-dependent transcriptional elongation. *Cell* **138:**129–145.

17. Saccani S, Pantano S, Natoli G. 2002. p38-Dependent marking of inflammatory genes for increased NF-kappa B recruitment. *Nat Immunol* **3:**69–75.

18. Foster SL, Hargreaves DC, Medzhitov R. 2007. Gene-specific control of inflammation by TLR-induced chromatin modifications. *Nature* **447:**972–978 *CORRIGENDUM Nature* **451:**102.

19. Chang PV, Hao L, Offermanns S, Medzhitov R. 2014. The microbial metabolite butyrate regulates intestinal macrophage function via histone deacetylase inhibition. *Proc Natl Acad Sci USA* **111:**2247–2252.

20. Fellows R, Denizot J, Stellato C, Cuomo A, Jain P, Stoyanova E, Balázsi S, Hajnády Z, Liebert A, Kazakevych J, Blackburn H, Corrêa RO, Fachi JL, Sato FT, Ribeiro WR, Ferreira CM, Perée H, Spagnuolo M, Mattiuz R, Matolcsi C, Guedes J, Clark J, Veldhoen M, Bonaldi T, Vinolo MAR, Varga-Weisz P. 2018. Microbiota derived short chain fatty acids promote histone crotonylation in the colon through histone deacetylases. *Nat Commun* **9:**105.

21. Haberland M, Montgomery RL, Olson EN. 2009. The many roles of histone deacetylases in development and physiology: implications for disease and therapy. *Nat Rev Genet* **10:**32–42.

22. Yarbrough VL, Winkle S, Herbst-Kralovetz MM. 2015. Antimicrobial peptides in the female reproductive tract: a critical component of the mucosal immune barrier with physiological and clinical implications. *Hum Reprod Update* **21:**353–377.

23. Bandyopadhaya A, Tsurumi A, Maura D, Jeffrey KL, Rahme LG. 2016. A quorum-sensing signal promotes host tolerance training through HDAC1-mediated epigenetic reprogramming. *Nat Microbiol* **1:**16174.

24. Alto NM, Orth K. 2012. Subversion of cell signaling by pathogens. *Cold Spring Harb Perspect Biol* **4:**a006114.

25. Wang Y, Curry HM, Zwilling BS, Lafuse WP. 2005. Mycobacteria inhibition of IFN-gamma induced HLA-DR gene expression by up-regulating histone deacetylation

at the promoter region in human THP-1 monocytic cells. *J Immunol* **174**:5687–5694.

26. Pennini ME, Pai RK, Schultz DC, Boom WH, Harding CV. 2006. *Mycobacterium tuberculosis* 19-kDa lipoprotein inhibits IFN-gamma-induced chromatin remodeling of MHC2TA by TLR2 and MAPK signaling. *J Immunol* **176**:4323–4330.

27. Cossart P. 2011. Illuminating the landscape of host-pathogen interactions with the bacterium *Listeria monocytogenes*. *Proc Natl Acad Sci USA* **108**:19484–19491.

28. Ireton K, Payrastre B, Cossart P. 1999. The *Listeria monocytogenes* protein InlB is an agonist of mammalian phosphoinositide 3-kinase. *J Biol Chem* **274**:17025–17032.

29. Bosse T, Ehinger J, Czuchra A, Benesch S, Steffen A, Wu X, Schloen K, Niemann HH, Scita G, Stradal TE, Brakebusch C, Rottner K. 2007. Cdc42 and phosphoinositide 3-kinase drive Rac-mediated actin polymerization downstream of c-Met in distinct and common pathways. *Mol Cell Biol* **27**:6615–6628.

30. Eskandarian HA, Impens F, Nahori MA, Soubigou G, Coppée JY, Cossart P, Hamon MA. 2013. A role for SIRT2-dependent histone H3K18 deacetylation in bacterial infection. *Science* **341**:1238858.

31. Pereira JM, Chevalier C, Chaze T, Gianetto Q, Impens F, Matondo M, Cossart P, Hamon MA. 2018. Infection reveals a modification of SIRT2 critical for chromatin association. *Cell Reports* **23**:1124–1137.

32. Kusters JG, van Vliet AHM, Kuipers EJ. 2006. Pathogenesis of *Helicobacter pylori* infection. *Clin Microbiol Rev* **19**:449–490.

33. Wang F, Meng W, Wang B, Qiao L. 2014. *Helicobacter pylori*-induced gastric inflammation and gastric cancer. *Cancer Lett* **345**:196–202.

34. Fehri LF, Rechner C, Janssen S, Mak TN, Holland C, Bartfeld S, Brüggemann H, Meyer TF. 2009. *Helicobacter pylori*-induced modification of the histone H3 phosphorylation status in gastric epithelial cells reflects its impact on cell cycle regulation. *Epigenetics* **4**:577–586.

35. Ding SZ, Fischer W, Kaparakis-Liaskos M, Liechti G, Merrell DS, Grant PA, Ferrero RL, Crowe SE, Haas R, Hatakeyama M, Goldberg JB. 2010. *Helicobacter pylori*-induced histone modification, associated gene expression in gastric epithelial cells, and its implication in pathogenesis. *PLoS One* **5**:e9875.

36. Dal Peraro M, van der Goot FG. 2016. Pore-forming toxins: ancient, but never really out of fashion. *Nat Rev Microbiol* **14**:77–92.

37. Hamon MA, Batsché E, Régnault B, Tham TN, Seveau S, Muchardt C, Cossart P. 2007. Histone modifications induced by a family of bacterial toxins. *Proc Natl Acad Sci USA* **104**:13467–13472 CORRECTION *Proc Natl Acad Sci USA* **104**:17555.

38. Hamon MA, Cossart P. 2011. K+ efflux is required for histone H3 dephosphorylation by *Listeria monocytogenes* listeriolysin O and other pore-forming toxins. *Infect Immun* **79**:2839–2846.

39. Dortet L, Lombardi C, Cretin F, Dessen A, Filloux A. 2018. Pore-forming activity of the *Pseudomonas aerugi-*nosa type III secretion system translocon alters the host epigenome. *Nat Microbiol* **3**:378–386.

40. Yaseen I, Kaur P, Nandicoori VK, Khosla S. 2015. Mycobacteria modulate host epigenetic machinery by Rv1988 methylation of a non-tail arginine of histone H3. *Nat Commun* **6**:8922.

41. The HC, Thanh DP, Holt KE, Thomson NR, Baker S. 2016. The genomic signatures of *Shigella* evolution, adaptation and geographical spread. *Nat Rev Microbiol* **14**: 235–250.

42. Arbibe L, Kim DW, Batsche E, Pedron T, Mateescu B, Muchardt C, Parsot C, Sansonetti PJ. 2007. An injected bacterial effector targets chromatin access for transcription factor NF-κB to alter transcription of host genes involved in immune responses. *Nat Immunol* **8**:47–56.

43. Li H, Xu H, Zhou Y, Zhang J, Long C, Li S, Chen S, Zhou JM, Shao F. 2007. The phosphothreonine lyase activity of a bacterial type III effector family. *Science* **315**: 1000–1003.

44. Harouz H, Rachez C, Meijer BM, Marteyn B, Donnadieu F, Cammas F, Muchardt C, Sansonetti P, Arbibe L. 2014. *Shigella flexneri* targets the HP1γ subcode through the phosphothreonine lyase OspF. *EMBO J* **33**:2606–2622.

45. Lebreton A, Lakisic G, Job V, Fritsch L, Tham TN, Camejo A, Matteï PJ, Regnault B, Nahori MA, Cabanes D, Gautreau A, Ait-Si-Ali S, Dessen A, Cossart P, Bierne H. 2011. A bacterial protein targets the BAHD1 chromatin complex to stimulate type III interferon response. *Science* **331**:1319–1321.

46. Dillon SC, Zhang X, Trievel RC, Cheng X. 2005. The SET-domain protein superfamily: protein lysine methyltransferases. *Genome Biol* **6**:227.

47. Mujtaba S, Winer BY, Jaganathan A, Patel J, Sgobba M, Schuch R, Gupta YK, Haider S, Wang R, Fischetti VA. 2013. Anthrax SET protein: a potential virulence determinant that epigenetically represses NF-κB activation in infected macrophages. *J Biol Chem* **288**: 23458–23472.

48. Pennini ME, Perrinet S, Dautry-Varsat A, Subtil A. 2010. Histone methylation by NUE, a novel nuclear effector of the intracellular pathogen *Chlamydia trachomatis*. *PLoS Pathog* **6**:e1000995.

49. Rolando M, Sanulli S, Rusniok C, Gomez-Valero L, Bertholet C, Sahr T, Margueron R, Buchrieser C. 2013. *Legionella pneumophila* effector RomA uniquely modifies host chromatin to repress gene expression and promote intracellular bacterial replication. *Cell Host Microbe* **13**: 395–405.

50. Elwell C, Mirrashidi K, Engel J. 2016. *Chlamydia* cell biology and pathogenesis. *Nat Rev Microbiol* **14**: 385–400.

51. Liu S, Moayeri M, Leppla SH. 2014. Anthrax lethal and edema toxins in anthrax pathogenesis. *Trends Microbiol* **22**:317–325.

52. Pacis A, Tailleux L, Morin AM, Lambourne J, MacIsaac JL, Yotova V, Dumaine A, Danckaert A, Luca F, Grenier JC, Hansen KD, Gicquel B, Yu M, Pai A, He C, Tung J, Pastinen T, Kobor MS, Pique-Regi R, Gilad Y, Barreiro LB. 2015. Bacterial infection remodels the DNA methyl-

ation landscape of human dendritic cells. *Genome Res* 25:1801–1811.

53. Sharma G, Upadhyay S, Srilalitha M, Nandicoori VK, Khosla S. 2015. The interaction of mycobacterial protein Rv2966c with host chromatin is mediated through non-CpG methylation and histone H3/H4 binding. *Nucleic Acids Res* 43:3922–3937.

54. Niwa T, Tsukamoto T, Toyoda T, Mori A, Tanaka H, Maekita T, Ichinose M, Tatematsu M, Ushijima T. 2010. Inflammatory processes triggered by *Helicobacter pylori* infection cause aberrant DNA methylation in gastric epithelial cells. *Cancer Res* 70:1430–1440.

55. Woo HD, Fernandez-Jimenez N, Ghantous A, Degli Esposti D, Cuenin C, Cahais V, Choi IJ, Kim YI, Kim J, Herceg Z. 2018. Genome-wide profiling of normal gastric mucosa identifies *Helicobacter pylori*- and cancer-associated DNA methylome changes. *Int J Cancer* 143:597–609.

56. Shin CM, Kim N, Jung Y, Park JH, Kang GH, Kim JS, Jung HC, Song IS. 2010. Role of *Helicobacter pylori* infection in aberrant DNA methylation along multistep gastric carcinogenesis. *Cancer Sci* 101:1337–1346.

57. Shin CM, Kim N, Jung Y, Park JH, Kang GH, Park WY, Kim JS, Jung HC, Song IS. 2011. Genome-wide DNA methylation profiles in noncancerous gastric mucosae with regard to *Helicobacter pylori* infection and the presence of gastric cancer. *Helicobacter* 16:179–188.

58. Zhang Y, Zhang XR, Park JL, Kim JH, Zhang L, Ma JL, Liu WD, Deng DJ, You WC, Kim YS, Pan KF. 2016. Genome-wide DNA methylation profiles altered by *Helicobacter pylori* in gastric mucosa and blood leukocyte DNA. *Oncotarget* 7:37132–37144.

59. Pero R, Peluso S, Angrisano T, Tuccillo C, Sacchetti S, Keller S, Tomaiuolo R, Bruni CB, Lembo F, Chiariotti L. 2011. Chromatin and DNA methylation dynamics of *Helicobacter pylori*-induced COX-2 activation. *Int J Med Microbiol* 301:140–149.

60. Maeda M, Moro H, Ushijima T. 2017. Mechanisms for the induction of gastric cancer by Helicobacter pylori infection: aberrant DNA methylation pathway. *Gastric Cancer* 20(Suppl 1):8–15.

61. Maekita T, Nakazawa K, Mihara M, Nakajima T, Yanaoka K, Iguchi M, Arii K, Kaneda A, Tsukamoto T, Tatematsu M, Tamura G, Saito D, Sugimura T, Ichinose M, Ushijima T. 2006. High levels of aberrant DNA methylation in *Helicobacter pylori*-infected gastric mucosae and its possible association with gastric cancer risk. *Clin Cancer Res* 12:989–995.

62. Chumduri C, Gurumurthy RK, Zadora PK, Mi Y, Meyer TF. 2013. *Chlamydia* infection promotes host DNA damage and proliferation but impairs the DNA damage response. *Cell Host Microbe* 13:746–758.

63. Vielfort K, Söderholm N, Weyler L, Vare D, Löfmark S, Aro H. 2013. *Neisseria gonorrhoeae* infection causes DNA damage and affects the expression of p21, p27 and p53 in non-tumor epithelial cells. *J Cell Sci* 126:339–347.

64. Strickertsson JA, Desler C, Martin-Bertelsen T, Machado AM, Wadstrøm T, Winther O, Rasmussen LJ, Friis-Hansen L. 2013. *Enterococcus faecalis* infection causes

inflammation, intracellular oxphos-independent ROS production, and DNA damage in human gastric cancer cells. *PLoS One* 8:e63147.

65. Samba-Louaka A, Pereira JM, Nahori MA, Villiers V, Deriano L, Hamon MA, Cossart P. 2014. *Listeria monocytogenes* dampens the DNA damage response. *PLoS Pathog* 10:e1004470.

66. Toller IM, Neelsen KJ, Steger M, Hartung ML, Hottiger MO, Stucki M, Kalali B, Gerhard M, Sartori AA, Lopes M, Müller A. 2011. Carcinogenic bacterial pathogen *Helicobacter pylori* triggers DNA double-strand breaks and a DNA damage response in its host cells. *Proc Natl Acad Sci USA* 108:14944–14949.

67. Lara-Tejero M, Galán JE. 2000. A bacterial toxin that controls cell cycle progression as a deoxyribonuclease I-like protein. *Science* 290:354–357.

68. Lara-Tejero M, Galán JE. 2001. CdtA, CdtB, and CdtC form a tripartite complex that is required for cytolethal distending toxin activity. *Infect Immun* 69:4358–4365.

69. Elwell CA, Dreyfus LA. 2000. DNase I homologous residues in CdtB are critical for cytolethal distending toxin-mediated cell cycle arrest. *Mol Microbiol* 37:952–963.

70. NešiX D, Hsu Y, Stebbins CE. 2004. Assembly and function of a bacterial genotoxin. *Nature* 429:429–433.

71. Shenker BJ, Boesze-Battaglia K, Scuron MD, Walker LP, Zekavat A, DlakiX M. 2016. The toxicity of the *Aggregatibacter actinomycetemcomitans* cytolethal distending toxin correlates with its phosphatidylinositol-3,4,5-triphosphate phosphatase activity. *Cell Microbiol* 18:223–243.

72. Nishikubo S, Ohara M, Ueno Y, Ikura M, Kurihara H, Komatsuzawa H, Oswald E, Sugai M. 2003. An N-terminal segment of the active component of the bacterial genotoxin cytolethal distending toxin B (CDTB) directs CDTB into the nucleus. *J Biol Chem* 278:50671–50681.

73. Frisan T, Cortes-Bratti X, Chaves-Olarte E, Stenerlöw B, Thelestam M. 2003. The *Haemophilus ducreyi* cytolethal distending toxin induces DNA double-strand breaks and promotes ATM-dependent activation of RhoA. *Cell Microbiol* 5:695–707.

74. Elwell C, Chao K, Patel K, Dreyfus L. 2001. *Escherichia coli* CdtB mediates cytolethal distending toxin cell cycle arrest. *Infect Immun* 69:3418–3422.

75. Guidi R, Guerra L, Levi L, Stenerlöw B, Fox JG, Josenhans C, Masucci MG, Frisan T. 2013. Chronic exposure to the cytolethal distending toxins of Gram-negative bacteria promotes genomic instability and altered DNA damage response. *Cell Microbiol* 15:98–113.

76. Ge Z, Rogers AB, Feng Y, Lee A, Xu S, Taylor NS, Fox JG. 2007. Bacterial cytolethal distending toxin promotes the development of dysplasia in a model of microbially induced hepatocarcinogenesis. *Cell Microbiol* 9:2070–2080.

77. Graillot V, Dormoy I, Dupuy J, Shay JW, Huc L, Mirey G, Vignard J. 2016. Genotoxicity of cytolethal distending toxin (CDT) on isogenic human colorectal cell lines: potential promoting effects for colorectal carcinogenesis. *Front Cell Infect Microbiol* 6:34.

78. Nougayrède J-P, Homburg S, Taieb F, Boury M, Brzuszkiewicz E, Gottschalk G, Buchrieser C, Hacker J, Dobrindt U, Oswald E. 2006. *Escherichia coli* induces DNA double-strand breaks in eukaryotic cells. *Science* 313:848–851.

79. Homburg S, Oswald E, Hacker J, Dobrindt U. 2007. Expression analysis of the colibactin gene cluster coding for a novel polyketide in *Escherichia coli*. *FEMS Microbiol Lett* 275:255–262.

80. Vizcaino MI, Crawford JM. 2015. The colibactin warhead crosslinks DNA. *Nat Chem* 7:411–417.

81. Vizcaino MI, Engel P, Trautman E, Crawford JM. 2014. Comparative metabolomics and structural characterizations illuminate colibactin pathway-dependent small molecules. *J Am Chem Soc* 136:9244–9247.

82. Bossuet-Greif N, Vignard J, Taieb F, Mirey G, Dubois D, Petit C, Oswald E, Nougayrède JP. 2018. The colibactin genotoxin generates DNA interstrand cross-links in infected cells. *mBio* 9:e02393-17.

83. Buc E, Dubois D, Sauvanet P, Raisch J, Delmas J, Darfeuille-Michaud A, Pezet D, Bonnet R. 2013. High prevalence of mucosa-associated E. coli producing cyclomodulin and genotoxin in colon cancer. *PLoS One* 8: e56964.

84. Netea MG, Joosten LA, Latz E, Mills KH, Natoli G, Stunnenberg HG, O'Neill LA, Xavier RJ. 2016. Trained immunity: A program of innate immune memory in health and disease. *Science* 352:aaf1098.

85. Netea MG, Quintin J, van der Meer JW. 2011. Trained immunity: a memory for innate host defense. *Cell Host Microbe* 9:355–361.

86. Netea MG, van Crevel R. 2014. BCG-induced protection: effects on innate immune memory. *Semin Immunol* 26:512–517.

87. Grode L, Seiler P, Baumann S, Hess J, Brinkmann V, Nasser Eddine A, Mann P, Goosmann C, Bandermann S, Smith D, Bancroft GJ, Reyrat JM, van Soolingen D, Raupach B, Kaufmann SH. 2005. Increased vaccine efficacy against tuberculosis of recombinant *Mycobacterium bovis* bacille Calmette-Guérin mutants that secrete listeriolysin. *J Clin Invest* 115:2472–2479.

88. Arts RJW, Moorlag SJCFM, Novakovic B, Li Y, Wang SY, Oosting M, Kumar V, Xavier RJ, Wijmenga C, Joosten LAB, Reusken CBEM, Benn CS, Aaby P, Koopmans MP, Stunnenberg HG, van Crevel R, Netea MG. 2018. BCG vaccination protects against experimental viral infection in humans through the induction of cytokines associated with trained immunity. *Cell Host Microbe* 23:89–100.e5.

Bacteria and Intracellularity
Edited by Pascale Cossart, Craig R. Roy, and Philippe Sansonetti
© 2019 American Society for Microbiology, Washington, DC
doi:10.1128/microbiolspec.BAI-0020-2019

Cell Biology of Intracellular Adaptation of *Mycobacterium leprae* in the Peripheral Nervous System

16

Samuel Hess[1] and Anura Rambukkana[1,2]

INTRODUCTION

Bacterial Infection of the Adult Nervous System

The nervous system comprises the central nervous system (CNS) and the peripheral nervous system (PNS). Although many bacterial pathogens are known to invade the CNS and cause associated neuropathologies, much less is known about their intracellular manipulation of neural cells, particularly early events of bacterial infections, and how such bacterium-induced neural cell alterations could lead to bacterial survival, persistence, and the progression of infection as well as pathogenesis. A majority of the studies with these bacterial pathogens are immune-centric and focused on inflammatory aspects of nervous system diseases, and many reviews are available elsewhere with more detail on inflammatory and immune mechanisms of this bacteria-induced neurodegeneration (1–3).

Bacterial Infections of the Adult PNS

Because the PNS connects CNS communication with the organs and limbs in order to effectively coordinate the body functions, the PNS is as important as the CNS when it comes to motor, sensory, and autonomous neuronal functions (Fig. 1). Thus, the bacterial pathogens that preferentially invade the PNS provide a model to dissect how they naturally target nerves and initiate and induce nerve degeneration by deregulating neural cell functions, most of which are yet to be identified.

Virtually all tissues of the body are innervated by peripheral nerves, supplied with a neuronal network along with the supporting glial cells (i.e., Schwann cells), which form myelin sheaths around larger axons and do not form myelin sheaths around smaller-diameter axons; the nerves and glial cells collectively serve as the functional units of the PNS (4, 5). Their peripheral location and ubiquitous presence give rise to a potential susceptibility of the peripheral nerves to invading pathogens; nerve terminals are present close to external sites on the body, including the skin and nasal cavity, and nerves frequently run close to blood vessels carrying systemic infectious agents. Considering this unprotected nature and close proximity of the PNS to the exterior, peripheral nerves are expected to be vulnerable even to environmental pathogens. Surprisingly, however, only a few bacterial pathogens have the capacity to invade the PNS and establish a productive infection. This level of defense against pathogens may be due to the privileged nature of the peripheral nerves, which are protected and surrounded by a connective tissue-rich perineurium and the blood-nerve barrier (BNB), akin to the blood-brain barrier of the CNS (6, 7).

MYCOBACTERIUM LEPRAE AS A MODEL FOR NEUROPATHOGENESIS

A classic example of an intracellular bacterial pathogen that breaches the BNB and preferentially enters the glial cells of the peripheral nerves (Schwann cells) is *Mycobacterium leprae*. Leprosy causes one of the most common infectious neuropathies, leprosy neuropathy, which is currently prevalent in low- and middle-income countries on three continents (8, 9). With the number of new cases detected exceeding 200,000 annually, leprosy remains a major public health problem in countries where

---

[1]Medical Research Council (MRC) Centre for Regenerative Medicine; [2]Centre for Edinburgh Infectious Diseases, University of Edinburgh, Edinburgh, United Kingdom.

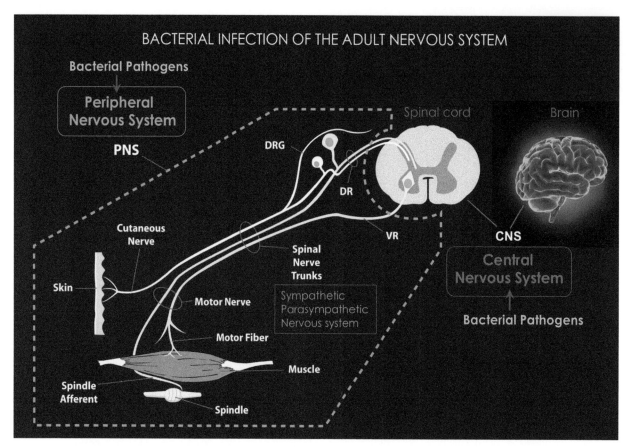

Figure 1   The adult nervous system comprises the PNS and CNS. The CNS is connected to the organs and limbs by the PNS, which also includes a sympathetic and parasympathetic nervous system. Infection of both the PNS and CNS by bacterial pathogens often leads to neurodegenerative diseases. Understanding how such bacterial pathogens target the nervous system and naturally cause disease not only provides insights into combating infectious neurodegenerative diseases but also sheds light on common themes of how neurodegenerative diseases are initiated. Some details of the adult PNS with innervation of skin and muscles are shown; these nerves are usually affected during PNS infections, leading to sensory loss and muscle atrophy, as in leprosy neuropathy.

it is endemic. Due to a lack of early diagnosis and an extremely long incubation period, most newly diagnosed leprosy patients clinically present with some form of neuropathy (8, 9). However, it remains unknown how this pathogen causes neuropathy.

M. *leprae*, the causative organism of human leprosy, preferentially invades the glial cells of the PNS (Schwann cells). This unique capacity for Schwann cell invasion by M. *leprae* and the subsequent neuropathy with sensory and motor neuronal impairment in humans demonstrate that M. *leprae* is an excellent model to dissect how bacteria initiate neuropathic conditions by targeting differentiated glial cells in the adult PNS. Such studies will provide new insights which will be useful for developing early intervention not only for

leprosy neuropathy but also perhaps for other neuropathic diseases with unknown etiologies but similar neuropathological features whose early events are completely unknown.

Pathology Caused by Leprosy Bacilli

Leprosy has been known to humankind since biblical times, having been described since about 600 BCE in texts originating from India, China, and Egypt (10). It is perhaps the most feared archetype of stigmatizing disease, to the extent that the term "leper" has become a generic term for a person shunned by others. The disease was highly prevalent in Europe, and the Norwegian physician Armauer Hansen was the first to identify the causative agent, M. *leprae*, in 1873 (11). Leprosy was the first human disease known to be caused by a microorganism (11). The first effective antibacterial therapies for leprosy were introduced in the 1940s, and the current standard therapy involves multidrug treatment regimens with dapsone, clofazimine, and rifampin (12). However, leprosy remains endemic in low- and middle-income countries on three continents, with a stable annual rate of new-case detection (13). If not diagnosed or treated early, *M. leprae* infection in humans develops into neuropathic conditions and stigmatizing skin conditions as a result of uncontrolled bacterial propagation in the skin and the peripheral nerves. The hallmark of leprosy is its effect on sensory and motor neurons; loss of sensation is associated with complications in the extremities and subsequent formation of ulcers, known as neuropathic ulcers, which can proceed to destroy other structures underlying the skin, including cartilage and bones, if untreated, causing severe disability. Indeed, at the time of diagnosis, most patients manifest some form of disability due to neurological injuries as a result of extremely long incubation. Facial disfiguration and bone loss are common in the late stage of the disease, and damage to the nerves controlling blinking can lead to blindness. Interestingly, most of these unusual pathologies occur in multibacillary leprosy patients (i.e., those harboring high loads of bacteria in the tissues), suggesting that direct host tissue responses to *M. leprae* may be associated with pathogenesis.

M. leprae Infection in Animal Models and Humans

Entirely dependent on host cells for bacterial survival, *M. leprae* is a strictly obligately intracellular bacterium (9, 14). This strictly intracellular lifestyle is directly linked to the bacterial genome, which comprises more pseudogenes and noncoding genes than protein-coding genes, rendering *M. leprae* dependent on host cell functions and metabolism for bacterial survival and replication (15, 16). In addition to humans, two animal hosts which are susceptible to naturally occurring systemic infections are known so far; *M. leprae* causes multibacillary leprosy-like disease in nine-banded armadillos (17, 18) and red squirrels in the wild (19), as well as in experimentally infected armadillos. The majority of the human population generally does not develop clinical leprosy following *M. leprae* infection (20, 21). Human leprosy could also be acquired by zoonotic transmission via nine-banded armadillos infected in the wild in the southern United States (22). The association of genetic factors with human leprosy was exemplified by the findings that genes PARK2 and PACRG are risk factors for leprosy (23–25). Interestingly, mutation of

the PARK2 gene, which encodes a ubiquitin E3 ligase, has been shown to be the cause of autosomal recessive early-onset Parkinson's disease, and this finding connects leprosy susceptibility to other neurodegenerative diseases with unknown etiology (26). Interestingly, potential environmental factors like bacterial and viral infections have been implicated in triggering Parkinson's and other neurodegenerative diseases (27, 28). Therefore, a better understanding of early molecular events during *M. leprae* infection could provide new insights into how other neurodegenerative diseases with unknown etiology might be triggered.

Temperature Sensitivity in Intracellular Bacterial Growth

Apart from the strictly obligate intracellular lifestyle, leprosy bacilli also require lower body temperature for survival and replication, and thus, in humans, preferential bacterial growth can be seen in peripheral tissues like peripheral nerves, skin, and testis, where peripheral body temperature is relatively low (20, 29, 30). Experimental evidence has shown that a temperature of 37°C is unfavorable for intracellular *M. leprae* viability, while in the footpads of immunocompromised nude mice, prolific bacterial growth can be achieved locally without disseminated infection due to the lower temperature in the extremities (31). The latter provides a valuable resource for the provision of *in vivo*-grown bacteria for basic leprosy research (31, 32). Interestingly, in nine-banded armadillos, the core body temperature is 33 to 35°C, and *M. leprae* propagates in both peripheral tissues and internal organs, such as the liver (33, 34).

M. leprae Infection in Humans

In humans, *M. leprae* infection of Schwann cells in the PNS is primarily responsible for developing neuropathic conditions. In multibacillary leprosy, a large number of intracellular *M. leprae* organisms can be seen in Schwann cells in peripheral nerves (20, 35). *M. leprae* rarely infects the axons, although axonal degeneration eventually contributes to neuropathic conditions which cause not only disability but also stigmatized conditions, including bone loss and muscle atrophy due to loss of sensation and associated complications that affect tissues underneath the skin. These conditions have caused leprosy to be one of the most feared and stigmatized diseases known to humankind. Humans show a wide spectrum of clinical immunological and histological presentations of leprosy, from tuberculoid leprosy, which entails a strong immune response and minimal detectable bacilli (paucibacillary leprosy), to lepromatous leprosy, with more widespread bacterial presence in peripheral tissues like the PNS and skin (multibacillary leprosy) and low or absent cell-mediated immune responses (9, 29, 36, 37), with intermediate classifications between these polar groups. Regardless of the clinical spectrum, nerve damage is widely seen in all groups of leprosy patients.

Although nerve damage in tuberculoid leprosy is expected to be caused by immune-mediated tissue destruction due to strong cell-mediated immune responses (38, 39), it is unknown how multibacillary leprosy with high numbers of bacteria in Schwann cells and minimal or no cell-mediated immune response causes neurological damage. In this context, previous research on the biology of multibacillary leprosy was designed to address several important questions. (i) How does *M. leprae* target and manipulate the functions of Schwann cells in the adult peripheral nerves? (ii) How does it hijack Schwann cell properties once inside the cells? (iii) How does it propagate and disseminate infection? (iv) How does preferential *M. leprae* infection in Schwann cells initiate and cause neurological injury?

SIGNIFICANCE OF MODELING *M. LEPRAE* INTERACTION

During human infection, *M. leprae* preferentially resides and replicates within adult Schwann cells for a long period before immune cell recruitment and immune-mediated attack, which over a long incubation period eventually manifests clinically as sensory or sensorimotor loss (29, 35, 40–42). We know nothing about what occurs early in human infection, from initial infection of Schwann cells to the first symptoms of nerve damage. This is a critical initial phase for the propagation of *M. leprae* within this privileged niche, including evasion of immune surveillance and the establishment of productive infection within the PNS. Although host immune responses to *M. leprae* play a decisive role in developing the clinical state of leprosy, it is the leprosy bacillus itself and its propagation in the preferred peripheral tissue niches, such as the PNS and the skin, that establish the productive infection that sets the stage for subsequent infectious processes. However, how *M. leprae* establishes infection in the PNS and what strategies it uses to achieve this are largely unknown. Also, tissue cell responses directly to high bacterial load, independent of or under the partial influence of immune responses, could give rise to pathological conditions, especially when bacilli reside in privileged niches like Schwann cells, where immune cell trafficking is minimal. This is the case in patients with multibacillary leprosy, who harbor a high load of bacteria in the tissues which cause the pathology independent

of cell-mediated immune responses. Thus, multibacillary leprosy provides an excellent disease model to study how a neurotrophic bacterial pathogen directly causes nervous system pathology. Therefore, mimicking multibacillary leprosy in model systems and searching for detailed mechanisms of how leprosy bacilli target the PNS are warranted.

M. leprae Targeting of the Peripheral Nerves
Molecular details of specific *M. leprae*-peripheral nerve interaction require model systems that mimic the unique PNS niche environment, since the anatomy of the PNS is critical for studying the specific interaction of *M. leprae* with cells in the PNS. This is because the way in which *M. leprae* might interact with the structural PNS components is distinct from the way in which it might interact with the CNS, both the brain and spinal cord. *M. leprae* interacts specifically with the mature glia of the human PNS (Schwann cells) (43), and clinical presentations involve peripheral nerves and tissues (9, 29, 42) and not the glia of the CNS (oligodendrocytes or astrocytes). Although some phenotypic similarities exist between myelin-producing Schwann cells and oligodendrocytes, these two cell types are distinct in terms of functional and signaling properties, developmental origin, and their interactions with axons (4, 44–48). Most importantly, the anatomical differences between the PNS and CNS are critical for the initial *in vivo* interaction of *M. leprae* with Schwann cells, which are the specific target of leprosy bacilli in the nervous system of humans.

Differences between glia of the adult PNS and CNS
The functional units that facilitate rapid nerve conduction of the PNS and CNS comprise glia-axon units: Schwann cell–axon units in the PNS and oligodendrocyte-axon units in the CNS. In the adult PNS, there are two functional units; some Schwann cells wrap around a single larger-diameter axon to form myelinated Schwann cell–axon units, and other Schwann cells make nonmyelinating Schwann cells by enclosing multiple smaller-diameter axons. Depending on the type of nerves, i.e., motor or sensory neurons, the ratio of myelinated to nonmyelinated axons varies (4, 5). In both cases, Schwann cell–axon units in the PNS are completely surrounded by the basal lamina (also called basement membrane when associated with epithelial cells, e.g., skin and intestine), which is composed of tissue-specific isoforms of matrix components secreted by Schwann cells (Fig. 2). These extracellular matrix (ECM) proteins on the outer surface of

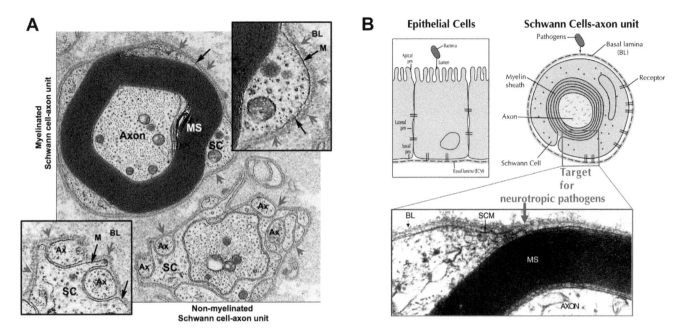

Figure 2 (**A**) Functional units of the adult human peripheral nerves, i.e., myelinated and nonmyelinated Schwann cell–axon units, depicting the distinct basal lamina that surrounds each Schwann cell–axon unit *in situ*. Red arrows indicate the basal lamina (BL) completely surrounding both myelinated (top inset) and nonmyelinated (bottom inset) Schwann cell–axon units. The Schwann cell membrane (M) is shown by black arrows. SC, Schwann cells; Ax, axons; MS, myelin sheath. (**B**) Sites of bacterial pathogens' targets and entry into epithelia and peripheral nerves. Pathogenic bacteria enter epithelia at the apical side of the cells which anchor the basal lamina, whereas neurotrophic bacterial pathogens (e.g., *M. leprae*) must cross the basal lamina barrier, and thus attach to the basal lamina matrix proteins deposited around Schwann cell–axon units. The micrograph (adapted from reference 70) shows myelinated Schwann cell–axon units with the basal lamina (BL), Schwann cell membrane (SCM), and the axons ensheathed by the myelin sheath (MS).

Schwann cells are anchored to the cell membrane via ECM receptors on the Schwann cell membrane (Fig. 2).

This characteristic feature of the basement membrane around each glia-axon unit is not present in the oligodendrocytes, astrocytes, or microglia in the CNS. Oligodendrocytes form highly complex network-like connections with multiple axons by extending oligodendrocyte processes, enclosing multiple axons and forming myelin sheaths with each encountered axon, thus elaborating a highly complex myelinated nerve network in the CNS (48, 49). On the other hand, in nonneural tissues, cell types such as epithelia anchor to the basal lamina and/or basement membrane only through the basal side of the cells and are not surrounded completely by basal lamina or basement membranes (Fig. 2B). Also, macrophages in the PNS and both microglia and macrophages in the CNS, which usually engulf many bacterial and viral pathogens in the nervous system, are not surrounded by basal lamina or basement

membranes. These facts indicate that the basal lamina that completely surrounds Schwann cell–axon units is a distinct anatomical feature in the PNS, and leprosy bacilli must cross the structural components of the basal lamina in order to invade Schwann cells. Perhaps the tropism of this bacterium to the adult peripheral nerves lies within this distinct bacterium–host component interaction, as immune cells such as ubiquitous macrophages are unlikely to exhibit such specific neural tropism.

DRG neuron and Schwann cell coculture model system

A model of the initial interaction of *M. leprae* with the native basal lamina components that surround both myelinated and nonmyelinated nerve fibers has been established using an *ex vivo* coculture system of purified primary rodent Schwann cells with purified dorsal root ganglion (DRG) neurons (50–54). In this model, as in peripheral nerve development, Schwann cells naturally wrap around DRG neuronal axons and establish a 1:1 relationship with larger-diameter axons and produce a myelin sheath, whereas other Schwann cells form non-myelinated Schwann cell–axon units on smaller-diameter axons. As in adult peripheral nerves, both Schwann cell–axon units in these cultures are surrounded by the basal lamina comprising ECM components. The major components of the basal lamina are laminin-2 isoform, collagen IV, heparin sulfate proteoglycan, and nidogen (also known as entactin) (55–57). Among them, the tissue restriction of ECM components lies within the laminin-2 isoform, which is formed by assembling three subunits of laminin chains, the $\beta1$, $\gamma1$, and $\alpha2$ chains (51).

Role of neural laminin $\alpha2$ chain

Laminins are large glycoproteins composed of three polypeptide chains, α, β, and γ, which are assembled in different combinations to form asymmetrical cruciform structures to give rise to various laminin isoforms with restricted tissue distribution (58–60). These laminin isoforms are major structural and functional components of the basal lamina and/or basement membrane to which cells from different tissue types anchor via various extracellular ligands and cellular receptors (43, 61–64). Such specific cell-ECM component interactions are critical for cell differentiation and survival within specialized tissue niches; for example in the gut, cells anchor to the basal lamina that is secreted specifically by gut epithelial cells, and in the Schwann cell–axon units, the basal lamina that surrounds the units is secreted by Schwann cells (43, 65).

Likewise, combinations of laminin α, β, and γ chains that are assembled to form different isoforms vary in different tissues. It is believed the α chain determines this restricted tissue distribution, because the same α chain is rarely found in different tissues; for example, the α chain of laminin-2 is expressed predominantly in the basal lamina of Schwann cells and muscle cells, whereas the laminin $\beta1$ and $\gamma1$ chains have a wider tissue distribution (43, 61, 63, 64). Importantly, the tissue specificity of the laminin α chain is relevant to its characteristic larger globular (G) domain at the carboxyl terminus, and this G domain is responsible for the binding through which cells anchor to the basal lamina (43) (Fig. 3B and 4). In the basal lamina of Schwann cell–axon units, the tissue specificity lies within the laminin $\alpha2$ chain and not within the $\beta1$ and $\gamma1$ chains, which are shared with other laminin isoforms, such as laminin-1, with a much broader tissue distribution (43, 51, 61, 63, 64). In the DRG Schwann cell–neuron coculture system, this tissue-restricted laminin $\alpha2$ chain is specifically secreted by Schwann cells, particularly under the influence of axons,

and thus contributes to the basal lamina that surrounds each nerve fiber, as in peripheral nerves *in vivo*.

Role of globular (G) domain of laminin $\alpha2$ in neural tropism

Molecular analysis of the laminin $\alpha2$ chain in relation to the tissue specificity of the basal lamina of Schwann cell–axon units in the PNS provides evidence that the neural tropism of *M. leprae* is determined by the G domain of the laminin $\alpha2$ chain ($\alpha2$LG), which is also the cell binding site of the laminin-2 isoform (43, 51). The $\alpha2$LG modules are integral components of the basal lamina that surrounds the Schwann cell–axon units and interacts with host cell receptors such as α-dystroglycan, a laminin-2 receptor in both PNS and muscles (64, 66) (Fig. 3 and 4). Several of these receptor binding sites have been mapped to various $\alpha2$LG modules (67). The resolved crystal structures of $\alpha2$LG modules reveal a compact β-sandwich fold and a novel calcium-binding site architecture (68, 69) (Fig. 3). The fact that *M. leprae* interacts specifically with $\alpha2$LG modules but cannot bind to the G domain of the $\alpha1$ chain of the laminin-1 isoform, which in contrast shows wider tissue distribution, is consistent with the high sequence divergence between the G domains of the $\alpha1$ and $\alpha2$ chains (43, 51) (Fig. 3 and 4). In terms of tissue tropism, the limited sequence identity of the G domains of different laminin α chains (20 to 40%) appears to contribute to the restricted tissue distribution of a given laminin isoform (reference 51 and references therein). Based on the findings that $\alpha2$LG specifically mediates the *M. leprae*–Schwann cell interaction and that *in vivo*, *M. leprae* failed to adhere to peripheral nerves of laminin-$\alpha2$-deficient mice, which also lack $\alpha2$LG, it was concluded that the tissue-restricted $\alpha2$LG of the laminin-2 isoform is largely responsible for the peripheral-nerve tropism of *M. leprae* (51, 70).

It should be noted that the neural tropism of *M. leprae* could be demonstrated only by using $\alpha2$LG modules and laminin $\alpha2$-deficient mice, not with total laminin-2, simply because of the fact that total laminin-2 contains both laminin $\beta1$ and $\gamma1$ chains with wider tissue distribution (43, 51), and many bacterial pathogens, including mycobacterial species, have been shown to bind to these common laminin isoforms. Therefore, the use of commercially available total laminin-2 or -4 alone containing several common laminin chains does not confirm the tissue specificity; previous studies using such total laminin without molecular details showed binding of mycobacterial species other than *M. leprae* (71). Considering these crucial factors determining general versus specific binding, it is important to clarify

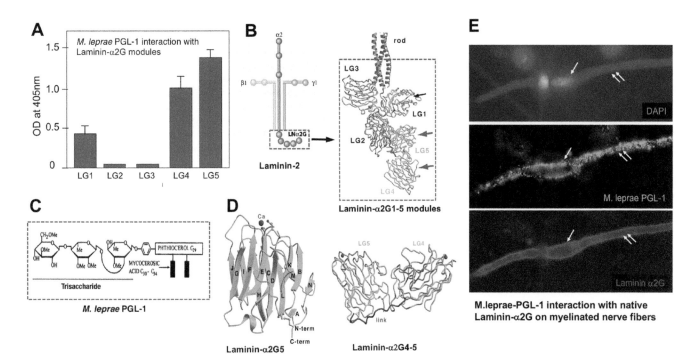

Figure 3 Molecular basis of neural tropism of *M. leprae*. Interaction of *M. leprae*-specific PGL-1 on the bacterial cell wall with the tissue-specific α2LG domain on the basal lamina. (**A**) PGL-1 binding to the recombinant G modules of the α2LG domain. OD, optical density. (**B**) Subunits of the laminin-2 isoform comprising α, β, and γ chains with the cell-binding α2G domain and its modules α2LG1 to α2LG5. (**C**) Composition of *M. leprae* PGL-1. (**D**) Crystal structure of PGL-1-binding α2LG5 and α2LG4-5 modules of the α2LG domain. (**E**) *M. leprae* PGL-1 binding (green) to the native α2LG domain (red) on the basal lamina surrounding a myelinated Schwann cell–axon unit (outer surface of nerve fiber is labeled in red to demarcate the α2G domain) colocalized with PGL-1 (green) when cultures were incubated with a PGL-1 suspension.

these molecular details for future studies of tissue-specific interaction of *M. leprae* with the peripheral nerves.

CONTRIBUTION OF BACTERIAL FACTORS TO NEURAL TROPISM

Although the peculiar affinity of leprosy bacilli for the peripheral nerve has been known since the histopathological study of leprosy began after the discovery by Armauer Hansen of *M. leprae* as the causative organism of leprosy (11), and early scientists were curious about the basis for the neural affinity of this organism, it remained unexplained until studies published in 1997 and 2000 which detailed a mechanism for neural tropism of leprosy bacilli (50, 51). Once the host molecules responsible for neural tropism in leprosy bacilli had been identified, the next studies were launched to delineate the *M. leprae*-specific molecules that determined such host-pathogen interaction at the molecular level.

Role of PGL-1 and Proteins in the *M. leprae* Cell Wall

The overall tissue tropism of a bacterial pathogen is determined by both host and bacterial components. In the case of pathogenic mycobacteria, it has long been proposed that the bacterial cell wall contains most of the elements that are associated with pathogenesis (72). These elements may include the specific cell wall components that direct these pathogens to their favored niches. The cell wall of *M. leprae* contains an extensive electron-transparent outer layer that is largely composed of phthiocerol dimycocerosic acid and related glycolipids, which mainly comprise *M. leprae*-specific phenolic glycolipid-1 (PGL-1) (73–76). These complex cell wall lipid structures, including PGL-1, are commonly thought of in the context of resistance to intracellular killing by macrophages (77), serological analysis (78), and complement fixation (79). Detailed analysis related to the role of bacterial cell wall components showed evidence that PGL-1 is involved in determining the unique

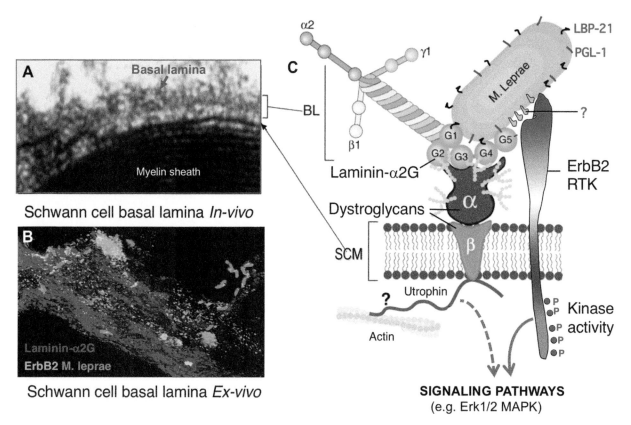

Figure 4 Schwann cell receptors α/β-dystroglycan and receptor tyrosine kinase ErbB2 serve as receptors for *M. leprae* on the Schwann cell membrane (SCM) in an α2LG domain-dependent and -independent manner. (**A**) Basal lamina (BL) and cell membrane of myelinated Schwann cells *in vivo*. Their molecular assembly is shown in the schematic (**C**). (**B**) *M. leprae* infection in an *ex vivo* Schwann cell–neuron coculture system, where *M. leprae* (blue) associates with α2LG in the basal lamina (red) and ErbB2 on the Schwann cell membrane (green). (**C**) Schematic showing the molecular basis of *M. leprae* interaction with α2LG, α/β-dystroglycan, and ErbB2 of Schwann cell–axon units in the peripheral nerves and potential activation of kinase domain of ErbB2, which initiate signaling cascades like phosphorylation of the Erk1/2 mitogen-activated protein kinase pathway.

affinity of *M. leprae* for peripheral nerves (50). PGL-1 is specific for *M. leprae* because it contains an antigenically distinct trisaccharide, which consists of 3,6-di-O-methylglucose linked α1→4 to 2,3-di-O-methylrhamnose, linked β1→2 to 3-O-methylrhamnose, that has not been found in any other bacterium (73, 74). Purified PGL-1 specifically binds to the laminin α2 chain in the basal lamina of Schwann cell–axon units in *ex vivo* tissue cultures, and this binding is mediated by the *M. leprae*-specific trisaccharide portion of PGL-1 (50).

Contribution of *M. leprae* PGL-1 to Neural Tropism

The finding that PGL-1 binding to the basal lamina of Schwann cell–axon units is mediated by the naturally cleaved fragments of the peripheral nerve laminin α2

chain encouraged the concept of neural tropism, as this is a rare bacterium-specific and host tissue-restricted interaction (43, 50, 80). In peripheral nerves, the proteolytic cleavage of the α2 chain occurs at the carboxy-terminal G domain, resulting in an 80-kDa fragment and a large (~300-kDa) amino-terminal fragment (81–83). PGL-1 binds to both peripheral-nerve-derived 80-kDa and 300-kDa fragments (50). Characterization of this binding using individual recombinant α2LG modules demonstrated that the activity to the 80-kDa fragment is associated with PGL-1 binding to the tissue-restricted α2LG4 and α2LG5 modules (50) (Fig. 3A and E). On the other hand, the lack of binding of lipoarabinomannan, another carbohydrate-containing cell wall component in *M. leprae* and *Mycobacterium tuberculosis*, to α2LG modules underscores the specific interaction of *M. leprae* PGL-1 trisaccharides with α2LG modules (50). The specificity of this interaction may be explained by the limited sequence identity of the LG modules of the laminin α2 and α1 chains. Sequence identities of the LG1, LG4, and LG5 modules of the laminin α2 and α1 chains are 45.7%, 36.1%, and 49.7%, respectively (84, 85). Thus, PGL-1 binding to α2LG modules corresponding to a highly divergent region of the α2 chain (α2LG1, α2LG4, and α2LG5) was found be the key to the neural affinity of *M. leprae* and thus establishes that these host and bacterial factors are responsible for neural tropism (50, 61, 86, 87) (Fig. 3).

SCHWANN CELL SIGNALING PATHWAYS ACTIVATED BY *M. LEPRAE*

α-Dystroglycan as a Receptor for *M. leprae*

In Schwann cell–axon units, the basal lamina anchors to the Schwann cell membrane via ECM receptors (61, 63, 64). One such receptor is dystroglycan, a highly glycosylated component of the dystrophin-glycoprotein complex (DGC) which is involved in the pathogenesis of muscular dystrophies (70, 88). The DGC is encoded by a single gene and serves as a receptor for Schwann cell–laminin-2 interaction and signaling (89). The encoded gene product is cleaved into two proteins, peripheral membrane α-dystroglycan and transmembrane β-dystroglycan, by posttranslational processing (90). Yamada et al. (91) have shown that the laminin α2 chain in the Schwann cell basal lamina binds peripheral membrane α-dystroglycan and that laminin α2 links to the Schwann cell cytoskeleton via the DGC (92). *M. leprae* binds to native α-dystroglycan purified from peripheral nerves only in the presence of α2LG (89), suggesting that α2LG has two binding sites, one for *M. leprae* and the other for α-dystroglycan; i.e., α2LG forms a bridge between *M. leprae* and the α-dystroglycan (89) (Fig. 3 and 4).

ErbB2 in Activation of Erk1/2 Mitogen-Activated Protein Kinase Signaling

Schwann cells, both during development and after acquisition of terminal differentiation, interact with neuronal (axonal) ligands for communication, as they are interdependent for maintaining their survival and functional properties (49, 93). This is mediated mainly by neuregulins, the axonal ligands, by binding to the receptor tyrosine kinase complex, ErbB2/ErbB3, on the Schwann cell membrane, which leads to the initiation of intracellular signaling pathways to drive prolifera-

tion and differentiation of Schwann cells, particularly the myelination of axons (94, 95). The ErbB family receptor ErbB2 is one of the major receptor tyrosine kinases expressed on Schwann cells and plays an important role in glial cell functions (95–98). Among the members of the ErbB family, ErbB2 is considered a "ligandless" receptor that transduces strong signals by avid dimerization with other ErbB members (99, 100). In Schwann cells, ErbB2 is known to process the signaling by dimerization with ErbB3 after neuregulin binds to ErbB3, which lacks a kinase domain (97). Strikingly, *M. leprae* directly binds to and activates ErbB2 without ErbB3 heterodimerization (53). This binding is sufficient to induce early demyelination, following activation of ErbB2 by a novel route that bypasses the classical signaling ErbB2-ErbB3 heterodimerization induced by growth factors including neuregulin, and subsequently induces a downstream MEK-dependent Erk1/2 signaling pathway, leading to myelin breakdown (53, 97) (Fig. 4 and 5). It is likely that *M. leprae* takes advantage of the existing Erk1/2 signaling that is involved in both nerve degeneration and regeneration (101).

M. LEPRAE-INDUCED DEMYELINATION OF SCHWANN CELLS

Myelin damage is known to be caused by immune-mediated inflammatory responses, as in many neurodegenerative diseases (102). However, whether such demyelination events also occur in the earliest stage of neurodegenerative diseases where inflammation is minimal or absent is unknown. *M. leprae* is known to initiate neurodegenerative conditions in humans and in susceptible animal models like nine-banded armadillos (9, 29, 33). Therefore, underlying mechanisms by which *M. leprae* initiates neurodegenerative conditions provide valuable insights into early events of neurodegeneration.

The initial interaction of *M. leprae* with the basal lamina of Schwann cell–axon units appears to deregulate the delicate Schwann cell–axon communication system, leading to the breakdown of the myelin sheath (80, 101). Although such early demyelination *in vivo* may not initially lead to clinical manifestation, as peripheral nerves possess a remarkable capacity to regenerate following injury, it may lead to activation of additional signaling from Schwann cells similar to nerve injury (101). Functional consequences like demyelination provide a survival advantage for *M. leprae*, as it induces dedifferentiation and proliferation and generates myelin-free Schwann cells with high plasticity, which naturally promote remyelination and nerve regeneration and are also highly susceptible to *M. leprae*

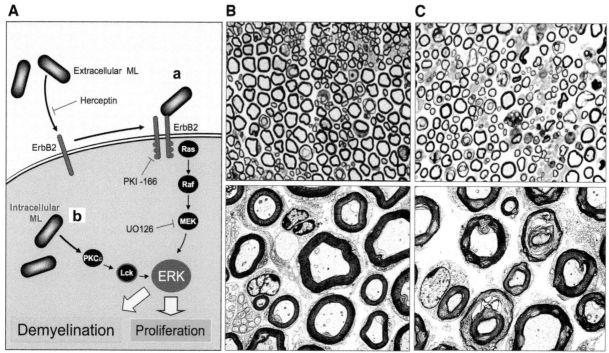

Figure 5 *In vivo* induction of demyelination by direct *M. leprae* injection into sciatic nerves of adult Rag-1 knockout mice, suggesting that early demyelination can be caused by the activation of signaling pathways in the absence of immune responses. (**A**) Schematic showing the activation of Erk1/2 MAPK signaling pathways by extracellular (a) and intracellular (b) *M. leprae* via two different pathways and their role in proliferation and demyelination. *M. leprae* binds to the ErbB2 receptor to induce Schwann cell demyelination and proliferation. (a) The binding of *M. leprae* (ML) to ErbB2 on the surface of myelinated Schwann cells triggers demyelination through the Ras-Raf-MEK-ERK pathway. ErbB2 inhibitors such as herceptin, PKI166, and U0126 block activation of this pathway in response to *M. leprae*. (b) Intracellular *M. leprae* induces proliferation of nonmyelinated Schwann cells through a different route to ERK that involves PKCε and Lck and that is independent of signaling through the Ras-Raf-MEK pathway. (**B** and **C**) Direct injection of *M. leprae* into sciatic nerves of Rag[−/−] knockout mice induces demyelination (**C**), in contrast to injection of phosphate-buffered saline alone, which shows almost intact myelinated Schwann cell–axon units (**B**).

invasion (103). This suggests that initial interactions with and activation of Schwann cells are crucial, as these events set the stage for subsequent intracellular survival and replication within the peripheral nerves.

From Signaling-Mediated Demyelination to Nerve Damage

Although nerve degeneration in the early phase of *M. leprae* infection in both *in vitro* and *in vivo* mouse models does not involve immune cells or macrophages, such nerve injury is likely to cause the destabilization of the neural microenvironment. This might subsequently lead to a cascade of cellular responses that eventually recruit immune cells. Evidence from studies with Rag-1[−/−] knockout mice, which lack mature B and

T cells and are thus unable to mount an adaptive immune response, showed the induction of significant demyelination in sciatic nerves 3 days after intraneural administration of *M. leprae* and its cell wall fraction (52) (Fig. 5). It is likely that the sequential recruitment and propagation of immune cell populations, preceded by non-immune-mediated demyelination and axonal damage at the site of infection, could eventually cause further aggravation of neurological injury to the peripheral nerves during *M. leprae* infection.

Zebrafish Spinal Cord Model

Recent studies have attempted to recapitulate myelin damage in response to *M. leprae* in zebrafish larvae using spinal cord injection of *M. leprae* as a CNS model

(104). Since the study of spinal cord injection of *M. leprae* examines the initial events in CNS cells, it is unlikely that a zebrafish CNS model exhibits the specific peripheral nerve pathology which is so distinctive of *M. leprae* infection in humans (9, 29, 42) due to the nervous systems' fundamental and functional differences as described above (Fig. 2). The underlying pathology of PNS diseases is distinct from that of CNS diseases, and as such, no studies to our knowledge use CNS models for insights into PNS damage.

M. leprae infects Schwann cell–axon units in the PNS, but not the oligodendrocyte-axon units in the spinal cord. Schwann cell–axon units are completely surrounded by the basal lamina (43, 51, 55, 65) (Fig. 2 and 4), providing barriers to *M. leprae* (Fig. 2). In contrast, the axon-oligodendrocyte and astrocyte units of the CNS are not surrounded by such a basal lamina, so it is not surprising that *M. leprae* could bind directly and cause subsequent demyelination when it is injected directly into the zebrafish larvae with immature myelin sheaths (93). Thus, the bacterial tropism for the PNS is difficult to evaluate with such a CNS model. Furthermore, without the PNS barriers, macrophages may have more straightforward access to oligodendrocytes in the zebrafish CNS model, causing the defects seen in the immature larval myelin sheath (104). Such findings indicating that an innate macrophage reaction to bacterial PGL-1 causes early nerve damage and neural tropism should be interpreted with caution, as the macrophage-mediated innate immune responses are ubiquitous and are unlikely to determine neural tropism.

Hijacking of Nerve Injury Responses by Leprosy Bacilli

Unlike CNS neurons, the neurons in the PNS can regenerate effectively when damaged; this differential response to injury is due largely to the proliferative and regenerative properties of adult Schwann cells (105, 106). Following demyelination and nerve injury, terminally differentiated Schwann cells undergo proliferation, and one of the key regulators of the cell cycle, cyclin D1, plays a role in this re-entry into the cell division cycle (107, 108). These nerve injury responses lead to the generation of new dedifferentiated Schwann cells, which serve as repair cells to facilitate the remyelination and regeneration of the damaged axons by initiating a Schwann cell redifferentiation program (106, 108, 109). *M. leprae* appears to mimic the events following nerve injury, since intracellular *M. leprae* induces the accumulation of cyclin D1 in infected human Schwann cells and subsequently increases the cell division (107). When newly generated Schwann cells or similar dedifferentiated Schwann cells are infected

by *M. leprae*, they turn off myelination-associated genes (110) and myelin protein expression, the integral components of the compact myelin sheath. These findings suggest that intracellular *M. leprae* turns off the Schwann cell differentiation program and maintains the infected cells in an undifferentiated stage.

M. leprae appears to hijack multiple pathways of injury repair processes during infection. At the signaling level, mitogen-activated protein kinase pathway Erk1/2 signaling is strongly activated in Schwann cells undergoing dedifferentiation during nerve injury *in vivo* (111). Similarly, once inside the cells, *M. leprae* also activates Erk1/2 signaling in dedifferentiated human Schwann cells (107). However, *M. leprae* activates Erk1/2 intracellularly, not via the Ras-MEK-dependent canonical pathway, but by a novel signaling pathway using a noncanonical MEK-independent and protein kinase Cε- and lymphocyte kinase (Lck)-dependent pathway (107). Therefore, it is possible that sustained activation of noncanonical Erk1/2 signaling in infected Schwann cells maintains cells in a dedifferentiated state and thus prevents remyelination.

M. LEPRAE REPROGRAMMING OF SCHWANN CELLS

The extremely long incubation period of *M. leprae* within Schwann cells during human infection provides *M. leprae* with ample time to alter host cell behavior for its strictly obligate intracellular lifestyle. This is likely to occur in peripheral nerves in multibacillary leprosy, where a high load of bacteria resides in Schwann cells for a long period (9, 29). What the fate of these bacteria-laden Schwann cells is and whether these cells retain or change Schwann cell identity were unknown until recently. It was also unknown how these bacteria disseminate from this privileged niche to other tissues. Intriguingly, in a study by Masaki et al. (110), it was discovered that leprosy bacteria hijack the notable plasticity and regenerative properties of adult Schwann cells for the establishment of infection within the PNS (52, 53, 101).

Masaki et al. (110) demonstrated that *M. leprae* can transcriptionally reprogram Schwann cells to a progenitor stem-like cell (pSLC) state by changing epigenetic modification of key genes (110). By reprogramming adult Schwann cells to stem cell-like cells with migratory properties, *M. leprae* facilitates its spread to other tissues (110) (Fig. 6). This strategy is highly favorable for spread of a strictly obligately intracellular pathogen like *M. leprae* via cell-to-cell transfer, as it was shown that bacteria-laden reprogrammed cells effectively

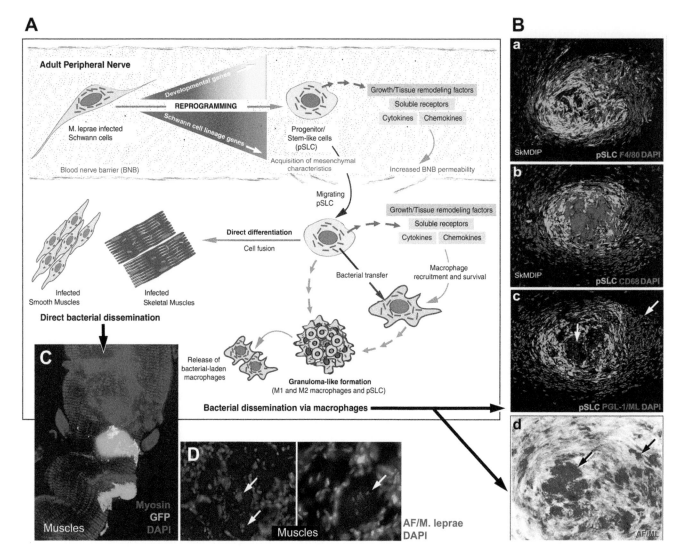

Figure 6   Proposed model of how adult Schwann cell reprogramming to stem cell-like cells by intracellular *M. leprae* promotes dissemination of infection. (**A**) Infected Schwann cells in the adult peripheral nerves undergo a reprogramming process whereby Schwann cell differentiation and myelination program-associated genes are turned off and embryonic genes of mesenchymal and neural crest development are turned on. The resulting pSLC acquire migratory properties and immunomodulatory characteristics and thus release immune factors, chemokines, cytokines, and growth and remodeling factors, which not only increase the permeability of the BNB but also recruit macrophages. (**B**) Acquired migratory properties promote *M. leprae*-laden pSLC to exit by breaching the BNB and disseminate to other preferred tissue niches, such as smooth muscles and skeletal muscles, where they are exposed to respective tissue microenvironments and undergo direct differentiation and thus transfer bacteria passively to these tissues. (**C**) By recruiting macrophages, pSLC can transfer *M. leprae* and form typical granuloma-like structures, which then release bacterium-laden macrophages, a mechanism by which reprogrammed cells may channel bacterial dissemination via systemic routes. DAPI, 4′,6-diamidino-2-phenylindole; GFP, green fluorescent protein-tagged pSLC; AF, acid-fast labeling of *M. leprae*.

rediffentiate to other tissues like muscles and directly transfer infection to muscle fibers, another host niche for leprosy bacilli in humans (110, 112, 113). Moreover, reprogrammed cells also have the capacity to transfer infection more effectively to fibroblasts than nonreprogrammed Schwann cells (114), permitting dissemination of infection to multiple tissues through intermediate cells like fibroblasts, which are abundant in most of the tissue milieu.

Bacterial Usage of Transcription Factors for Reprogramming

By recapitulating an injury-like response where *M. leprae* dedifferentiates adult Schwann cells following demyelination of infected nerves at the early stage of infection, Masaki et al. (110) purified dedifferentiated Schwann cells from wild-type adult mouse peripheral nerves and then infected them with *M. leprae* at a high bacterial load, mimicking the conditions in multibacillary leprosy. Over time, it was found that the transcriptional and proteomic profile underwent radical alterations, including loss of Schwann cell-specific lineage markers such as Sox10 and ErbB3 and myelin genes including that encoding myelin basic protein, suggesting turning off of the differentiation-myelination program (95, 115–118). Concordantly, infection upregulated a range of early developmental and embryonic markers, particularly mesenchymal and neural crest stem cell transcripts (110). A key early event appears to be the loss of the Sox10 transcription factor from the nuclei of Schwann cells after infection (110). As a master regulator of Schwann cell identity and lineage specificity, Sox10 is present throughout Schwann development and the adult stage (4, 115, 116, 119), and thus the bacterial removal of Sox10 clears the way for loss of Schwann cell lineage identity and the ability of these reprogrammed cells to convert to other cell types. Change in Sox10 gene expression appears to be regulated epigenetically, as *M. leprae* causes DNA methylation at the *Sox10* locus (110), which is associated with gene silencing.

On the other hand, the transcription factor Sox2, which is activated in dedifferentiated Schwann cells during injury but not in intact adult peripheral nerves and is known to be a repressor of myelination (120–122), is retained after reprogramming by *M. leprae*. Sox2 is an embryonic stem cell marker known to function in regulating gene networks and phenotype in embryonic stem and neural progenitor cells (123–140). Indeed, a transgenic mouse model in which overexpression of Sox2 was sustained in adult nerves was shown to inhibit myelination and cause subsequent neuropathic conditions (122). Taken together, these observations indicate that it is possible that the bacteria use this stem cell factor in the switch between a Schwann cell program and a progenitor cell program, aided by the loss of Sox10. However, such mechanistic possibilities need further investigation.

Epithelial-Mesenchymal Transition during Schwann Cell Reprogramming

Schwann cell reprogramming by *M. leprae* also involves the epithelial-mesenchymal transition (EMT) program, a key developmental program which also occurs during neural crest cell specification and epithelial and endothelial cell transition to mesenchymal phenotypes as well as in metastatic epithelial cancers (110, 141). EMT genes upregulated after infection, including *Twist, Snail1/2*, and *Msx2*, may enforce such inherent phenotypic plasticity to change Schwann cell fate, as dedifferentiated Schwann cells appear to behave as mesenchymal-type cells. Upregulation of these EMT genes is also regulated by epigenetic mechanisms, as further analysis of Schwann cell reprogramming revealed that there are widespread changes in DNA methylation status arising from bacterial influence (110). More research will undoubtedly yield further knowledge of how this pathogen uses sophisticated approaches to alter the host cell transcriptional and epigenetic networks.

Schwann Cell Reprogramming and Neuropathy

Reprogramming of functional adult Schwann cells means that these cells reactivate their developmental program to convert to an immature-like state that lacks mature-cell properties necessary to maintain functional nerves. Certainly, such reprogramming would contribute to the pathology observed in patients, since disruption of the well-structured Schwann cell–axon unit would undoubtedly lead to Schwann cell dedifferentiation. These events lead to reduced conduction of action potentials and exposition of the axon to damage and degeneration over time during extremely long-term infection in multibacillary leprosy patients, consistent with sensory and motor loss of leprosy neuropathy. Although ultimately detrimental to the host, reprogramming of Schwann cells appears to bring a range of survival advantages to the bacteria, as it might provide a favorable microenvironment for bacterial propagation within the PNS.

Schwann Cell Reprogramming and Bacterial Dissemination

The reprogrammed Schwann cells have expression patterns resembling a neural crest/stem cell-like phenotype and display multipotency to differentiate not only to muscles but also to bone and adipose tissues (110). This, alongside acquired migratory and immunomodulatory properties as in mesenchymal stem cells (142), may enable the bacteria to exit peripheral nerves, potentially breaching the BNB by immunomodulatory agents that reprogrammed cells can release and that can thus enter the bloodstream, recruit macrophages, or directly transdifferentiate into desired tissue cell types once reaching other preferred target cells like muscles, bone, and adipose tissues (Fig. 6) (103, 110). An additional bacterial advantage is that reprogrammed Schwann cells, but not normal Schwann cells, show more efficient cell-cell transfer of the bacteria to fibroblasts from both skin and peripheral nerve origins (114). As such, bacterial retention in Schwann cells during early infection may permit a period of survival and growth of the extremely slowly dividing bacteria prior to onward invasion of surrounding nerve tissue and beyond.

Granuloma formation

As another route of bacterial spread, reprogrammed cells, which release chemokines/cytokines, also contribute to granuloma formation by recruiting macrophages, which in turn contribute to bacterial propagation and dissemination. Indeed, granulomas are a commonly observed pathological feature in leprosy and other mycobacterial diseases (110, 143–145). Such granuloma formation is facilitated by many innate immune chemokines and cytokines produced by reprogrammed Schwann cells that can recruit macrophages to produce granulomatous formations (Fig. 6) (110, 142, 146, 147). So, by invading the Schwann cells and subsequent reprogramming, *M. leprae* has acquired a number of advantages to promote its survival, persistence, and dissemination. The combination of these strategies is quite distinct from the strategies of many other bacterial pathogens that have shorter life cycles and cause more acute damage to host cells and tissues. It is possible that the long evolutionary history of *M. leprae* within human and animal hosts, the complete reliance on host cells for replication, and the extremely long bacterial replication time have contributed to the special coexistence of this intracellular bacterium with long-lived host cells, particularly the nervous system cells.

CONCLUDING REMARKS

Pathogen interactions with nervous system cells are crucial in the establishment and pathogenesis of infectious diseases affecting the nervous system. We describe, using leprosy bacilli as an example, how intracellular bacterial pathogens can make use of or subvert host cell molecules and pathways and their functions for bacterial invasion with selective tropisms with underlying mechanisms, and how they can hijack the unique properties of cell plasticity once they are inside the nervous system cells for survival, establishment of infection, and dissemination. The sustained abilities of the bacterial pathogens to coexist with nervous system cells and develop subsequent innate and inflammatory responses can lead to neuropathologies causing neurodegeneration. Thus, neurotrophic pathogen interactions with nerve cells can be used as models to gain insights into how neurodegeneration is initiated following infectious triggers and to translate such knowledge to the understanding of potential common themes of early events in neurodegenerative diseases whose causes or triggers are unknown. Despite limited available information for many of these changes due to the short period of studies of neurotrophic bacteria, the long life of *M. leprae* demonstrates how bacteria can have a long-term influence on their host cells and manipulate cellular plasticity to reprogram cells in a way that is beneficial for their persistence and that helps achieve the most difficult task of dissemination despite their strictly obligately intracellular lifestyle. This unexpected link between host cell reprogramming and natural bacterial infection presents a previously unseen degree of sophistication in cell manipulation by the hijacking of the genomic plasticity of host cells by a human bacterial pathogen and thus opens up a new premise in host-pathogen interactions as well as a novel theme of intersection of infection biology with stem cell and regeneration biology. Understanding detailed mechanisms regarding these bacterial processes will help us to develop new tools for cellular reprogramming in stem cell biology and regenerative medicine and provide us with new targets not only for combating bacterial pathogens but also for developing treatments and cures for neurodegenerative diseases. In particular, this understanding can help us learn how neurotrophic pathogens naturally manipulate the nervous system cells by hijacking endogenous pathways and thus understand better how the nervous system works normally.

Acknowledgments. We thank present and past members of the Rambukkana laboratory at the University of Edinburgh and the Rockefeller University in New York and collaborators who contributed for many years of work, which are described and cited here. Research presented was funded in part by grants from NINDS (NS45187), NIAID (AI45816), the Rockefeller University, the University of Edinburgh, the Wellcome Trust Institutional Strategic Support Funds, and the Medical Research Council (MRC), UK.

Citation. Hess S, Rambukkana A. 2019. Cell biology of intracellular adaptation of *Mycobacterium leprae* in the peripheral nervous system. Microbiol Spectrum 7(4):BAI-0020-2019.

REFERENCES

1. **Drevets DA, Leenen PJM, Greenfield RA.** 2004. Invasion of the central nervous system by intracellular bacteria. *Clin Microbiol Rev* 17:323–347.

2. **Deigendesch N, Stenzel W.** 2018. Acute and chronic bacterial infections and sarcoidosis, p 217–226. *In Handbook of Clinical Neurology.* Elsevier, New York, NY.

3. **Suthar R, Sankhyan N.** 2018. Bacterial infections of the central nervous system. *Indian J Pediatr* 86:60–69.

4. **Jessen KR, Mirsky R.** 2005. The origin and development of glial cells in peripheral nerves. *Nat Rev Neurosci* 6:671–682.

5. **Jessen KR, Mirsky R, Lloyd AC.** 2015. Schwann cells: development and role in nerve repair. *Cold Spring Harb Perspect Biol* 7:a020487.

6. **Peltonen S, Alanne M, Peltonen J.** 2013. Barriers of the peripheral nerve. *Tissue Barriers* 1:e24956.

7. **Reinhold AK, Rittner HL.** 2017. Barrier function in the peripheral and central nervous system—a review. *Pflugers Arch* 469:123–134.

8. **World Health Organization.** 2017. Global leprosy update, 2016: accelerating reduction of disease burden. *Wkly Epidemiol Rec* 92:501–519.

9. **van Brakel WH, Post E, Saunderson PR, Gopal PK.** 2017. Leprosy, p 391–401. *In* Quah SR (ed), *International Encyclopedia of Public Health*, 2nd ed. Academic Press, New York, NY.

10. **Browne SG.** 1985. The history of leprosy, p 1–14. *In* Hastings RC (ed), *Leprosy*. Churchill Livingstone, Edinburgh, United Kingdom.

11. **Hansen GHA.** 1874. Undersøgelser angående spedalskhedens årsager (investigations concerning the etiology of leprosy). *Nor Mag Laegervidenskaben* 4:1–88.

12. **Suzuki K, Akama T, Kawashima A, Yoshihara A, Yotsu RR, Ishii N.** 2012. Current status of leprosy: epidemiology, basic science and clinical perspectives. *J Dermatol* 39:121–129.

13. **World Health Organization.** 2017. *Global Leprosy Strategy 2016-2020.* World Health Organization, Geneva, Switzerland.

14. **Cruz RCDS, Bührer-Sékula S, Penna MLF, Penna GO, Talhari S.** 2017. Leprosy: current situation, clinical and laboratory aspects, treatment history and perspective of the uniform multidrug therapy for all patients. *An Bras Dermatol* 92:761–773.

15. **Cole ST, et al.** 2001. Massive gene decay in the leprosy bacillus. *Nature* 409:1007–1011.

16. **Singh P, Cole ST.** 2011. *Mycobacterium leprae*: genes, pseudogenes and genetic diversity. *Future Microbiol* 6:57–71.

17. **Truman R.** 2005. Leprosy in wild armadillos. *Lepr Rev* 76:198–208.

18. **Balamayooran G, Pena M, Sharma R, Truman RW.** 2015. The armadillo as an animal model and reservoir host for *Mycobacterium leprae*. *Clin Dermatol* 33:108–115.

19. **Avanzi C, Del-Pozo J, Benjak A, Stevenson K, Simpson VR, Busso P, McLuckie J, Loiseau C, Lawton C, Schoening J, Shaw DJ, Piton J, Vera-Cabrera L, Velarde-Felix JS, McDermott F, Gordon SV, Cole ST, Meredith AL.** 2016. Red squirrels in the British Isles are infected with leprosy bacilli. *Science* 354:744–747.

20. **Scollard DM, Truman RW, Ebenezer GJ.** 2015. Mechanisms of nerve injury in leprosy. *Clin Dermatol* 33:46–54.

21. **Lázaro FP, Werneck RI, Mackert CCO, Cobat A, Prevedello FC, Pimentel RP, Macedo GMM, Eleutério MAM, Vilar G, Abel L, Xavier MB, Alcaïs A, Mira MT.** 2010. A major gene controls leprosy susceptibility in a hyperendemic isolated population from north of Brazil. *J Infect Dis* 201:1598–1605.

22. **Truman RW, Singh P, Sharma R, Busso P, Rougemont J, Paniz-Mondolfi A, Kapopoulou A, Brisse S, Scollard DM, Gillis TP, Cole ST.** 2011. Probable zoonotic leprosy in the southern United States. *N Engl J Med* 364:1626–1633.

23. **Chopra R, Ali S, Srivastava AK, Aggarwal S, Kumar B, Manvati S, Kalaiarasan P, Jena M, Garg VK, Bhattacharya SN, Bamezai RNK.** 2013. Mapping of PARK2 and PACRG overlapping regulatory region reveals LD structure and functional variants in association with leprosy in unrelated Indian population groups. *PLoS Genet* 9:e1003578.

24. **Chopra R, Kalaiarasan P, Ali S, Srivastava AK, Aggarwal S, Garg VK, Bhattacharya SN, Bamezai RNK.** 2014. PARK2 and proinflammatory/anti-inflammatory cytokine gene interactions contribute to the susceptibility to leprosy: a case-control study of North Indian population. *BMJ Open* 4:e004239.

25. **Mira MT, Alcaïs A, Nguyen VT, Moraes MO, Di Flumeri C, Vu HT, Mai CP, Nguyen TH, Nguyen NB, Pham XK, Sarno EN, Alter A, Montpetit A, Moraes ME, Moraes JR, Doré C, Gallant CJ, Lepage P, Verner A, Van De Vosse E, Hudson TJ, Abel L, Schurr E.** 2004. Susceptibility to leprosy is associated with PARK2 and PACRG. *Nature* 427:636–640.

26. **Domingo A, Klein C.** 2018. Genetics of Parkinson disease, p 211–227. *In Handbook of Clinical Neurology.* Elsevier, New York, NY.

27. **Meng L, Shen L, Ji HF.** 2019. Impact of infection on risk of Parkinson's disease: a quantitative assessment of case-control and cohort studies. *J Neurovirol* 25:221–228.

28. **De Chiara G, Marcocci ME, Sgarbanti R, Civitelli L, Ripoli C, Piacentini R, Garaci E, Grassi C, Palamara AT.** 2012. Infectious agents and neurodegeneration. *Mol Neurobiol* 46:614–638.

29. **Masaki T, Rambukkana A.** 2014. Neurodegeneration in leprosy: insights from model systems and patients, p 217–232. *In* Bentivoglio M, Cavalheiro EA, Kristensson K, Patel NB (ed), *Neglected Tropical Diseases and Conditions of the Nervous System*. Springer, New York, NY.

30. Scollard DM, Adams LB, Gillis TP, Krahenbuhl JL, Truman RW, Williams DL. 2006. The continuing challenges of leprosy. *Clin Microbiol Rev* **19**:338–381.

31. Truman RW, Krahenbuhl JL. 2001. Viable *M. leprae* as a research reagent. *Int J Lepr Other Mycobact Dis* **69**:1–12.

32. Colston MJ, Hilson GRF. 1976. Growth of *Mycobacterium leprae* and *M. marinum* in congenitally athymic (nude) mice. *Nature* **262**:399–401.

33. Truman RW, Ebenezer GJ, Pena MT, Sharma R, Balamayooran G, Gillingwater TH, Scollard DM, McArthur JC, Rambukkana A. 2014. The armadillo as a model for peripheral neuropathy in leprosy. *ILAR J* **54**:304–314.

34. Sharma R, Lahiri R, Scollard DM, Pena M, Williams DL, Adams LB, Figarola J, Truman RW. 2013. The armadillo: a model for the neuropathy of leprosy and potentially other neurodegenerative diseases. *Dis Model Mech* **6**:19–24.

35. Job CK. 1989. Nerve damage in leprosy. *Int J Lepr Other Mycobact Dis* **57**:532–539.

36. Jennekens FG, van Brakel WH. 1998. Neuropathy in leprosy, p 319–339. *In* Latov N, Wokke JHJ, Kelly JJ Jr (ed), *Immunological and Infectious Diseases of the Peripheral Nerves*. Cambridge University Press, Cambridge, United Kingdom.

37. Rodrigues LC, Lockwood DN. 2011. Leprosy now: epidemiology, progress, challenges, and research gaps. *Lancet Infect Dis* **11**:464–470.

38. Chen L, Deng H, Cui H, Fang J, Zuo Z, Deng J, Li Y, Wang X, Zhao L. 2017. Inflammatory responses and inflammation-associated diseases in organs. *Oncotarget* **9**:7204–7218.

39. Ransohoff RM. 2016. How neuroinflammation contributes to neurodegeneration. *Science* **353**:777–783.

40. Stoner GL. 1979. Importance of the neural predilection of *Mycobacterium leprae* in leprosy. *Lancet* **ii**:994–996.

41. Miko TL, Le Maitre C, Kinfu Y. 1993. Damage and regeneration of peripheral nerves in advanced treated leprosy. *Lancet* **342**:521–525.

42. Ooi WW, Srinivasan J. 2004. Leprosy and the peripheral nervous system: basic and clinical aspects. *Muscle Nerve* **30**:393–409.

43. Rambukkana A. 2001. Molecular basis for the peripheral nerve predilection of *Mycobacterium leprae*. *Curr Opin Microbiol* **4**:21–27.

44. Nave K-A, Werner HB. 2014. Myelination of the nervous system: mechanisms and functions. *Annu Rev Cell Dev Biol* **30**:503–533.

45. Pereira JA, Lebrun-Julien F, Suter U. 2012. Molecular mechanisms regulating myelination in the peripheral nervous system. *Trends Neurosci* **35**:123–134.

46. Taveggia C, Feltri ML, Wrabetz L. 2010. Signals to promote myelin formation and repair. *Nat Rev Neurol* **6**:276–287.

47. Ahrendsen JT, Macklin W. 2013. Signaling mechanisms regulating myelination in the central nervous system. *Neurosci Bull* **29**:199–215.

48. Mitew S, Hay CM, Peckham H, Xiao J, Koenning M, Emery B. 2014. Mechanisms regulating the development of oligodendrocytes and central nervous system myelin. *Neuroscience* **276**:29–47.

49. Nave KA. 2010. Myelination and support of axonal integrity by glia. *Nature* **468**:244–252.

50. Ng V, Zanazzi G, Timpl R, Talts JF, Salzer JL, Brennan PJ, Rambukkana A. 2000. Role of the cell wall phenolic glycolipid-1 in the peripheral nerve predilection of *Mycobacterium leprae*. *Cell* **103**:511–524.

51. Rambukkana A, Salzer JL, Yurchenco PD, Tuomanen EI. 1997. Neural targeting of *Mycobacterium leprae* mediated by the G domain of the laminin-α2 chain. *Cell* **88**:811–821.

52. Rambukkana A, Zanazzi G, Tapinos N, Salzer JL. 2002. Contact-dependent demyelination by *Mycobacterium leprae* in the absence of immune cells. *Science* **296**:927–931.

53. Tapinos N, Ohnishi M, Rambukkana A. 2006. ErbB2 receptor tyrosine kinase signaling mediates early demyelination induced by leprosy bacilli. *Nat Med* **12**:961–966. CORRIGENDUM *Nat Med* **12**:1100.

54. Einheber S, Milner TA, Giancotti F, Salzer JL. 1993. Axonal regulation of Schwann cell integrin expression suggests a role for alpha 6 beta 4 in myelination. *J Cell Biol* **123**:1223–1236.

55. Cornbrooks CJ, Carey DJ, McDonald JA, Timpl R, Bunge RP. 1983. In vivo and in vitro observations on laminin production by Schwann cells. *Proc Natl Acad Sci USA* **80**:3850–3854.

56. Jaakkola S, Peltonen J, Riccardi V, Chu ML, Uitto J. 1989. Type 1 neurofibromatosis: selective expression of extracellular matrix genes by Schwann cells, perineurial cells, and fibroblasts in mixed cultures. *J Clin Invest* **84**:253–261.

57. Sanes JR, Engvall E, Butkowski R, Hunter DD. 1990. Molecular heterogeneity of basal laminae: isoforms of laminin and collagen IV at the neuromuscular junction and elsewhere. *J Cell Biol* **111**:1685–1699.

58. Burgeson RE, Chiquet M, Deutzmann R, Ekblom P, Engel J, Kleinman H, Martin GR, Meneguzzi G, Paulsson M, Sanes J, Timpl R, Tryggvason K, Yamada Y, Yurchenco PD. 1994. A new nomenclature for the laminins. *Matrix Biol* **14**:209–211.

59. Engvall E, Wewer UM. 1996. Domains of laminin. *J Cell Biochem* **61**:493–501.

60. Timpl R, Brown JC. 1994. The laminins. *Matrix Biol* **14**:275–281.

61. Leivo I, Engvall E. 1988. Merosin, a protein specific for basement membranes of Schwann cells, striated muscle, and trophoblast, is expressed late in nerve and muscle development. *Proc Natl Acad Sci USA* **85**:1544–1548.

62. Yurchenco PD, O'Rear JJ. 1994. Basal lamina assembly. *Curr Opin Cell Biol* **6**:674–681.

63. Aumailley M, Smyth N. 1998. The role of laminins in basement membrane function. *J Anat* **193**:1–21.

64. Sasaki T, Timpl R. 1999. Laminins, p 434–443. *In* Kreis T, Vale R (ed), *Guidebook to the Extracellular*

Matrix, Anchor and Adhesion Proteins, 3rd ed. Oxford University Press, Oxford, United Kingdom.

65. Bunge MB, Bunge RP. 1986. Linkage between Schwann cell extracellular matrix production and ensheathment function. *Ann N Y Acad Sci* **486**(1 Neurofibromat): 241–247.

66. Henry MD, Campbell KP. 1999. Dystroglycan inside and out. *Curr Opin Cell Biol* **11**:602–607.

67. Talts JF, Andac Z, Göhring W, Brancaccio A, Timpl R. 1999. Binding of the G domains of laminin α1 and α2 chains and perlecan to heparin, sulfatides, α-dystroglycan and several extracellular matrix proteins. *EMBO J* **18**: 863–870.

68. Hohenester E, Tisi D, Talts JF, Timpl R. 1999. The crystal structure of a laminin G-like module reveals the molecular basis of α-dystroglycan binding to laminins, perlecan, and agrin. *Mol Cell* **4**:783–792.

69. Tisi D, Talts JF, Timpl R, Hohenester E. 2000. Structure of the C-terminal laminin G-like domain pair of the laminin α2 chain harbouring binding sites for α-dystroglycan and heparin. *EMBO J* **19**:1432–1440.

70. Rambukkana A. 2000. How does *Mycobacterium leprae* target the peripheral nervous system? *Trends Microbiol* **8**: 23–28.

71. Marques MAM, Antônio VL, Sarno EN, Brennan PJ, Pessolani MCV. 2001. Binding of α2-laminins by pathogenic and non-pathogenic mycobacteria and adherence to Schwann cells. *J Med Microbiol* **50**:23–28.

72. Anderson RJ. 1932. The chemistry of the lipoids of tubercle bacilli. *Physiol Rev* **12**:166–189.

73. Hunter SW, Brennan PJ. 1981. A novel phenolic glycolipid from *Mycobacterium leprae* possibly involved in immunogenicity and pathogenicity. *J Bacteriol* **147**: 728–735.

74. Hunter SW, Fujiwara T, Brennan PJ. 1982. Structure and antigenicity of the major specific glycolipid antigen of *Mycobacterium leprae*. *J Biol Chem* **257**:15072–15078.

75. Brennan PJ. 1989. Structure of mycobacteria: recent developments in defining cell wall carbohydrates and proteins. *Rev Infect Dis* **11**(Suppl 2):S420–S430.

76. Rastogi N, Frehel C, David HL. 1986. Triple-layered structure of mycobacterial cell wall: evidence for the existence of a polysaccharide-rich outer layer in 18 mycobacterial species. *Curr Microbiol* **13**:237–242.

77. Neill MA, Klebanoff SJ. 1988. The effect of phenolic glycolipid-1 from *Mycobacterium leprae* on the antimicrobial activity of human macrophages. *J Exp Med* **167**: 30–42.

78. Young DB, Buchanan TM. 1983. A serological test for leprosy with a glycolipid specific for *Mycobacterium leprae*. *Science* **221**:1057–1059.

79. Schlesinger LS, Horwitz MA. 1991. Phenolic glycolipid-1 of *Mycobacterium leprae* binds complement component C3 in serum and mediates phagocytosis by human monocytes. *J Exp Med* **174**:1031–1038.

80. Rambukkana A. 2004. *Mycobacterium leprae*-induced demyelination: a model for early nerve degeneration. *Curr Opin Immunol* **16**:511–518.

81. Ehrig K, Leivo I, Argraves WS, Ruoslahti E, Engvall E. 1990. Merosin, a tissue-specific basement membrane protein, is a laminin-like protein. *Proc Natl Acad Sci USA* **87**:3264–3268.

82. Talts JF, Timpl R. 1999. Mutation of a basic sequence in the laminin α2LG3 module leads to a lack of proteolytic processing and has different effects on β1 integrin-mediated cell adhesion and α-dystroglycan binding. *FEBS Lett* **458**:319–323.

83. Talts JF, Mann K, Yamada Y, Timpl R. 1998. Structural analysis and proteolytic processing of recombinant G domain of mouse laminin α2 chain. *FEBS Lett* **426**: 71–76.

84. Bernier SM, Utani A, Sugiyama S, Doi T, Polistina C, Yamada Y. 1995. Cloning and expression of laminin α2 chain (M-chain) in the mouse. *Matrix Biol* **14**:447–455.

85. Sasaki M, Kleinman HK, Huber H, Deutzmann R, Yamada Y. 1988. Laminin, a multidomain protein. The A chain has a unique globular domain and homology with the basement membrane proteoglycan and the laminin B chains. *J Biol Chem* **263**:16536–16544.

86. Engvall E, Earwicker D, Haaparanta T, Ruoslahti E, Sanes JR. 1990. Distribution and isolation of four laminin variants; tissue restricted distribution of heterotrimers assembled from five different subunits. *Cell Regul* **1**:731–740.

87. Patton BL, Miner JH, Chiu AY, Sanes JR. 1997. Distribution and function of laminins in the neuromuscular system of developing, adult, and mutant mice. *J Cell Biol* **139**:1507–1521.

88. Campbell KP. 1995. Three muscular dystrophies: loss of cytoskeleton-extracellular matrix linkage. *Cell* **80**: 675–679.

89. Rambukkana A, Yamada H, Zanazzi G, Mathus T, Salzer JL, Yurchenco PD, Campbell KP, Fischetti VA. 1998. Role of alpha-dystroglycan as a Schwann cell receptor for *Mycobacterium leprae*. *Science* **282**:2076–2079.

90. Ibraghimov-Beskrovnaya O, Ervasti JM, Leveille CJ, Slaughter CA, Sernett SW, Campbell KP. 1992. Primary structure of dystrophin-associated glycoproteins linking dystrophin to the extracellular matrix. *Nature* **355**: 696–702.

91. Yamada H, Denzer AJ, Hori H, Tanaka T, Anderson LVB, Fujita S, Fukuta-Ohi H, Shimizu T, Ruegg MA, Matsumura K. 1996. Dystroglycan is a dual receptor for agrin and laminin-2 in Schwann cell membrane. *J Biol Chem* **271**:23418–23423.

92. Saito F, Masaki T, Kamakura K, Anderson LVB, Fujita S, Fukuta-Ohi H, Sunada Y, Shimizu T, Matsumura K. 1999. Characterization of the transmembrane molecular architecture of the dystroglycan complex in Schwann cells. *J Biol Chem* **274**:8240–8246.

93. Nave K-A, Trapp BD. 2008. Axon-glial signaling and the glial support of axon function. *Annu Rev Neurosci* **31**:535–561.

94. Nave K-A, Salzer JL. 2006. Axonal regulation of myelination by neuregulin 1. *Curr Opin Neurobiol* **16**:492–500.

95. Lemke G. 2006. Neuregulin-1 and myelination. *Sci STKE* **2006**:pe11.

96. Riethmacher D, Sonnenberg-Riethmacher E, Brinkmann V, Yamaai T, Lewin GR, Birchmeier C. 1997. Severe neuropathies in mice with targeted mutations in the ErbB3 receptor. *Nature* 389:725–730.

97. Garratt AN, Britsch S, Birchmeier C. 2000. Neuregulin, a factor with many functions in the life of a Schwann cell. *BioEssays* 22:987–996.

98. Guertin AD, Zhang DP, Mak KS, Alberta JA, Kim HA. 2005. Microanatomy of axon/glial signaling during Wallerian degeneration. *J Neurosci* 25:3478–3487.

99. Yarden Y, Sliwkowski MX. 2001. Untangling the ErbB signalling network. *Nat Rev Mol Cell Biol* 2:127–137.

100. Hynes NE, Lane HA. 2005. ERBB receptors and cancer: the complexity of targeted inhibitors. *Nat Rev Cancer* 5:341–354.

101. Rambukkana A. 2010. Usage of signaling in neurodegeneration and regeneration of peripheral nerves by leprosy bacteria. *Prog Neurobiol* 91:102–107.

102. Waxman SG. 1998. Demyelinating diseases—new pathological insights, new therapeutic targets. *N Engl J Med* 338:323–325.

103. Hess S, Rambukkana A. 2015. Bacterial-induced cell reprogramming to stem cell-like cells: new premise in host-pathogen interactions. *Curr Opin Microbiol* 23:179–188.

104. Madigan CA, Cambier CJ, Kelly-Scumpia KM, Scumpia PO, Cheng TY, Zailaa J, Bloom BR, Moody DB, Smale ST, Sagasti A, Modlin RL, Ramakrishnan L. 2017. A macrophage response to *Mycobacterium leprae* phenolic glycolipid initiates nerve damage in leprosy. *Cell* 170: 973–985.E10.

105. Kim HA, Mindos T, Parkinson DB. 2013. Plastic fantastic: Schwann cells and repair of the peripheral nervous system. *Stem Cells Transl Med* 2:553–557.

106. Jessen KR, Mirsky R. 2016. The repair Schwann cell and its function in regenerating nerves. *J Physiol* 594: 3521–3531.

107. Tapinos N, Rambukkana A. 2005. Insights into regulation of human Schwann cell proliferation by Erk1/2 via a MEK-independent and p56Lck-dependent pathway from leprosy bacilli. *Proc Natl Acad Sci USA* 102:9188–9193.

108. Kim HA, Pomeroy SL, Whoriskey W, Pawlitzky I, Benowitz LI, Sicinski P, Stiles CD, Roberts TM. 2000. A developmentally regulated switch directs regenerative growth of Schwann cells through cyclin D1. *Neuron* 26: 405–416.

109. Stoll G, Jander S, Myers RR. 2002. Degeneration and regeneration of the peripheral nervous system: From Augustus Waller's observations to neuroinflammation. *J Peripher Nerv Syst* 7:13–27.

110. Masaki T, Qu J, Cholewa-Waclaw J, Burr K, Raaum R, Rambukkana A. 2013. Reprogramming adult Schwann cells to stem cell-like cells by leprosy bacilli promotes dissemination of infection. *Cell* 152:51–67.

111. Harrisingh MC, Perez-Nadales E, Parkinson DB, Malcolm DS, Mudge AW, Lloyd AC. 2004. The Ras/Raf/ERK signalling pathway drives Schwann cell dedifferentiation. *EMBO J* 23:3061–3071.

112. Pearson JM, Rees RJ, Weddell AG. 1970. *Mycobacterium leprae* in the striated muscle of patients with leprosy. *Lepr Rev* 41:155–166.

113. Werneck LC, Teive HA, Scola RH. 1999. Muscle involvement in leprosy. Study of the anterior tibial muscle in 40 patients. *Arq Neuropsiquiatr* 57(3B):723–734.

114. Masaki T, McGlinchey A, Tomlinson SR, Qu J, Rambukkana A. 2013. Reprogramming diminishes retention of *Mycobacterium leprae* in Schwann cells and elevates bacterial transfer property to fibroblasts. *F1000 Res* 2:198.

115. Finzsch M, Schreiner S, Kichko T, Reeh P, Tamm ER, Bösl MR, Meijer D, Wegner M. 2010. Sox10 is required for Schwann cell identity and progression beyond the immature Schwann cell stage. *J Cell Biol* 189: 701–712.

116. Bremer M, Fröb F, Kichko T, Reeh P, Tamm ER, Suter U, Wegner M. 2011. Sox10 is required for Schwann-cell homeostasis and myelin maintenance in the adult peripheral nerve. *Glia* 59:1022–1032.

117. Britsch S, Goerich DE, Riethmacher D, Peirano RI, Rossner M, Nave KA, Birchmeier C, Wegner M. 2001. The transcription factor Sox10 is a key regulator of peripheral glial development. *Genes Dev* 15:66–78.

118. Mirsky R, Woodhoo A, Parkinson DB, Arthur-Farraj P, Bhaskaran A, Jessen KR. 2008. Novel signals controlling embryonic Schwann cell development, myelination and dedifferentiation. *J Peripher Nerv Syst* 13:122–135.

119. Fröb F, Bremer M, Finzsch M, Kichko T, Reeh P, Tamm ER, Charnay P, Wegner M. 2012. Establishment of myelinating Schwann cells and barrier integrity between central and peripheral nervous systems depend on Sox10. *Glia* 60:806–819.

120. Le N, Nagarajan R, Wang JYT, Araki T, Schmidt RE, Milbrandt J. 2005. Analysis of congenital hypomyelinating Egr2Lo/Lo nerves identifies Sox2 as an inhibitor of Schwann cell differentiation and myelination. *Proc Natl Acad Sci USA* 102:2596–2601.

121. Jessen KR, Mirsky R. 2008. Negative regulation of myelination: relevance for development, injury, and demyelinating disease. *Glia* 56:1552–1565.

122. Roberts SL, Dun XP, Doddrell RDS, Mindos T, Drake LK, Onaitis MW, Florio F, Quattrini A, Lloyd AC, D'Antonio M, Parkinson DB. 2017. Sox2 expression in Schwann cells inhibits myelination *in vivo* and induces influx of macrophages to the nerve. *Development* 144: 3114–3125.

123. Chambers I, Tomlinson SR. 2009. The transcriptional foundation of pluripotency. *Development* 136:2311–2322.

124. Wang J, Rao S, Chu J, Shen X, Levasseur DN, Theunissen TW, Orkin SH. 2006. A protein interaction network for pluripotency of embryonic stem cells. *Nature* 444:364–368.

125. Miyagi S, Masui S, Niwa H, Saito T, Shimazaki T, Okano H, Nishimoto M, Muramatsu M, Iwama A, Okuda A. 2008. Consequence of the loss of Sox2 in the developing brain of the mouse. *FEBS Lett* 582:2811–2815.

126. Favaro R, Valotta M, Ferri ALM, Latorre E, Mariani J, Giachino C, Lancini C, Tosetti V, Ottolenghi S, Taylor V, Nicolis SK. 2009. Hippocampal development and neural stem cell maintenance require Sox2-dependent regulation of Shh. *Nat Neurosci* **12:**1248–1256.

127. Komitova M, Eriksson PS. 2004. Sox-2 is expressed by neural progenitors and astroglia in the adult rat brain. *Neurosci Lett* **369:**24–27.

128. Cavallaro M, Mariani J, Lancini C, Latorre E, Caccia R, Gullo F, Valotta M, DeBiasi S, Spinardi L, Ronchi A, Wanke E, Brunelli S, Favaro R, Ottolenghi S, Nicolis SK. 2008. Impaired generation of mature neurons by neural stem cells from hypomorphic Sox2 mutants. *Development* **135:**541–557.

129. Gómez-López S, Wiskow O, Favaro R, Nicolis SK, Price DJ, Pollard SM, Smith A. 2011. Sox2 and Pax6 maintain the proliferative and developmental potential of gliogenic neural stem cells in vitro. *Glia* **59:**1588–1599.

130. Cimadamore F, Fishwick K, Giusto E, Gnedeva K, Cattarossi G, Miller A, Pluchino S, Brill LM, Bronner-Fraser M, Terskikh AV. 2011. Human ESC-derived neural crest model reveals a key role for SOX2 in sensory neurogenesis. *Cell Stem Cell* **8:**538–551.

131. Taranova OV, Magness ST, Fagan BM, Wu Y, Surzenko N, Hutton SR, Pevny LH. 2006. SOX2 is a dose-dependent regulator of retinal neural progenitor competence. *Genes Dev* **20:**1187–1202.

132. Surzenko N, Crowl T, Bachleda A, Langer L, Pevny L. 2013. SOX2 maintains the quiescent progenitor cell state of postnatal retinal Muller glia. *Development* **140:**1445–1456.

133. Jaenisch R, Young R. 2008. Stem cells, the molecular circuitry of pluripotency and nuclear reprogramming. *Cell* **132:**567–582.

134. Kim J, Chu J, Shen X, Wang J, Orkin SH. 2008. An extended transcriptional network for pluripotency of embryonic stem cells. *Cell* **132:**1049–1061.

135. Young RA. 2011. Control of the embryonic stem cell state. *Cell* **144:**940–954.

136. De Los Angeles A, Ferrari F, Xi R, Fujiwara Y, Benvenisty N, Deng H, Hochedlinger K, Jaenisch R, Lee S, Leitch HG, Lensch MW, Lujan E, Pei D, Rossant J, Wernig M, Park PJ, Daley GQ. 2015. Hallmarks of pluripotency. *Nature* **525:**469–478. *CORRIGENDUM Nature* **531:**400.

137. Lodato MA, Ng CW, Wamstad JA, Cheng AW, Thai KK, Fraenkel E, Jaenisch R, Boyer LA. 2013. SOX2 co-occupies distal enhancer elements with distinct POU factors in ESCs and NPCs to specify cell state. *PLoS Genet* **9:**e1003288.

138. Avilion AA, Nicolis SK, Pevny LH, Perez L, Vivian N, Lovell-Badge R. 2003. Multipotent cell lineages in early mouse development depend on SOX2 function. *Genes Dev* **17:**126–140.

139. Arnold K, Sarkar A, Yram MA, Polo JM, Bronson R, Sengupta S, Seandel M, Geijsen N, Hochedlinger K. 2011. Sox2+ adult stem and progenitor cells are important for tissue regeneration and survival of mice. *Cell Stem Cell* **9:**317–329.

140. Ellis P, Fagan BM, Magness ST, Hutton S, Taranova O, Hayashi S, McMahon A, Rao M, Pevny L. 2004. SOX2, a persistent marker for multipotential neural stem cells derived from embryonic stem cells, the embryo or the adult. *Dev Neurosci* **26:**148–165.

141. Lim J, Thiery JP. 2012. Epithelial-mesenchymal transitions: insights from development. *Development* **139:**3471–3486.

142. Masaki T, McGlinchey A, Cholewa-Waclaw J, Qu J, Tomlinson SR, Rambukkana A. 2014. Innate immune response precedes *Mycobacterium leprae*-induced reprogramming of adult Schwann cells. *Cell Reprogram* **16:**9–17.

143. Modlin RL, Rea TH. 1988. Immunopathology of leprosy granulomas. *Springer Semin Immunopathol* **10:**359–374.

144. Chan J, Flynn J. 2004. The immunological aspects of latency in tuberculosis. *Clin Immunol* **110:**2–12.

145. Bold TD, Ernst JD. 2009. Who benefits from granulomas, mycobacteria or host? *Cell* **136:**17–19.

146. Qiu B, Frait KA, Reich F, Komunniecki E, Chensue SW. 2001. Chemokine expression dynamics in mycobacterial (type-1) and schistosomal (type-2) antigen-elicited pulmonary granuloma formation. *Am J Pathol* **158:**1503–1515.

147. Chiu B-C, Freeman CM, Stolberg VR, Hu JS, Komunniecki E, Chensue SW. 2004. The innate pulmonary granuloma: characterization and demonstration of dendritic cell recruitment and function. *Am J Pathol* **164:**1021–1030.

Bacteria and Intracellularity
Edited by Pascale Cossart, Craig R. Roy, and Philippe Sansonetti
© 2019 American Society for Microbiology, Washington, DC
doi:10.1128/microbiolspec.BAI-0002-2019

Multifaceted Roles of MicroRNAs in Host-Bacterial Pathogen Interaction

17

Carmen Aguilar,[1] Miguel Mano,[2] and Ana Eulalio[1,3]

INTRODUCTION

MicroRNAs (miRNAs) are a class of small noncoding RNAs (typically 20 to 22 nucleotides long) that post-transcriptionally regulate the expression of target mRNAs exhibiting partially complementary binding sites (1). miRNAs are found in a wide range of organisms, including animals, plants, and viruses. According to the latest release of miRBase (http://www.mirbase.org/; release 22 March 2018), a total of 48,885 mature miRNAs are currently annotated in 271 species; 2,694 mature miRNAs are annotated in the human genome.

miRNA biogenesis is a well-described multistep process (reviewed in reference 2) (Fig. 1). Typically, the primary miRNA transcripts (pri-miRNAs) are long, capped, and polyadenylated RNA molecules containing hairpin structures transcribed by RNA polymerase II. The pri-miRNA is then processed in the nucleus by the microprocessor complex (comprising the RNase III enzyme Drosha and the double-stranded RNA binding protein DGCR8) into a 60- to 100-nucleotide hairpin precursor miRNA. Exportin-5 mediates the transport of the precursor miRNA from the nucleus to the cytoplasm, where it is further processed into a miRNA duplex of approximately 20 bp by Dicer, an enzyme that also belongs to the RNase III family, in complex with the RNA binding protein TRBP. One of the strands of the miRNA is then loaded into the miRNA-induced silencing complex, which contains, among multiple components, an Argonaute (AGO) protein that binds to the mature miRNA. Target mRNAs are identified by base-pairing between the miRNA and mRNA, usually involving nucleotides 2 to 7/8 of the 5′ end of the miRNA (known as the seed-region). miRNAs repress target gene expression by a combination of mechanisms involving translation repression and target mRNA degradation following deadenylation and decapping (reviewed in reference 3).

Based on the high number of miRNAs identified in the human genome, bioinformatic predictions, and experimental identification of hundreds of target mRNAs for a number of individual miRNAs, it has been suggested that approximately 60% of the human genome is under the regulation of miRNAs (4), though this may be an underestimation. Consistent with a pervasive role of miRNAs in the control of gene expression, miRNAs have been shown to regulate countless fundamental biological processes (e.g., cellular proliferation, differentiation, apoptosis [5–7]), and miRNA dysregulation has been implicated in a wide spectrum of human diseases (e.g., cancer, cardiovascular disorders [8, 9]).

In addition to these functions, it is now clear that miRNAs have a preponderant role during infections caused by viruses, parasites, fungi, and bacterial pathogens. Initial work addressing miRNA function in the context of infection focused on viruses (reviewed in reference 10). In these seminal studies, the expression of miRNAs encoded by DNA viruses (herpesvirus, polyomavirus, and adenovirus) was revealed; this was first shown for Epstein-Barr virus (11). Equally important, the repertoire of host miRNAs is vastly changed in response to viral infections. Indeed, viral and host miRNAs modulate multiple processes relevant to infection, ranging from virus replication and propagation to host antiviral responses and/or promotion of the viral life cycle through complex regulatory pathways.

During the past decade, miRNAs have also emerged as powerful players in the interaction of bacterial pathogens with the host. It has become clear that bacteria

[1]Host RNA Metabolism Group, Institute for Molecular Infection Biology (IMIB), University of Würzburg, Würzburg, Germany; [2]Functional Genomics and RNA-Based Therapeutics Group, Center for Neuroscience and Cell Biology (CNC), University of Coimbra, Coimbra, Portugal; [3]RNA & Infection Group, Center for Neuroscience and Cell Biology (CNC), University of Coimbra, Coimbra, Portugal.

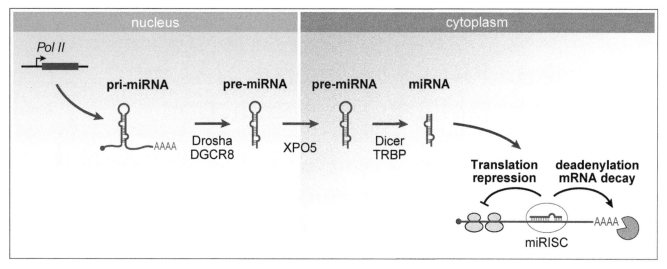

Figure 1   Overview of the canonical miRNA biogenesis pathway. miRNA genes are transcribed as pri-miRNAs by RNA polymerase II. The main proteins involved in the multistep miRNA processing are indicated. Repression of target gene expression occurs through inhibition of translation and mRNA degradation.

have evolved sophisticated mechanisms of harnessing host miRNAs to create an immune-tolerant environment and/or to modulate host pathways for their own benefit, promoting pathogen survival, replication, and latency/persistence. From the host perspective, miRNAs are an integral part of an effective immunological response, relevant for the control and clearance of infection.

In this chapter, we summarize a growing body of literature on the modulation and function of host miRNAs in the context of infection by bacterial pathogens.

miRNA RESPONSE TO BACTERIAL INFECTION

The first evidence of the regulatory role of miRNAs in response to bacterial infections was obtained in 2006 from studies performed with plants. In this seminal work, Navarro and colleagues described the increased expression of miR-393a as an important mediator of the resistance of *Arabidopsis thaliana* to infection by the extracellular pathogen *Pseudomonas syringae* (12). Specifically, the authors showed that recognition of a flagellin-derived peptide from *P. syringae* by the FLS2 receptor of *A. thaliana* induces the transcription of miR-393a, which in turn represses the expression of three F-box auxin receptors. This blunts signaling by auxin, a plant hormone that negatively regulates the plant immune system, ultimately restraining bacterial spreading and enhancing plant resistance to *P. syringae* infection (12). Interestingly, the authors later demonstrated that *P. syringae* is able to counteract this miRNA-

mediated antibacterial response through the secretion into host cells of effector proteins that suppress transcription, biogenesis, stability, and activity of pathogen-associated molecular pattern-responsive miRNAs (13).

In mammalian cells, the first report implicating miRNAs in the innate immune response to bacterial components resulted from the pioneering study of Taganov and colleagues (14). These authors investigated the expression of a panel of 200 miRNAs in human monocytes stimulated with lipopolysaccharide (LPS), a major component of the outer membrane of Gram-negative bacteria that is sensed by the Toll-like receptor 4 (TLR4). This work led to the identification of the first three endotoxin-responsive miRNAs (miR-146a/b, miR-132, and miR-155). Interestingly, the characterization of miR-146a/b targets uncovered several components of the TLR4 signaling cascade, suggesting the existence of a negative-feedback loop that might protect host cells from an excessive inflammatory response.

Subsequent studies established miRNA regulation upon infection as a common phenomenon (summarized in Table 1), with implications for multiple host cell functions ranging from the control of the immune response and autophagy to cell cycle and cell death, among others (Fig. 2). The main findings obtained in this context are described below, grouped by bacterial pathogen.

Salmonella enterica

S. enterica remains a leading cause of gastroenteritis worldwide, with *S. enterica* subspecies *enterica* serovar Typhimurium (*S.* Typhimurium) being one of the most

TABLE 1   Host cell miRNAs regulated upon infection by bacterial pathogens[a]

Bacterium	miRNA	Regulation	Cell/tissue	Reference
Salmonella enterica	let-7 family	Down	HeLa, RAW264.7	17
	miR-1, miR-125a/b, miR-130, miR-148	Down	Piglet MLN	28
	miR-15 family	Down	HeLa	22
	miR-21, miR-29a/b, miR-146a/b	Up	Zebrafish embryos	25
	miR-21, miR-146a/b, miR-155	Up	RAW264.7	17
	miR-26, miR-143	Up	Pig whole blood	30
	miR-29a	Up	Piglet ileal tissue	27
	miR-30c/e	Up	HeLa, J774	24
	miR-34a-5p, miR-215-5p, miR-1662	Down	Chicken cecum	32
	miR-101-3p	Down	Chicken spleen tissue	19
	miR-125b-5p, miR-1416-5p	Up	Chicken cecum	32
	miR-128	Up	HT-29, murine small intestine and colon tissue	31
	miR-146a/b	Up	THP-1	18
	miR-155	Up	Chicken spleen tissue	19
	miR-193a-5p, miR-3525	Up	Chicken cecum	26
	miR-214	Down	Piglet whole blood	29
	miR-331-3p	Up	Piglet whole blood	29
	miR-1308	Up	HeLa	17
Helicobacter pylori	let-7 family, miR-103, miR-125a, miR-130a, miR-491-5p, miR-500, miR-532	Down	AZ-521, human gastric mucosa	58
	let-7b	Down	AGS, GES-1, human gastric mucosa	57
	miR-21	Up	AGS, human gastric mucosa	35
	miR-30b	Up	AGS, human gastric mucosa	62
	miR-30d	Up	AGS, GES-1	63
	miR-101	Down	GES-1, MKN-45, SGC-7901, primary gastric cells	38
	miR-143-3p	Up	Human gastric mucosa	47
	miR-146a	Up	MNK-45, GES-1, HGC-27, AGS, human gastric mucosa	56
	miR-146a	Up	GES-1	55
	miR-146a	Up	HGC-27	54
	miR-146a, miR-16	Up	GES-1	52
	miR-146a, miR-155	Up	Human gastric mucosa	50
	miR-152, miR-200b	Down	AGS, human gastric mucosa	59
	miR-155	Up	AGS, GES-1, MKN-45, human gastric mucosa	52
	miR-155	Up	Jurkat, CCRF-CEM, AGS, MKN-74, J774A, murine BMDMs, human gastric mucosa	48
	miR-155	Up	Human gastric mucosa	56
	miR-155	Up	Murine gastric mucosa	51
	miR-155	Up	AZ-521	58
	miR-155	Up	J774A.1, murine BMDMs	49
	miR-210	Down	Mongolian gerbil and human gastric mucosa	39
	miR-212-3p, miR-361-3p	Down	Human esophagus tissue, HET-1A, OE33	45
	miR-222	Up	HGC-27, AGS, BGC-823, SGC-7901, GES-1	36
	miR-222	Up	Human gastric mucosa	37
	miR-223	Up	Human gastric mucosa	58
	miR-223	Up	THP-1, AGS	53

(Continued)

TABLE 1 *(Continued)*

Bacterium	miRNA	Regulation	Cell/tissue	Reference
	miR-320	Down	MKN-28, AGS	40
	miR-370	Down	AGS, human and murine gastric mucosa	41
	miR-371, miR-372, miR-373	Down	AGS	46
	miR-584, miR-1290	Up	AGS	42
	miR-1289	Up	AGS, human gastric mucosa	64
	miR-4270, miR-4459	Down	Human MDMs	61
Mycobacterium spp.	let-7e, miR-29a, miR-146a, miR-155, miR-886-5p	Up	Human MDMs	75
	let-7f	Down	RAW264.7; human MDMs; murine BMDMs; lung, spleen, and lymph node tissue	79
	miR-15a, miR-21-3p, miR-22-3p, miR-23a, miR-30b-5p, miR-142-5p, miR-146a/b	Up	Bovine alveolar macrophages	100
	miR-17-5p	Down	RAW264.7; murine BMDMs; lung, spleen, and lymph node tissue	90
	miR-17-5p	Up	RAW264.7	91
	miR-20a	Up	RAW264.7	98
	miR-20b	Down	Human MDMs, murine lung tissue	88
	miR-21	Up	RAW264.7	86
	miR-21	Up	Human PBMCs, skin samples	82
	miR-21, miR-26a, miR-29a, miR-142-3p	Down	Human T-cells, peripheral blood	84
	miR-26a	Down	RAW264.7; THP1; human MDMs; murine BMDMs; lung, spleen, and lymph nodes	101
	miR-27a	Up	Human PBMCs, murine lung tissue, peritoneal macrophages	95
	miR-27b	Up	RAW264.7, murine BMDMs, lung and spleen tissue	78
	miR-29a	Up	Human serum, sputum	83
	miR-29a/b	Down	Murine splenocytes, T-cells	85
	miR-30a	Up	THP1, human alveolar macrophages	92
	miR-30a/e, miR-155, miR-1275, miR-3178, miR-3665, miR-4484, miR-4497, miR-4668-5p	Up	THP1	68
	miR-33, miR-33*	Up	Murine peritoneal and alveolar macrophages, THP1, BMDMs	94
	miR-106b-5p	Up	Human MDMs	102
	miR-125a-3p	Up	RAW264.7, murine BMDMs	93
	miR-125b, miR-146a, miR-155	Up	RAW264.7, THP1, murine peritoneal macrophages	72
	miR-125b, miR-155	Up	Human MDMs	73
	miR-142-3p	Up	J774A.1, human MDMs	81
	miR-144-3p	Up	RAW264.7	97
	miR-144-5p	Up	THP1, human MDMs, lung and lymph nodes tissue	96
	miR-155	Up	Human PBMCs, murine spleen, lymph node and peritoneal macrophages	66
	miR-155	Up	RAW264.7, murine BMDMs	67
	miR-155	Up	RAW264.7, murine lung tissue and BMDMs	76
	miR-155	Up	THP1, human PMBCs	71
	miR-155	Up	Human dendritic cells	70

(Continued)

TABLE 1   *(Continued)*

Bacterium	miRNA	Regulation	Cell/tissue	Reference
	miR-155	Up	Murine BMDMs	74
	miR-155	Up	RAW264.7	77
	miR-199a	Up	J774A.1, murine BMDMs, lung and spleen tissue	99
	miR-223	Up	Murine whole blood and lung tissue, human peripheral blood and lung tissue	80
	miR-582-5p	Up	Human PBMCs	87
Listeria	miR-16, miR-146b, miR-155	Up	Caco-2	107
monocytogenes	miR-21	Up	Murine BMDMs	106
	miR-29a/b	Down	Murine splenocytes and NK cells	85
	miR-125a-3p/-5p, miR-146a, miR-155, miR-149	Up	Murine BMDMs	104
	miR-143, miR-148a, miR-194, miR-200b/c, miR-378	Down	Murine ileal tissue	113
	miR-145, let-7a1	Down	Caco-2	107
	miR-192, miR-200b, miR-215	Down	Murine ileal tissue	112
Francisella spp.	miR-133a, miR-146a, miR-150, miR-155, miR-886-5p	Up	Human MDMs	114
	miR-155	Up	Human PBMCs, murine lung, liver and spleen tissue	115
Citrobacter rodentium	miR-7a, miR-17, miR-20a, miR-21, miR-142-3p, miR-203	Up	Murine colonic crypts	117
Staphylococcus aureus	miR-15b-5p	Up	Human and porcine skin tissue	121
	miR-20b, miR-31, miR-155, miR-182, miR-222	Up	Murine lung monocytes	118
	miR-24	Down	U937, RAW264.7	119
Pseudomonas aeruginosa	miR-26a-5p, miR-155, miR-182-5p, miR-200c-3p, miR-294-3p, miR-302b-3p, miR-495-3p, miR-669k-3p	Up	MH-S	124
	miR-302b	Up	MLE-12, MH-S, murine lung tissue	124
Chlamydia spp.	miR-16, miR-23b, miR-30c/e, miR-125b-5p, miR-135a, miR-182, miR-183, miR-214	Down	Murine genital tract tissue	130
	miR-30c-5p	Up	HUVEC, hFIMB, HFF	127
	miR-100-5p, miR-200a-3p, miR-200b-3p/-5p, miR-411-5p	Down	Murine genital tract tissue	131
	miR-132, miR-142-3p, miR-147-3p, miR-149-3p, miR-212-3p	Up	Murine genital tract tissue	131
	miR-146, miR-451	Up	Murine genital tract tissue	130
	miR-155	Up	Murine dendritic cells	129
	miR-182, miR-183	Up	Murine splenic T-cells	129
	miR-214	Down	Murine genital tract tissue	128
Brucella spp.	let-7b, miR-92a, miR-99a, miR-142-5p, miR-181b, miR-1981	Up	RAW264.7	132
	miR-93, miR-151-3p	Down	RAW264.7	132
	miR-125b-5p	Down	RAW264.7	133
	miR-130a-3p	Up	PAM	134
	miR-146a, miR-181a/b, miR-301a-3p	Up	RAW264.7, PAM	134
	miR-351-5p	Up	RAW264.7	134
Shigella flexneri	miR-29b-2-5p	Down	HeLa	135

[a]Abbreviations: BMDM, bone marrow-derived macrophages; HFF, primary human foreskin fibroblasts; hFIMB, human fallopian tube fimbriae cells; HUVEC, human umbilical vein endothelial cells; MDM, monocyte-derived macrophages; MLN, mesenteric lymph node; PAM, porcine alveolar macrophages; PBMC, peripheral blood mononuclear cells.

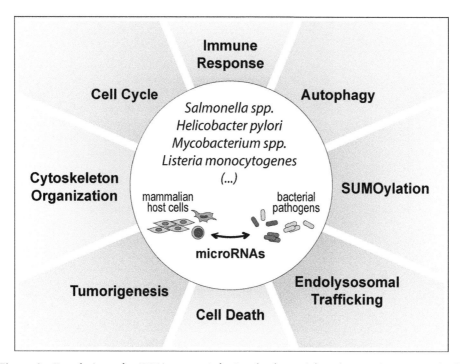

Figure 2 Regulation of miRNAs upon infection by bacterial pathogens impacts multiple crucial host cell functions. miRNA modulation upon infection has been shown to be an integral part of the host response or a mechanism exploited by bacteria to promote infection.

frequent serovars causing foodborne disease (15). *Salmonella* spp. can infect phagocytic and nonphagocytic cells in humans as well as in a wide range of domestic and wild animals (16).

Host miRNA regulation of *S.* Typhimurium infection was first shown in mouse macrophages, where miR-155, miR-146a/b, and miR-21 were strongly induced (17). Interestingly, regulation of these miRNAs was also observed with *S.* Typhimurium mutant strains defective in cell invasion (ΔSPI-1) and replication (ΔSPI-2), as well as upon treatment with purified *Salmonella* LPS, showing that sensing of extracellular stimuli triggers the regulation of these miRNAs. Similar results were obtained in human monocytes (18). These studies and additional findings have singled miR-155 as a key immune miRNA supporting the proinflammatory host response against infection (17, 19). However, miR-155 also participates in negative-feedback regulation of the proinflammatory signaling, ultimately protecting the host from a potentially damaging inflammation overreaction (20). Moreover, this miRNA was shown to be essential for normal immune function, particularly of dendritic cells and B and T lymphocytes, and as part of immunization with attenuated *S.* Typhimurium (21).

By comparing miRNome (the full spectrum of expressed miRNAs) changes in macrophages and epi-thelial cells, Schulte et al. showed that members of the let-7 miRNA family are downregulated in both cell types, revealing a common denominator of the phagocytic and nonphagocytic cell response to *S.* Typhimurium infection (17). Interestingly, the let-7 family was shown to target two major cytokines—the anti-inflammatory cytokine interleukin 10 (IL-10) and the proinflammatory cytokine IL-6. The decreased let-7 expression upon infection and consequent derepression of cytokines with opposing effects likely contributes to a balanced inflammatory response to *S.* Typhimurium infection.

In addition to participating in the host response to *S.* Typhimurium infection, miRNA regulation can be harnessed to modulate host physiology, ultimately rendering host cells more permissive to bacterial infection. By employing a high-content screening approach in which the individual effect of ca. 1,000 miRNAs was tested on *S.* Typhimurium replication in epithelial cells, our group has identified multiple miRNAs controlling bacterial interaction with host cells (22). Among the strongest inhibitors of *S.* Typhimurium infection, we identified the miR-15 family, which blocks host G_1/S cell cycle transition through the repression of cyclin D1. Interestingly, expression of the miR-15 miRNA family is downregulated upon *S.* Typhimurium infection, thus favoring cell cycle progression and, ultimately, bacterial replication.

SUMOylation, a posttranslational modification pathway central for cell homeostasis (23), is essential for *Salmonella* intracellular survival, and it has also been shown to be subverted by modulation of host miRNAs. Indeed, *S.* Typhimurium survival inside host cells relies on the depletion of Ubc-9, a crucial enzyme of the SUMO pathway, which is achieved by the increased levels of miR-30c and miR-30e upon infection (24).

The effect of *Salmonella* infection on miRNAs has been also studied *in vivo* in different models of infection, including zebrafish, chicken, and especially pig. In zebrafish embryos, several miRNAs were shown to be upregulated upon *S.* Typhimurium infection, including the two miR-146 family members, miR-146a/b (25). Interestingly, combined knockdown of these miRNAs in zebrafish embryos infected with *S.* Typhimurium had a minor effect on the proinflammatory response, but it induced apolipoprotein-mediated lipid transport genes, suggesting a possible function of these miRNAs in regulating lipid metabolism during inflammation (25). In the chicken model, 14 miRNAs were shown to be differentially expressed upon *S.* Typhimurium infection. From these, the most strongly induced miRNAs were miR-3525 and miR-193a-5p, which might impact the immune response against *S.* Typhimurium by targeting IL-6 signal transducer and interferon-γ (IFN-γ), respectively (26). In the ileum of piglets, *S.* Typhimurium upregulated miR-29a expression (27). This miRNA was shown to target Caveolin-2, an inhibitor of the small Rho GTPase Cdc42, thus favoring *S.* Typhimurium invasion of epithelial cells. In a recent study, Herrera-Uribe et al. identified 110 dysregulated miRNAs in mesenteric lymph nodes of *S.* Typhimurium-infected piglets (28). Among these, the authors highlighted several miRNAs with predicted and validated targets among major histocompatibility complex class I and II antigen presentation pathways. The miRNA expression profile of whole-blood samples of pigs challenged with *S.* Typhimurium has also been analyzed, revealing 62 differentially expressed miRNAs (29). From these, the decrease of miR-214 was shown to increase expression of SLC11A1 and LILR-like expression, potentially regulating bacterial replication by actively removing iron from the phagosomal space and by negatively regulating TLR-mediated responses to maintain a balanced inflammatory response, respectively. Induction of miR-331-3p was also validated and suggested to contribute to blocking *S.* Typhimurium uptake by suppressing the activity of Rho GTPase family members (e.g., RhoA, Cdc42, and Rac1) through targeting of VAV2 (29).

Similarly, Yao et al. demonstrated that miR-143, miR-26, and miR-4335 are differentially expressed in whole-blood samples of *S.* Typhimurium-infected pigs (30).

Although to a lesser extent, the miRNA regulation by other *Salmonella* serovars, specifically *S. enterica* subsp. *enterica* serovar Enteritidis (*S.* Enteritidis), has also been investigated. Analysis of the miRNome of colon epithelial cells infected with two strains of *S.* Enteritidis revealed 22 differentially regulated miRNAs (31). miR-128 was shown to be consistently upregulated in *S.* Enteritidis-infected samples *in vitro* and *in vivo*, through a mechanism likely involving activation of the p53 signaling pathway by bacterial secreted proteins. miR-128 was shown to target macrophage colony-stimulating factor (M-CSF), leading to impaired M-CSF-mediated macrophage recruitment and thus benefiting bacterial survival. In chicken, 37 and 32 miRNAs were shown to be differentially regulated between noninfected and *S.* Enteritidis-infected cecum (32) and spleen (19) samples, respectively. Through integrated analysis of miRNA and transcriptome datasets obtained from spleen samples, two miRNAs were identified in hub positions of the regulatory network—miR-155 and miR-101-3p—likely with important consequences to the immune response upon infection (19).

Helicobacter pylori

H. pylori is a Gram-negative bacterium estimated to chronically colonize the gastric mucosa of more than half of the human population. Unless treated, colonization persists lifelong and represents a key factor in the etiology of gastritis, peptic ulcer, and gastric cancer (33). Similar to other pathogens, *H. pylori* pathogenesis depends on its bacterial virulence factors, such as the cytotoxin-associated gene A (CagA) and vacuolating cytotoxin A (VacA), which affect a multitude of host cell pathways (34).

The first evidence that bacterial pathogens can affect the expression of mammalian host miRNAs was obtained in a pioneering study by Zhang and colleagues, who used *H. pylori* as a model pathogen (35). This study demonstrated that miR-21 is upregulated in gastric epithelium tissue samples of *H. pylori*-infected patients compared to noninfected samples; similar results were reported *in vitro* in the human gastric cancer cell line AGS. Interestingly, miR-21 overexpression was shown to promote cellular proliferation and invasion by targeting RECK, a known tumor suppressor. These results suggested a strong link between miR-21 regulation upon *H. pylori* infection and the development of gastric cancers (35). Other studies have further explored the connection between regulation of host miRNA expression upon *H. pylori* infection and the ability of this pathogen to induce tumorigenesis. In one of these studies, *H. pylori* infection was shown to induce the expression of miR-222, another oncomiR (oncogenic miRNA) that also targets RECK (36). Recently, miR-222 was also shown to directly target the homeodomain-interacting protein kinase-2, promoting cell proliferation and invasion and inhibiting apoptosis of gastric cancer cells (37). Along the same line, miR-101 was shown to be downregulated in *H. pylori*-infected samples and cultured cells, with similar consequences for cell growth and tumorigenesis, elicited by the derepression of its direct target, the oncogene SOCS2 (38). In addition, DNA methylation of the miR-210 gene promoter was shown to be increased in *H. pylori*-infected human gastric mucosa samples compared to negative controls, promoting cell proliferation through derepression of STMN1 (involved in the initiation of tumor development) and DIMT1 (a member of the *S*-adenosylmethionine-dependent methyltransferase superfamily) (39).

Mechanistically, the *H. pylori* virulence factor CagA was shown to be an important player in *H. pylori*-induced miRNA expression changes, with 61 miRNAs differentially expressed in a CagA-dependent manner (40). CagA-dependent downregulation of miR-320 upon *H. pylori* infection results in increased expression of its target MCL1, an antiapoptotic gene, likely contributing to an increased risk of tumorigenesis (40). Similarly, the downregulation of miR-370, in a CagA-dependent manner, leads to increased expression of FoxM1, a transcription factor involved in promoting cell cycle progression (41). CagA was also shown to stimulate expression of miRNAs, specifically of miR-584 and miR-1290. These miRNAs have as a common target FOXA1, which is an important negative regulator of epithelial-mesenchymal transition, critical for the development of cancer metastasis (42).

Although *H. pylori* primarily affects the stomach mucosa, its presence has also been associated with other pathological conditions, such as Barrett's esophageal disease and esophagus adenocarcinoma (43, 44). In the context of esophageal epithelial cells, Teng et al. showed that *H. pylori* decreases miR-212-3p and miR-361-3p expression, leading to derepression of their targets, COX2 and CDX2, respectively, two oncoproteins associated with transformation of esophageal epithelial cells (45).

Although a large body of literature coherently supports the involvement of miRNA regulation during *H. pylori* infection to promote cell proliferation and, ultimately, favor tumorigenesis, *H. pylori* has also been shown to block cell cycle progression and cell prolifera-

tion in gastric epithelial cells through the regulation of miRNAs (46, 47). Indeed, CagA-dependent downregulation of miR-372 and miR-373 in *H. pylori*-infected cells increases expression of their target LATS2, a tumor suppressor, leading to G_1 cell cycle arrest (46). Recently, Wang et al. analyzed miRNA expression in gastric cancer patients, comparing *H. pylori*-positive and -negative subgroups. Among the 53 miRNAs differentially expressed in these samples, the authors focused on miR-143-3p, which was the most upregulated miRNA in *H. pylori*-positive gastric cancer tissues. The authors demonstrated that high levels of miR-143-3p dampen cell growth, migration, and invasion through the direct targeting of AKT2 (47), a pro-survival protein that is frequently overexpressed in cancer. Although these studies reveal an unexpected facet of *H. pylori*, i.e., bacterial-induced host cell cycle arrest and inhibition of cell proliferation, it is conceivable that this can be relevant to inhibit gastric epithelium renewal and therefore constitute a host defense mechanism against infection.

H. pylori infection elicits a strong immune response, triggering the expression of diverse cytokines and chemokines by gastric epithelial cells. Along the same line, several studies have reported the deregulation of immune-related miRNAs in response to *H. pylori* infection. For example, miR-155 is strongly upregulated upon *H. pylori* infection, both *in vitro* (epithelial cells, macrophages, and lymphocytes) and *in vivo* (human biopsies from infected gastric mucosa) (48–52). Upregulation of miR-155 was shown to be dependent on sensing of *H. pylori* LPS by TLR4 and subsequent NF-κB pathway activation (49, 52), as well as on the secretion of bacterial proteins by the type-IV secretion system, particularly VacA and γ-glutamyl transpeptidase (48). miR-155 inhibits the release of the proinflammatory cytokines IL-8 and GRO-α, resulting in attenuated NF-κB activity and weakened inflammatory response against *H. pylori* (52). In macrophages, upregulation of miR-155 was also shown to inhibit DNA damage-induced apoptosis, a mechanism that might increase cell survival upon DNA damage induced by *H. pylori* (49). Interestingly, miR-155 knockout mice are unable to control *H. pylori* infection, owing to a deficient pathogen-specific Th1 and Th17 response (51). Pachathundikandi et al. showed that in infected THP-1 monocytes, the inflammasome-forming NLRP3 protein is downregulated upon *H. pylori* infection through the upregulation of miR-223-3p (53). The immune-related miRNA miR-146a is also upregulated by *H. pylori* infection, both *in vitro* and *in vivo* (52, 54–56). miR-146a negatively regulates TRAF6, PTGS2, and IRAK1 and, consequently, blunts the inflammatory response against *H. pylori* (54–56). Similar to *Salmonella* spp., *H. pylori* infection downregulates the let-7 miRNA family both *in vitro* and *in vivo* through its major virulence factor CagA (57, 58). Decreased expression of let-7 family members leads to the derepression of their target TLR4 and to the consequent activation of the NF-κB-dependent inflammatory response. In addition to classical immune-related miRNAs, other miRNAs have been implicated in the regulation of immune function in the context of *H. pylori* infection. In a recent study, Xie and colleagues showed that *H. pylori* induces the expression of B7-H1 by decreasing the levels of miR-152 and miR-200b (59). Indeed, B7-H1 functions as a negative regulator of cell-mediated immune response by inhibiting proliferation and inducing apoptosis of activated T-cells (60). In a recent study, Pagliari et al. described that *H. pylori* can alter miR-4270 expression as a strategy to persist in macrophages and thus evade the immune system (61). miR-4270 controls the expression of the plasma membrane receptor CD300E, compromising the ability of macrophages to expose major histocompatibility complex class II molecules, ultimately compromising recognition by T-cells, and providing a survival niche for the bacterium.

Beyond immune-related functions, *H. pylori* subverts other cellular processes for its own benefit through miRNA regulation. Upregulation of miR-30b was shown to occur in AGS cells and gastric tissues infected with *H. pylori* (62). miR-30b negatively regulates the autophagy pathway by targeting Beclin-1 and ATG12, two proteins involved in the formation and maturation of autophagosomes, likely contributing to preventing *H. pylori* clearance by autophagy. The expression of these two autophagy proteins (along with ATG2B, ATG5, and BNIP3L) was also shown to be repressed by the upregulation of miR-30d induced during *H. pylori* infection (63). *H. pylori* can also decrease the gastric acidity by inducing the expression of miR-1289 in a CagA- and soluble lytic transglycolase-dependent manner. miR-1289 represses HKα, a subunit of the gastric H$^+$/K$^+$ ATPase (64), leading to a transient hypochlorhydria that favors *H. pylori* colonization of the gastric mucosa.

Mycobacterium Species

The genus *Mycobacterium* includes highly pathogenic species responsible for diseases that remain major public health challenges, such as tuberculosis (caused by *Mycobacterium tuberculosis*) and leprosy (caused by *Mycobacterium leprae*). In addition, it also encompasses opportunistic pathogens, such as *Mycobacterium avium*, that can infect immunocompromised patients. Not surprisingly, miRNAs play relevant roles in the

modulation of the host response to mycobacterial infection (reviewed in reference 65).

Several studies have examined the regulation and role of miR-155 in mycobacterial infection using different cellular models, experimental conditions, and *Mycobacterium* species (66–77). These studies have generated divergent results, particularly regarding the function of miR-155 during infection, though the majority underlined the recurrent function of miR-155 in the regulation of the innate immune response. Adding to the body of knowledge on the role of miR-155 in infection, a recent study by Rothchild and colleagues applied an integrative approach to analyze the miRNA network in infected macrophages, revealing a critical and dual role for miR-155 in *M. tuberculosis* infection (74): on the one hand, miR-155 promotes the survival of infected macrophages, providing a bacterial niche during the early stages of infection, while on the other hand, it promotes the survival and function of specific T-cells, enabling an effective adaptive immune response. miR-27b, another miRNA with a dual role in mycobacterial infection, has recently been shown to be induced upon infection. miR-27b targets the Bcl-2-associated athanogene 2 protein (Bag2)—which inhibits the production of proinflammatory factors by blunting NF-κB activity but also increases p53-dependent apoptosis and reactive oxygen species production—thus increasing bacterial clearance (78). Other miRNAs have been shown to blunt the proinflammatory response against *Mycobacterium* to favor bacterial survival. For example, downregulation of let-7f in macrophages infected with *M. tuberculosis* was shown to derepress the expression of A20 deubiquitinase, a negative regulator of the NF-κB pathway (79). Along the same line, induction of miR-223 reduces the expression of the cytokine IL6 and chemokines CXCL2 and CCL3 upon infection, inhibiting proper recruitment of neutrophils to the infection site and increasing bacterial survival (80).

The miRNA response against *Mycobacterium* spp. has been shown to be highly dependent on the cell context and bacterial species. For example, while miR-21, miR-29a, and miR-142-3p levels were shown to increase in infected macrophages and serum of tuberculosis patients (75, 81–83), they are downregulated in CD4$^+$ T-cells and samples of peripheral blood of tuberculosis patients (84). Similar to the observations in *Listeria* (see "*Listeria monocytogenes*" below), miR-29 is downregulated in natural killer (NK) cells upon *M. bovis* infection (85), which was shown to enhance bacterial clearance by derepressing IFN-γ expression. In contrast, in macrophages infected with *M. avium*, miR-29a expression, along with let-7e, is upregulated, resulting in inhibition of apoptosis through a decrease of caspase-3 and caspase-7 (75). Regulation of host cell death is emerging as a recurrent target of miRNAs regulated during mycobacterial infection. Along this line, upon *M. tuberculosis* infection, upregulation of miR-582-5p, miR-155, and miR-21 was also shown to inhibit apoptosis, by targeting FOX1, FOX3, and NF-κB/Bcl-2, respectively (71, 86, 87). On the other hand, a decrease of miR-20b in *M. tuberculosis*-infected macrophages derepresses NLRP3, leading to the activation of the NRLP3/caspase-1/IL-1β pathway and, consequently, enhancing inflammation and pyroptosis (88).

Autophagy is a process by which intracellular components are targeted for degradation, and it plays a crucial role in the host defense against intracellular pathogens, including mycobacteria (89). *Mycobacterium* spp. have evolved strategies based on host miRNA modulation to subvert the autophagy pathway and ensure intracellular survival. Figure 3 illustrates the impact of mycobacteria-regulated miRNAs on autophagy and lysosomal trafficking. The role of miR-155 as a positive or negative regulator of autophagy in the context of mycobacterial infection is still controversial, and it likely depends on cell context and bacterial strain. A proautophagic function of miR-155 through the repression of the negative autophagy regulator RHEB was shown in macrophages (76), compromising *M. tuberculosis* survival. Con-

versely, upon *M. tuberculosis* infection of dendritic cells, upregulated miR-155 was shown to directly target ATG3 and reduce the lipidated form of LC3 in the autophagosomes, indicating negative regulation of autophagy (70). In addition to miR-155, other miRNAs were shown to impinge on autophagic regulation during *M. tuberculosis* infection. Downregulation of miR-17 leads to an increase of STAT3, a transcriptional activator of the autophagy regulator MCL-1 (90), impairing autophagy and contributing to mycobacterial survival. In the context of *M. bovis* bacillus Calmette-Guérin (BCG) infection, upregulation of miR-17 has been reported to repress ULK1, an essential autophagy initiation protein, ultimately favoring BCG growth (91). This apparently contradictory result on miR-17 expression might be linked to the different *Mycobacterium* spp. used. *Mycobacterium* was also shown to block autophagy by increasing the levels of miR-30a and miR-125a-3p, which target Beclin-1 and UVRAG, respectively, two essential players in autophagy induction (92, 93). *M. tuberculosis* also induces the expression of miR-33 and miR-33*, which target several players in the autophagy and lysosomal pathways (ATG5, ATG12, LC3B, LAMP1, AMPK, FOXO3, and TFEB) (94). Recently, Liu et al. showed that induction of miR-27a upon infection represses the expression of the endoplasmic reticulum-located calcium transporter CAC-NA2D3,

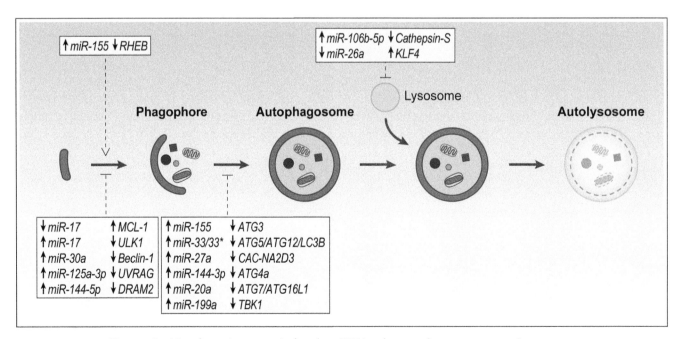

Figure 3 *Mycobacterium* spp.-induced miRNA changes have a strong impact on autophagy. The autophagic flux is controlled by multiple miRNAs that are regulated as a consequence of mycobacterial infection. Most studies report that miRNA modulation inhibits specific steps of the autophagy pathway, thus impairing bacterial degradation.

impairing the calcium signaling required for autophagosome formation (95). miR-144-5p and miR-144-3p have also been implicated in the control of autophagy: miR-144-5p is upregulated during *M. tuberculosis* infection, suppressing autophagy by targeting the autophagy regulator DRAM2 (96), while an increase of miR-144-3p upon BCG infection inhibits autophagy by targeting ATG4a (97). miR-20a and miR-199a are also upregulated upon *M. bovis* infection and inhibit autophagy through downregulation of ATG7, ATG16L1 (98), and TBK1 (99), respectively. Overall, the majority of the studies reported above support a model in which mycobacteria-modulated host miRNAs have a predominant effect on dampening the autophagic process, with positive consequences for bacterial survival.

Mycobacterium spp. can also modulate phagosomal trafficking for their own benefit by modulating several miRNAs. Vegh et al. found a set of miRNAs regulated in bovine macrophages upon infection with *M. bovis* (6 miRNAs at 24 h postinfection and 40 miRNAs at 48 h postinfection); analysis of the predicted targets of the upregulated miRNAs showed an enrichment for genes related to the lysosome and endocytosis, including members of the membrane trafficking Rab family (100). Downregulation of miR-26a during *M. tuberculosis* infection was shown to derepress KLF4, preventing bacterial trafficking to lysosomes and reducing inducible nitric oxide synthase production (101). Recently, it was also shown that *M. tuberculosis* upregulates miR-106b-5p expression, which directly represses cathepsin-S, decreasing the lysosomal enzymatic activity and consequently increasing bacterial intracellular survival (102). miRNAs have also been shown to negatively modulate bacterial uptake, likely as part of the host response to counteract infection. Specifically, an increase of miR-142-3p in response to *M. tuberculosis* infection represses N-WASP, an actin binding protein essential for phagocytosis (81).

Listeria monocytogenes

L. monocytogenes is a Gram-positive facultative intracellular bacterium that is the causative agent of human listeriosis, a foodborne disease. *Listeria* can cause gastroenteritis in healthy adults and severe illness in children, the elderly, and other immunocompromised individuals (103).

Genome-wide miRNA profiling in murine bone marrow-derived macrophages infected with *L. monocytogenes* identified 13 miRNAs that were significantly upregulated, including miRNAs known to regulate the inflammatory response (e.g., miR-155 and miR-146a) (104). In addition, miR-155 has been shown to be es-

sential for the CD8$^+$ T-cell response to *L. monocytogenes* (105). Recently, the immune-related miRNA miR-21 was also shown to be upregulated following *L. monocytogenes* infection of bone marrow-derived macrophages (106). Interestingly, miR-21 knockout macrophages showed an increased bacterial burden at early times postinfection (30 min). The identification of the actin-modulating proteins RHOB and MARCKS as putative miR-21 targets suggests a possible role for this miRNA in the negative regulation of phagocytosis during infection.

The effect of *L. monocytogenes* infection on host miRNA expression has also been addressed in human intestinal epithelial Caco-2 cells (107); in this study, five miRNAs (miR-146b, miR-16, let-7a1, miR-145, and miR-155) were found to be dysregulated upon *L. monocytogenes* infection. Similar to what has been described in macrophages (104), in Caco-2 cells the expression of miR-155 was induced to a comparable extent by infection with wild-type *L. monocytogenes* or with a mutant deficient for listeriolysin, a secreted toxin that is essential for bacterial vacuolar escape, among other functions, in *L. monocytogenes* virulence. Strikingly, upregulation of miR-155 also occurs following incubation of cells with purified listeriolysin (107). Among the miRNAs dysregulated by *L. monocytogenes* in Caco-2 cells, Izar and colleagues showed the downregulation of miR-145 (107). This miRNA exerts a proinflammatory effect by potentiating the production of the proinflammatory cytokines IL-5 and IL-13 (108) and by decreasing the levels of the anti-inflammatory cytokine IFN-β (109), a cytokine shown to be beneficial to *L. monocytogenes* infection (reviewed in 110). However, a recent study by Li and colleagues revealed an anti-inflammatory effect of miR-145 by reducing ARF6 expression and downstream signal transduction via NF-κB (111). Taken together, these studies suggest that downregulation of miR-145 could play an essential role in balancing the inflammatory response during *Listeria* infection.

In vivo, challenge with *L. monocytogenes* has also been shown to induce significant host miRNome changes. Systemic infection of mice with *L. monocytogenes* downregulates miR-29 expression in NK cells, CD4$^+$ T-cells, and CD8$^+$ T-cells (85). Ma et al. (85) suggested that decreased miR-29 expression upon infection facilitates IFN-γ production, promoting bacterial clearance and host resistance to *L. monocytogenes* infection. miR-192, miR-215, and miR-200b were shown to be downregulated in the ileum of orally infected gnotobiotic humanized mice (112). Interestingly, pretreatment with *Lactobacillus casei* prevented the decrease of expression of these miRNAs upon *L. monocytogenes* infection. In another study, Archambaud et al. reported the decreased expression of six miRNAs (miR-143, miR-148a, miR-194, miR-200b, miR-200c, and miR-378) in the ileum of conventional mice infected with *L. monocytogenes* (113). Interestingly, regulation of four of these miRNAs (miR-143, miR-148a, miR-200b, and miR-200c) occurs only in the presence of a normal microbiota, whereas miR-194 is decreased in both the presence and absence of gut microbiota and miR-378 expression is increased in germ-free mice. Overall, these studies reveal an interesting microbiota-dependent regulation of miRNA expression during *Listeria* infection, suggesting that the microbiota plays an important role in the miRNA host cell response, with relevant implications for infection with bacterial pathogens.

Other Bacterial Pathogens

As described above, analysis of miRNA expression and the characterization of the role of miRNAs are well under way for certain bacterial pathogens. For most bacterial pathogens, however, this analysis has not yet been performed or is just at its inception. We provide below a nonexhaustive review of what is known concerning the role of miRNAs in infection by other bacterial pathogens. Of note, most of these studies have focused on immune response-related miRNAs, most prominently miR-155. For example, miR-155 was shown to be differentially induced upon infection with *Francisella tularensis* (114, 115), a Gram-negative facultative intracellular bacterium that causes turalemia. Interestingly, miR-155 is strongly induced in an LPS-dependent manner upon infection with *F. tularensis* subsp. *novicida*, a low-virulence *F. tularensis* subspecies, while infection with the highly virulent *F. tularensis* subsp. *tularensis* leads to significantly lower miR-155 induction, probably due to the low bioactivity of its LPS. This might contribute to explaining the higher bacterial dissemination and more severe disease caused by *F. tularensis* subsp. *tularensis* (114, 115). Indeed, the increase of miR-155 upon *F. tularensis* subsp. *novicida* infection represses SHIP (a key negative regulator of the PI3K/Akt pathway), similarly to what was described for *Mycobacterium* infection (67), thus enhancing the proinflammatory cytokine response and contributing to infection clearance (115). Clare and colleagues demonstrated that miR-155 knockout mice are unable to clear infection by *Citrobacter rodentium* (116), a murine pathogen that is used as a model for understanding enteropathogenic and enterohemorrhagic *Escherichia coli* *in vivo* since it shares several pathogenic mechanisms with these two important human gastrointestinal pathogens. In addition to miR-155, the increased expression of miR-203 in colonic crypts of *C. rodentium*-infected mice was detected and shown to deregulate Wnt/β-catenin signaling through the direct repression of the Wnt antagonist WIF1 (117). This may contribute to the observed Wnt/β-catenin-dependent crypt hyperplasia in response to *C. rodentium* infection.

Staphylococcus aureus is another example of a pathogen for which the role of miRNAs during infection is starting to be addressed. Initial reports investigated the impact of staphylococcal enterotoxin B (SEB), an exotoxin responsible for food poisoning and toxic shock, on miRNA expression in lung-infiltrating mononuclear cells isolated from mice exposed to SEB (118). miR-155, the most upregulated miRNA, was shown to enhance the accumulation of IFN-γ by targeting SOCS1, leading to an exacerbated inflammatory response. Interestingly, miR-155 knockout mice are protected against the overinflammation and lung injury elicited by SEB (118), further supporting the relevance of this miRNA on SEB toxicity and, arguably, on *S. aureus* pathogenicity. Decreased expression of miR-24 has been described in *S. aureus*-infected macrophages (119). In these cells, reduced miR-24 levels were shown to contribute to a macrophage M1 polarization phenotype via increased CHI3L1 expression. Colonization by *S. aureus* is frequently linked to chronic skin wounds, particularly in diabetic patients and obese or immunosuppressed individuals (120). The presence of *S. aureus* in wounds increases miR-15b-5p expression, impairing DNA repair and the inflammatory response, with likely negative consequences to wound healing (121). Using an miR-142 knockout mouse, miR-142-3p and miR-142-5p were also shown to contribute to healing of *S. aureus*-infected skin wounds (122). Indeed, this phenotype was related to impaired neutrophil chemotactic and phagocytic behavior due to abnormal expression of Rac and Rho GTPases. Recently, the therapeutic potential of miRNA modulation was shown in a model of *S. aureus*-infected wounds (123). Mice with a specific deletion of miR-223 showed enhanced repair of *S. aureus*-infected wounds compared to wild-type mice. Similar improvement of wound healing was observed in wild-type mice transplanted with neutrophils lacking miR-223 or treated with inhibitors of miR-223. Interestingly, miR-223 was identified as one of the most highly expressed miRNAs at wound sites during the inflammatory phase.

More systematic studies of miRNA expression have also been performed for a number of pathogens. For example, infection of mouse alveolar macrophages with the opportunistic pathogen *Pseudomonas aeruginosa* was shown to upregulate eight miRNAs, miR-302b being the most prominently increased (124). Upregulation of this miRNA results in a dampened inflammatory response via targeting of IRAK4, a component of the MyD88 signaling complex critical for NF-κB activation.

The effect of infection with *Chlamydia trachomatis*, an obligate intracellular pathogen that is the causative agent of trachoma and sexually transmitted infections, on host miRNA expression has been analyzed (reviewed in reference 125). Derrick et al. analyzed miRNA expression profiles of trachoma disease patients, including conjunctival scarring with and without inflammation, revealing 82 differentially expressed miRNAs (126). Pathway analysis revealed an enrichment of genes related to fibrosis and epithelial cell differentiation among the predicted targets of these miRNAs. A recent study by Chowdhury and colleagues analyzed differentially expressed miRNAs in primary human umbilical vein endothelial cells infected with *C. trachomatis*, revealing miR-30c-5p as one of the most upregulated miRNAs (127). miR-30c-5p upregulation leads to p53-mediated downregulation of Drp1, a mitochondrial fission regulator, thereby inhibiting stress-induced mitochondrial fission and promoting cell survival during infection. In addition, several groups used the mouse pathogen *Chlamydia muridarum*, a model organism to study human *C. trachomatis* urogenital tract infections, to investigate miRNA expression changes (128–131). Interestingly, Yeruva et al. showed that *C. muridarum* infection decreases the protein levels of two components of the miRNA machinery, Dicer and Ago2 (131). Although the consequence of these changes to infection is not yet clear, this suggests a broad effect of *C. muridarum* in blunting host miRNA responses.

In macrophages, infection by the Gram-negative bacterium *Brucella melitensis*, the causative agent of brucellosis, was shown to regulate the expression of 57 miRNAs (132). Putative targets of the six most abundant differentially expressed miRNAs (miR-92a, miR-93, miR-151-3p, miR-181b, miR-1981, and let7-b) revealed enrichment for apoptosis, autophagy, and immune response-related pathways. Recent studies have demonstrated that the related pathogen *Brucella abortus* is also able to modulate host miRNA expression to increase its intracellular survival in macrophages. Indeed, downregulation of miR-125b-5p by *B. abortus* was shown to diminish the proinflammatory host response via derepression of the inhibitor of NF-κB activation A20 (133). miRNA expression upon *Brucella suis* infection of porcine and murine macrophages revealed that a common set of five miRNAs (miR-130a-3p, miR-146a, miR-181a, miR-301a-3p, and miR-351-5p)

are upregulated. By controlling these miRNAs, *B. suis* negatively regulates TNFα to promote bacterial intracellular survival (134).

High-throughput functional screenings have recently started to be applied to identify miRNAs controlling different biological processes. We have pioneered the application of this approach to infections by bacterial pathogens, specifically S. Typhimurium (cf. section above [22]) and *Shigella flexneri* (135). *S. flexneri* is a major causative agent of shigellosis in humans (136). Using an unbiased functional screening approach, we identified miR-29b-2-5p as a miRNA with a dual regulatory effect on *S. flexneri* infection, enhancing both bacterial binding to host cells and intracellular bacterial replication (135). miR-29b-2-5p leads to increased filopodia formation through the direct regulation of UNC5C, ultimately enhancing *S. flexneri* binding to host cells. Interestingly, *S. flexneri* intracellular replication decreases miR-29b-2-5p expression at late times postinfection by specific degradation of the mature miRNA by the exonuclease PNPT1. A decrease of miR-29b-2-5p may constitute a bacterial strategy to promote balanced intracellular replication, avoiding premature host cell death and favoring spreading to neighboring cells or, alternatively, may be part of the host response to counteract *Shigella* infection.

PERSPECTIVES

Advances in RNA sequencing have contributed to the extensive analysis of the host miRNome and contributed to demonstrating that infection by various bacterial pathogens induces major miRNome changes. Of note, these studies highlighted that even closely related species (e.g., *M. tuberculosis* versus *M. bovis* versus *M. avium*, or *F. tularensis* subsp. *tularensis* versus *F. tularensis* subsp. *novicida*) lead to widely different host miRNA profiles. However, a common set of miRNAs regulated as part of the host immune response (e.g., miR-155, miR-146, and let-7) has been described for a wide spectrum of pathogens. Along this line, a recent analysis of miRNA response to infection of dendritic cells by six bacteria revealed a core of 49 miRNAs with consistently altered expression (137). Interestingly, this study also showed that the relative abundance of miRNA duplex arms (−3p and −5p miRNAs) and the expression dynamics of miRNA isoforms (isomiRs) are strongly impacted by bacterial infection, although the consequences of these phenomena to infection are yet to be determined.

In addition to the identity of the pathogen, the regulation of host miRNAs upon infection is dependent on the cellular context (e.g., epithelial cells versus macrophages).

Added to this, the majority of the miRNA expression analysis in the context of infection has been performed in bulk cell populations comprising both cells with internalized bacteria and bystander cells. The heterogeneity of the miRNA response of individual cells to infection and its dependency on the extent of bacterial internalization and/or replication still require further investigation. With the improvement of single-cell RNA sequencing, reliable analysis of miRNA profiles with sufficient coverage will be attainable (138). One additional interesting point concerns differences in the response of cells with internalized bacteria and bystander cells. Initial reports in sorted populations of infected and bystander cells suggest that although miRNA changes in the bystander population generally echo those observed in infected cells, a portion of the changes appear to be specific to bystander cells (22). The relevance of the miRNA reprogramming in bystander cells and their consequences to infection clearly deserve further investigation. Importantly, the molecular mechanisms underlying most of the observed miRNA regulations, irrespective of whether these occur in infected or bystander cells, remain poorly understood. In this regard, the direct manipulation of the miRNA pathway by secreted bacterial factors remains a fascinating hypothesis prompted by the discovery of RNA silencing suppressor proteins in viruses and plant bacterial pathogens.

The impacts of microbiota on host miRNA expression and their implications for organ/tissue homeostasis and/or infections are also an exciting subject. In this regard, the resident gut microbiota has been shown to modulate host miRNA expression (139, 140), and a recent report suggests that the host might influence the gut microbiome through miRNAs (141). Moreover, analysis of the host miRNA response to *L. monocytogenes* infection in conventional versus germ-free mice identified five miRNAs that were downregulated upon infection in a microbiota-dependent manner (113).

Overall, miRNAs are now considered major players in the infection process. As summarized in this chapter, a growing number of studies are uncovering host miRNAs as part of the defense strategies mounted by the host to fight infection but also as pathogen strategies to subvert host functions and promote virulence. The study of miRNAs in the context of infection and, equally importantly, the identification and characterization of downstream targets and underlying mechanisms of action will continue to provide important insights into the intricate interplay between pathogens and host.

Acknowledgments. Work in the M.M. and A.E. laboratories on microRNAs and infection was supported by the ERA-NET Infect-ERA CampyRNA and grants from the Portuguese Science Foundation (FCT, #POCI-01-0145-FEDER-029999 and IF/01105/2015).

Citation. Aguilar C, Mano M, Eulalio A. 2019. Multifaceted roles of microRNAs in host-bacterial pathogen interaction. Microbiol Spectrum 7(3):BAI-0002-2019.

References

1. Bartel DP. 2018. Metazoan MicroRNAs. *Cell* **173:** 20–51.

2. Krol J, Loedige I, Filipowicz W. 2010. The widespread regulation of microRNA biogenesis, function and decay. *Nat Rev Genet* **11:**597–610.

3. Jonas S, Izaurralde E. 2015. Towards a molecular understanding of microRNA-mediated gene silencing. *Nat Rev Genet* **16:**421–433.

4. Friedman RC, Farh KK, Burge CB, Bartel DP. 2009. Most mammalian mRNAs are conserved targets of microRNAs. *Genome Res* **19:**92–105.

5. Bueno MJ, Pérez de Castro I, Malumbres M. 2008. Control of cell proliferation pathways by microRNAs. *Cell Cycle* **7:**3143–3148.

6. Jovanovic M, Hengartner MO. 2006. miRNAs and apoptosis: RNAs to die for. *Oncogene* **25:**6176–6187.

7. Shenoy A, Blelloch RH. 2014. Regulation of microRNA function in somatic stem cell proliferation and differentiation. *Nat Rev Mol Cell Biol* **15:**565–576.

8. Croce CM. 2009. Causes and consequences of microRNA dysregulation in cancer. *Nat Rev Genet* **10:** 704–714.

9. Small EM, Olson EN. 2011. Pervasive roles of microRNAs in cardiovascular biology. *Nature* **469:**336–342.

10. Bruscella P, Bottini S, Baudesson C, Pawlotsky JM, Feray C, Trabucchi M. 2017. Viruses and miRNAs: more friends than foes. *Front Microbiol* **8:**824.

11. Pfeffer S, Zavolan M, Grässer FA, Chien M, Russo JJ, Ju J, John B, Enright AJ, Marks D, Sander C, Tuschl T. 2004. Identification of virus-encoded microRNAs. *Science* **304:**734–736.

12. Navarro L, Dunoyer P, Jay F, Arnold B, Dharmasiri N, Estelle M, Voinnet O, Jones JD. 2006. A plant miRNA contributes to antibacterial resistance by repressing auxin signaling. *Science* **312:**436–439.

13. Navarro L, Jay F, Nomura K, He SY, Voinnet O. 2008. Suppression of the microRNA pathway by bacterial effector proteins. *Science* **321:**964–967.

14. Taganov KD, Boldin MP, Chang KJ, Baltimore D. 2006. NF-kappaB-dependent induction of microRNA miR-146, an inhibitor targeted to signaling proteins of innate immune responses. *Proc Natl Acad Sci U S A* **103:**12481–12486.

15. Majowicz SE, Musto J, Scallan E, Angulo FJ, Kirk M, O'Brien SJ, Jones TF, Fazil A, Hoekstra RM, International Collaboration on Enteric Disease 'Burden of Illness' Studies. 2010. The global burden of nontyphoidal *Salmonella* gastroenteritis. *Clin Infect Dis* **50:**882–889.

16. Herrero-Fresno A, Olsen JE. 2018. *Salmonella* Typhimurium metabolism affects virulence in the host: a mini-review. *Food Microbiol* **71:**98–110.

17. Schulte LN, Eulalio A, Mollenkopf HJ, Reinhardt R, Vogel J. 2011. Analysis of the host microRNA response to *Salmonella* uncovers the control of major cytokines by the let-7 family. *EMBO J* 30:1977–1989.

18. Sharbati S, Sharbati J, Hoeke L, Bohmer M, Einspanier R. 2012. Quantification and accurate normalisation of small RNAs through new custom RT-qPCR arrays demonstrates *Salmonella*-induced microRNAs in human monocytes. *BMC Genomics* 13:23.

19. Li P, Fan W, Li Q, Wang J, Liu R, Everaert N, Liu J, Zhang Y, Zheng M, Cui H, Zhao G, Wen J. 2017. Splenic microRNA expression profiles and integration analyses involved in host responses to *Salmonella enteritidis* infection in chickens. *Front Cell Infect Microbiol* 7:377.

20. Schulte LN, Westermann AJ, Vogel J. 2013. Differential activation and functional specialization of miR-146 and miR-155 in innate immune sensing. *Nucleic Acids Res* 41:542–553.

21. Rodriguez A, Vigorito E, Clare S, Warren MV, Couttet P, Soond DR, van Dongen S, Grocock RJ, Das PP, Miska EA, Vetrie D, Okkenhaug K, Enright AJ, Dougan G, Turner M, Bradley A. 2007. Requirement of bic/microRNA-155 for normal immune function. *Science* 316:608–611.

22. Maudet C, Mano M, Sunkavalli U, Sharan M, Giacca M, Förstner KU, Eulalio A. 2014. Functional high-throughput screening identifies the miR-15 microRNA family as cellular restriction factors for *Salmonella* infection. *Nat Commun* 5:4718.

23. Flotho A, Melchior F. 2013. Sumoylation: a regulatory protein modification in health and disease. *Annu Rev Biochem* 82:357–385.

24. Verma S, Mohapatra G, Ahmad SM, Rana S, Jain S, Khalsa JK, Srikanth CV. 2015. *Salmonella* engages host microRNAs to modulate SUMOylation: a new arsenal for intracellular survival. *Mol Cell Biol* 35:2932–2946.

25. Ordas A, Kanwal Z, Lindenberg V, Rougeot J, Mink M, Spaink HP, Meijer AH. 2013. MicroRNA-146 function in the innate immune transcriptome response of zebrafish embryos to *Salmonella* Typhimurium infection. *BMC Genomics* 14:696.

26. Chen Q, Tong C, Ma S, Zhou L, Zhao L, Zhao X. 2017. Involvement of MicroRNAs in probiotics-induced reduction of the cecal inflammation by *Salmonella* Typhimurium. *Front Immunol* 8:704.

27. Hoeke L, Sharbati J, Pawar K, Keller A, Einspanier R, Sharbati S. 2013. Intestinal *Salmonella* Typhimurium infection leads to miR-29a induced caveolin 2 regulation. *PLoS One* 8:e67300.

28. Herrera-Uribe J, Zaldívar-López S, Aguilar C, Luque C, Bautista R, Carvajal A, Claros MG, Garrido JJ. 2018. Regulatory role of microRNA in mesenteric lymph nodes after *Salmonella* Typhimurium infection. *Vet Res (Faisalabad)* 49:9.

29. Bao H, Kommadath A, Liang G, Sun X, Arantes AS, Tuggle CK, Bearson SM, Plastow GS, Stothard P, Guan L. 2015. Genome-wide whole blood microRNAome and transcriptome analyses reveal miRNA-mRNA regu-lated host response to foodborne pathogen *Salmonella* infection in swine. *Sci Rep* 5:12620.

30. Yao M, Gao W, Tao H, Yang J, Liu G, Huang T. 2016. Regulation signature of miR-143 and miR-26 in porcine *Salmonella* infection identified by binding site enrichment analysis. *Mol Genet Genomics* 291:789–799.

31. Zhang T, Yu J, Zhang Y, Li L, Chen Y, Li D, Liu F, Zhang CY, Gu H, Zen K. 2014. *Salmonella enterica* serovar Enteritidis modulates intestinal epithelial miR-128 levels to decrease macrophage recruitment via macrophage colony-stimulating factor. *J Infect Dis* 209:2000–2011.

32. Wu G, Qi Y, Liu X, Yang N, Xu G, Liu L, Li X. 2017. Cecal MicroRNAome response to *Salmonella enterica* serovar Enteritidis infection in white leghorn layer. *BMC Genomics* 18:77.

33. Cover TL, Blaser MJ. 2009. *Helicobacter pylori* in health and disease. *Gastroenterology* 136:1863–1873.

34. Jones KR, Whitmire JM, Merrell DS. 2010. A tale of two toxins: *Helicobacter pylori* CagA and VacA modu-late host pathways that impact disease. *Front Microbiol* 1:115.

35. Zhang Z, Li Z, Gao C, Chen P, Chen J, Liu W, Xiao S, Lu H. 2008. miR-21 plays a pivotal role in gastric can-cer pathogenesis and progression. *Lab Invest* 88:1358–1366.

36. Li N, Tang B, Zhu ED, Li BS, Zhuang Y, Yu S, Lu DS, Zou QM, Xiao B, Mao XH. 2012. Increased miR-222 in *H. pylori*-associated gastric cancer correlated with tu-mor progression by promoting cancer cell proliferation and targeting RECK. *FEBS Lett* 586:722–728.

37. Tan X, Tang H, Bi J, Li N, Jia Y. 2018. MicroRNA-222-3p associated with *Helicobacter pylori* targets HIPK2 to promote cell proliferation, invasion, and in-hibits apoptosis in gastric cancer. *J Cell Biochem* 119:5153–5162.

38. Zhou X, Xia Y, Li L, Zhang G. 2015. MiR-101 inhibits cell growth and tumorigenesis of *Helicobacter pylori* re-lated gastric cancer by repression of SOCS2. *Cancer Biol Ther* 16:160–169.

39. Kiga K, Mimuro H, Suzuki M, Shinozaki-Ushiku A, Kobayashi T, Sanada T, Kim M, Ogawa M, Iwasaki YW, Kayo H, Fukuda-Yuzawa Y, Yashiro M, Fukayama M, Fukao T, Sasakawa C. 2014. Epigenetic silencing of miR-210 increases the proliferation of gas-tric epithelium during chronic *Helicobacter pylori* infec-tion. *Nat Commun* 5:4497.

40. Noto JM, Piazuelo MB, Chaturvedi R, Bartel CA, Thatcher EJ, Delgado A, Romero-Gallo J, Wilson KT, Correa P, Patton JG, Peek RM Jr. 2013. Strain-specific suppression of microRNA-320 by carcinogenic *Helicobacter pylori* promotes expression of the antiapoptotic protein Mcl-1. *Am J Physiol Gastrointest Liver Physiol* 305:G786–G796.

41. Feng Y, Wang L, Zeng J, Shen L, Liang X, Yu H, Liu S, Liu Z, Sun Y, Li W, Chen C, Jia J. 2013. FoxM1 is overexpressed in *Helicobacter pylori*-induced gastric carcinogenesis and is negatively regulated by miR-370. *Mol Cancer Res* 11:834–844.

42. Zhu Y, Jiang Q, Lou X, Ji X, Wen Z, Wu J, Tao H, Jiang T, He W, Wang C, Du Q, Zheng S, Mao J, Huang J. 2012. MicroRNAs up-regulated by CagA of *Helicobacter pylori* induce intestinal metaplasia of gastric epithelial cells. *PLoS One* 7:e35147.

43. Chu YX, Wang WH, Dai Y, Teng GG, Wang SJ. 2014. Esophageal *Helicobacter pylori* colonization aggravates esophageal injury caused by reflux. *World J Gastroenterol* 20:15715–15726.

44. Liu FX, Wang WH, Wang J, Li J, Gao PP. 2011. Effect of *Helicobacter pylori* infection on Barrett's esophagus and esophageal adenocarcinoma formation in a rat model of chronic gastroesophageal reflux. *Helicobacter* 16:66–77.

45. Teng G, Dai Y, Chu Y, Li J, Zhang H, Wu T, Shuai X, Wang W. 2018. *Helicobacter pylori* induces caudal-type homeobox protein 2 and cyclooxygenase 2 expression by modulating microRNAs in esophageal epithelial cells. *Cancer Sci* 109:297–307.

46. Belair C, Baud J, Chabas S, Sharma CM, Vogel J, Staedel C, Darfeuille F. 2011. *Helicobacter pylori* interferes with an embryonic stem cell micro RNA cluster to block cell cycle progression. *Silence* 2:7.

47. Wang F, Liu J, Zou Y, Jiao Y, Huang Y, Fan L, Li X, Yu H, He C, Wei W, Wang H, Sun G. 2017. MicroRNA-143-3p, up-regulated in *H. pylori*-positive gastric cancer, suppresses tumor growth, migration and invasion by directly targeting AKT2. *Oncotarget* 8:28711–28724.

48. Fassi Fehri L, Koch M, Belogolova E, Khalil H, Bolz C, Kalali B, Mollenkopf HJ, Beigier-Bompadre M, Karlas A, Schneider T, Churin Y, Gerhard M, Meyer TF. 2010. *Helicobacter pylori* induces miR-155 in T cells in a cAMP-Foxp3-dependent manner. *PLoS One* 5:e9500.

49. Koch M, Mollenkopf HJ, Klemm U, Meyer TF. 2012. Induction of microRNA-155 is TLR- and type IV secretion system-dependent in macrophages and inhibits DNA-damage induced apoptosis. *Proc Natl Acad Sci U S A* 109:E1153–E1162.

50. Lario S, Ramírez-Lázaro MJ, Aransay AM, Lozano JJ, Montserrat A, Casalots Á, Junquera F, Álvarez J, Segura F, Campo R, Calvet X. 2012. microRNA profiling in duodenal ulcer disease caused by *Helicobacter pylori* infection in a Western population. *Clin Microbiol Infect* 18:E273–E282.

51. Oertli M, Engler DB, Kohler E, Koch M, Meyer TF, Müller A. 2011. MicroRNA-155 is essential for the T cell-mediated control of *Helicobacter pylori* infection and for the induction of chronic gastritis and colitis. *J Immunol* 187:3578–3586.

52. Xiao B, Liu Z, Li BS, Tang B, Li W, Guo G, Shi Y, Wang F, Wu Y, Tong WD, Guo H, Mao XH, Zou QM. 2009. Induction of microRNA-155 during *Helicobacter pylori* infection and its negative regulatory role in the inflammatory response. *J Infect Dis* 200:916–925.

53. Pachathundikandi SK, Backert S. 2018. *Helicobacter pylori* controls NLRP3 expression by regulating hsa-miR-223-3p and IL-10 in cultured and primary human immune cells. *Innate Immun* 24:11–23.

54. Li N, Xu X, Xiao B, Zhu ED, Li BS, Liu Z, Tang B, Zou QM, Liang HP, Mao XH. 2012. *H. pylori* related proinflammatory cytokines contribute to the induction of miR-146a in human gastric epithelial cells. *Mol Biol Rep* 39:4655–4661.

55. Liu Z, Wang D, Hu Y, Zhou G, Zhu C, Yu Q, Chi Y, Cao Y, Jia C, Zou Q. 2013. MicroRNA-146a negatively regulates PTGS2 expression induced by *Helicobacter pylori* in human gastric epithelial cells. *J Gastroenterol* 48:86–92.

56. Liu Z, Xiao B, Tang B, Li B, Li N, Zhu E, Guo G, Gu J, Zhuang Y, Liu X, Ding H, Zhao X, Guo H, Mao X, Zou Q. 2010. Up-regulated microRNA-146a negatively modulate *Helicobacter pylori*-induced inflammatory response in human gastric epithelial cells. *Microbes Infect* 12:854–863.

57. Teng GG, Wang WH, Dai Y, Wang SJ, Chu YX, Li J. 2013. Let-7b is involved in the inflammation and immune responses associated with *Helicobacter pylori* infection by targeting Toll-like receptor 4. *PLoS One* 8: e56709.

58. Matsushima K, Isomoto H, Inoue N, Nakayama T, Hayashi T, Nakayama M, Nakao K, Hirayama T, Kohno S. 2011. MicroRNA signatures in *Helicobacter pylori*-infected gastric mucosa. *Int J Cancer* 128: 361–370.

59. Xie G, Li W, Li R, Wu K, Zhao E, Zhang Y, Zhang P, Shi L, Wang D, Yin Y, Deng R, Tao K. 2017. *Helicobacter pylori* promote B7-H1 expression by suppressing miR-152 and miR-200b in gastric cancer cells. *PLoS One* 12:e0168822.

60. Chen J, Li G, Meng H, Fan Y, Song Y, Wang S, Zhu F, Guo C, Zhang L, Shi Y. 2012. Upregulation of B7-H1 expression is associated with macrophage infiltration in hepatocellular carcinomas. *Cancer Immunol Immunother* 61:101–108.

61. Pagliari M, Munari F, Toffoletto M, Lonardi S, Chemello F, Codolo G, Millino C, Della Bella C, Pacchioni B, Vermi W, Fassan M, de Bernard M, Cagnin S. 2017. *Helicobacter pylori* affects the antigen presentation activity of macrophages modulating the expression of the immune receptor CD300E through miR-4270. *Front Immunol* 8:1288.

62. Tang B, Li N, Gu J, Zhuang Y, Li Q, Wang HG, Fang Y, Yu B, Zhang JY, Xie QH, Chen L, Jiang XJ, Xiao B, Zou QM, Mao XH. 2012. Compromised autophagy by MIR30B benefits the intracellular survival of *Helicobacter pylori*. *Autophagy* 8:1045–1057.

63. Yang XJ, Si RH, Liang YH, Ma BQ, Jiang ZB, Wang B, Gao P. 2016. Mir-30d increases intracellular survival of *Helicobacter pylori* through inhibition of autophagy pathway. *World J Gastroenterol* 22:3978–3991.

64. Zhang YM, Noto JM, Hammond CE, Barth JL, Argraves WS, Backert S, Peek RM Jr, Smolka AJ. 2014. *Helicobacter pylori*-induced posttranscriptional regulation of H-K-ATPase α-subunit gene expression by miRNA. *Am J Physiol Gastrointest Liver Physiol* 306: G606–G613.

65. Abdalla AE, Duan X, Deng W, Zeng J, Xie J. 2016. MicroRNAs play big roles in modulating macrophages

response toward mycobacteria infection. *Infect Genet Evol* 45:378–382.

66. Ghorpade DS, Leyland R, Kurowska-Stolarska M, Patil SA, Balaji KN. 2012. MicroRNA-155 is required for *Mycobacterium bovis* BCG-mediated apoptosis of macrophages. *Mol Cell Biol* 32:2239–2253.

67. Kumar R, Halder P, Sahu SK, Kumar M, Kumari M, Jana K, Ghosh Z, Sharma P, Kundu M, Basu J. 2012. Identification of a novel role of ESAT-6-dependent miR-155 induction during infection of macrophages with *Mycobacterium tuberculosis*. *Cell Microbiol* 14:1620–1631.

68. Das K, Saikolappan S, Dhandayuthapani S. 2013. Differential expression of miRNAs by macrophages infected with virulent and avirulent *Mycobacterium tuberculosis*. *Tuberculosis (Edinb)* 93(Suppl):S47–S50.

69. Ahluwalia PK, Pandey RK, Sehajpal PK, Prajapati VK. 2017. Perturbed microRNA expression by *Mycobacterium tuberculosis* promotes macrophage polarization leading to pro-survival foam cell. *Front Immunol* 8:107.

70. Etna MP, Sinigaglia A, Grassi A, Giacomini E, Romagnoli A, Pardini M, Severa M, Cruciani M, Rizzo F, Anastasiadou E, Di Camillo B, Barzon L, Fimia GM, Manganelli R, Coccia EM. 2018. *Mycobacterium tuberculosis*-induced miR-155 subverts autophagy by targeting ATG3 in human dendritic cells. *PLoS Pathog* 14:e1006790.

71. Huang J, Jiao J, Xu W, Zhao H, Zhang C, Shi Y, Xiao Z. 2015. MiR-155 is upregulated in patients with active tuberculosis and inhibits apoptosis of monocytes by targeting FOXO3. *Mol Med Rep* 12:7102–7108.

72. Qin Y, Wang Q, Zhou Y, Duan Y, Gao Q. 2016. Inhibition of IFN-γ-induced nitric oxide dependent antimycobacterial activity by miR-155 and C/EBPβ. *Int J Mol Sci* 17:535.

73. Rajaram MV, Ni B, Morris JD, Brooks MN, Carlson TK, Bakthavachalu B, Schoenberg DR, Torrelles JB, Schlesinger LS. 2011. *Mycobacterium tuberculosis* lipomannan blocks TNF biosynthesis by regulating macrophage MAPK-activated protein kinase 2 (MK2) and microRNA miR-125b. *Proc Natl Acad Sci U S A* 108:17408–17413.

74. Rothchild AC, Sissons JR, Shafiani S, Plaisier C, Min D, Mai D, Gilchrist M, Peschon J, Larson RP, Bergthaler A, Baliga NS, Urdahl KB, Aderem A. 2016. MiR-155-regulated molecular network orchestrates cell fate in the innate and adaptive immune response to *Mycobacterium tuberculosis*. *Proc Natl Acad Sci U S A* 113:E6172–E6181.

75. Sharbati J, Lewin A, Kutz-Lohroff B, Kamal E, Einspanier R, Sharbati S. 2011. Integrated microRNA-mRNA-analysis of human monocyte derived macrophages upon *Mycobacterium avium* subsp. *hominissuis* infection. *PLoS One* 6:e20258.

76. Wang J, Yang K, Zhou L, Minhaowu, Wu Y, Zhu M, Lai X, Chen T, Feng L, Li M, Huang C, Zhong Q, Huang X. 2013. MicroRNA-155 promotes autophagy to eliminate intracellular mycobacteria by targeting Rheb. *PLoS Pathog* 9:e1003697.

77. Yang S, Li F, Jia S, Zhang K, Jiang W, Shang Y, Chang K, Deng S, Chen M. 2015. Early secreted antigen ESAT-6 of *Mycobacterium tuberculosis* promotes apoptosis of macrophages via targeting the microRNA155-SOCS1 interaction. *Cell Physiol Biochem* 35:1276–1288.

78. Liang S, Song Z, Wu Y, Gao Y, Gao M, Liu F, Wang F, Zhang Y. 2018. MicroRNA-27b modulates inflammatory response and apoptosis during *Mycobacterium tuberculosis* infection. *J Immunol* 200:3506–3518.

79. Kumar M, Sahu SK, Kumar R, Subuddhi A, Maji RK, Jana K, Gupta P, Raffetseder J, Lerm M, Ghosh Z, van Loo G, Beyaert R, Gupta UD, Kundu M, Basu J. 2015. MicroRNA let-7 modulates the immune response to *Mycobacterium tuberculosis* infection via control of A20, an inhibitor of the NF-κB pathway. *Cell Host Microbe* 17:345–356.

80. Dorhoi A, Iannaccone M, Farinacci M, Faé KC, Schreiber J, Moura-Alves P, Nouailles G, Mollenkopf HJ, Oberbeck-Müller D, Jörg S, Heinemann E, Hahnke K, Löwe D, Del Nonno F, Goletti D, Capparelli R, Kaufmann SH. 2013. MicroRNA-223 controls susceptibility to tuberculosis by regulating lung neutrophil recruitment. *J Clin Invest* 123:4836–4848.

81. Bettencourt P, Marion S, Pires D, Santos LF, Lastrucci C, Carmo N, Blake J, Benes V, Griffiths G, Neyrolles O, Lugo-Villarino G, Anes E. 2013. Actin-binding protein regulation by microRNAs as a novel microbial strategy to modulate phagocytosis by host cells: the case of N-Wasp and miR-142-3p. *Front Cell Infect Microbiol* 3:19.

82. Liu PT, Wheelwright M, Teles R, Komisopoulou E, Edfeldt K, Ferguson B, Mehta MD, Vazirnia A, Rea TH, Sarno EN, Graeber TG, Modlin RL. 2012. MicroRNA-21 targets the vitamin D-dependent antimicrobial pathway in leprosy. *Nat Med* 18:267–273.

83. Fu Y, Yi Z, Wu X, Li J, Xu F. 2011. Circulating microRNAs in patients with active pulmonary tuberculosis. *J Clin Microbiol* 49:4246–4251.

84. Kleinsteuber K, Heesch K, Schattling S, Kohns M, Sander-Jülch C, Walzl G, Hesseling A, Mayatepek E, Fleischer B, Marx FM, Jacobsen M. 2013. Decreased expression of miR-21, miR-26a, miR-29a, and miR-142-3p in CD4+ T cells and peripheral blood from tuberculosis patients. *PLoS One* 8:e61609.

85. Ma F, Xu S, Liu X, Zhang Q, Xu X, Liu M, Hua M, Li N, Yao H, Cao X. 2011. The microRNA miR-29 controls innate and adaptive immune responses to intracellular bacterial infection by targeting interferon-γ. *Nat Immunol* 12:861–869.

86. Wang Q, Liu S, Tang Y, Liu Q, Yao Y. 2014. MPT64 protein from *Mycobacterium tuberculosis* inhibits apoptosis of macrophages through NF-kB-miRNA21-Bcl-2 pathway. *PLoS One* 9:e100949.

87. Liu Y, Jiang J, Wang X, Zhai F, Cheng X. 2013. miR-582-5p is upregulated in patients with active tuberculosis and inhibits apoptosis of monocytes by targeting FOXO1. *PLoS One* 8:e78381.

88. Lou J, Wang Y, Zhang Z, Qiu W. 2017. MiR-20b inhibits mycobacterium tuberculosis induced inflammation in the lung of mice through targeting NLRP3. *Exp Cell Res* 358:120–128.

89. Jo EK, Yuk JM, Shin DM, Sasakawa C. 2013. Roles of autophagy in elimination of intracellular bacterial pathogens. *Front Immunol* 4:97.

90. Kumar R, Sahu SK, Kumar M, Jana K, Gupta P, Gupta UD, Kundu M, Basu J. 2016. MicroRNA 17-5p regulates autophagy in *Mycobacterium tuberculosis*-infected macrophages by targeting Mcl-1 and STAT3. *Cell Microbiol* 18:679–691.

91. Duan X, Zhang T, Ding S, Wei J, Su C, Liu H, Xu G. 2015. microRNA-17-5p modulates bacille Calmette-Guerin growth in RAW264.7 cells by targeting ULK1. *PLoS One* 10:e0138011.

92. Chen Z, Wang T, Liu Z, Zhang G, Wang J, Feng S, Liang J. 2015. Inhibition of autophagy by MiR-30A induced by *Mycobacteria tuberculosis* as a possible mechanism of immune escape in human macrophages. *Jpn J Infect Dis* 68:420–424.

93. Kim JK, Yuk JM, Kim SY, Kim TS, Jin HS, Yang CS, Jo EK. 2015. MicroRNA-125a inhibits autophagy activation and antimicrobial responses during mycobacterial infection. *J Immunol* 194:5355–5365.

94. Ouimet M, Koster S, Sakowski E, Ramkhelawon B, van Solingen C, Oldebeken S, Karunakaran D, Portal-Celhay C, Sheedy FJ, Ray TD, Cecchini K, Zamore PD, Rayner KJ, Marcel YL, Philips JA, Moore KJ. 2016. *Mycobacterium tuberculosis* induces the miR-33 locus to reprogram autophagy and host lipid metabolism. *Nat Immunol* 17:677–686.

95. Liu F, Chen J, Wang P, Li H, Zhou Y, Liu H, Liu Z, Zheng R, Wang L, Yang H, Cui Z, Wang F, Huang X, Wang J, Sha W, Xiao H, Ge B. 2018. MicroRNA-27a controls the intracellular survival of *Mycobacterium tuberculosis* by regulating calcium-associated autophagy. *Nat Commun* 9:4295.

96. Kim JK, Lee HM, Park KS, Shin DM, Kim TS, Kim YS, Suh HW, Kim SY, Kim IS, Kim JM, Son JW, Sohn KM, Jung SS, Chung C, Han SB, Yang CS, Jo EK. 2017. MIR144* inhibits antimicrobial responses against *Mycobacterium tuberculosis* in human monocytes and macrophages by targeting the autophagy protein DRAM2. *Autophagy* 13:423–441.

97. Guo L, Zhou L, Gao Q, Zhang A, Wei J, Hong D, Chu Y, Duan X, Zhang Y, Xu G. 2017. MicroRNA-144-3p inhibits autophagy activation and enhances bacillus Calmette-Guérin infection by targeting ATG4a in RAW264.7 macrophage cells. *PLoS One* 12:e0179772.

98. Guo L, Zhao J, Qu Y, Yin R, Gao Q, Ding S, Zhang Y, Wei J, Xu G. 2016. microRNA-20a inhibits autophagic process by targeting ATG7 and ATG16L1 and favors mycobacterial survival in macrophage cells. *Front Cell Infect Microbiol* 6:134.

99. Wang J, Hussain T, Yue R, Liao Y, Li Q, Yao J, Song Y, Sun X, Wang N, Xu L, Sreevatsan S, Zhao D, Zhou X. 2018. MicroRNA-199a inhibits cellular autophagy and downregulates IFN-β expression by targeting TBK1 in *Mycobacterium bovis* infected cells. *Front Cell Infect Microbiol* 8:238.

100. Vegh P, Magee DA, Nalpas NC, Bryan K, McCabe MS, Browne JA, Conlon KM, Gordon SV, Bradley DG, MacHugh DE, Lynn DJ. 2015. MicroRNA profiling of the bovine alveolar macrophage response to *Mycobacterium bovis* infection suggests pathogen survival is enhanced by microRNA regulation of endocytosis and lysosome trafficking. *Tuberculosis (Edinb)* 95:60–67.

101. Sahu SK, Kumar M, Chakraborty S, Banerjee SK, Kumar R, Gupta P, Jana K, Gupta UD, Ghosh Z, Kundu M, Basu J. 2017. MicroRNA 26a (miR-26a)/KLF4 and CREB-C/EBPβ regulate innate immune signaling, the polarization of macrophages and the trafficking of *Mycobacterium tuberculosis* to lysosomes during infection. *PLoS Pathog* 13:e1006410.

102. Pires D, Bernard EM, Pombo JP, Carmo N, Fialho C, Gutierrez MG, Bettencourt P, Anes E. 2017. *Mycobacterium tuberculosis* modulates miR-106b-5p to control cathepsin S expression resulting in higher pathogen survival and poor T-cell activation. *Front Immunol* 8:1819.

103. Cossart P. 2011. Illuminating the landscape of host-pathogen interactions with the bacterium *Listeria monocytogenes*. *Proc Natl Acad Sci U S A* 108:19484–19491.

104. Schnitger AK, Machova A, Mueller RU, Androulidaki A, Schermer B, Pasparakis M, Krönke M, Papadopoulou N. 2011. *Listeria monocytogenes* infection in macrophages induces vacuolar-dependent host miRNA response. *PLoS One* 6:e27435.

105. Lind EF, Elford AR, Ohashi PS. 2013. Micro-RNA 155 is required for optimal CD8+ T cell responses to acute viral and intracellular bacterial challenges. *J Immunol* 190:1210–1216.

106. Johnston DGW, Kearney J, Zasłona Z, Williams MA, O'Neill LAJ, Corr SC. 2017. MicroRNA-21 limits uptake of *Listeria monocytogenes* by macrophages to reduce the intracellular niche and control infection. *Front Cell Infect Microbiol* 7:201.

107. Izar B, Mannala GK, Mraheil MA, Chakraborty T, Hain T. 2012. microRNA response to *Listeria monocytogenes* infection in epithelial cells. *Int J Mol Sci* 13:1173–1185.

108. Collison A, Mattes J, Plank M, Foster PS. 2011. Inhibition of house dust mite-induced allergic airways disease by antagonism of microRNA-145 is comparable to glucocorticoid treatment. *J Allergy Clin Immunol* 128:160–167e164.

109. Witwer KW, Sisk JM, Gama L, Clements JE. 2010. MicroRNA regulation of IFN-beta protein expression: rapid and sensitive modulation of the innate immune response. *J Immunol* 184:2369–2376.

110. Dussurget O, Bierne H, Cossart P. 2014. The bacterial pathogen *Listeria monocytogenes* and the interferon family: type I, type II and type III interferons. *Front Cell Infect Microbiol* 4:50.

111. Li R, Shen Q, Wu N, He M, Liu N, Huang J, Lu B, Yao Q, Yang Y, Hu R. 2018. MiR-145 improves macrophage-mediated inflammation through targeting Arf6. *Endocrine* 60:73–82.

112. Archambaud C, Nahori MA, Soubigou G, Bécavin C, Laval L, Lechat P, Smokvina T, Langella P, Lecuit M,

Cossart P. 2012. Impact of lactobacilli on orally acquired listeriosis. *Proc Natl Acad Sci U S A* 109:16684–16689.

113. Archambaud C, Sismeiro O, Toedling J, Soubigou G, Bécavin C, Lechat P, Lebreton A, Ciaudo C, Cossart P. 2013. The intestinal microbiota interferes with the microRNA response upon oral *Listeria* infection. *MBio* 4:e00707-13.

114. Bandyopadhyay S, Long ME, Allen LA. 2014. Differential expression of microRNAs in *Francisella tularensis*-infected human macrophages: miR-155-dependent downregulation of MyD88 inhibits the inflammatory response. *PLoS One* 9:e109525.

115. Cremer TJ, Ravneberg DH, Clay CD, Piper-Hunter MG, Marsh CB, Elton TS, Gunn JS, Amer A, Kanneganti TD, Schlesinger LS, Butchar JP, Tridandapani S. 2009. MiR-155 induction by *F. novicida* but not the virulent *F. tularensis* results in SHIP down-regulation and enhanced pro-inflammatory cytokine response. *PLoS One* 4:e8508.

116. Clare S, John V, Walker AW, Hill JL, Abreu-Goodger C, Hale C, Goulding D, Lawley TD, Mastroeni P, Frankel G, Enright AJ, Vigorito E, Dougan G. 2013. Enhanced susceptibility to *Citrobacter rodentium* infection in microRNA-155-deficient mice. *Infect Immun* 81:723–732.

117. Roy BC, Subramaniam D, Ahmed I, Jala VR, Hester CM, Greiner KA, Haribabu B, Anant S, Umar S. 2015. Role of bacterial infection in the epigenetic regulation of Wnt antagonist WIF1 by PRC2 protein EZH2. *Oncogene* 34:4519–4530.

118. Rao R, Rieder SA, Nagarkatti P, Nagarkatti M. 2014. Staphylococcal enterotoxin B-induced microRNA-155 targets SOCS1 to promote acute inflammatory lung injury. *Infect Immun* 82:2971–2979. (Erratum, 82:3986.)

119. Jingjing Z, Nan Z, Wei W, Qinghe G, Weijuan W, Peng W, Xiangpeng W. 2017. MicroRNA-24 modulates *Staphylococcus aureus*-induced macrophage polarization by suppressing CHI3L1. *Inflammation* 40:995–1005.

120. Wolcott RD, Hanson JD, Rees EJ, Koenig LD, Phillips CD, Wolcott RA, Cox SB, White JS. 2016. Analysis of the chronic wound microbiota of 2,963 patients by 16S rDNA pyrosequencing. *Wound Repair Regen* 24: 163–174.

121. Ramirez HA, Pastar I, Jozic I, Stojadinovic O, Stone RC, Ojeh N, Gil J, Davis SC, Kirsner RS, Tomic-Canic M. 2018. *Staphylococcus aureus* triggers induction of miR-15B-5P to diminish DNA repair and deregulate inflammatory response in diabetic foot ulcers. *J Invest Dermatol* 138:1187–1196.

122. Tanaka K, Kim SE, Yano H, Matsumoto G, Ohuchida R, Ishikura Y, Araki M, Araki K, Park S, Komatsu T, Hayashi H, Ikematsu K, Tanaka K, Hirano A, Martin P, Shimokawa I, Mori R. 2017. MiR-142 is required for *Staphylococcus aureus* clearance at skin wound sites via small GTPase-mediated regulation of the neutrophil actin cytoskeleton. *J Invest Dermatol* 137:931–940.

123. de Kerckhove M, Tanaka K, Umehara T, Okamoto M, Kanematsu S, Hayashi H, Yano H, Nishiura S, Tooyama S, Matsubayashi Y, Komatsu T, Park S, Okada Y, Takahashi R, Kawano Y, Hanawa T,

Iwasaki K, Nozaki T, Torigoe H, Ikematsu K, Suzuki Y, Tanaka K, Martin P, Shimokawa I, Mori R. 2018. Targeting *miR-223* in neutrophils enhances the clearance of *Staphylococcus aureus* in infected wounds. *EMBO Mol Med* 10:e9024.

124. Zhou X, Li X, Ye Y, Zhao K, Zhuang Y, Li Y, Wei Y, Wu M. 2014. MicroRNA-302b augments host defense to bacteria by regulating inflammatory responses via feedback to TLR/IRAK4 circuits. *Nat Commun* 5:3619. (Erratum, 6:8679.)

125. Eledge MR, Yeruva L. 2018. Host and pathogen interface: microRNAs are modulators of disease outcome. *Microbes Infect* 20:410–415.

126. Derrick T, Roberts C, Rajasekhar M, Burr SE, Joof H, Makalo P, Bailey RL, Mabey DC, Burton MJ, Holland MJ. 2013. Conjunctival MicroRNA expression in inflammatory trachomatous scarring. *PLoS Negl Trop Dis* 7:e2117.

127. Chowdhury SR, Reimer A, Sharan M, Kozjak-Pavlovic V, Eulalio A, Prusty BK, Fraunholz M, Karunakaran K, Rudel T. 2017. *Chlamydia* preserves the mitochondrial network necessary for replication via microRNA-dependent inhibition of fission. *J Cell Biol* 216:1071–1089.

128. Arkatkar T, Gupta R, Li W, Yu JJ, Wali S, Neal Guentzel M, Chambers JP, Christenson LK, Arulanandam BP. 2015. Murine MicroRNA-214 regulates intracellular adhesion molecule (ICAM1) gene expression in genital *Chlamydia muridarum* infection. *Immunology* 145:534–542.

129. Gupta R, Arkatkar T, Keck J, Koundinya GK, Castillo K, Hobel S, Chambers JP, Yu JJ, Guentzel MN, Aigner A, Christenson LK, Arulanandam BP. 2016. Antigen specific immune response in *Chlamydia muridarum* genital infection is dependent on murine microRNAs-155 and -182. *Oncotarget* 7:64726–64742.

130. Gupta R, Arkatkar T, Yu JJ, Wali S, Haskins WE, Chambers JP, Murthy AK, Bakar SA, Guentzel MN, Arulanandam BP. 2015. *Chlamydia muridarum* infection associated host MicroRNAs in the murine genital tract and contribution to generation of host immune response. *Am J Reprod Immunol* 73:126–140.

131. Yeruva L, Pouncey DL, Eledge MR, Bhattacharya S, Luo C, Weatherford EW, Ojcius DM, Rank RG. 2016. MicroRNAs modulate pathogenesis resulting from chlamydial infection in mice. *Infect Immun* 85:e00768-16.

132. Zheng K, Chen DS, Wu YQ, Xu XJ, Zhang H, Chen CF, Chen HC, Liu ZF. 2012. MicroRNA expression profile in RAW264.7 cells in response to *Brucella melitensis* infection. *Int J Biol Sci* 8:1013–1022.

133. Liu N, Wang L, Sun C, Yang L, Sun W, Peng Q. 2016. MicroRNA-125b-5p suppresses *Brucella abortus* intracellular survival via control of A20 expression. *BMC Microbiol* 16:171.

134. Luo X, Zhang X, Wu X, Yang X, Han C, Wang Z, Du Q, Zhao X, Liu SL, Tong D, Huang Y. 2018. *Brucella* downregulates tumor necrosis factor-α to promote intracellular survival via Omp25 regulation of different MicroRNAs in porcine and murine macrophages. *Front Immunol* 8:2013.

135. **Sunkavalli U, Aguilar C, Silva RJ, Sharan M, Cruz AR, Tawk C, Maudet C, Mano M, Eulalio A.** 2017. Analysis of host microRNA function uncovers a role for miR-29b-2-5p in *Shigella* capture by filopodia. *PLoS Pathog* **13**:e1006327.

136. **Kotloff KL, Riddle MS, Platts-Mills JA, Pavlinac P, Zaidi AKM.** 2018. Shigellosis. *Lancet* **391**:801–812.

137. **Siddle KJ, Tailleux L, Deschamps M, Loh YH, Deluen C, Gicquel B, Antoniewski C, Barreiro LB, Farinelli L, Quintana-Murci L.** 2015. Bacterial infection drives the expression dynamics of microRNAs and their isomiRs. *PLoS Genet* **11**:e1005064.

138. **Faridani OR, Abdullayev I, Hagemann-Jensen M, Schell JP, Lanner F, Sandberg R.** 2016. Single-cell sequencing of the small-RNA transcriptome. *Nat Biotechnol* **34**: 1264–1266.

139. **Dalmasso G, Nguyen HT, Yan Y, Laroui H, Charania MA, Ayyadurai S, Sitaraman SV, Merlin D.** 2011. Microbiota modulate host gene expression via microRNAs. *PLoS One* **6**:e19293.

140. **Singh N, Shirdel EA, Waldron L, Zhang RH, Jurisica I, Comelli EM.** 2012. The murine caecal microRNA signature depends on the presence of the endogenous microbiota. *Int J Biol Sci* **8**:171–186.

141. **Liu S, da Cunha AP, Rezende RM, Cialic R, Wei Z, Bry L, Comstock LE, Gandhi R, Weiner HL.** 2016. The host shapes the gut microbiota via fecal MicroRNA. *Cell Host Microbe* **19**:32–43.

Bacteria and Intracellularity
Edited by Pascale Cossart, Craig R. Roy, and Philippe Sansonetti
© 2019 American Society for Microbiology, Washington, DC
doi:10.1128/microbiolspec.BAI-0012-2019

Modulation of Host Cell Metabolism by *Chlamydia trachomatis*

18

Marion Rother,[1,2,3] Ana Rita Teixeira da Costa,[3] Rike Zietlow,[3] Thomas F. Meyer,[3] and Thomas Rudel[4]

INTRODUCTION

The human obligate intracellular pathogen *Chlamydia trachomatis* is the most frequent cause of sexually transmitted bacterial infection, with over 130 million cases per year (1). *C. trachomatis* causes blinding trachoma and pelvic inflammatory disease, the latter being causally connected with infertility and ectopic pregnancy (2, 3). Pelvic inflammatory disease has further been linked to the occurrence of ovarian cancer (4); likewise, direct associations of *C. trachomatis* to ovarian and cervical carcinoma have been reported (5–7).

Uncomplicated *C. trachomatis* infections are treatable with antibiotics (azithromycin, doxycycline). However, while initially often asymptomatic, *C. trachomatis* infections frequently turn into a chronic state that is refractory to antibiotic treatment. Reinfections are common, as are relapses, due to the inability of antibiotics to completely eradicate bacteria under persistent infection conditions, leading to severe chronic pathology. The therapeutic failure is estimated to be ~10% (1). Since such chronic *C. trachomatis* infections are very difficult to treat with conventional antibiotic regimens, there is an urgency for the development of therapeutics with improved efficacy.

The complex life cycle of *C. trachomatis* is divided into two stages. Elementary bodies (EBs) represent the infectious form, which is adapted for survival outside the host cell due to a highly condensed nucleoid and a rigid cell wall. Once attached to the host cell, *C. trachomatis* translocates Tarp (translocated actin-recruiting phosphoprotein) into the cell, which mediates actin rearrangement to facilitate EB entry via phagocytosis. Further, *C. trachomatis* proteins drive the conversion of the developing phagocytic compartment into a replicative niche, termed inclusion, inside of which EBs differentiate into the replicative reticulate bodies (RBs) (8–11). RBs undergo several rounds of replication before differentiating back into EBs, which are finally released from the host cell, by extrusion or cell lysis, to start a new round of infection (12–14).

The success of *C. trachomatis* is based on superb adaptation to its host, from which it obtains nucleotides, amino acids, lipids, iron, and additional nutrients (8, 15). During evolution, its exclusive intracellular lifestyle has enabled *C. trachomatis* to minimize its genome size, thereby becoming strictly dependent on its host. For replication, *C. trachomatis* depends entirely on the supply of nutrients from the host cytoplasm. If metabolic provision is suboptimal, e.g., during tryptophan starvation, it can slow down its developmental cycle and halt replication, resulting in the formation of so-called aberrant bodies, which can persist for prolonged periods inside an inclusion (16–18). Evolving strategies that enable efficient capture of almost all required metabolites from the host cytoplasm thus allowed *C. trachomatis* to reduce its genome to 1.04 Mb, containing ~894 tentative protein-coding sequences (19). In addition, some isolates harbor an extrachromosomal plasmid of 7 kb, which contains 8 coding sequences. Because *C. trachomatis* cannot replicate outside host cells, manipulating the chlamydial genome has been inherently difficult, and the biological functions of these plasmid-encoded genes have not been conclusively assigned. Nonetheless, it has been shown that the development of *C. trachomatis* is accompanied by shifts in gene expression, with early genes expressed upon host cell entry,

[1]Steinbeis Innovation Center for Systems Biomedicine, 14612 Berlin-Falkensee, Germany; [2]Institute of Experimental Internal Medicine, Otto von Guericke University Magdeburg, 39120 Magdeburg, Germany; [3]Max Planck Institute for Infection Biology, Department of Molecular Biology, 10117 Berlin, Germany; [4]Department of Microbiology, Biocenter, University of Wuerzburg, 97074 Wuerzburg, Germany.

followed about 18 h later by activation of mid-cycle genes that encode structural and intermediary metabolism genes, followed by late genes transcribed by a second form of RNA polymerase containing an alternative sigma factor (11, 20–22).

Entry of host metabolites into the inclusion is mediated through active transporters located in the inclusion membrane and potentially also via passive diffusion of molecules smaller than 520 daltons, such as sugars, amino acids, and nucleotides (23). In addition, *C. trachomatis* obtains lipids by vesicular and nonvesicular trafficking from the endoplasmic reticulum, the Golgi apparatus, multivesicular bodies, and lipid droplets (24, 25).

GLOBAL CHANGES IN HOST CELL METABOLISM

It has become increasingly clear that to ensure its survival, *C. trachomatis* does not merely take up available metabolites from the host cell; instead, it actively modulates the host metabolism to optimize the supply of required nutrients. However, so far, few studies have attempted to gain a comprehensive understanding of the metabolic changes induced in host cells or the host pathways required to support *C. trachomatis* development. In a recent study to identify host factors that are essential for successful *C. trachomatis* growth, Rother et al. (26) carried out a genome-wide RNA interference screen targeting 23,000 human genes. Three days after transfection with small interfering RNAs (siRNAs), HeLa cells were infected with *C. trachomatis* for 2 days. Infectious progeny was then assessed by titrating the lysate onto fresh cells and quantifying the formation of inclusions. In a subsequent validation screen with four independent siRNAs per gene, 171 hits were confirmed as high-confidence host factors that are essential for *C. trachomatis* infection and propagation. Using gene ontology, these genes were classified according to the biological processes they participate in, revealing that 113 of them had a known role in metabolic processes (Fig. 1), including several human enzymes involved in the regulation of energy and precursor metabolites of the central carbon metabolism, as well as biosynthesis of guanosine-containing compounds. These findings confirmed the extensive dependence of *C. trachomatis* on host metabolites to meet its energy requirements and the supply of biosynthetic substrates required to fuel bacterial growth and replication. Importantly, this study revealed which specific host genes and isoforms—while being essential for *C. trachomatis* infection—are dispensable for the host cells, at least for the period of interference, and thus could be blocked without

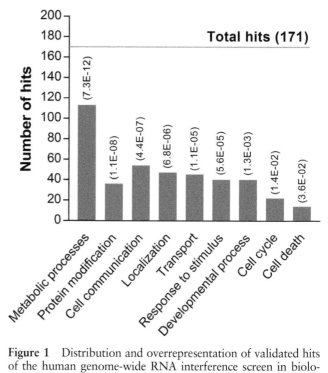

Figure 1 Distribution and overrepresentation of validated hits of the human genome-wide RNA interference screen in biological processes of the host cell. Numbers in parentheses indicate the *p* values for each overrepresented biological process (determined with the PANTHER Overrepresentation Test).

displaying cytotoxic effects. The identified targets therefore represent candidates for pharmacological intervention to block *C. trachomatis* infection.

CARBOHYDRATE METABOLISM

Chlamydia

C. trachomatis contains a number of genes that can potentially drive a minimal electron transport chain through oxidative phosphorylation, which may serve to fuel transport processes dependent on electrochemical membrane potential (27). The nonreplicative, extracellular EBs utilize *de novo* protein synthesis and generate ATP by converting glucose-6-phosphate (G6P) to pyruvate via glycolysis. Several studies have shown that along with their metabolic activity, the gene expression profile of the replicative RBs is substantially different, because they are unable to meet the increased energy demands by ATP synthesis during their replication. ATP generation therefore requires supplementation by direct import from the host cell, rendering RBs entirely dependent on host-derived ATP as an energy source (27–30).

Insight into *C. trachomatis*'s restricted metabolic activity has been gleaned from analysis of its genome and experimental observations (19, 30–32) (Fig. 2A). *C. tra-*

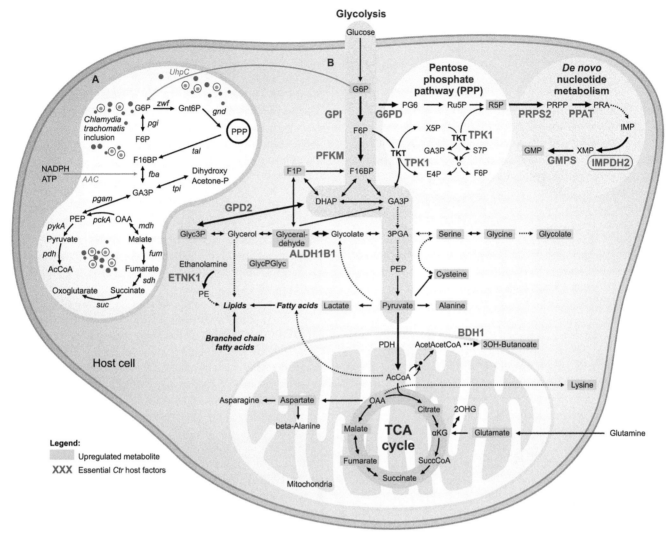

Figure 2 Pathway map representing modulated metabolites and related host factors essential for *C. trachomatis* (*Ctr*) infection. See text for explanation. Abbreviations for metabolites: 2OHG, 2-hydroxyglutarate; 3OH-butanoate, D-3-hydroxybutyrate; 3PGA, 3-phosphoglyceric acid; AcCoA, acetyl coenzyme A; AcetAcetCoA, acetoacetyl-CoA; aKg, alpha-ketoglutaric acid; DHAP, dihydroxyacetone phosphate; E4P, erythrose 4-phosphate; F16BP, fructose-1-6-bisphosphate; F6P, fructose-6-phosphate; G6P, glucose-6-phosphate; GA3P, glyceraldehyde 3-phosphate; Glyc3P, glycerol-3-phosphate; GlycPGlyc, glycerophosphoglycerol; GMP, guanosine monophosphate; IMP, inosine monophosphate; OAA, oxaloacetic acid; PE, phosphatidylethanolamine; PEP, phosphoenolpyruvate; PG6, phosphogluconolactone; PRA, 5′-phosphoribosylamine; PRPP, 5-phospho-D-ribose α-1-pyrophosphate; R5P, ribose-5-phosphate; Ru5P, ribulose-5-phosphate; S7P, D-sedo heptulose 7-P; SuccCoA, succinyl coenzyme A; X5P, xylulose 5-phosphate; XMP, xanthine monophosphate. RNA interference screen hits: ALDH1B1, aldehyde dehydrogenase 1 family member B1; BDH1, 3-hydroxybutyrate dehydrogenase, type 1; ETNK1, ethanolamine kinase 1; G6PD, glucose-6-phosphate dehydrogenase; GMPS, guanosine monophosphate synthetase; GPD2, mitochondrial glycerol-3-phosphate dehydrogenase; GPI, glucose-6-phosphate isomerase; IMPDH2, inosine-5′-monophosphate dehydrogenase 2; PDH, pyruvate dehydrogenase; PDK2, pyruvate dehydrogenase kinase isoform 2; PFKM, 6-phosphofructokinase; PPAT, phosphoribosyl pyrophosphate amidotransferase; PRPS2, phosphoribosyl pyrophosphate synthetase 2; TKT, transketolase; TPK1, thiamine pyrophosphokinase 1. Chlamydial metabolic genes: *AAC*, ATP/ADP translocase; *fba*, fructose 1,6-bisphosphate aldolase; *fum*, fumarate hydratase; *gnd*, 6-phosphogluconate dehydrogenase; *mdh*, malate dehydrogenase; *pdh*, pyruvate dehydrogenase; *pgam*, phosphoglycerate mutase; *pgi*, glucose-6-phosphate isomerase; *pykA*, pyruvate kinase; *sdh*, succinate dehydrogenase; *suc*, succinyl-CoA ligase; *UhpC*, G6P transporter; *tal*, transaldolase; *tpi*, triosephosphate isomerase; *zwf*, glucose-6-phosphate 1-dehydrogenase.

chomatis lacks the gene for hexokinase, which converts glucose, the major energy source of the host cell, into G6P. G6P is taken up by *C. trachomatis* via the *C. trachomatis*-produced UhpC antiporter (27, 33) and channeled directly into the bacterial metabolism. Analysis of ^{13}C-labeled substrate has shown that the imported G6P is mainly shuttled into cell wall synthesis in RBs (32). *C. trachomatis* encodes all the enzymes required for the pentose phosphate pathway (PPP), allowing it to generate both NADPH and pentose phosphates. It also encodes a complete gluconeogenesis pathway, as well as the enzymes required for glycogen synthesis and degradation. During active replication, UDP-glucose is imported into the inclusion and converted to glycogen by chlamydial glycogen metabolic enzymes secreted from RBs into the inclusion lumen (34). Once the RBs convert to EBs, G6P becomes the central energy source. EBs obtain G6P directly from the cell or from luminal glycogen via degradation into G1P and subsequent conversion to G6P by the phosphoglucomutase MrsA. Nonetheless, experimental evidence suggests that these pathways are not fully functional: although *C. trachomatis* can grow in infected cells supplied only with glutamate, malate, 2-oxoglutarate, or oxaloacetate as the major carbon source, the replication rate is greatly reduced compared to conditions where glucose is available (35).

C. trachomatis is also capable of generating acetyl-coenzyme A (acetyl-CoA) through glycolysis and fatty acid degradation, although its incomplete tricarboxylic acid (TCA) cycle does not utilize it as a substrate (36). Instead, the TCA cycle of *C. trachomatis* appears to rely on the import of other substrates directly from the host, for example, glutamate, which is converted to oxoglutarate. *C. trachomatis* can also directly take up dicarboxylates of the TCA, such as malate, which is converted to fumarate and succinate in the bacteria (32). The TCA cycle of *C. trachomatis* is further compromised by two frame-shift mutations that result in impaired function of the succinate dehydrogenase subunit C (*SdhC*) and fumarate hydratase (*FumC*). Despite the high degree of sequence homology of some central metabolic enzymes, several of the many genes with unknown function in *C. trachomatis* may be involved in catalyzing additional metabolic reactions (27).

Host

In the wake of technological advances, new approaches to unravel metabolic host-pathogen interactions have been developed. Rother et al. (26) employed one such approach to comprehensively examine the changes in host metabolism following *C. trachomatis* infection. To obtain a detailed picture of how *C. trachomatis* infec-

tion influences the flow of metabolites from glucose, gas chromatography-mass spectrometry analysis was performed in this study to profile the central carbon metabolism upon infection. Numerous metabolites were upregulated in infected compared to noninfected cells. Figure 2B shows an interactive pathway map highlighting metabolites that were upregulated by *C. trachomatis* 48 h post-infection. Strikingly, many of the corresponding enzymes were essential host factors identified in the genome-wide siRNA screen performed in the same study. In brief, *C. trachomatis* infection caused a marked increase in G6P and relied on the host glycolytic enzymes glucose-6-phosphate isomerase and 6-phosphofructokinase for successful propagation. Further, *C. trachomatis* infection induced strong upregulation of pyruvate, lactate, and glutamate, features that are reminiscent of Warburg metabolism (37). This metabolic state is associated with high proliferative activity, as observed in cancer cells, and is characterized by increased utilization of glucose by aerobic glycolysis, resulting in the generation of lactate. In congruence, one of the mitochondrial enzymes regulating this metabolic shift, pyruvate dehydrogenase kinase 2 (PDK2), was identified as an essential host factor in the RNA interference screen. PDK2 blocks the conversion of pyruvate, the end product of glycolysis, to acetyl-coenzyme A for entry into the TCA cycle. As a result, pyruvate is converted into lactate, while at the same time more glycolytic intermediates can be shunted into the PPP to be converted into ribonucleotides. Interestingly, TCA cycle metabolites were found to increase in parallel, likely due to utilization of substrates that are not derived from glycolysis, such as glutamate, which was also found to be strongly elevated upon *C. trachomatis* infection. In fact, glucose utilization via Warburg metabolism is known to be more effective for the generation of anabolic substrates. Thus, *C. trachomatis* is capable of switching the host cell into a hypermetabolic state to meet the high metabolic demand imposed by the replicating bacteria (37). The necessity for shunting glycolytic intermediates into anabolic pathways was further confirmed by the observed upregulation of carbon flux through the PPP, which is required for the synthesis of nucleotides and serine.

In addition, four enzymes of the *de novo* nucleotide metabolism were identified as essential host factors: PRPS2 (phosphoribosyl pyrophosphate synthetase 2), PPAT (phosphoribosyl pyrophosphate amidotransferase), IMPDH2 (inosine-5′-monophosphate dehydrogenase 2), and GMPS (guanosine monophosphate synthetase). In this study, HeLa cells were chosen as a robust screenable model for *C. trachomatis* infection, allowing for strong siRNA knockdown efficiencies. Since cancer cells such as HeLa cells are known to have altered metabolic requirements, key metabolic host factors for *C. trachomatis* infection were validated in primary epithelial cells from the ectocervix. Follow-up gas chromatography-mass spectrometry experiments in primary cells from the fallopian tube confirmed the upregulation of several metabolites.

It was further evaluated if host targets essential for *C. trachomatis* infection could provide valid targets for pharmacological intervention. Based on this newly identified collection of *C. trachomatis*-relevant host factors, Rother et al. (26) performed target prioritization using databases for chemical compounds and safety profiles of selected compounds inhibiting these host targets. Thereby, IMPDH2, the rate-limiting enzyme in the *de novo* GMP biosynthesis pathway leading to GTP production, was identified as a promising therapeutic target against *C. trachomatis* infection. IMPDH2 can be specifically inhibited by the clinically approved and well-referenced compound mycophenolate mofetil (38, 39). In accordance with the known drug mechanism of mycophenolate mofetil and the fact that *C. trachomatis* specifically relies on the supply of GTP from its host, it was demonstrated that pharmacologic inhibition of IMPDH2 results in efficient blocking of *C. trachomatis* infection both in cell cultures and *in vivo* in a mouse infection model. Thus, these results provide a proof-of-concept for the validity of a host-directed approach against *C. trachomatis* infections.

MITOCHONDRIA AT THE CROSSROAD OF METABOLISM AND APOPTOSIS INHIBITION

Preventing Host Cell Apoptosis

Mitochondria are highly dynamic organelles that play a central role in energy metabolism and constitute a hub for biosynthetic processes. They are the main source of ATP production via oxidative phosphorylation and are essential in the biosynthesis of macromolecules, such as nucleotides and lipids. Beyond metabolism, mitochondria are also central in orchestrating signals for inducing or preventing cell death. Their dual function in metabolism and cell death regulation makes them primary targets for *C. trachomatis*, since its high demand for metabolites induces massive stress in the host cell, which eventually leads to the induction of apoptotic cell death as a cell autonomous defense mechanism (40). However, competition for and depletion of metabolites is not the only stress factor for infected host cells. *C. trachomatis* infection also induces the production of reactive oxygen species (ROS) in the host cell (41). ROS

cause oxidative DNA damage, producing single strand breaks, which if unrepaired, are converted to double strand breaks (42). This creates a dangerous situation for the bacteria, since ROS generally not only have anti-microbial activity but can severely damage the host cell and thereby also *C. trachomatis* growing inside it. Paradoxically, chlamydial growth and development require ROS production within the host cell (41, 43). Irrespective of the severe metabolic or oxidative stress and extensive DNA damage resulting from infection (44), *C. trachomatis*-infected cells are protected from apoptotic cell death (45, 46). Recently, an interesting connection between metabolic signaling and cell death regulation in infected cells was described. Human cells have two hexokinase isoforms, which phosphorylate glucose to G6P, the glucose derivative taken up by *C. trachomatis*. The hexokinase II isoform (HKII) is strongly upregulated during *C. trachomatis* infection via 3-phosphoinositide-dependent protein kinase-1 (PDPK1)-Myc signaling pathways and translocates to the mitochondria (47). Previous work has shown that HKII associates with the mitochondrial voltage-dependent anion channel (VDAC), an interaction that increased glycolysis and oxidative metabolism and inhibited apoptosis (48). Interestingly, interfering with the interaction between HKII and VDAC triggered apoptosis in infected cells, indicating that the HKII-mitochondria interaction is crucial for maintaining intrinsic apoptosis resistance (47). Interrupting HKII-VDAC interactions or interfering with PDPK1-Myc signaling also affected normal chlamydial development, underlining the importance of this pathway for cell death regulation and likely also metabolic adaptation of the infected cell.

The mitochondrial architecture is governed by a fine-tuned mechanism that responds to stress, nutritional deprivation, survival, and apoptotic signals (49–51). In each of these cases, the fusion and fission machinery reacts by either promoting the branching and elongation of the mitochondrial fragments or by inducing fragmentation of the network. Mitochondrial function is tightly connected to their morphology, and alterations in the mitochondrial architecture have a direct impact on their metabolic capacity and the induction of cell death (52, 53). However, not only the function but also the increase or loss of mitochondrial mass is influenced by their architecture. ROS-mediated mitochondrial fragmentation is catalyzed by Drp1-dependent mitochondrial fission, which creates smaller mitochondrial particles that can be targeted for mitophagy. Alternatively, under nutritional stress, indiscriminate autophagy may lead to organelle loss. Under such conditions, Drp1 is phosphorylated to prevent mitochondrial fragmentation, and fusion is promoted to elongate the mitochondrial fragments (54–56). However, our own studies showed that mitochondrial architecture is well preserved upon *C. trachomatis* infection, even upon challenge with excess peroxide, which normally causes severe fragmentation of mitochondria (57) (Fig. 3). This clearly points to active protection of mitochondria in infected cells.

Maintaining the Energy Supply

Besides preventing apoptosis, one of the primary reasons for *C. trachomatis* to protect the mitochondrial integrity is to ensure the supply of metabolites necessary for chlamydial development, especially ATP. By shifting the glycolytic metabolism toward anaerobic glycolysis (as outlined above), *C. trachomatis* ensures increased production of ATP. In addition, during the replication phase the bacteria compete with the host cell for G6P. However, G6P in the bacteria is mainly channeled into cell wall biosynthesis and thus is not available for ATP production via bacterial glycolysis (32). Under such conditions, *C. trachomatis* depends entirely on ATP as an energy

source from the host cell, and the supply of ATP from host cell glycolysis may not suffice under conditions of increased bacterial replication. This may be especially relevant in the nondividing epithelial cells of the urogenital tract, which like all nondividing cells generate ATP mostly via oxidative phosphorylation.

The mechanism of infection-induced stabilization of mitochondrial architecture turns out to involve the central tumor suppressor p53. In normal cells, DNA damage causes immediate activation of p53 as a vital element of the DNA damage response, which initiates DNA repair or cell death in case of severe damage. *C. trachomatis* infection can cause DNA damage (44) yet severely downregulates p53 protein levels, preventing DNA damage-induced cell death (58, 59). Intriguingly, a key function of p53 is metabolic regulation (60). As p53 represents one of the most important inhibitors of glycolysis in tumor cells, its inhibition enhances the Warburg effect. Downregulation of p53 upon *C. trachomatis* infection increases the metabolism of G6P via the host PPP—a crucial pathway for the synthesis of

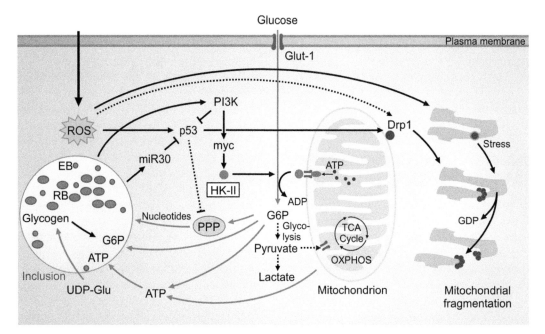

Figure 3 Regulation of glucose metabolism and mitochondrial architecture in *C. trachomatis*-infected cells. Glucose is taken up by the host cell and converted to glucose-6-P (G6P) by hexokinase II (HKII). G6P is then channeled into the PPP and increased nucleotide biosynthesis or is directly taken up by *C. trachomatis*. ATP from the host cell is directly used by *C. trachomatis* as an energy source during active replication. UDP-glucose (UDP-Glu) from the host cell is converted to glycogen in the inclusion lumen and serves as a source for G6P in the EB. PI3 kinase (PI3K)-dependent upregulation of c-Myc and PI3K/miR30-induced downregulation of p53 pathways increase glycolysis and the G6P flux to the host PPP. P53 downregulation also prevents the transcription of Drp1, the major factor involved in mitochondrial fission. Prevention of mitochondrial fragmentation preserves the ATP supply from mitochondria.

NADPH and other nucleotides required by the bacteria for their growth (59). Stabilized p53 interferes with chlamydial development, which could be overcome by artificially overexpressing the p53 target and PPP key enzyme glucose-6-phosphate dehydrogenase, demonstrating the central role p53 has in the metabolic control of infected cells.

The connection to a role of p53 in mitochondrial architecture regulation came from the investigation of host cell microRNAs that are upregulated during chlamydial infection. One of these, miR-30c, provoked severe mitochondrial fragmentation in infected cells upon experimental downregulation. p53 was identified as the critical target of miR-30c, which strongly decreases p53 protein levels in infected cells. MiR-30c modulation can deplete the mitochondrial fission regulator Drp1, since p53 is an essential transcription factor responsible for the stress-induced transcription of the Drp1 mRNA (61, 62). Drp1-mediated fission is essential not only for the healthy recycling of mitochondrial particles and mitochondrial biogenesis but also for the pre-apoptotic fragmentation of mitochondria (63–65). The presence of oxidative stress or any general pro-apoptotic stimuli promotes Drp1-dependent mitochondrial fragmentation, which is essential for the proper execution of the apoptotic cascade. Inhibition of mitochondrial fission via blockage or depletion of Drp1 stalls the release of cytochrome c and apoptotic processes (66, 67) and therefore likely supports the overall anti-apoptotic properties of C. trachomatis-infected cells.

A decrease in the fusion/fission ratio due to elevation of Drp1 leads to a fragmented mitochondrial architecture, which is less efficient in producing ATP (52, 53). Therefore, the effect of ROS generated during the growth of C. trachomatis must somehow be neutralized to maintain unrestricted production of ATP. Upon comparing the levels of ATP in cells transfected with Drp1 and p53 siRNAs and treated with H_2O_2, it was demonstrated that depletion of either protein protected the cells against the disruptive effects of H_2O_2-derived ROS on cellular ATP production. These results indicate that upregulation of miR-30c upon infection serves to partially ameliorate the effects of infection-induced oxidative stress on mitochondrial integrity and metabolism.

The involvement of signaling pathways in C. trachomatis-infected cells that are central to oncogenic transformation is intriguing. Both the pro-oncogenic c-Myc and the tumor-suppressive p53 pathway are involved in metabolic reprogramming and cell survival control. Their activation and inactivation, respectively, convert the host cell into an infection-supportive phenotype reprogrammed to provide nutrients for chlamydial replication and insensitive to pro-apoptotic signaling to survive the immense infection-induced stress. It is tempting to speculate that the evolutionary pressure put on obligate intracellular Chlamydiae to metabolically reprogram their host and render their host cells apoptosis resistant may support oncogenic transformation of the infected tissue.

CONCLUSION: EXPLOITING HOST METABOLISM CHANGES FOR HOST-DIRECTED THERAPY

Comprehensive investigation of the host determinants and targeted metabolic pathways utilized by C. trachomatis not only lends important insight into our understanding of the mechanisms underlying infections with this highly prevalent human pathogen, but it further reveals a repository of host targets that are potentially suitable for pharmacological intervention. In addition to acute infections, C. trachomatis often causes chronic infections that are refractory to conventional antibiotic treatment and lead to severe sequelae, including pelvic inflammatory disease, ectopic pregnancy, and infertility. This, taken together with the fact that C. trachomatis strictly depends on the functional contribution of the host for successful propagation, renders it an excellent candidate pathogen for the investigation of host-pathogen interactions and the development of host-directed therapies based on those interactions. Notably, host-directed therapy also offers an advantage over conventional antibiotic treatment, since drugs act in the background of the host, and thus, development of resistances is widely avoided.

High-throughput RNA interference screens are an efficient tool for the discovery of host factors that are essential for infection processes. With the identification of infection-related host factors, well-characterized and approved drugs could be used to specifically block such infection-related targets and for anti-infective treatments. The major advantages of this powerful drug repositioning strategy are the following: (i) Existing drugs, already approved for the treatment of other clinical conditions and demonstrated to be safe in late-stage clinical trials, present a significantly reduced risk for application in new clinical settings. (ii) Since repositioned drugs rely on already existing data, including efficacy and safety studies, the process of development until use in new clinical indications is significantly faster than in the de novo drug development (3 to 12 years versus 10 to 17 years). (iii) The costs of the development of a repositioned drug are significantly lower compared to the development of a new chemical entity.

So far, screening-based drug repositioning strategies have mainly been applied for viruses (68, 69). It has been shown that host factor targeting of the enzyme IMPDH2 using such a drug repositioning strategy is effective against *C. trachomatis* infection both *in vitro* and *in vivo* in a mouse infection model (26). This provided the initial proof-of-concept for the feasibility of metabolic interference as a host-directed therapeutic approach against *C. trachomatis* infections. In fact, for the treatment of chronic *C. trachomatis* infections refractory to currently available antibiotics, host-directed approaches affecting critical metabolic routes may be therapeutically beneficial, especially in combination with conventional antibiotic regimens. Future work along these lines will pave the way for a better way to treat chronically infected *C. trachomatis* patients.

Citation. Rother M, Teixeira da Costa AR, Zietlow R, Meyer TF, Rudel T. 2019. Modulation of host cell metabolism by *Chlamydia trachomatis*. Microbiol Spectrum 7(3):BAI-0012-2019.

References

1. **WHO.** 2016. *WHO guidelines for the treatment of* Chlamydia trachomatis. https://www.ncbi.nlm.nih.gov/books/NBK379707/.

2. **Cates W Jr, Wasserheit JN.** 1991. Genital chlamydial infections: epidemiology and reproductive sequelae. *Am J Obstet Gynecol* 164:1771–1781.

3. **Weström L, Joesoef R, Reynolds G, Hagdu A, Thompson SE.** 1992. Pelvic inflammatory disease and fertility. A cohort study of 1,844 women with laparoscopically verified disease and 657 control women with normal laparoscopic results. *Sex Transm Dis* 19:185–192.

4. **Lin HW, Tu YY, Lin SY, Su WJ, Lin WL, Lin WZ, Wu SC, Lai YL.** 2011. Risk of ovarian cancer in women with pelvic inflammatory disease: a population-based study. *Lancet Oncol* 12:900–904.

5. **Shanmughapriya S, Senthilkumar G, Vinodhini K, Das BC, Vasanthi N, Natarajaseenivasan K.** 2012. Viral and bacterial aetiologies of epithelial ovarian cancer. *Eur J Clin Microbiol Infect Dis* 31:2311–2317.

6. **Koskela P, Anttila T, Bjørge T, Brunsvig A, Dillner J, Hakama M, Hakulinen T, Jellum E, Lehtinen M, Lenner P, Luostarinen T, Pukkala E, Saikku P, Thoresen S, Youngman L, Paavonen J.** 2000. *Chlamydia trachomatis* infection as a risk factor for invasive cervical cancer. *Int J Cancer* 85:35–39.

7. **Zhu H, Shen Z, Luo H, Zhang W, Zhu X.** 2016. *Chlamydia trachomatis* infection-associated risk of cervical cancer: a meta-analysis. *Medicine (Baltimore)* 95:e3077.

8. **Bastidas RJ, Elwell CA, Engel JN, Valdivia RH.** 2013. Chlamydial intracellular survival strategies. *Cold Spring Harb Perspect Med* 3:a010256.

9. **Bauler LD, Hackstadt T.** 2014. Expression and targeting of secreted proteins from *Chlamydia trachomatis*. *J Bacteriol* 196:1325–1334.

10. **Elwell C, Mirrashidi K, Engel J.** 2016. *Chlamydia* cell biology and pathogenesis. *Nat Rev Microbiol* 14:385–400.

11. **Valdivia RH.** 2008. *Chlamydia* effector proteins and new insights into chlamydial cellular microbiology. *Curr Opin Microbiol* 11:53–59.

12. **Beatty WL, Morrison RP, Byrne GI.** 1994. Persistent chlamydiae: from cell culture to a paradigm for chlamydial pathogenesis. *Microbiol Rev* 58:686–699.

13. **Engel J.** 2004. Tarp and Arp: how *Chlamydia* induces its own entry. *Proc Natl Acad Sci U S A* 101:9947–9948.

14. **Matsumoto A, Manire GP.** 1970. Electron microscopic observations on the effects of penicillin on the morphology of *Chlamydia psittaci*. *J Bacteriol* 101:278–285.

15. **Saka HA, Valdivia RH.** 2010. Acquisition of nutrients by *Chlamydiae*: unique challenges of living in an intracellular compartment. *Curr Opin Microbiol* 13:4–10.

16. **Peters J, Wilson DP, Myers G, Timms P, Bavoil PM.** 2007. Type III secretion à la *Chlamydia*. *Trends Microbiol* 15:241–251.

17. **Skilton RJ, Cutcliffe LT, Barlow D, Wang Y, Salim O, Lambden PR, Clarke IN.** 2009. Penicillin induced persistence in *Chlamydia trachomatis*: high quality time lapse video analysis of the developmental cycle. *PLoS One* 4:e7723.

18. **Wang Y, Cutcliffe LT, Skilton RJ, Persson K, Bjartling C, Clarke IN.** 2013. Transformation of a plasmid-free, genital tract isolate of *Chlamydia trachomatis* with a plasmid vector carrying a deletion in CDS6 revealed that this gene regulates inclusion phenotype. *Pathog Dis* 67:100–103.

19. **Stephens RS, Kalman S, Lammel C, Fan J, Marathe R, Aravind L, Mitchell W, Olinger L, Tatusov RL, Zhao Q, Koonin EV, Davis RW.** 1998. Genome sequence of an obligate intracellular pathogen of humans: *Chlamydia trachomatis*. *Science* 282:754–759.

20. **Nicholson TL, Olinger L, Chong K, Schoolnik G, Stephens RS.** 2003. Global stage-specific gene regulation during the developmental cycle of *Chlamydia trachomatis*. *J Bacteriol* 185:3179–3189.

21. **Rosario CJ, Tan M.** 2012. The early gene product EUO is a transcriptional repressor that selectively regulates promoters of *Chlamydia* late genes. *Mol Microbiol* 84:1097–1107.

22. **Shaw EI, Dooley CA, Fischer ER, Scidmore MA, Fields KA, Hackstadt T.** 2000. Three temporal classes of gene expression during the *Chlamydia trachomatis* developmental cycle. *Mol Microbiol* 37:913–925.

23. **Heinzen RA, Hackstadt T.** 1997. The *Chlamydia trachomatis* parasitophorous vacuolar membrane is not passively permeable to low-molecular-weight compounds. *Infect Immun* 65:1088–1094.

24. **Cocchiaro JL, Kumar Y, Fischer ER, Hackstadt T, Valdivia RH.** 2008. Cytoplasmic lipid droplets are translocated into the lumen of the *Chlamydia trachomatis* parasitophorous vacuole. *Proc Natl Acad Sci U S A* 105:9379–9384.

25. **Elwell CA, Engel JN.** 2012. Lipid acquisition by intracellular *Chlamydiae*. *Cell Microbiol* 14:1010–1018.

26. **Rother M, Gonzalez E, Teixeira da Costa AR, Wask L, Gravenstein I, Pardo M, Pietzke M, Gurumurthy RK, Angermann J, Laudeley R, Glage S, Meyer M, Chumduri**

C, Kempa S, Dinkel K, Unger A, Klebl B, Klos A, Meyer TF. 2018. Combined human genome-wide RNAi and metabolite analyses identify IMPDH as a host-directed target against *Chlamydia* infection. *Cell Host Microbe* 23:661–671.e8.

27. Iliffe-Lee ER, McClarty G. 1999. Glucose metabolism in *Chlamydia trachomatis*: the 'energy parasite' hypothesis revisited. *Mol Microbiol* 33:177–187.

28. Hatch TP, Miceli M, Silverman JA. 1985. Synthesis of protein in host-free reticulate bodies of *Chlamydia psittaci* and *Chlamydia trachomatis*. *J Bacteriol* 162: 938–942.

29. Omsland A, Sager J, Nair V, Sturdevant DE, Hackstadt T. 2012. Developmental stage-specific metabolic and transcriptional activity of *Chlamydia trachomatis* in an axenic medium. *Proc Natl Acad Sci U S A* 109:19781–19785. (Erratum, 110:1970.)

30. Omsland A, Sixt BS, Horn M, Hackstadt T. 2014. Chlamydial metabolism revisited: interspecies metabolic variability and developmental stage-specific physiologic activities. *FEMS Microbiol Rev* 38:779–801.

31. Fuchs TM, Eisenreich W, Heesemann J, Goebel W. 2012. Metabolic adaptation of human pathogenic and related nonpathogenic bacteria to extra- and intracellular habitats. *FEMS Microbiol Rev* 36:435–462.

32. Mehlitz A, Eylert E, Huber C, Lindner B, Vollmuth N, Karunakaran K, Goebel W, Eisenreich W, Rudel T. 2017. Metabolic adaptation of *Chlamydia trachomatis* to mammalian host cells. *Mol Microbiol* 103:1004–1019.

33. Weiss E. 1965. Adenosine triphosphate and other requirements for the utilization of glucose by agents of the psittacosis-trachoma group. *J Bacteriol* 90:243–253.

34. Gehre L, Gorgette O, Perrinet S, Prevost MC, Ducatez M, Giebel AM, Nelson DE, Ball SG, Subtil A. 2016. Sequestration of host metabolism by an intracellular pathogen. *eLife* 5:e12552.

35. Iliffe-Lee ER, McClarty G. 2000. Regulation of carbon metabolism in *Chlamydia trachomatis*. *Mol Microbiol* 38: 20–30.

36. Weiss E. 1967. Transaminase activity and other enzymatic reactions involving pyruvate and glutamate in *Chlamydia* (psittacosis-trachoma group). *J Bacteriol* 93: 177–184.

37. Asgari Y, Zabihinpour Z, Salehzadeh-Yazdi A, Schreiber F, Masoudi-Nejad A. 2015. Alterations in cancer cell metabolism: the Warburg effect and metabolic adaptation. *Genomics* 105:275–281.

38. Markham GD, Bock CL, Schalk-Hihi C. 1999. Acid-base catalysis in the chemical mechanism of inosine monophosphate dehydrogenase. *Biochemistry* 38:4433–4440.

39. Morath C, Schwenger V, Beimler J, Mehrabi A, Schmidt J, Zeier M, Muranyi W. 2006. Antifibrotic actions of mycophenolic acid. *Clin Transplant* 20(Suppl 17):25–29.

40. Fischer A, Rudel T. 2016. Subversion of cell-autonomous host defense by *Chlamydia* infection. *Curr Top Microbiol Immunol* 412:81–106.

41. Abdul-Sater AA, Saïd-Sadier N, Lam VM, Singh B, Pettengill MA, Soares F, Tattoli I, Lipinski S, Girardin SE, Rosenstiel P, Ojcius DM. 2010. Enhancement of reactive oxygen species production and chlamydial infection by the mitochondrial Nod-like family member NLRX1. *J Biol Chem* 285:41637–41645.

42. Kuzminov A. 2001. Single-strand interruptions in replicating chromosomes cause double-strand breaks. *Proc Natl Acad Sci U S A* 98:8241–8246.

43. Boncompain G, Schneider B, Delevoye C, Kellermann O, Dautry-Varsat A, Subtil A. 2010. Production of reactive oxygen species is turned on and rapidly shut down in epithelial cells infected with *Chlamydia trachomatis*. *Infect Immun* 78:80–87.

44. Chumduri C, Gurumurthy RK, Zadora PK, Mi Y, Meyer TF. 2013. *Chlamydia* infection promotes host DNA damage and proliferation but impairs the DNA damage response. *Cell Host Microbe* 13:746–758.

45. Fan T, Lu H, Hu H, Shi L, McClarty GA, Nance DM, Greenberg AH, Zhong G. 1998. Inhibition of apoptosis in *Chlamydia*-infected cells: blockade of mitochondrial cytochrome c release and caspase activation. *J Exp Med* 187: 487–496.

46. Sharma M, Rudel T. 2009. Apoptosis resistance in *Chlamydia*-infected cells: a fate worse than death? *FEMS Immunol Med Microbiol* 55:154–161.

47. Al-Zeer MA, Xavier A, Abu Lubad M, Sigulla J, Kessler M, Hurwitz R, Meyer TF. 2017. *Chlamydia trachomatis* prevents apoptosis via activation of PDPK1-MYC and enhanced mitochondrial binding of hexokinase II. *EBioMedicine* 23:100–110.

48. Robey RB, Hay N. 2006. Mitochondrial hexokinases, novel mediators of the antiapoptotic effects of growth factors and Akt. *Oncogene* 25:4683–4696.

49. Dahlmans D, Houzelle A, Schrauwen P, Hoeks J. 2016. Mitochondrial dynamics, quality control and miRNA regulation in skeletal muscle: implications for obesity and related metabolic disease. *Clin Sci (Lond)* 130:843–852.

50. Suen DF, Norris KL, Youle RJ. 2008. Mitochondrial dynamics and apoptosis. *Genes Dev* 22:1577–1590.

51. Wang S, Mao Y, Xi S, Wang X, Sun L. 2017. Nutrient starvation sensitizes human ovarian cancer SKOV3 cells to BH3 mimetic via modulation of mitochondrial dynamics. *Anat Rec (Hoboken)* 300:326–339.

52. Sarin M, Wang Y, Zhang F, Rothermund K, Zhang Y, Lu J, Sims-Lucas S, Beer-Stolz D, Van Houten BE, Vockley J, Goetzman ES, Graves JA, Prochownik EV. 2013. Alterations in c-Myc phenotypes resulting from dynamin-related protein 1 (Drp1)-mediated mitochondrial fission. *Cell Death Dis* 4:e670.

53. Touvier T, De Palma C, Rigamonti E, Scagliola A, Incerti E, Mazelin L, Thomas JL, D'Antonio M, Politi L, Schaeffer L, Clementi E, Brunelli S. 2015. Muscle-specific Drp1 overexpression impairs skeletal muscle growth via translational attenuation. *Cell Death Dis* 6:e1663.

54. Frank M, Duvezin-Caubet S, Koob S, Occhipinti A, Jagasia R, Petcherski A, Ruonala MO, Priault M, Salin B, Reichert AS. 2012. Mitophagy is triggered by mild oxidative stress in a mitochondrial fission dependent manner. *Biochim Biophys Acta* 1823:2297–2310.

55. Gomes LC, Di Benedetto G, Scorrano L. 2011. During autophagy mitochondria elongate, are spared from

degradation and sustain cell viability. *Nat Cell Biol* **13:** 589–598.

56. Lee J, Giordano S, Zhang J. 2012. Autophagy, mitochondria and oxidative stress: cross-talk and redox signalling. *Biochem J* 441:523–540.

57. Chowdhury SR, Reimer A, Sharan M, Kozjak-Pavlovic V, Eulalio A, Prusty BK, Fraunholz M, Karunakaran K, Rudel T. 2017. *Chlamydia* preserves the mitochondrial network necessary for replication via microRNA-dependent inhibition of fission. *J Cell Biol* 216:1071–1089.

58. González E, Rother M, Kerr MC, Al-Zeer MA, Abu-Lubad M, Kessler M, Brinkmann V, Loewer A, Meyer TF. 2014. *Chlamydia* infection depends on a functional MDM2-p53 axis. *Nat Commun* 5:5201.

59. Siegl C, Prusty BK, Karunakaran K, Wischhusen J, Rudel T. 2014. Tumor suppressor p53 alters host cell metabolism to limit *Chlamydia trachomatis* infection. *Cell Reports* 9: 918–929.

60. Vousden KH, Ryan KM. 2009. p53 and metabolism. *Nat Rev Cancer* 9:691–700.

61. Li J, Donath S, Li Y, Qin D, Prabhakar BS, Li P. 2010. miR-30 regulates mitochondrial fission through targeting p53 and the dynamin-related protein-1 pathway. *PLoS Genet* 6:e1000795.

62. Wang J, Jiao Y, Cui L, Jiang L. 2017. miR-30 functions as an oncomiR in gastric cancer cells through regulation of P53-mediated mitochondrial apoptotic pathway. *Biosci Biotechnol Biochem* 81:119–126.

63. Frank S, Gaume B, Bergmann-Leitner ES, Leitner WW, Robert EG, Catez F, Smith CL, Youle RJ. 2001. The role of dynamin-related protein 1, a mediator of mitochondrial fission, in apoptosis. *Dev Cell* 1:515–525.

64. Röth D, Krammer PH, Gülow K. 2014. Dynamin related protein 1-dependent mitochondrial fission regulates oxidative signalling in T cells. *FEBS Lett* 588:1749–1754.

65. Smirnova E, Griparic L, Shurland DL, van der Bliek AM. 2001. Dynamin-related protein Drp1 is required for mitochondrial division in mammalian cells. *Mol Biol Cell* 12:2245–2256.

66. Qi X, Qvit N, Su YC, Mochly-Rosen D. 2013. A novel Drp1 inhibitor diminishes aberrant mitochondrial fission and neurotoxicity. *J Cell Sci* 126:789–802.

67. Su YC, Chiu HW, Hung JC, Hong JR. 2014. Beta-nodavirus B2 protein induces hydrogen peroxide production, leading to Drp1-recruited mitochondrial fragmentation and cell death via mitochondrial targeting. *Apoptosis* 19:1457–1470.

68. Karlas A, Berre S, Couderc T, Varjak M, Braun P, Meyer M, Gangneux N, Karo-Astover L, Weege F, Raftery M, Schönrich G, Klemm U, Wurzlbauer A, Bracher F, Merits A, Meyer TF, Lecuit M. 2016. A human genome-wide loss-of-function screen identifies effective chikungunya antiviral drugs. *Nat Commun* 7:11320.

69. Tripathi S, Pohl MO, Zhou Y, Rodriguez-Frandsen A, Wang G, Stein DA, Moulton HM, DeJesus P, Che J, Mulder LC, Yángüez E, Andenmatten D, Pache L, Manicassamy B, Albrecht RA, Gonzalez MG, Nguyen Q, Brass A, Elledge S, White M, Shapira S, Hacohen N, Karlas A, Meyer TF, Shales M, Gatorano A, Johnson JR, Jang G, Johnson T, Verschueren E, Sanders D, Krogan N, Shaw M, König R, Stertz S, García-Sastre A, Chanda SK. 2015. Meta- and orthogonal integration of influenza "OMICs" data defines a role for UBR4 in virus budding. *Cell Host Microbe* 18:723–735.

Autonomous Defense Pathways in the Cell

III

Bacteria and Intracellularity
Edited by Pascale Cossart, Craig R. Roy, and Philippe Sansonetti
© 2019 American Society for Microbiology, Washington, DC
doi:10.1128/microbiolspec.BAI-0011-2019

Host-Encoded Sensors of Bacteria: Our Windows into the Microbial World

19

Charlotte Odendall[1] and Jonathan C. Kagan[2]

INTRODUCTION

Outside a mammalian host, bacteria face numerous challenges that can result in life-threatening risks. These challenges include variations in temperature and osmolarity, predation, desiccation, and nutrient shortage. For bacteria with the ability to survive within a mammalian host, several of these threats are less severe, as host cells exist at a fixed temperature, osmolarity, and water and nutrient content. However, there is a cost associated with the benefits of an intracellular lifestyle. That cost is the threat of host-encoded immune defenses. Here, we describe the molecular mechanisms used by mammalian hosts to detect bacterial infection. We discuss the receptors encoded by the host immune system that recognize infection and the bacterial molecules that these receptors detect. Finally, we illustrate how these detection strategies, which have diverse mechanisms of action, share a thematically similar goal. This goal is to induce inflammatory responses that are typified by the recruitment of the biggest threat to bacterial viability to the sites of infection—polymorphonuclear leukocytes, also known as neutrophils.

BACTERIAL MOLECULES THAT INDUCE HOST DEFENSE

All multicellular organisms face the threat of microbial colonization, which poses a threat to the viability of the host. Studies over the last two decades, first by the late Charles Janeway, Jr., and subsequently by many others, established a common strategy used by multicellular organisms to detect bacterial encounters. This common strategy of bacterial detection comes from the use of germ line-encoded host proteins that recognize molecules present within large classes of bacteria. The microbial molecules sensed by the host include structural components of the bacterial cell wall, such as lipopolysaccharides (LPS), lipoproteins, peptidoglycan fragments, and flagellin subunits (Table 1). Additional microbial molecules include nucleic acids—DNA and RNA. As mammalian cells lack a cell wall, the presence of LPS and other cell wall components in the host provides a high-fidelity indicator of a bacterial encounter. Thus, the host-encoded sensors of cell wall components, referred to as pattern recognition receptors (PRRs), most certainly evolved under the selective pressure to rapidly detect bacterial encounters. Nucleic acids, in contrast, are not exclusively bacterial and can be found in all living cells and viruses. Thus, while PRRs that detect nucleic acids can detect bacteria, the true selective pressure that drove the evolution of these receptors may have been based on the need to detect viral infection. There is one exception to this statement, as recent studies revealed that a specific sequence found in bacterial rRNA is a potent inducer of host defenses (1, 2). This rRNA sequence is highly conserved and is not found in eukaryotic rRNAs or viral genomes. Therefore, the receptors that detect bacterial rRNA likely evolved to detect these microorganisms.

The evolutionary focus of this discussion prompts consideration of the selective pressures placed on hosts and bacteria that directed the design of PRRs and their aforementioned microbial ligands. These microbial ligands are collectively referred to as pathogen-associated molecular patterns (PAMPs) (Table 1). Within the human genome, there are genes encoding

[1]Kings College, Department of Infectious Diseases, Guy's Hospital, London, United Kingdom; [2]Harvard Medical School and Division of Gastroenterology, Boston Children's Hospital, Boston, MA.

TABLE 1 Mammalian PRRs and their targets[a]

Family	Sensor	PAMP	Localization
TLR	TLR2/1, TLR2/6	Lipoproteins	Plasma membrane
	TLR4	LPS	Plasma membrane
	TLR3	dsRNA	Endosomes
	TLR5	Flagellin	Plasma membrane
	TLR7	ssRNA	Endosomes
	TLR8	ssRNA	Endosomes
	TLR9	CpG DNA	Endosomes
	TLR13	rRNA with specific sequence	Endosomes
NLR	Nod1	iE-DAP	Cytosol
	Nod2	Muramyl dipeptide	Cytosol
	NLRP3	Peptidoglycan	Cytosol
	NAIP2	T3SS rod	Cytosol
	NAIP5	Flagellin	Cytosol
	NAIP6	Flagellin	Cytosol
	CGAS	DNA	Cytosol
ALR	AIM2	DNA	Cytosol
RNA	RIG-I	Short dsRNA with 5′ terminus	Cytosol
	MDA5	Long branched chains of dsRNA	Cytosol

[a]ALR, AIM2-like receptor; ss, single stranded; ds, double stranded; iE-DAP, γ-D-glutamyl-*meso*-diaminopimelic acid.

proteins that regulate numerous activities, including tissue development, body patterning, and neurological, cardiac, and hormonal activities. The molecular cues (ligands) that control these processes are encoded by the same genome that encodes the receptors and pathways that these cues stimulate. Thus, in developmental and metabolic systems, receptors and ligands are under positive selection to reinforce the fidelity of the network. In contrast, PRRs and their microbial ligands are synthesized by different organisms. Moreover, robust detection of a PAMP by a PRR drives defensive responses that eliminate the bacterium that produced the very ligand that the receptor evolved to detect. Based on the separation of genomes that encode PAMPs and PRRs, and the antagonistic outcome of the receptor-ligand interaction, it is logical that host proteins involved in immune defense are encoded by some of the most rapidly evolving genes present in the human genome. Probably due to the rapid evolving nature of the receptors that inform our understanding of host-bacterium encounters, different multicellular organisms encode different repertoires of PRRs. These receptors, consequently, can induce defensive responses to infection that are tailored to suit the needs of the

host. For example, PRRs that operate in humans link microbial detection to the initiation of T and B cell-mediated adaptive immunity (3). As the fruit fly *Drosophila melanogaster* does not contain T and B cells, PRRs within this organism link bacterial detection to the production of antimicrobial peptides. Despite this diversity of receptor design and defensive strategy, multicellular organisms from every kingdom of life appear to have evolved to use a similar set of PAMPs as indicators of infection. Below, we focus on the best-characterized experimental systems to study PRR activities in the context of bacterial encounters—the human and the mouse. We refer the reader to several excellent reviews that describe host defense strategies that operate in insects and plants (4–6).

HOST-ENCODED SENSORS OF BACTERIAL MOLECULES

Several families of PRRs exist in humans and mice. Within each family are proteins that exhibit significant structural similarity, but there is limited similarity across PRR families. Thus, the unifying feature that links these diverse families of proteins is function—the ability to detect and respond to bacterial encounters. The first-described and best-characterized family of PRRs consists of the Toll-like receptors (TLRs) (7–11). TLRs are type I transmembrane proteins that are structurally characterized as containing a large extracellular leucine-rich repeat domain that recognizes PAMPs and an intracellular signaling domain that shares homology with the intracellular domain of the interleukin 1 (IL-1) receptor and various plant resistance proteins. Consequently, the cytosolic tail of TLRs is classified as a Toll–IL-1 receptor resistance domain (7). Several TLRs are considered specific sensors of bacteria, in that they recognize specific components of the cell wall. These cell wall components include LPSs, which are detected by TLR4 (8–11), lipoproteins (detected by TLR2/1 or TLR2/6 heterodimers) (12, 13), and flagellin (TLR5) (14). TLR9, the receptor for unmethylated CpG-containing DNA, is also implicated in the detection of bacteria (15). However, as described above, TLR9, along with the other nucleic acid-sensing TLRs (TLR3, -7, and -8), probably evolved to detect viruses. TLR13 is the most recently defined member of this family and perhaps the most intriguing, in the context of bacterial detection. TLR13 recognizes an RNA sequence that corresponds to that found in bacterial rRNA (1, 2). In contrast, all other RNA-sensing TLRs do not detect their cognate PAMPs in a sequence specific manner. Interestingly, the sequence detected by TLR13 corresponds to the sequence targeted by several naturally occurring fungal metabolites that display potent antibacterial activity. This sequence of RNA is highly conserved across bacteria, which may explain why it is targeted by mammalian TLRs and fungal metabolites. Further evidence in support of the unusual nature of the target of TLR13 is based on the surprising finding that TLR13 is found only in mice. Despite the lack of TLR13, humans mount potent inflammatory responses to the RNA ligands that activate this receptor. Based on these findings, one must conclude that there is substantial selective pressure to detect bacterial encounters, and multiple PRRs likely evolved independently in diverse species to serve this purpose.

Whereas most TLRs detect bacterial PAMPs directly, one notable exception derives from studies of LPS detection by TLR4. TLR4 interacts weakly with LPS, yet picomolar concentrations of this PAMP can induce TLR4-dependent inflammatory responses (16). This high degree of sensitivity to LPS has been explained by the finding that TLR4 is not the sole sensor of extracellular LPS. Indeed, three LPS-binding proteins act upstream of TLR4 to promote high-efficiency detection. The extracellular LPS-binding protein is the first of these receptors to act, as it binds directly to the outer membrane of Gram-negative bacteria, bacterial outer membrane vesicles, or micelles. These interactions somehow disrupt the tight packaging of LPS and facilitate the extraction of a monomer of LPS by the glycosylphosphatidylinositol-anchored protein CD14. CD14 then transfers LPS to the small molecule MD-2, which is constitutively associated with the extracellular domain of TLR4. Only upon binding MD-2 can LPS form contacts with TLR4, which results in its dimerization. The dimerized ectodomain is the first step in the signaling process, whereby the intracellular Toll–IL-1 receptor resistance domains also dimerize and promote NF-κB-dependent inflammatory responses. The directionality of LPS transfer to TLR4 is ensured by the increasing affinity of LPS-binding protein, CD14, and MD-2 for LPS (17–22).

Interestingly, despite the symmetrical operation of many stages of microbial detection and inflammation induction across different PRR families, this complex process of PAMP binding is unique to TLR4. All other well-characterized PRRs detect their ligands directly, with high affinity. One possible explanation why PAMP detection by TLR4 is so complex is based on the nature of the ligand itself. Like other PAMPs derived from the bacterial cell wall, LPS is surface exposed. However, it is not the exposed substructure of LPS that is bound by MD-2 and TLR4, but rather the hydrophobic acyl chains that are buried in the membrane. Thus,

the nonexposed structures within LPS must be extracted by CD14 and presented to downstream PRRs. But why extract LPS in the first place? Why not simply couple initial detection of the exposed LPS substructures with inflammation-inducing activities? While the answer to this question is unknown, it is worth noting that the very nature of LPS detection by TLR4 involves a single molecule of LPS being extracted by a bacterium that contains thousands of such molecules. Importantly, it has been estimated that 1,000 molecules of LPS can be extracted from an individual *Escherichia coli* cell, each of which could (in principle) be used to activate TLR4-induced inflammatory responses on 1,000 different macrophages (16). The use of the term "overwhelming force," which is often associated with military dominance, is appropriate for this discussion, as we can consider the unusual strategy of LPS detection a means to amplify the number of cells that respond to a single bacterial encounter.

In recent years, new LPS receptors have been identified, as well as new functions for known LPS receptors. For example, caspase-11 in mice and caspase-4 and -5 in humans are now known to bind directly to LPS (23, 24). Recent biophysical analysis illustrated that, unlike the aforementioned receptors that bind monomers of LPS, caspase-4 (and likely the functional orthologues) do not bind monomers. Rather, these caspases appear to bind large aggregates of LPS (25). Additionally, the G-protein-coupled receptor BAI-1 was identified as a protein that binds the surface-exposed core oligosaccharides of LPS. Finally, CD14, in addition to transferring LPS to TLR4, acts to promote endocytosis, thereby promoting the transfer of TLR4 dimers into endosomes, which is an important site of inflammatory signal transduction (26).

Whereas the TLRs are the primary sensors of extracellular bacteria, several PRRs detect cytosolic bacteria. In terms of number of receptors that participate in cytosolic bacteria detection, the nucleotide-binding leucine-rich repeat proteins (NLRs) are most notable. Among the NLRs, NOD1 detects γ-D-glutamyl-*meso*-diaminopimelic acid (27, 28), NOD2 detects muramyl dipeptide, and NLRP3 detects the activities of the *N*-acetylglucosamine fragment of peptidoglycan (29, 30). The NLRs NAIP2, -5, and -6 also detect bacterial products directly, with NAIP2 detecting a bacterial secretion system structure and NAIP5 and NAIP6 detecting a substructure within flagellin distinct from that detected by TLR5 (31). Members of the RIG-I-like receptor (RLR) family also detect bacteria, as do the DNA sensors cGAS and AIM2. Each of these receptors surveys the cytosol for nucleic acid ligands. The first-described

RLR, RIG-I, detects short double-stranded RNA sequences with a di- or triphosphorylated 5′ terminus, and the RLR MDA5 detects long branched chains of double-stranded RNA (32–36).

Genetic analysis has implicated RLRs in the detection of bacterial infections, most notably those caused by the cytosolic pathogen *Listeria monocytogenes* (37, 38). Rather than sensing RNA sequences in the cytosol, cGAS and AIM2 detect DNA in this subcellular compartment (39, 40). The presence of DNA in the cytosol is unusual, as all cellular sources of DNA should be confined to the nucleus of mitochondria. cGAS and AIM2 each contain high-affinity DNA-binding domains, which can detect any DNA that leaks into the cytosol, such as during genotoxic stress or mitochondrial dysfunction of bacterial lysis. While bacteriolysis in the cytosol would be considered a rare event, the number of infections known to activate cGAS is increasing. For example, cGAS appears to detect *Mycobacterium tuberculosis*, *Chlamydia* species, and *Legionella pneumophila* (41, 42). Several of the aforementioned studies proposed that the DNA detected during these infections is derived from living (not lysed) intracellular bacteria. At present, it is unclear how DNA would be released from bacteria without lysis, although bacterial type III, IV, and VII secretion systems (T3SS, T4SS, and T7SS) may provide conduits to the cytosol.

HOST-ENCODED SENSORS OF PATHOGEN ACTIVITIES

While most PRRs detect microbes by directly sensing the presence of PAMPs, others detect infection through sensing of activities carried out by bacteria as part of their virulence strategies. The consequences of these activities can be cellular stress, damage, and biochemical modification of host factors. Inflammasomes are sensors that detect pathogen activities, and they are discussed in greater detail in other articles. Of note, the NLRP3 inflammasome detects disturbances in cellular homeostasis, including damage to membranes caused by bacterial toxins and secretion systems, including T3SSs and T4SSs. Secretion systems are a common virulence mechanism of many bacterial pathogens of plants and animals. Bacteria use these organelles to inject factors (known as effector proteins) into target cells. T3SSs and T4SSs are molecular syringes that span bacterial membranes and insert themselves into the host cell membrane (and cell wall in the case of plant cells). The pore formed by the insertion of translocon components into host membranes causes activation of the NLRP3 inflammasome, leading to pyroptosis via caspase-1 activation (43).

In addition to the physical disruption caused by the presence of bacteria and their secretion systems, the biochemical activities of secreted effectors themselves are signals detected by host PRRs. Translocated effectors carry out a number of biochemical functions to manipulate host cell functions, including affecting membrane trafficking, affecting cytoskeletal dynamics, and inhibiting the host immune response. The injection of this arsenal of toxins does not go unnoticed, and we now know that host cells are able to detect certain modification of host targets. This phenomenon of "indirect interaction" was long thought to be unique to plant innate immunity and is often discussed in that context under the name "guard hypothesis." This theory stipulates that important host proteins that are targeted by bacterial effectors are "guarded" by sensors. Sensor activation leads to the activation of an innate response (4, 44). For example, *Arabidopsis thaliana* RIN4 is an important negative regulator of plant immunity. It is phosphorylated and inhibited by a number of bacterial factors, including the *Pseudomonas syringae* effectors AvrB and AvrRpm1 (45). This phosphorylation event is detected by two plant proteins, the guards RPM1 and RPS2, activating an immune response (46–48).

Such a relationship has now been described in metazoans, including insects and vertebrates. In both cases, the guarded targets identified are small GTPases of the Rho family (RhoA, Rac1/2, and Cdc42). Rho GTPases sit at the apex of a number of signaling pathways that regulate critical cellular functions, including cytoskeletal dynamics and activation of inflammation. As such, they are targeted by a range of bacterial factors. For example, *E. coli* cytotoxic necrotizing factor 1 activates the Rho GTPase Rac2. This modification is detected by the immune adaptor IMD in flies and Rip1-Rip2 in mammalian cells, leading to the expression of proinflammatory cytokines (49). Similarly, the intracellular pathogen *Salmonella* activates Rac1 and Cdc42 in order to induce its internalization into nonphagocytic cells. This process of Rac1 manipulation is detected by Nod1, in a complex with Hsp90 and Rip2 (50). Finally, RhoA inhibition by a number of pathogens is sensed by the cytosolic protein pyrin, leading to subsequent activation of pyroptosis mediated by the inflammasome (51).

NEUTROPHIL RECRUITMENT TO THE SITES OF INFECTION—A COMMON OUTCOME OF BACTERIAL DETECTION

The varying sensors of bacterial molecules or virulence factor activities lead to the activation of defense responses that can be generally classified as inflammatory (Fig. 1). These responses involve the upregulation of genes that promote numerous aspects of host defense. Many downstream host defense responses are context dependent, but a common response associated with all innate immune responses is the induction of inflammation at the site of bacteria detection. Upon bacterial detection, all of the PRR pathways described herein induce the production of chemokines that promote the recruitment of large numbers of neutrophils to infected tissues. Many neutrophil chemokines are expressed by the action of the transcription factors NF-κB and AP-1, which are commonly activated by transcription-inducing PRR pathways and inflammasome pathways via the release of IL-1 (3, 52). In most cases

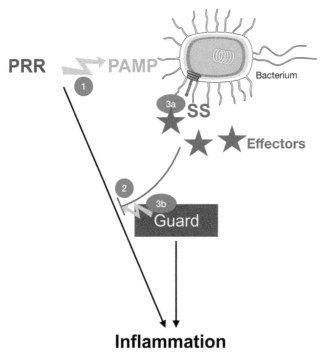

Inflammation

Figure 1 Evolutionary arms race between the host immune system and bacterial virulence mechanisms. (1) PRRs recognize PAMPs and activate conserved signaling pathways that induce transcriptional activation of inflammation with expression of cytokines and interferons. (2) Pathogenic bacteria use secretion systems (SS) to inject effector proteins into host cells. The diverse functions of these effectors include the ability to block different components of PRR-induced pathways. (3) The activities of pathogenic bacteria are detected by guard proteins. In vertebrates, these are mostly NLRs and other inflammasome stimulators. They detect the presence of T3SSs and T4SSs, usually through the formation of pores in host membranes (3a) and posttranslational modification of host proteins (3b). Consequently, NLRs and inflammasomes induce inflammation at the transcriptional and posttranslational levels through caspase-dependent activation of pyroptosis.

of bacterial encounters, neutrophils are the first cells recruited from the bloodstream to the infected tissue. Neutrophils are the most potent antibacterial phagocytes known to operate in the human body. Unlike dendritic cells, monocytes, and macrophages, which are also professional phagocytes, neutrophils rarely live longer than 24 hours and are not thought to play a role in antigen presentation to T lymphocytes (53, 54). Rather, the primary function of neutrophils is to kill bacteria and other microorganisms. These cells display several activities supporting such an antibacterial function, including potent phagocytic activity and the ability to produce copious amounts of reactive oxygen species. Neutrophils also contain secretory granules and lysosome-like organelles that are rich in antimicrobial peptides and enzymes that operate to degrade virtually every component of the bacterial cell wall. Finally, neutrophils are adept at undergoing an unusual form of cell death known as NETosis, where the cells release genomic DNA into the extracellular space to ensnare bacteria. Not only do these DNA-rich nets capture bacteria and prevent bacterial spread, but the associated histones display potent antibacterial activity (55, 56).

It is worth noting that several of the activities described here are also observed in other phagocytic cells, such as the ability to produce reactive oxygen species and ingest bacteria. However, these antibacterial activities appear to be most active in neutrophils and, in the case of NETosis, appear to be unique to this cell type. When this is considered in the context of the rapid accumulation of large numbers of these cells in infected tissues, it is reasonable to suggest that the biggest threat to bacterial survival in the host is the antimicrobial activities of neutrophils. Consistent with this suggestion are numerous findings that bacteria that have the ability to replicate within other phagocytes are readily killed by neutrophils. Thus, the mechanisms that link bacterial detection by PRRs to antibacterial activity of neutrophils are of prime importance for host defense. Other aspects of immunity, such as the activation of antigen-specific T lymphocytes and production of antigen-specific antibodies, are also important, but these activities are induced after neutrophil-mediated activities are mobilized to contain the infection.

PERSPECTIVES

In this essay, we discuss several means by which mammalian cells detect and respond to bacterial encounters. These means include the use of structurally diverse receptors and mechanistically distinct signaling pathways. Despite this diversity, the evolutionary pressures to develop these detection systems are likely constant, as they must meet the need to ensure host survival by preventing bacterial replication. It is worth noting that much of our knowledge in this area derives from studies that have focused on the interactions between bacteria and phagocytes or fibroblasts, neither of which are the first cells to encounter bacteria in the natural course of events. Epithelial cells in the skin, airway, and digestive tract represent the barrier to the environment. As such, these cells are poised for rapid detection of bacterial infection, and the innate immune pathways that operate in epithelial cells likely influence many downstream innate and adaptive responses to infection. Indeed, there is ample evidence that epithelia are the first cells that experience the activities of bacterial T3SSs, in particular, those involved in invasion. Studies over the next several years will likely expand our knowledge of the innate immune system in phagocytes and fibroblasts to include similar inquiries into the biology of barrier tissues. This broadening of the scope of host-microbe analysis will allow the classification of innate immune responses as being either common to all cell types or tissue specific. The emergence of human and mouse organoid models that represent an increasingly diverse set of tissues should facilitate such inquiries and may allow a more detailed view of the earliest stages of any host-bacterium interaction to emerge.

Acknowledgments. We thank the members of the Kagan and Odendall labs for helpful discussions. This work was supported by NIH grants AI133524, AI093589, AI116550, and P30DK34854 to J.C.K. J.C.K. holds an Investigators in the Pathogenesis of Infectious Disease Award from the Burroughs Wellcome Fund. C.O. is supported by a King's College London Prize Fellowship and a Sir Henry Dale Fellowship from the Royal Society and the Wellcome Trust (grant number 206200/Z/17/Z).

Citation. Odendall C, Kagan JC. 2019. Host-encoded sensors of bacteria: our windows into the microbial world. Microbiol Spectrum 7(3):BAI-0011-2019.

References

1. Oldenburg M, Krüger A, Ferstl R, Kaufmann A, Nees G, Sigmund A, Bathke B, Lauterbach H, Suter M, Dreher S, Koedel U, Akira S, Kawai T, Buer J, Wagner H, Bauer S, Hochrein H, Kirschning CJ. 2012. TLR13 recognizes bacterial 23S rRNA devoid of erythromycin resistance-forming modification. *Science* 337:1111–1115.

2. Li X-D, Chen ZJ. 2012. Sequence specific detection of bacterial 23S ribosomal RNA by TLR13. *eLife* 1:e00102.

3. Palm NW, Medzhitov R. 2009. Pattern recognition receptors and control of adaptive immunity. *Immunol Rev* 227:221–233.

4. Jones JDG, Dangl JL. 2006. The plant immune system. *Nature* 444:323–329.

5. Padmanabhan M, Cournoyer P, Dinesh-Kumar SP. 2009. The leucine-rich repeat domain in plant innate immunity: a wealth of possibilities. *Cell Microbiol* 11:191–198.

6. Buchon N, Silverman N, Cherry S. 2014. Immunity in *Drosophila melanogaster*—from microbial recognition to whole-organism physiology. *Nat Rev Immunol* 14:796–810.

7. Dunne A, O'Neill LAJ. 2003. The interleukin-1 receptor/Toll-like receptor superfamily: signal transduction during inflammation and host defense. *Sci STKE* 2003:re3.

8. Medzhitov R, Preston-Hurlburt P, Janeway CA Jr. 1997. A human homologue of the *Drosophila* Toll protein signals activation of adaptive immunity. *Nature* 388:394–397.

9. Poltorak A, He X, Smirnova I, Liu MY, Van Huffel C, Du X, Birdwell D, Alejos E, Silva M, Galanos C, Freudenberg M, Ricciardi-Castagnoli P, Layton B, Beutler B. 1998. Defective LPS signaling in C3H/HeJ and C57BL/10ScCr mice: mutations in Tlr4 gene. *Science* 282:2085–2088.

10. Poltorak A, Smirnova I, He X, Liu MY, Van Huffel C, Birdwell D, Alejos E, Silva M, Du X, Thompson P, Chan EK, Ledesma J, Roe B, Clifton S, Vogel SN, Beutler B. 1998. Genetic and physical mapping of the Lps locus: identification of the Toll-4 receptor as a candidate gene in the critical region. *Blood Cells Mol Dis* 24:340–355.

11. Hoshino K, Takeuchi O, Kawai T, Sanjo H, Ogawa T, Takeda Y, Takeda K, Akira S. 1999. Cutting edge: Toll-like receptor 4 (TLR4)-deficient mice are hyporesponsive to lipopolysaccharide: evidence for TLR4 as the Lps gene product. *J Immunol* 162:3749–3752.

12. Takeuchi O, Hoshino K, Kawai T, Sanjo H, Takada H, Ogawa T, Takeda K, Akira S. 1999. Differential roles of TLR2 and TLR4 in recognition of gram-negative and gram-positive bacterial cell wall components. *Immunity* 11:443–451.

13. Aliprantis AO, Yang RB, Mark MR, Suggett S, Devaux B, Radolf JD, Klimpel GR, Godowski P, Zychlinsky A. 1999. Cell activation and apoptosis by bacterial lipoproteins through Toll-like receptor-2. *Science* 285:736–739.

14. Hayashi F, Smith KD, Ozinsky A, Hawn TR, Yi EC, Goodlett DR, Eng JK, Akira S, Underhill DM, Aderem A. 2001. The innate immune response to bacterial flagellin is mediated by Toll-like receptor 5. *Nature* 410:1099–1103.

15. Hemmi H, Takeuchi O, Kawai T, Kaisho T, Sato S, Sanjo H, Matsumoto M, Hoshino K, Wagner H, Takeda K, Akira S. 2000. A Toll-like receptor recognizes bacterial DNA. *Nature* 408:740–745.

16. Gioannini TL, Weiss JP. 2007. Regulation of interactions of Gram-negative bacterial endotoxins with mammalian cells. *Immunol Res* 39:249–260.

17. Tobias PS, Soldau K, Ulevitch RJ. 1986. Isolation of a lipopolysaccharide-binding acute phase reactant from rabbit serum. *J Exp Med* 164:777–793.

18. Wright SD, Ramos RA, Tobias PS, Ulevitch RJ, Mathison JC. 1990. CD14, a receptor for complexes of

lipopolysaccharide (LPS) and LPS binding protein. *Science* 249:1431–1433.

19. Tobias PS, Soldau K, Kline L, Lee JD, Kato K, Martin TP, Ulevitch RJ. 1993. Cross-linking of lipopolysaccharide (LPS) to CD14 on THP-1 cells mediated by LPS-binding protein. *J Immunol* 150:3011–3021.

20. Haziot A, Ferrero E, Köntgen F, Hijiya N, Yamamoto S, Silver J, Stewart CL, Goyert SM. 1996. Resistance to endotoxin shock and reduced dissemination of gram-negative bacteria in CD14-deficient mice. *Immunity* 4:407–414.

21. Shimazu R, Akashi S, Ogata H, Nagai Y, Fukudome K, Miyake K, Kimoto M. 1999. MD-2, a molecule that confers lipopolysaccharide responsiveness on Toll-like receptor 4. *J Exp Med* 189:1777–1782.

22. Viriyakosol S, Tobias PS, Kitchens RL, Kirkland TN. 2001. MD-2 binds to bacterial lipopolysaccharide. *J Biol Chem* 276:38044–38051.

23. Kayagaki N, Wong MT, Stowe IB, Ramani SR, Gonzalez LC, Akashi-Takamura S, Miyake K, Zhang J, Lee WP, MuszyXski A, Forsberg LS, Carlson RW, Dixit VM. 2013. Noncanonical inflammasome activation by intracellular LPS independent of TLR4. *Science* 341:1246–1249.

24. Hagar JA, Powell DA, Aachoui Y, Ernst RK, Miao EA. 2013. Cytoplasmic LPS activates caspase-11: implications in TLR4-independent endotoxic shock. *Science* 341:1250–1253.

25. Lagrange B, Benaoudia S, Wallet P, Magnotti F, Provost A, Michal F, Martin A, Di Lorenzo F, Py BF, Molinaro A, Henry T. 2018. Human caspase-4 detects tetra-acylated LPS and cytosolic *Francisella* and functions differently from murine caspase-11. *Nat Commun* 9:242.

26. Zanoni I, Ostuni R, Marek LR, Barresi S, Barbalat R, Barton GM, Granucci F, Kagan JC. 2011. CD14 controls the LPS-induced endocytosis of Toll-like receptor 4. *Cell* 147:868–880.

27. Chamaillard M, Hashimoto M, Horie Y, Masumoto J, Qiu S, Saab L, Ogura Y, Kawasaki A, Fukase K, Kusumoto S, Valvano MA, Foster SJ, Mak TW, Nuñez G, Inohara N. 2003. An essential role for NOD1 in host recognition of bacterial peptidoglycan containing diaminopimelic acid. *Nat Immunol* 4:702–707.

28. Girardin SE, Boneca IG, Carneiro LAM, Antignac A, Jéhanno M, Viala J, Tedin K, Taha M-K, Labigne A, Zähringer U, Coyle AJ, DiStefano PS, Bertin J, Sansonetti PJ, Philpott DJ. 2003. Nod1 detects a unique muropeptide from gram-negative bacterial peptidoglycan. *Science* 300:1584–1587.

29. Inohara N, Ogura Y, Fontalba A, Gutierrez O, Pons F, Crespo J, Fukase K, Inamura S, Kusumoto S, Hashimoto M, Foster SJ, Moran AP, Fernandez-Luna JL, Nuñez G. 2003. Host recognition of bacterial muramyl dipeptide mediated through NOD2. Implications for Crohn's disease. *J Biol Chem* 278:5509–5512.

30. Girardin SE, Boneca IG, Viala J, Chamaillard M, Labigne A, Thomas G, Philpott DJ, Sansonetti PJ. 2003. Nod2 is a general sensor of peptidoglycan through muramyl dipeptide (MDP) detection. *J Biol Chem* 278:8869–8872.

31. Kofoed EM, Vance RE. 2011. Innate immune recognition of bacterial ligands by NAIPs determines inflammasome specificity. *Nature* 477:592–595.

32. Kang D-C, Gopalkrishnan RV, Wu Q, Jankowsky E, Pyle AM, Fisher PB. 2002. *mda-5*: an interferon-inducible putative RNA helicase with double-stranded RNA-dependent ATPase activity and melanoma growth-suppressive properties. *Proc Natl Acad Sci USA* 99:637–642.

33. Yoneyama M, Kikuchi M, Natsukawa T, Shinobu N, Imaizumi T, Miyagishi M, Taira K, Akira S, Fujita T. 2004. The RNA helicase RIG-I has an essential function in double-stranded RNA-induced innate antiviral responses. *Nat Immunol* 5:730–737.

34. Kato H, Takeuchi O, Sato S, Yoneyama M, Yamamoto M, Matsui K, Uematsu S, Jung A, Kawai T, Ishii KJ, Yamaguchi O, Otsu K, Tsujimura T, Koh C-S, Reis e Sousa C, Matsuura Y, Fujita T, Akira S. 2006. Differential roles of MDA5 and RIG-I helicases in the recognition of RNA viruses. *Nature* 441:101–105.

35. Hornung V, Ellegast J, Kim S, Brzózka K, Jung A, Kato H, Poeck H, Akira S, Conzelmann K-K, Schlee M, Endres S, Hartmann G. 2006. 5′-triphosphate RNA is the ligand for RIG-I. *Science* 314:994–997.

36. Pichlmair A, Schulz O, Tan CP, Näslund TI, Liljeström P, Weber F, Reis e Sousa C. 2006. RIG-I-mediated antiviral responses to single-stranded RNA bearing 5′-phosphates. *Science* 314:997–1001.

37. Hagmann CA, Herzner AM, Abdullah Z, Zillinger T, Jakobs C, Schuberth C, Coch C, Higgins PG, Wisplinghoff H, Barchet W, Hornung V, Hartmann G, Schlee M. 2013. RIG-I detects triphosphorylated RNA of *Listeria monocytogenes* during infection in non-immune cells. *PLoS One* 8:e62872.

38. Odendall C, Dixit E, Stavru F, Bierne H, Franz KM, Durbin AF, Boulant S, Gehrke L, Cossart P, Kagan JC. 2014. Diverse intracellular pathogens activate type III interferon expression from peroxisomes. *Nat Immunol* 15:717–726.

39. Hornung V, Ablasser A, Charrel-Dennis M, Bauernfeind F, Horvath G, Caffrey DR, Latz E, Fitzgerald KA. 2009. AIM2 recognizes cytosolic dsDNA and forms a caspase-1-activating inflammasome with ASC. *Nature* 458:514–518.

40. Sun L, Wu J, Du F, Chen X, Chen ZJ. 2013. Cyclic GMP-AMP synthase is a cytosolic DNA sensor that activates the type I interferon pathway. *Science* 339:786–791.

41. Prantner D, Darville T, Nagarajan UM. 2010. Stimulator of IFN gene is critical for induction of IFN-beta during *Chlamydia muridarum* infection. *J Immunol* 184:2551–2560.

42. Lippmann J, Müller HC, Naujoks J, Tabeling C, Shin S, Witzenrath M, Hellwig K, Kirschning CJ, Taylor GA, Barchet W, Bauer S, Suttorp N, Roy CR, Opitz B. 2011. Dissection of a type I interferon pathway in controlling bacterial intracellular infection in mice. *Cell Microbiol* 13:1668–1682.

43. Brodsky IE, Palm NW, Sadanand S, Ryndak MB, Sutterwala FS, Flavell RA, Bliska JB, Medzhitov R.

2010. A *Yersinia* effector protein promotes virulence by preventing inflammasome recognition of the type III secretion system. *Cell Host Microbe* **7:**376–387.

44. Marathe R, Dinesh-Kumar SP. 2003. Plant defense: one post, multiple guards?! *Mol Cell* **11:**284–286.

45. Lee D, Bourdais G, Yu G, Robatzek S, Coaker G. 2015. Phosphorylation of the plant immune regulator RPM1-INTERACTING PROTEIN4 enhances plant plasma membrane H⁺-ATPase activity and inhibits flagellin-triggered immune responses in *Arabidopsis*. *Plant Cell* **27:**2042–2056.

46. Chung E-H, da Cunha L, Wu A-J, Gao Z, Cherkis K, Afzal AJ, Mackey D, Dangl JL. 2011. Specific threonine phosphorylation of a host target by two unrelated type III effectors activates a host innate immune receptor in plants. *Cell Host Microbe* **9:**125–136.

47. Mackey D, Belkhadir Y, Alonso JM, Ecker JR, Dangl JL. 2003. Arabidopsis RIN4 is a target of the type III virulence effector AvrRpt2 and modulates RPS2-mediated resistance. *Cell* **112:**379–389.

48. Mackey D, Holt BF III, Wiig A, Dangl JL. 2002. RIN4 interacts with *Pseudomonas syringae* type III effector molecules and is required for RPM1-mediated resistance in *Arabidopsis*. *Cell* **108:**743–754.

49. Boyer L, Magoc L, Dejardin S, Cappillino M, Paquette N, Hinault C, Charriere GM, Ip WKE, Fracchia S, Hennessy E, Erturk-Hasdemir D, Reichhart J-M, Silverman N, Lacy-Hulbert A, Stuart LM. 2011. Pathogen-derived effectors trigger protective immunity via activation of the Rac2 enzyme and the IMD or Rip kinase signaling pathway. *Immunity* **35:**536–549.

50. Keestra AM, Winter MG, Auburger JJ, Frässle SP, Xavier MN, Winter SE, Kim A, Poon V, Ravesloot MM, Waldenmaier JFT, Tsolis RM, Eigenheer RA, Bäumler AJ. 2013. Manipulation of small Rho GTPases is a pathogen-induced process detected by NOD1. *Nature* **496:**233–237.

51. Xu H, Yang J, Gao W, Li L, Li P, Zhang L, Gong Y-N, Peng X, Xi JJ, Chen S, Wang F, Shao F. 2014. Innate immune sensing of bacterial modifications of Rho GTPases by the pyrin inflammasome. *Nature* **513:**237–241.

52. Vijay K. 2018. Toll-like receptors in immunity and inflammatory diseases: past, present, and future. *Int Immunopharmacol* **59:**391–412. *CORRIGENDUM Int Immunopharmacol* **62:**338.

53. Kolaczkowska E, Kubes P. 2013. Neutrophil recruitment and function in health and inflammation. *Nat Rev Immunol* **13:**159–175.

54. Galli SJ, Borregaard N, Wynn TA. 2011. Phenotypic and functional plasticity of cells of innate immunity: macrophages, mast cells and neutrophils. *Nat Immunol* **12:**1035–1044.

55. Brinkmann V, Reichard U, Goosmann C, Fauler B, Uhlemann Y, Weiss DS, Weinrauch Y, Zychlinsky A. 2004. Neutrophil extracellular traps kill bacteria. *Science* **303:**1532–1535.

56. Amulic B, Cazalet C, Hayes GL, Metzler KD, Zychlinsky A. 2012. Neutrophil function: from mechanisms to disease. *Annu Rev Immunol* **30:**459–489.

Bacteria and Intracellularity
Edited by Pascale Cossart, Craig R. Roy, and Philippe Sansonetti
© 2019 American Society for Microbiology, Washington, DC
doi:10.1128/microbiolspec.BAI-0003-2019

Recognition of Intracellular Bacteria by Inflammasomes

20

Petr Broz[1]

INTRODUCTION

The innate immune system comprises different mechanisms that recognize, restrict, and even kill intracellular bacteria. While most of these mechanisms aim at eradicating the infecting pathogen while maintaining cellular integrity, some also result in the concomitant death of the infected cell. The latter mechanism is exemplified by the assembly and activation of inflammasome complexes (1). The term "inflammasome" was coined in the early 2000s to describe multiprotein complexes that are assembled in the cytosol of activated macrophages and that serve as activation platforms for the cysteine protease caspase-1 (2). They are assembled by cytosolic sensor proteins that detect the presence of pathogen- or microbe-derived molecular patterns in the host cell cytosol, endogenous danger signals, or even disturbances of cellular homeostasis, so-called homeostasis-altering processes (1, 3).

Since their discovery over 15 years ago, intense research revealed the nature and mode of action of these complexes in the context of infection but also their contribution to (auto)inflammatory disorders. To date, five distinct types of inflammasome complexes have been identified; they are formed by either the nucleotide-binding oligomerization domain, leucine-rich repeat (LRR)-containing protein (NLR) family members, or the proteins AIM2 (absent in melanoma 2) and pyrin (Fig. 1A). They all feature death fold domains (either a PYD [pyrin domain] or CARD [caspase recruitment domain]), which allow the activated sensor protein to oligomerize and recruit a signaling adaptor known as ASC (1). ASC oligomerizes via its PYD into long cross-linked filaments, a process that acts as a signal amplification step (4, 5). ASC filaments aggregate via CARD-CARD interactions to form the micrometer-sized ASC speck, a macromolecular inflammasome, which recruits caspase-1,

the zymogen of the cysteine protease caspase-1 (Fig. 1B). Homodimerization and autoproteolysis activate the caspase, which then cleaves protein substrates to initiate immune defenses (6). The best-studied of these substrates are the "pro-" forms of the interleukin 1 (IL-1) family cytokines IL-1b and IL-18 (6) and gasdermin-D (GSDMD) (7, 8), a member of the extended gasdermin protein family (Fig. 1C).

Caspase cleavage removes an inhibitory C-terminal domain of GSDMD, allowing the N-terminal fragment to target and permeabilize the plasma membrane (7, 8). This fragment is inserted into and oligomerizes in the plasma membrane to form pores with diameters of up to 15 nm (9–12), which disrupt the electrochemical gradient and cause a type of necrotic cell death known as pyroptosis (13). GSDMD pore formation and pyroptosis also promote the release of mature IL-1b and IL-18 cytokines (7, 8, 14, 15), which are generated by caspase-1 cleavage. These cytokines promote the inflammatory response and, in the case of IL-18, engage additional antimicrobial effectors by stimulating gamma interferon (IFN-γ) production (16). In this chapter, I focus on the ligands and activation mechanism of inflammasome-forming pattern recognition receptors (PRRs) in the context of infections with intracellular bacteria and discuss different strategies that the host uses to detect infection and avoid bacterial immune evasion. Finally, I also highlight the role of pyroptosis in restricting bacterial replication in *in vitro* and *in vivo* infection models.

INFLAMMASOME-FORMING SENSORS

To date, five cytosolic sensor proteins have been confirmed to assemble inflammasomes, among them the NLR family members NLRP1, NLRP3, and NLRC4 as well as the proteins absent in AIM2 and pyrin (Fig. 1A).

---

[1]Department of Biochemistry, University of Lausanne, Switzerland.

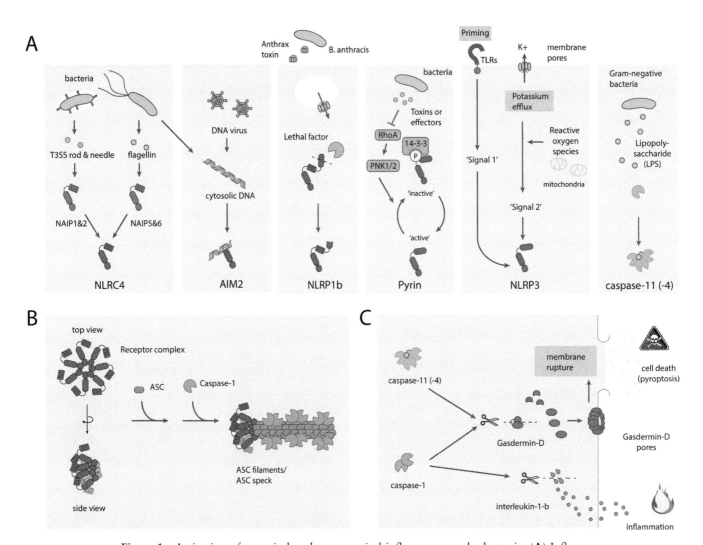

Figure 1 Activation of canonical and noncanonical inflammasomes by bacteria. (**A**) Inflammasome receptors use different recognition mechanisms to sense bacterial infections. The NAIP-NLRC4 and AIM2 pathways involve direct binding of the respective ligands (flagellin, T3SS structural proteins, or DNA). Nlrp1b recognizes the proteolytic activity of the metalloprotease lethal factor from *B. anthracis* by serving as a decoy substrate. Pyrin uses a guard mechanism to detect the inactivation of RhoA. The kinase activities of RhoA and PNK1/2 are required to keep pyrin in an inactive state, in which it is phosphorylated and bound by 14-3-3 proteins. NLRP3 activation involves priming by signal 1, followed by activation by signal 2. The nature of signal 2 and the mechanism of recognition are yet unknown, but they are linked to membrane permeabilization, K^+ efflux, and mitochondrial dysfunction. The noncanonical pathway involves direct detection of LPS by caspase-11 in mice or caspase-4 (or caspase-5) in humans. (**B**) Following activation, inflammasome receptors oligomerize and recruit the bipartite adaptor ASC, which forms long filaments that cluster to form the ASC speck. Procaspase-1 is recruited to the filaments by CARD-CARD interaction and activated by dimerization and autoproteolysis. (**C**) Active caspase-1 and caspase-11 process GSDMD, removing the regulatory C-terminal domain and unleashing the cytotoxic activity of the N-terminal fragment. The GSDMD N terminus is inserted into the plasma membrane and forms large pores, which disrupt the electrochemical gradient and induce pyroptosis. Caspase-1 also processes IL-1 family cytokines (like IL-1b) and promotes their release from cells in a pathway that is at least partially GSDMD dependent.

These proteins promote caspase-1 activation and are thus classified as canonical inflammasomes, in order to distinguish them from the noncanonical inflammasome pathway, which targets caspase-11 in mice and caspase-4 and/or caspase-5 in human cells. In the sections below, I highlight the distinct mode of activation of these pathways and the potential microbial strategies to escape the respective sensing mechanisms. Additional PRRs have also been shown to promote caspase-1 activation; however, these pathways are less well characterized and require independent confirmation, and they are therefore not discussed here.

The NAIP-NLRC4 Inflammasome

NLRC4 (or IPAF) was first shown to assemble an inflammasome and activate caspase-1 in macrophages infected with the intracellular bacterium *Salmonella enterica* serovar Typhimurium (17). Follow-up studies showed that NLRC4 is also engaged during infection with many other intracellular bacteria, among them *Legionella pneumophila* and *Shigella flexneri*, and that activation of NLRC4 was directly linked to the activity of bacterial secretion mechanisms like the type 3 and type 4 secretion systems (T3SS and T4SS) (18–22). Furthermore, studies using *Salmonella* identified bacterial flagellin as the critical factor that triggers NLRC4 activation, leading to the notion that activity of these secretion systems results in "accidental" injection of flagellin into the host cell cytosol (18, 19). However, since nonflagellated shigellae also triggered caspase-1 activation via NLRC4 (21), it became clear that additional ligands besides flagellin must exist. Consequently, Miao et al. demonstrated that NLRC4 was also engaged by flagellin-deficient *Salmonella* and that this required the injection of PrgJ, the rod component of the *Salmonella* SPI-1 T3SS (23). Despite the evolutionary similarities of the flagellum and T3S apparatus, it nevertheless remained unclear how NLRC4 detects these proteins, as no direct interaction could be found.

The mechanism by which NLRC4 detects its ligands became clear in studies that explored the function of a subfamily of NLRs, the apoptosis-inhibitory proteins (NAIPs). Early reports had shown that NLRC4-dependent caspase-1 activation during *L. pneumophila* infection also required NAIP5, while NAIP5 was only partially required for NLRC4 activation during *S. Ty*phimurium infection (22, 24). Given that *S. Typhimuri*um features a T3SS apparatus, while *L. pneumophila* has a T4SS, it became apparent that the NAIPs might confer specificity of NLRC4 for its different ligands. Work spearheaded by the Vance and Shao labs showed that binding of their cognate ligands—the T3SS rod

protein by NAIP2, the T3SS needle protein by NAIP1, and flagellin by NAIP5 and NAIP6—allows the NAIPs to interact with NLRC4 and initiate inflammasome complex assembly (25–28). Although humans feature only one NAIP gene, they express different NAIP isoforms in a cell type-specific manner. These NAIP isoforms can recognize different ligands, in that the full-length NAIP* isoform binds flagellin, while the shorter NAIP binds only the T3SS needle subunit (29).

Biochemical studies of mouse NAIPs revealed, somewhat unexpectedly, that ligand sensing is conferred not by the LRR, as previously assumed, but by the region surrounding the central NACHT domain of mouse NAIPs (30). Since the NAIPs employ a direct-binding mechanism to detect the presence of bacterial factors, bacteria could in theory easily escape immune surveillance by mutating the corresponding proteins, e.g., flagellin or T3SS structural components. This question was addressed by a recent study that performed an unbiased alanine scanning mutagenesis of the D0 domain of flagellin and the PrgJ protein of *S.* Typhimurium and then assayed NAIP5-flagellin and NAIP2-PrgJ recognition (31). This analysis revealed that NAIPs recognize multiple discrete surfaces or motifs on their cognate ligands and that the evasion of NAIP-mediated recognition required the combined mutation of several of these motifs. Even more remarkably, the authors found that these regions were essential for bacterial virulence in that combined mutation of these motifs abrogated bacterial motility or T3SS function. Thus, despite being highly specific for only a few ligands, the NAIP-NLRC4 inflammasome has evolved a strategy of multisurface recognition to limit the evolutionary paths that are available for bacterial pathogens to evade innate immune detection.

The AIM2 Inflammasome

AIM2 is a member of the HIN200 or AIM2-like receptor family of PRRs, which feature an N-terminal PYD and one or two DNA-binding hematopoietic IFN-inducible nuclear proteins with 200-amino-acid (HIN200) domains. In mice and several human cell types, AIM2 binds cytosolic DNA and assembles an inflammasome complex together with the adaptor ASC (32–37). AIM2 does not distinguish between DNA from viral, bacterial, and endogenous origins but requires at least 70-bp-long DNA molecules for efficient inflammasome assembly (38). To date, AIM2 appears to participate in the recognition of only a few intracellular bacterial pathogens, such as *Francisella tularensis*, *Listeria monocytogenes*, *Brucella abortus*, and *Mycobacterium* species (37, 39–43). It is, however, very likely that AIM2 is also engaged if other intracellular bacteria, such as *S.* Typhimurium or *L. pneu-mophila*, enter the cytosol but that in these cases, the AIM2 inflammasome response is undetectable by strong NLRC4/NAIP- and caspase-11-induced cell death and cy-tokine processing. Consistently, it was recently reported that flagellin-deficient *L. pneumophila* causes detectable AIM2 activation in *Casp11*$^{-/-}$ macrophages (44).

Importantly, AIM2 activation by intracellular bacteria requires that the bacterial DNA somehow reaches the cy-tosolic compartment. In the case of *Francisella novicida*, which replicates in the cytosol of phagocytes, AIM2 acti-vation is linked to bacteriolysis, and ASC specks can consistently be detected in close proximity to DNA ex-pelled by lysed bacteria (37). Interestingly, AIM2 activa-tion during bacterial infection was also found to be strictly linked to the preceding production of type I IFNs (45). Further investigation into the role of interferons re-vealed that they are necessary to drive IRF1 signaling and the expression of IFN-inducible GTPases, among them guanylate-binding proteins (GBPs) and the interferon-regulated GTPases (IRGs) (46, 47). These GTPases are part of a cytosolic antimicrobial defense mechanism and known to target pathogen-containing vacuoles and cy-tosolic bacteria (48). In the case of *F. novicida*, GBP and IRGB10 target cytosolic bacteria, thereby promoting the destabilization of the bacterial membranes and the release of bacterial DNA (46, 47, 49). The exact mechanism by which GBPs are recruited and mediate bacteriolysis is currently unknown, but it is likely that the GBPs only form a platform for the recruitment of additional anti-microbial mechanisms. How other intracellular bacteria introduce DNA into the cytosol is currently unknown, but it has been speculated that similar mechanisms could be involved or that the activity of bacterial secretion sys-tems introduces DNA into the cytosolic compartment. Immune evasion of AIM2 sensing is virtually impossible, since DNA is normally hidden within the bacterial cell. Thus, bacterial strategies to avoid recognition could be directed toward the upstream mechanisms, notably GBP recruitment. Indeed, several recent studies reported that the *S. flexneri* T3SS effector IpaH9.8, an E3 ubiquitin li-gase, ubiquitinates GBPs and thereby promotes their degradation (50–52).

The NLRP1 Inflammasome

Although human NLRP1 was the first NLR shown to assemble an inflammasome (2), its function in host de-fense remains largely uncharacterized. Humans feature only a single NLRP1 protein, while mice express up to three different isoforms of NLRP1, known as Nlrp1a, -1b, and -1c (53). Human NLRP1 also differs from the mouse proteins in that it also features an N-terminal

PYD. This PYD has a negative regulatory function, and thus both mouse and human NLRP1 proteins recruit ASC or caspase-1 via the CARD (54). Five different al-leles for mouse Nlrp1b exist, and two are associated with responsiveness to lethal toxin of *Bacillus anthracis*, an A/B toxin consisting of the protective antigen, a cell-binding protein, edema factor, and lethal factor (53). There are no reports suggesting that human NLRP1 al-so controls the response to anthrax toxin, but NLRP1 from Fisher rats was shown to mediate lethal factor-induced lethality (55). Lethal factor is a zinc metallo-protease that uses a channel formed by the protective antigen to translocate into the cell cytosol, where it inac-tivates immune signaling by cleaving mitogen-activated protein kinase kinases. Interestingly, the protease activi-ty of lethal factor is also necessary to activate Nlrp1b, as inactive lethal factor mutants do not trigger inflamma-some assembly (53). Based on these findings, it was hy-pothesized that NLRP1 does not detect lethal factor directly but monitors its activity in the cytosol, for ex-ample by serving as a substrate itself. This hypothesis was confirmed by several studies that demonstrated that lethal factor cleaves NLRP1 from Fisher rats or mouse NLRP1b and that this cleavage is required for NLRP1-dependent caspase-1 activation (55–57). Activation of human and mouse NLRP1 also requires an autoprocess-ing event in a unique "function to find" domain (FIIND) that lies between the C-terminal CARD and LRR motifs, but this processing is not carried out by lethal factor. How NLRP1 cleavage activates the protein is unknown, but most likely it relieves an intramolecular autoinhibi-tion conferred by its N terminus and/or induces confor-mational changes that allow oligomerization.

Nevertheless, it is now accepted that rodent NLRP1 proteins recognize anthrax toxin by acting as so-called decoy substrates for the protease lethal factor. A simi-lar decoy mechanism has also been reported for cer-tain plant R (resistance) gene products, for example, for *Arabidopsis* PBL2, which is uridylated and thus activated to drive immunity by the *Xanthomonas campestris* effector AvrAC, which normally dampens plant immune resistance by uridylating and inactivating BIK1 kinase (58, 59). Importantly, this mechanism limits the evasion of immune recognition, since any eva-sion strategy would require changing the substrate speci-ficity of the pathogen effector proteins and consequently result in a loss of its primary target activity.

The Pyrin Inflammasome

Pyrin (also known as marenostrin and TRIM20) is a TRIM family protein encoded by the gene *MEFV*. It features an N-terminal PYD followed by two B boxes and a coiled-coil region. Human pyrin also contains a C-terminal B30.2 domain (also known as a SPRY/PRY domain), which is not present in the mouse protein. Mutations within the B30.2 domain of human pyrin are associated with familial Mediterranean fever, an autoinflammatory disease (60). It was shown that these mutations result in excessive caspase-1 activation and IL-1β release, indicating that they confer a gain-of-function phenotype (61). The physiological function and activation mechanism of pyrin started to emerge following a seminal study that showed that pyrin initiates inflammasome assembly and caspase-1 activation in response to bacterial toxins, among them *Clostridioides* (formerly *Clostridium*) *difficile* toxin B/A and *Clostridium botulinum* C3 toxin, and bacterial effector proteins, such as VopS from *Vibrio parahaemolyticus* and IbpA from *Histophilus somni* (62). Mechanistically, pyrin is activated upon toxin-mediated modification of the Switch-I region of the small GTPase RhoA, which results in RhoA inactivation. In contrast, inactivation of other Rho GTPase family members like Rac1 and Cdc42 did not elicit pyrin activation. Since no direct interaction between pyrin and RhoA was observed, it was hypothesized that RhoA inactivation must be sensed in an indirect fashion and that pyrin might "guard" the activity of RhoA, similar to certain plant R proteins.

The activation mechanism was explored in several subsequent studies, which showed that RhoA effector kinases, notably PKN1 and PKN2, phosphorylate pyrin at critical serine residues (S208 and S242 in humans and S205 and S241 in mice) and that this results in the binding of 14-3-3 proteins to pyrin and inhibition of pyrin activity (63, 64). Based on these findings, it was proposed that when bacteria inactivate RhoA, PKN1/2 activity is lost, resulting in the dephosphorylation of pyrin, dissociation of 14-3-3 proteins, and thus pyrin activation (65). This mechanism supports that pyrin acts not as a direct sensor of pathogen infection but as a sensor of homeostasis-altering molecular processes, a sensing mechanism that allows the innate immune system to detect a wide variety of infectious agents and even evolutionary novel infections (3). At the same time, this mode of indirect sensing reduces the possibility of immune evasion, since targeting and manipulating small GTPases, in particular RhoA, constitute a critical step in the pathogenesis of many bacteria.

The NLRP3 Inflammasome

NLRP3 consists of an N-terminal PYD, a central NACHT domain, and C-terminal LRRs. It is activated by the widest set of stimuli by far, including many extra- and intracellular bacteria (66). Unlike the other inflammasomes, NLRP3 also requires a priming signal, or signal 1, such as the stimulation of Toll-like receptors for its activation. The priming signal results in transcriptional upregulation of NLRP3 and pro-IL-1b but also triggers nontranscriptional mechanisms that license NLRP3 activation (66). These include the dephosphorylation of residues within the N-terminal PYD (67), phosphorylation of a critical serine residue between the PYD and NACHT domains (68), and NLRP3 deubiquitination (69, 70). These priming events provide checkpoints in order to prevent unwanted and uncontrolled NLRP3 activation.

The actual activation of NLRP3 occurs upon the detection of so-called signal 2, which can be provided by noxious substances, crystalline matter, infection with microbial pathogens, lysosomal damage and the release of cathepsins, and the presence of extracellular endogenous danger signals or ionophores. The exact nature of signal 2, which is elicited by all these activators, is yet to be defined, but it appears to involve the permeabilization of the plasma membrane and the subsequent efflux of K$^+$ ions (71). In addition, mitochondrial production of reactive oxygen species, presumably upon mitochondrial dysfunction, has also been shown to provide a signal for NLRP3 activation (66). It is thus believed that NLRP3 functions also as a sensor for homeostasis-altering molecular processes and thus detects either the damage inflicted by pathogen infection upon the plasma membrane or disturbances in cellular homeostasis. While some bacteria trigger NLRP3 activation directly by releasing pore-forming proteins (*Staphylococcus aureus*, *Streptococcus pneumoniae*, and *L. monocytogenes*) (40), many others trigger it indirectly by activating the so-called noncanonical inflammasome (see below), whose activation can also provide signal 2 for NLRP3 engagement.

The Noncanonical Inflammasome

A noncanonical inflammasome pathway was identified in 2011 and shown to initiate the activation of caspase-11 in mouse cells and caspase-4 and caspase-5 in human cells upon infection with bacterial pathogens (72–74). In contrast to caspase-1, these caspases can cleave and activate GSDMD but cannot process cytokines like IL-1b and IL-18 efficiently. Nevertheless, caspase-11 or caspase-4 activation usually also results in concomitant IL-1b release, which depends on the NLRP3–ASC–caspase-1 axis. NLRP3 activation in this context is triggered in a cell-autonomous manner by K$^+$ efflux caused by the formation GSDMD plasma membrane pores (75).

Early reports showed that the noncanonical inflammasome is triggered only by Gram-negative intracellular bacteria and not Gram-positive pathogens (72, 76,

77), and it could be consistently demonstrated that the Gram-negative bacterial trigger is lipopolysaccharide (LPS; a component of the Gram-negative bacterial cell wall) (78, 79), specifically, its lipid A moiety. For LPS to trigger noncanonical inflammasome activation, it needs to reach the cytosolic compartment, be it by a bacterial infection, LPS transfection, or other delivery methods, since extracellular LPS by itself does not trigger the pathway (78). Interestingly, studies by the Shao lab showed that caspase-11 does not utilize a specific receptor to detect LPS but directly binds LPS via its N-terminal CARD (80).

LPS binding results in the oligomerization or aggregation of the caspase, which presumably results in its activation (80). Since LPS is very hydrophobic, accessory proteins or coreceptors might be necessary, analogous to Toll-like receptor 4-mediated LPS sensing, which is known to require additional LPS-binding proteins like LBP, CD14, and MD-2 (81). In that respect, it is important to note that caspase-11 activation during bacterial infection or upon LPS transfection requires IFN-induced GTPases (49, 82–84). Similarly to AIM2 activation, GBP family members (in particular GBP2) and IRGB10 play an important role, since Gbp^{chr3}- and $Irgb10$-deficient cells display delayed caspase-11 activation and reduced levels of LPS–caspase-11 interaction, suggesting that they modulate the access of caspase-11 to LPS (84–86). Furthermore, microscopy analysis found that these GTPases directly associate with bacterial membranes, transfected LPS, or intracellular outer membrane vesicles (84). However, additional studies are needed to determine if GBPs promote noncanonical inflammasome activation by destroying LPS-containing membranes or by directly binding LPS and presenting it to caspase-11.

Caspase-11 is triggered by intracellular bacteria upon entry into cytosol, such as S. Typhimurium, *Burkholderia thailandensis*, and *L. pneumophila*. However, it does not recognize the Gram-negative bacterium *F. novicida*, a professional cytosolic pathogen (78, 79). The molecular basis of this distinction is the fact that caspase-11 specifically recognizes hexa-acylated lipid A, while *F. novicida* features tetra-acylated lipid A. Interestingly, a recent study showed that caspase-4 functions differently from caspase-11, in that it efficiently recognizes the tetra-acylated lipid A from *F. novicida* (87). Despite this difference, GBPs were also found to be necessary to trigger caspase-4 activation in human cells upon infection with *F. novicida* or transfection with LPS from *F. novicida* or *Escherichia coli* (87). Finally, it is worth noting that the invasion of the cytosol is not an absolute prerequisite for caspase-11 activation. Several studies have reported that even some extracellular bacteria can activate caspase-1 and that this activation is conferred by bacterium-derived outer membrane vesicles, which reach the cytosol upon endocytosis (84, 88). The noncanonical pathway thus represents a versatile mechanism for the detection of both extra- and intracellular Gram-negative bacteria.

ANTIMICROBIAL FUNCTION OF PYROPTOSIS

Studies in the mid-1990s reported that infection with intracellular bacterial pathogens resulted in the death of macrophages with concurrent IL-1 release (89). Because of some morphological similarities, this cell death was initially referred to as apoptosis. In the early 2000s, however, it was recognized that this type of cell death was functionally distinct from apoptosis, since it required caspase-1 (13, 90). Given the necrotic and pro-inflammatory features of this cell death, it was named pyroptosis, from the Greek *pyro* (fire, fever) and *ptosis* (to fall).

While many studies show that inflammasome activation is essential for host defense against and clearance of bacterial infections, the individual contributions of pyroptosis and cytokine (IL-1b and -18) release are difficult to dissect. Deletion of the GSDMD gene abrogates pyroptosis partially (7, 8) but also reduces cytokine secretion, since formation of GSDMD pores is necessary to release IL-1 family cytokines (14, 15). Nevertheless, the picture that has emerged over the years is that the main functions of pyroptosis in infected phagocytes are to restrict the replication of intracellular bacteria by eliminating their replicative niche and to expose the pathogens to killing by extracellular immune responses (Fig. 2A). An elegant set of experiments using S. Typhimurium expressing flagellin under a doxycycline-inducible promoter showed that these organisms are rapidly cleared *in vivo* after doxycycline treatment, and that this process did not require IL-1 cytokine but depended on neutrophils (91).

Follow-up studies showed that intracellular bacteria remained associated with or trapped within the pyroptotic cell bodies, hence named pyroptosis- or pore-induced intracellular traps (PITs) (92, 93). These PITs induce innate immune responses via complement and scavenger receptors to drive recruitment of and efferocytosis by neutrophils and ultimately bacteria clearance. Intriguingly, several groups report that bacteria trapped within pyroptotic cells show signs of reduced membrane integrity and increased susceptibility to stressors or antibiotics (12, 92). Since cardiolipin, a component of the inner mitochondrial as well as bacterial membranes,

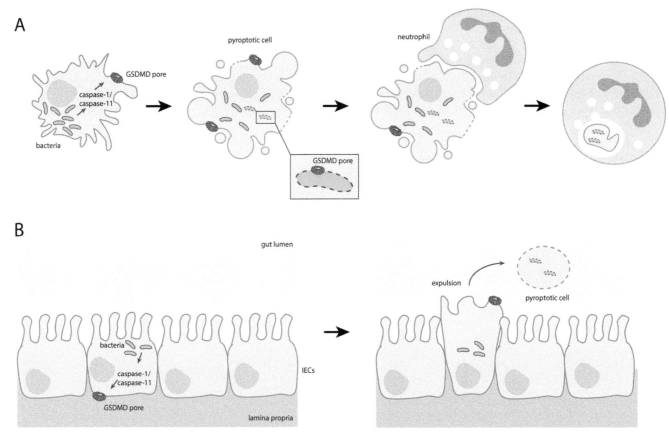

Figure 2 Antimicrobial effects of pyroptosis. (**A**) Activation of canonical or noncanonical inflammasomes in infected phagocytes results in the formation of GSDMD pores and pyroptosis. Intracellular bacteria are trapped within pyroptotic cell bodies, called PITs. GSDMD pores can potentially also damage intracellular bacteria. PITs are recognized and efferocytosed by neutrophils, which efficiently kill PIT-associated bacteria. (**B**) Engagement of pyroptosis in IECs promotes the expulsion of pyroptotic cells from the epithelial cell layer into the gut lumen. Any associated bacteria are removed with the dying cells and expelled from the intestines.

promotes the association of the GSDMD N-terminal fragment with liposomal membranes, it was speculated that GSDMD pores target and weaken intracellular bacteria during pyroptosis. Indeed, a recombinant GSDMD N terminus was found to associate with bacteria and reduce CFU counts *in vitro* (12). However, another study found that that GSDMD was not necessary for intracellular restriction of cytosolic *S.* Typhimurium (94). Therefore, defining the antimicrobial nature of pyroptosis and GSDMD will require additional studies.

Efferocytosis of pyroptotic cells may not always be necessary to restrict bacterial replication. Indeed, it has been recognized that inflammasome activation and cell death are not restricted to immune cells but also occur in a variety of epithelial cells, most notably in intestinal epithelial cells (IECs). The mechanism by which IEC pyroptosis restricts pathogen replication was highlighted by

two independent studies that observed that the NAIP-NLRC4 inflammasome in mice or the caspase-11 inflammasome in human cells was necessary to limit the intraepithelial growth of *Salmonella* and consequently the transcytosis of the bacteria to the lamina propria (95, 96) (Fig. 2B). Both studies found that pyroptosis quickly promoted the expulsion of the dying cells containing *Salmonella* into the gut lumen. This expulsion process was shown to be cell intrinsic, not requiring any additional cells, but was accompanied by major actin rearrangements in the neighboring IECs, which maintained the integrity of the epithelium (97). Furthermore, IEC expulsion is accompanied by epithelial cell production of IL-18 as well as of eicosanoid lipid mediators, such as PGE2, that trigger vascular leakage and fluid accumulation in the intestinal lumen (97), indicating that the eicosanoid-induced fluid response could act in concert with IEC expulsion to provide a mechanism for flushing expelled IEC from the intestines.

While infected cells can die as a result of many different cell death mechanisms, ranging from programmed cell death (apoptosis, necroptosis, and pyroptosis) to simple necrosis, pyroptosis most likely presents the best option for the host to not only restrict the replication of the pathogen but also prevent its spread to neighboring cells. A large proportion of intracellular bacteria remains trapped within the dying cells and is potentially exposed to the pore-forming activity of the GSDMD N terminus. Furthermore, since pyroptosis also results in concomitant cytokine release, it can drive the recruitment and activation of strong antimicrobial effector cells, in particular neutrophils, that efferocytose the dying cells and thus efficiently kill any trapped bacteria.

Citation. Broz P. 2019. Recognition of intracellular bacteria by inflammasomes. Microbiol Spectrum 7(2):BAI-0003-2019.

References

1. Broz P, Dixit VM. 2016. Inflammasomes: mechanism of assembly, regulation and signalling. *Nat Rev Immunol* **16**:407–420.

2. Martinon F, Burns K, Tschopp J. 2002. The inflammasome: a molecular platform triggering activation of inflammatory caspases and processing of proIL-beta. *Mol Cell* **10**:417–426.

3. Liston A, Masters SL. 2017. Homeostasis-altering molecular processes as mechanisms of inflammasome activation. *Nat Rev Immunol* **17**:208–214.

4. Dick MS, Sborgi L, Rühl S, Hiller S, Broz P. 2016. ASC filament formation serves as a signal amplification mechanism for inflammasomes. *Nat Commun* **7**:11929.

5. Lu A, Magupalli VG, Ruan J, Yin Q, Atianand MK, Vos MR, Schröder GF, Fitzgerald KA, Wu H, Egelman EH. 2014. Unified polymerization mechanism for the assembly of ASC-dependent inflammasomes. *Cell* **156**:1193–1206.

6. Thornberry NA, Bull HG, Calaycay JR, Chapman KT, Howard AD, Kostura MJ, Miller DK, Molineaux SM, Weidner JR, Aunins J, Elliston KO, Ayala JM, Casano FJ, Chin J, Ding GJ-F, Egger LA, Gaffney EP, Limjuco G, Palyha OC, Raju SM, Rolando AM, Salley JP, Yamin T-T, Lee TD, Shively JE, MacCross M, Mumford RA, Schmidt JA, Tocci MJ. 1992. A novel heterodimeric cysteine protease is required for interleukin-1 beta processing in monocytes. *Nature* **356**:768–774.

7. Shi J, Zhao Y, Wang K, Shi X, Wang Y, Huang H, Zhuang Y, Cai T, Wang F, Shao F. 2015. Cleavage of GSDMD by inflammatory caspases determines pyroptotic cell death. *Nature* **526**:660–665.

8. Kayagaki N, Stowe IB, Lee BL, O'Rourke K, Anderson K, Warming S, Cuellar T, Haley B, Roose-Girma M, Phung QT, Liu PS, Lill JR, Li H, Wu J, Kummerfeld S, Zhang J, Lee WP, Snipas SJ, Salvesen GS, Morris LX, Fitzgerald L, Zhang Y, Bertram EM, Goodnow CC, Dixit VM. 2015. Caspase-11 cleaves gasdermin D for non-canonical inflammasome signalling. *Nature* **526**:666–671.

9. Sborgi L, Rühl S, Mulvihill E, Pipercevic J, Heilig R, Stahlberg H, Farady CJ, Müller DJ, Broz P, Hiller S. 2016. GSDMD membrane pore formation constitutes the mechanism of pyroptotic cell death. *EMBO J* **35**:1766–1778.

10. Aglietti RA, Estevez A, Gupta A, Ramirez MG, Liu PS, Kayagaki N, Ciferri C, Dixit VM, Dueber EC. 2016. GsdmD p30 elicited by caspase-11 during pyroptosis forms pores in membranes. *Proc Natl Acad Sci USA* **113**:7858–7863.

11. Ding J, Wang K, Liu W, She Y, Sun Q, Shi J, Sun H, Wang DC, Shao F. 2016. Pore-forming activity and structural autoinhibition of the gasdermin family. *Nature* **535**:111–116. ERRATUM *Nature* **640**:150.

12. Liu X, Zhang Z, Ruan J, Pan Y, Magupalli VG, Wu H, Lieberman J. 2016. Inflammasome-activated gasdermin D causes pyroptosis by forming membrane pores. *Nature* **535**:153–158.

13. Bergsbaken T, Fink SL, Cookson BT. 2009. Pyroptosis: host cell death and inflammation. *Nat Rev Microbiol* **7**:99–109.

14. Evavold CL, Ruan J, Tan Y, Xia S, Wu H, Kagan JC. 2017. The pore-forming protein gasdermin D regulates interleukin-1 secretion from living macrophages. *Immunity* **48**:35–44.e6.

15. Heilig R, Dick MS, Sborgi L, Meunier E, Hiller S, Broz P. 2017. The gasdermin-D pore acts as a conduit for IL-1β secretion in mice. *Eur J Immunol* **48**:584–592.

16. Monteleone M, Stow JL, Schroder K. 2015. Mechanisms of unconventional secretion of IL-1 family cytokines. *Cytokine* **74**:213–218.

17. Mariathasan S, Newton K, Monack DM, Vucic D, French DM, Lee WP, Roose-Girma M, Erickson S, Dixit VM. 2004. Differential activation of the inflammasome by caspase-1 adaptors ASC and Ipaf. *Nature* **430**:213–218.

18. Franchi L, Amer A, Body-Malapel M, Kanneganti TD, Ozören N, Jagirdar R, Inohara N, Vandenabeele P, Bertin J, Coyle A, Grant EP, Núñez G. 2006. Cytosolic flagellin requires Ipaf for activation of caspase-1 and interleukin 1beta in salmonella-infected macrophages. *Nat Immunol* **7**:576–582.

19. Miao EA, Alpuche-Aranda CM, Dors M, Clark AE, Bader MW, Miller SI, Aderem A. 2006. Cytoplasmic flagellin activates caspase-1 and secretion of interleukin 1beta via Ipaf. *Nat Immunol* **7**:569–575.

20. Sutterwala FS, Mijares LA, Li L, Ogura Y, Kazmierczak BI, Flavell RA. 2007. Immune recognition of *Pseudomonas aeruginosa* mediated by the IPAF/NLRC4 inflammasome. *J Exp Med* **204**:3235–3245.

21. Suzuki T, Franchi L, Toma C, Ashida H, Ogawa M, Yoshikawa Y, Mimuro H, Inohara N, Sasakawa C, Nuñez G. 2007. Differential regulation of caspase-1 activation, pyroptosis, and autophagy via Ipaf and ASC in *Shigella*-infected macrophages. *PLoS Pathog* **3**:e111.

22. Zamboni DS, Kobayashi KS, Kohlsdorf T, Ogura Y, Long EM, Vance RE, Kuida K, Mariathasan S, Dixit VM, Flavell RA, Dietrich WF, Roy CR. 2006. The Birc1e cytosolic pattern-recognition receptor contributes to the detection

and control of *Legionella pneumophila* infection. *Nat Immunol* 7:318–325.

23. Miao EA, Mao DP, Yudkovsky N, Bonneau R, Lorang CG, Warren SE, Leaf IA, Aderem A. 2010. Innate immune detection of the type III secretion apparatus through the NLRC4 inflammasome. *Proc Natl Acad Sci USA* 107: 3076–3080.

24. Lightfield KL, Persson J, Brubaker SW, Witte CE, von Moltke J, Dunipace EA, Henry T, Sun YH, Cado D, Dietrich WF, Monack DM, Tsolis RM, Vance RE. 2008. Critical function for Naip5 in inflammasome activation by a conserved carboxy-terminal domain of flagellin. *Nat Immunol* 9:1171–1178.

25. Kofoed EM, Vance RE. 2011. Innate immune recognition of bacterial ligands by NAIPs determines inflammasome specificity. *Nature* 477:592–595.

26. Zhao Y, Yang J, Shi J, Gong YN, Lu Q, Xu H, Liu L, Shao F. 2011. The NLRC4 inflammasome receptors for bacterial flagellin and type III secretion apparatus. *Nature* 477:596–600.

27. Yang J, Zhao Y, Shi J, Shao F. 2013. Human NAIP and mouse NAIP1 recognize bacterial type III secretion needle protein for inflammasome activation. *Proc Natl Acad Sci USA* 110:14408–14413.

28. Suzuki S, Franchi L, He Y, Muñoz-Planillo R, Mimuro H, Suzuki T, Sasakawa C, Núñez G. 2014. *Shigella* type III secretion protein MxiI is recognized by Naip2 to induce Nlrc4 inflammasome activation independently of Pkcδ. *PLoS Pathog* 10:e1003926.

29. Kortmann J, Brubaker SW, Monack DM. 2015. Cutting edge: inflammasome activation in primary human macrophages is dependent on flagellin. *J Immunol* 195: 815–819.

30. Tenthorey JL, Kofoed EM, Daugherty MD, Malik HS, Vance RE. 2014. Molecular basis for specific recognition of bacterial ligands by NAIP/NLRC4 inflammasomes. *Mol Cell* 54:17–29.

31. Tenthorey JL, Haloupek N, López-Blanco JR, Grob P, Adamson E, Hartenian E, Lind NA, Bourgeois NM, Chacón P, Nogales E, Vance RE. 2017. The structural basis of flagellin detection by NAIP5: A strategy to limit pathogen immune evasion. *Science* 358:888–893.

32. Bürckstümmer T, Baumann C, Blüml S, Dixit E, Dürnberger G, Jahn H, Planyavsky M, Bilban M, Colinge J, Bennett KL, Superti-Furga G. 2009. An orthogonal proteomic-genomic screen identifies AIM2 as a cytoplasmic DNA sensor for the inflammasome. *Nat Immunol* 10:266–272.

33. Fernandes-Alnemri T, Yu JW, Datta P, Wu J, Alnemri ES. 2009. AIM2 activates the inflammasome and cell death in response to cytoplasmic DNA. *Nature* 458:509–513.

34. Fernandes-Alnemri T, Yu JW, Juliana C, Solorzano L, Kang S, Wu J, Datta P, McCormick M, Huang L, McDermott E, Eisenlohr L, Landel CP, Alnemri ES. 2010. The AIM2 inflammasome is critical for innate immunity to *Francisella tularensis. Nat Immunol* 11:385–393.

35. Hornung V, Ablasser A, Charrel-Dennis M, Bauernfeind F, Horvath G, Caffrey DR, Latz E, Fitzgerald KA. 2009. AIM2 recognizes cytosolic dsDNA and forms a caspase-

1-activating inflammasome with ASC. *Nature* 458: 514–518.

36. Rathinam VA, Jiang Z, Waggoner SN, Sharma S, Cole LE, Waggoner L, Vanaja SK, Monks BG, Ganesan S, Latz E, Hornung V, Vogel SN, Szomolanyi-Tsuda E, Fitzgerald KA. 2010. The AIM2 inflammasome is essential for host defense against cytosolic bacteria and DNA viruses. *Nat Immunol* 11:395–402.

37. Jones JW, Kayagaki N, Broz P, Henry T, Newton K, O'Rourke K, Chan S, Dong J, Qu Y, Roose-Girma M, Dixit VM, Monack DM. 2010. Absent in melanoma 2 is required for innate immune recognition of *Francisella tularensis. Proc Natl Acad Sci USA* 107:9771–9776.

38. Morrone SR, Matyszewski M, Yu X, Delannoy M, Egelman EH, Sohn J. 2015. Assembly-driven activation of the AIM2 foreign-dsDNA sensor provides a polymerization template for downstream ASC. *Nat Commun* 6:7827.

39. Sauer JD, Witte CE, Zemansky J, Hanson B, Lauer P, Portnoy DA. 2010. *Listeria monocytogenes* triggers AIM2-mediated pyroptosis upon infrequent bacteriolysis in the macrophage cytosol. *Cell Host Microbe* 7:412–419.

40. Kim S, Bauernfeind F, Ablasser A, Hartmann G, Fitzgerald KA, Latz E, Hornung V. 2010. *Listeria monocytogenes* is sensed by the NLRP3 and AIM2 inflammasome. *Eur J Immunol* 40:1545–1551.

41. Wassermann R, Gulen MF, Sala C, Perin SG, Lou Y, Rybniker J, Schmid-Burgk JL, Schmidt T, Hornung V, Cole ST, Ablasser A. 2015. *Mycobacterium tuberculosis* differentially activates cGAS- and inflammasome-dependent intracellular immune responses through ESX-1. *Cell Host Microbe* 17:799–810.

42. Saiga H, Kitada S, Shimada Y, Kamiyama N, Okuyama M, Makino M, Yamamoto M, Takeda K. 2012. Critical role of AIM2 in *Mycobacterium tuberculosis* infection. *Int Immunol* 24:637–644.

43. Marim FM, Franco MMC, Gomes MTR, Miraglia MC, Giambartolomei GH, Oliveira SC. 2017. The role of NLRP3 and AIM2 in inflammasome activation during *Brucella abortus* infection. *Semin Immunopathol* 39: 215–223.

44. Cunha LD, Silva ALN, Ribeiro JM, Mascarenhas DPA, Quirino GFS, Santos LL, Flavell RA, Zamboni DS. 2017. AIM2 engages active but unprocessed caspase-1 to induce noncanonical activation of the NLRP3 inflammasome. *Cell Reports* 20:794–805.

45. Henry T, Brotcke A, Weiss DS, Thompson LJ, Monack DM. 2007. Type I interferon signaling is required for activation of the inflammasome during *Francisella* infection. *J Exp Med* 204:987–994.

46. Meunier E, Wallet P, Dreier RF, Costanzo S, Anton L, Rühl S, Dussurgey S, Dick MS, Kistner A, Rigard M, Degrandi D, Pfeffer K, Yamamoto M, Henry T, Broz P. 2015. Guanylate-binding proteins promote activation of the AIM2 inflammasome during infection with *Francisella novicida. Nat Immunol* 16:476–484.

47. Man SM, Karki R, Malireddi RK, Neale G, Vogel P, Yamamoto M, Lamkanfi M, Kanneganti TD. 2015. The transcription factor IRF1 and guanylate-binding proteins

target activation of the AIM2 inflammasome by *Francisella infection. Nat Immunol* 16:467–475.

48. Meunier E, Broz P. 2016. Interferon-inducible GTPases in cell autonomous and innate immunity. *Cell Microbiol* 18: 168–180.

49. Man SM, Karki R, Sasai M, Place DE, Kesavardhana S, Temirov J, Frase S, Zhu Q, Malireddi RKS, Kuriakose T, Peters JL, Neale G, Brown SA, Yamamoto M, Kanneganti T-D. 2016. IRGB10 liberates bacterial ligands for sensing by the AIM2 and caspase-11-NLRP3 inflammasomes. *Cell* 167:382–396.e17.

50. Piro AS, Hernandez D, Luoma S, Feeley EM, Finethy R, Yirga A, Frickel EM, Lesser CF, Coers J. 2017. Detection of cytosolic *Shigella flexneri* via a C-terminal triple-arginine motif of GBP1 inhibits actin-based motility. *mBio* 8: e01979-17.

51. Wandel MP, Pathe C, Werner EI, Ellison CJ, Boyle KB, von der Malsburg A, Rohde J, Randow F. 2017. GBPs inhibit motility of *Shigella flexneri* but are targeted for degradation by the bacterial ubiquitin ligase IpaH9.8. *Cell Host Microbe* 22:507–518.e5.

52. Li P, Jiang W, Yu Q, Liu W, Zhou P, Li J, Xu J, Xu B, Wang F, Shao F. 2017. Ubiquitination and degradation of GBPs by a *Shigella* effector to suppress host defence. *Nature* 551:378–383.

53. Boyden ED, Dietrich WF. 2006. Nalp1b controls mouse macrophage susceptibility to anthrax lethal toxin. *Nat Genet* 38:240–244.

54. Zhong FL, Mamai O, Sborgi L, Boussofara L, Hopkins R, Robinson K, Szeverenyi I, Takeichi T, Balaji R, Lau A, Tye H, Roy K, Bonnard C, Ahl PJ, Jones LA, Baker P, Lacina L, Otsuka A, Fournie PR, Malecaze F, Lane EB, Akiyama M, Kabashima K, Connolly JE, Masters SL, Soler VJ, Omar SS, McGrath JA, Nedelcu R, Gribaa M, Denguezli M, Saad A, Hiller S, Reversade B. 2016. Germline NLRP1 mutations cause skin inflammatory and cancer susceptibility syndromes via inflammasome activation. *Cell* 167:187–202 e17.

55. Levinsohn JL, Newman ZL, Hellmich KA, Fattah R, Getz MA, Liu S, Sastalla I, Leppla SH, Moayeri M. 2012. Anthrax lethal factor cleavage of Nlrp1 is required for activation of the inflammasome. *PLoS Pathog* 8:e1002638.

56. Hellmich KA, Levinsohn JL, Fattah R, Newman ZL, Maier N, Sastalla I, Liu S, Leppla SH, Moayeri M. 2012. Anthrax lethal factor cleaves mouse nlrp1b in both toxin-sensitive and toxin-resistant macrophages. *PLoS One* 7:e49741.

57. Chavarría-Smith J, Vance RE. 2013. Direct proteolytic cleavage of NLRP1B is necessary and sufficient for inflammasome activation by anthrax lethal factor. *PLoS Pathog* 9:e1003452.

58. Wang G, Roux B, Feng F, Guy E, Li L, Li N, Zhang X, Lautier M, Jardinaud M-F, Chabannes M, Arlat M, Chen S, He C, Noël LD, Zhou J-M. 2015. The decoy substrate of a pathogen effector and a pseudokinase specify pathogen-induced modified-self recognition and immunity in plants. *Cell Host Microbe* 18:285–295.

59. van der Hoorn RA, Kamoun S. 2008. From guard to decoy: a new model for perception of plant pathogen effectors. *Plant Cell* 20:2009–2017.

60. Bernot A, Clepet C, Dasilva C, Devaud C, Petit J-L, Caloustian C, Cruaud C, Samson D, Pulcini F, Weissenbach J, Heilig R, Notanicola C, Domingo C, Rozenbaum M, Benchetrit E, Topaloglu R, Dewalle M, Dross C, Hadjari P, Dupont M, Demaille J, Touitou I, Smaoui N, Nedelec B, Méry J-P, Chaabouni H, Delpech M, Grateau G, French FMF Consortium. 1997. A candidate gene for familial Mediterranean fever. *Nat Genet* 17:25–31.

61. Chae JJ, Cho YH, Lee GS, Cheng J, Liu PP, Feigenbaum L, Katz SI, Kastner DL. 2011. Gain-of-function pyrin mutations induce NLRP3 protein-independent interleukin-1β activation and severe autoinflammation in mice. *Immunity* 34:755–768.

62. Xu H, Yang J, Gao W, Li L, Li P, Zhang L, Gong YN, Peng X, Xi JJ, Chen S, Wang F, Shao F. 2014. Innate immune sensing of bacterial modifications of Rho GTPases by the pyrin inflammasome. *Nature* 513:237–241.

63. Gao W, Yang J, Liu W, Wang Y, Shao F. 2016. Site-specific phosphorylation and microtubule dynamics control pyrin inflammasome activation. *Proc Natl Acad Sci USA* 113:E4857–E4866.

64. Park YH, Wood G, Kastner DL, Chae JJ. 2016. Pyrin inflammasome activation and RhoA signaling in the autoinflammatory diseases FMF and HIDS. *Nat Immunol* 17: 914–921.

65. Heilig R, Broz P. 2018. Function and mechanism of the pyrin inflammasome. *Eur J Immunol* 48:230–238.

66. Latz E, Xiao TS, Stutz A. 2013. Activation and regulation of the inflammasomes. *Nat Rev Immunol* 13:397–411.

67. Stutz A, Kolbe C-C, Stahl R, Horvath GL, Franklin BS, van Ray O, Brinkschulte R, Geyer M, Meissner F, Latz E. 2017. NLRP3 inflammasome assembly is regulated by phosphorylation of the pyrin domain. *J Exp Med* 214: 1725–1736.

68. Song N, Liu Z-S, Xue W, Bai Z-F, Wang Q-Y, Dai J, Liu X, Huang Y-J, Cai H, Zhan X-Y, Han Q-Y, Wang H, Chen Y, Li H-Y, Li A-L, Zhang X-M, Zhou T, Li T. 2017. NLRP3 phosphorylation is an essential priming event for inflammasome activation. *Mol Cell* 68:185–197.e6.

69. Juliana C, Fernandes-Alnemri T, Kang S, Farias A, Qin F, Alnemri ES. 2012. Non-transcriptional priming and deubiquitination regulate NLRP3 inflammasome activation. *J Biol Chem* 287:36617–36622.

70. Py BF, Kim MS, Vakifahmetoglu-Norberg H, Yuan J. 2013. Deubiquitination of NLRP3 by BRCC3 critically regulates inflammasome activity. *Mol Cell* 49:331–338.

71. Muñoz-Planillo R, Kuffa P, Martínez-Colón G, Smith BL, Rajendiran TM, Núñez G. 2013. K+ efflux is the common trigger of NLRP3 inflammasome activation by bacterial toxins and particulate matter. *Immunity* 38:1142–1153.

72. Kayagaki N, Warming S, Lamkanfi M, Vande Walle L, Louie S, Dong J, Newton K, Qu Y, Liu J, Heldens S, Zhang J, Lee WP, Roose-Girma M, Dixit VM. 2011. Non-canonical inflammasome activation targets caspase-11. *Nature* 479:117–121.

73. Baker PJ, Boucher D, Bierschenk D, Tebartz C, Whitney PG, D'Silva DB, Tanzer MC, Monteleone M, Robertson AA, Cooper MA, Alvarez-Diaz S, Herold MJ, Bedoui S, Schroder K, Masters SL. 2015. NLRP3 inflammasome

activation downstream of cytoplasmic LPS recognition by both caspase-4 and caspase-5. *Eur J Immunol* **45**: 2918–2926.

74. Schmid-Burgk JL, Gaidt MM, Schmidt T, Ebert TS, Bartok E, Hornung V. 2015. Caspase-4 mediates non-canonical activation of the NLRP3 inflammasome in human myeloid cells. *Eur J Immunol* **45**:2911–2917.

75. Rühl S, Broz P. 2015. Caspase-11 activates a canonical NLRP3 inflammasome by promoting K⁺ efflux. *Eur J Immunol* **45**:2927–2936.

76. Broz P, Ruby T, Belhocine K, Bouley DM, Kayagaki N, Dixit VM, Monack DM. 2012. Caspase-11 increases susceptibility to *Salmonella* infection in the absence of caspase-1. *Nature* **490**:288–291.

77. Rathinam VA, Vanaja SK, Waggoner L, Sokolovska A, Becker C, Stuart LM, Leong JM, Fitzgerald KA. 2012. TRIF licenses caspase-11-dependent NLRP3 inflammasome activation by gram-negative bacteria. *Cell* **150**: 606–619.

78. Kayagaki N, Wong MT, Stowe IB, Ramani SR, Gonzalez LC, Akashi-Takamura S, Miyake K, Zhang J, Lee WP, Muszynski A, Forsberg LS, Carlson RW, Dixit VM. 2013. Noncanonical inflammasome activation by intracellular LPS independent of TLR4. *Science* **341**:1246–1249.

79. Hagar JA, Powell DA, Aachoui Y, Ernst RK, Miao EA. 2013. Cytoplasmic LPS activates caspase-11: implications in TLR4-independent endotoxic shock. *Science* **341**: 1250–1253.

80. Shi J, Zhao Y, Wang Y, Gao W, Ding J, Li P, Hu L, Shao F. 2014. Inflammatory caspases are innate immune receptors for intracellular LPS. *Nature* **514**:187–192.

81. Beutler B, Jiang Z, Georgel P, Crozat K, Croker B, Rutschmann S, Du X, Hoebe K. 2006. Genetic analysis of host resistance: toll-like receptor signaling and immunity at large. *Annu Rev Immunol* **24**:353–389.

82. Meunier E, Dick MS, Dreier RF, Schürmann N, Kenzelmann Broz D, Warming S, Roose-Girma M, Bumann D, Kayagaki N, Takeda K, Yamamoto M, Broz P. 2014. Caspase-11 activation requires lysis of pathogen-containing vacuoles by IFN-induced GTPases. *Nature* **509**: 366–370.

83. Pilla DM, Hagar JA, Haldar AK, Mason AK, Degrandi D, Pfeffer K, Ernst RK, Yamamoto M, Miao EA, Coers J. 2014. Guanylate binding proteins promote caspase-11-dependent pyroptosis in response to cytoplasmic LPS. *Proc Natl Acad Sci USA* **111**:6046–6051.

84. Santos JC, Dick MS, Lagrange B, Degrandi D, Pfeffer K, Yamamoto M, Meunier E, Pelczar P, Henry T, Broz P. 2018. LPS targets host guanylate-binding proteins to the bacterial outer membrane for non-canonical inflammasome activation. *EMBO J* **37**:e98089.

85. Finethy R, Luoma S, Orench-Rivera N, Feeley EM, Haldar AK, Yamamoto M, Kanneganti T-D, Kuehn MJ, Coers J. 2017. Inflammasome activation by bacterial outer membrane vesicles requires guanylate binding proteins. *mBio* **8**: e01188-17.

86. Gu L, Meng R, Tang Y, Zhao K, Liang F, Zhang R, Xue Q, Chen F, Xiao X, Wang H, Wang H, Billiar TR, Lu B. 2018. Toll like receptor 4 signaling licenses the cytosolic transport of lipopolysaccharide from bacterial outer membrane vesicles. *Shock* **51**:256–265.

87. Lagrange B, Benaoudia S, Wallet P, Magnotti F, Provost A, Michal F, Martin A, Di Lorenzo F, Py BF, Molinaro A, Henry T. 2018. Human caspase-4 detects tetra-acylated LPS and cytosolic *Francisella* and functions differently from murine caspase-11. *Nat Commun* **9**:242.

88. Vanaja SK, Russo AJ, Behl B, Banerjee I, Yankova M, Deshmukh SD, Rathinam VAK. 2016. Bacterial outer membrane vesicles mediate cytosolic localization of LPS and caspase-11 activation. *Cell* **165**:1106–1119.

89. Zychlinsky A, Prevost MC, Sansonetti PJ. 1992. *Shigella flexneri* induces apoptosis in infected macrophages. *Nature* **358**:167–169.

90. Fink SL, Bergsbaken T, Cookson BT. 2008. Anthrax lethal toxin and *Salmonella* elicit the common cell death pathway of caspase-1-dependent pyroptosis via distinct mechanisms. *Proc Natl Acad Sci USA* **105**:4312–4317.

91. Miao EA, Leaf IA, Treuting PM, Mao DP, Dors M, Sarkar A, Warren SE, Wewers MD, Aderem A. 2010. Caspase-1-induced pyroptosis is an innate immune effector mechanism against intracellular bacteria. *Nat Immunol* **11**:1136–1142.

92. Jorgensen I, Zhang Y, Krantz BA, Miao EA. 2016. Pyroptosis triggers pore-induced intracellular traps (PITs) that capture bacteria and lead to their clearance by efferocytosis. *J Exp Med* **213**:2113–2128.

93. Jorgensen I, Lopez JP, Laufer SA, Miao EA. 2016. IL-1β, IL-18, and eicosanoids promote neutrophil recruitment to pore-induced intracellular traps following pyroptosis. *Eur J Immunol* **46**:2761–2766.

94. Thurston TL, Matthews SA, Jennings E, Alix E, Shao F, Shenoy AR, Birrell MA, Holden DW. 2016. Growth inhibition of cytosolic *Salmonella* by caspase-1 and caspase-11 precedes host cell death. *Nat Commun* **7**:13292.

95. Sellin ME, Müller AA, Felmy B, Dolowschiak T, Diard M, Tardivel A, Maslowski KM, Hardt WD. 2014. Epithelium-intrinsic NAIP/NLRC4 inflammasome drives infected enterocyte expulsion to restrict *Salmonella* replication in the intestinal mucosa. *Cell Host Microbe* **16**: 237–248.

96. Knodler LA, Crowley SM, Sham HP, Yang H, Wrande M, Ma C, Ernst RK, Steele-Mortimer O, Celli J, Vallance BA. 2014. Noncanonical inflammasome activation of caspase-4/caspase-11 mediates epithelial defenses against enteric bacterial pathogens. *Cell Host Microbe* **16**: 249–256.

97. Rauch I, Deets KA, Ji DX, von Moltke J, Tenthorey JL, Lee AY, Philip NH, Ayres JS, Brodsky IE, Gronert K, Vance RE. 2017. NAIP-NLRC4 inflammasomes coordinate intestinal epithelial cell expulsion with eicosanoid and IL-18 release via activation of caspase-1 and -8. *Immunity* **46**:649–659.

New Technologies To Move Cellular Microbiology to Organs and Tissues

IV

Bacteria and Intracellularity
Edited by Pascale Cossart, Craig R. Roy, and Philippe Sansonetti
© 2019 American Society for Microbiology, Washington, DC
doi:10.1128/microbiolspec.BAI-0019-2019

Modeling Infectious Diseases in Mice with a "Humanized" Immune System

21

Yan Li[1,2] and James P. Di Santo[1,2]

DEVELOPMENT OF IMMUNODEFICIENT MOUSE STRAINS

Immunocompetent mice harbor several layers of immune defense that can promote rejection of cell and tissue xenografts; these include innate mechanisms (mediated by complement, macrophage, and neutrophils) as well as adaptive immune responses (T cell-mediated and antibody-mediated rejection). In addition, resident tissues in the mouse harbor self-renewing stem cells and their differentiated progeny, which can effectively compete with human cells for endogenous tissue resources (physical space, nutrients, growth factors, etc.) that may play a role in sustaining human xenografts. As such, the development of "humanized" mouse models (human immune system [HIS] mice) is closely associated with the history of mutant mouse strains that harbor defects in hematopoietic system development and function. In recent decades, knowledge of the molecular mechanisms that regulate innate and adaptive immunity has led to the development of mouse models with an ever-increasing capacity to engraft human cells and tissues (reviewed in references 1–4). With respect to engraftment of the human hematopoietic system, as the severity of the immune deficiency in the mouse host has increased, the efficiency and durability of human hematopoietic cell "take" have improved remarkably, and importantly, a diverse compartment comprising many unique human immune subsets (including not only lymphocytes but also myeloid cells) has been achieved (Fig. 1).

Mice Deficient in Adaptive Lymphocytes (T and B Cells)

In 1962, a spontaneous mutation in mice causing hair loss (*nude*) was discovered; nude mice were also remarkable for the absence of a thymus (5). It was later shown that nude mice harbor a mutation in *Foxn1*, which encodes a transcription factor that is essential for thymic epithelial function; its absence results in a complete block in T cell development (6). The T cell immunodeficiency in *nude*-bearing mice allowed the earliest studies of patient-derived tumor xenografts (7). Nevertheless, other immune mechanisms were still operative in this strain, as nude mice were not able to support reconstitution of mononuclear cells from human bone marrow even after lethal irradiation (8).

In 1983, a spontaneous mutation was identified in mice that was involved in DNA repair and that severely affected development of B and T cells (9). This mutation was designated *scid* (for severe combined immune deficiency), and SCID mice were shown to carry a mutation in the gene *Prkdc* (protein kinase, DNA-activated, catalytic polypeptide), encoding a kinase which plays a critical role in nonhomologous end joining during double-strand-break repair. The B and T cell immunodeficiency in SCID mice arises from the inability of these mice to perform VDJ recombination to generate mature T and B lymphocytes (10); as a result, SCID mice lack both cell-mediated (T cell) and humoral (B cell and antibody) responses. Moreover, the defect in DNA repair that SCID mice manifest is not restricted to the adaptive immune system but is a generalized defect in DNA repair that affects all somatic cells (11).

Curiously, the *Prkdc* mutation in SCID mice appears to be leaky, meaning that in some SCID mutant mice, a low level of VDJ recombination can be detected, leading to a residual level of B and T cell differentiation (12). As such, a fraction of SCID mice show some immune competence and can elicit immune responses against various types of immunogens. In addition, leaky SCID mice have an increased incidence of thymic lymphoma formation, which unfortunately limits the use of SCID mice for long-term transplantation studies (11). Finally, due to

---

[1]Innate Immunity Unit, Immunology Department, Institut Pasteur, Paris, France; [2]Inserm U1223, Paris, France.

Development of Human Immune System (HIS) Mouse Models

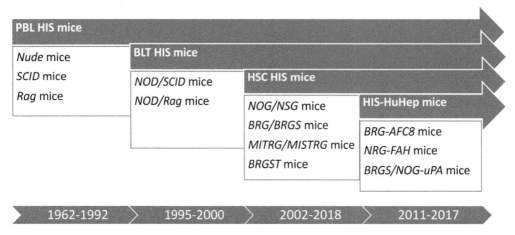

Figure 1 Timeline for development of immunodeficient mouse strains that form the basis for current HIS models. Indicated strains are described in the text.

their generalized DNA repair defects, SCID mice are highly sensitive to irradiation, and radiation doses must be carefully titrated for each colony (13).

In order to create a non-leaky SCID model, mouse strains with stable defects in T and B cell development were created by targeted mutation in the VDJ recombinase genes *Rag1* and *Rag2*, which together catalyze double-strand breaks that initiate VDJ recombination but are not involved in general DNA repair (14, 15). Compared with *Pkrdc*$^{-/-}$ and *Foxn1*$^{-/-}$ mice, *Rag*-deficient strains showed similar levels of cell engraftment following injection of human hematopoietic stem cells (HSC) and peripheral blood lymphocytes (PBL), while the formation of thymic lymphomas in *Rag*-deficient hosts is markedly decreased compared to that in SCID-based models, as *Rag*$^{-/-}$ mice have normal irradiation sensitivity profiles (16).

Mice with Compromised Macrophage Rejection of Human Xenografts

While nude, SCID, and *Rag*-deficient hosts demonstrate the importance of adaptive immunity as a mechanism of xenograft rejection, studies comparing SCID mice on different host backgrounds demonstrated that additional nonadaptive immune mechanisms also affected human xenograft take. SCID mice on the nonobese diabetic (NOD) background were superior hosts for human cell transplantation compared with SCID

mice on the C57BL/6 background (17). A seminal report published in 2007 illuminated the biology behind these differences (18). Signal regulatory protein α (Sirpa) is an inhibitory transmembrane receptor, mainly expressed on myeloid cells and macrophages. The ligand for Sirpa is the glycoprotein CD47, which is highly expressed by immune cells. Importantly, CD47 interaction with Sirpa delivers an inhibitory signal ("don't eat me" signal) to Sirpa-expressing macrophages. In NOD mice, the *Sirpa* allele differs from the one expressed in C57BL/6 mice. Takenaka et al. showed that the *Sirpa*^{NOD} allele could interact with human CD47, whereas *Sirpa*^{B6} could not (18). As a result, macrophages (and also myeloid cells) in NOD-based mice are more tolerant of human CD47-expressing cells, whereas C57BL/6 macrophages rapidly eliminate human cells via phagocytosis.

By extensive backcrossing of the *scid* and *Rag* mutations on the NOD background, novel immunodeficient mouse strains harboring the congenic *Sirpa*^{NOD} allele were developed that showed enhanced levels of human immune cell engraftment following transfer of PBL or CD34$^+$ HSC. Due to these properties, NOD/SCID and NOD/*Rag* mouse models rapidly became the gold standard for studies investigating *in vivo* human HSC biology in humanized mice (16, 17). Nevertheless, the immune subsets that differentiated from injected human HSC in NOD/SCID mice consisted mostly of transitional B cells, whereas T cell development was still largely underrepresented. As such, these first-generation NOD/SCID strains were not adequate models to study human innate and adaptive immune responses *in vivo*.

Mice with Deficiencies in Endogenous Lymphocyte Precursors

Engrafted human HSC generate hematopoietic precursor cells that must take up residence in primary lymphoid organs of the mouse (bone marrow and thymus), expand, and differentiate into mature human lymphocytes before exiting to seed peripheral lymphoid organs for immune responses. As mentioned above, human hematopoietic precursors will in many cases have to compete with endogenous mouse hematolymphoid precursors for niches that provide resources for survival and growth. Immunodeficient mice described thus far have defects in mature B and T cells, but the mutations (*Rag* and *Prkdc*) do not perturb early lymphoid precursor development or homeostasis, which depends on cytokines and other growth factors.

The common cytokine receptor γ chain (γc, encoded at the locus *Il2rg*) is a receptor subunit shared by interleukin 2 (IL-2), IL-4, IL-7, IL-9, IL-15, and IL-21 receptors. IL2RG is mutated in human X-linked SCID, a disease characterized by an absence of T cells and NK cells (19). *Il2rg*$^{-/-}$ mice have multiple defects in immune development, with few mature B or T cells and a complete absence of NK cells (20). Importantly, these immune phenotypes have been traced to the role of γc as a survival and expansion factor for early lymphoid precursors. As such, *Il2rg*$^{-/-}$ mice have severely depleted NK, B, and T cell precursors in the thymus and bone marrow (21).

The development of *Il2rg*$^{-/-}$ mice spawned a new series of immunodeficient mouse models that incorporated mutations in this shared cytokine receptor (22–25). These include NOD/SCID/*Il2rg* (*NSG* or *NOG*), NOD/*Rag*/*Il2rg* (*NRG*), BALB/c *Rag*/*Il2rg* (*BRG*), and BALB/c *Rag2*/*Il2rg*/*Sirpa*^{NOD} (*BRGS*) mice. Quite unexpectedly, mice with these different *Il2rg*-based immunodeficiencies showed robust development of human T cells after HSC engraftment that was achieved *in situ* in the residual mouse thymus (22–25). Human thymopoiesis that was achieved in *NSG* or *BRG* mice injected with human CD34$^+$ HSC was remarkably similar to that observed in human thymus, and mature T cells that developed in *NSG*- and *BRG*-based HIS mice appeared diverse in their T cell-receptor repertoire and in their capacity to be stimulated via the T cell receptor (26, 27), suggesting that they had undergone a normal process of differentiation. These "second-generation" *Il2rg*-based HIS models

(*NSG, NOG,* and *BRGS*) rapidly became the models of choice for studies of human immune responses, as both cell-mediated (T cell) and humoral (B cell) immunity could be elicited following infection or immunization (reviewed in references 1–4). The basis for the improved human thymopoiesis in *Il2rg*-based HIS mice is not fully understood, but it could relate to the absence of competition with mouse lymphoid precursors and/or to the absence of NK cell-mediated xenograft rejection.

Mice with Immune Deficiencies but Intact Innate Lymphoid Cell Function

Innate lymphoid cells (ILC) are a recently identified group of hematopoietic effector cells with lymphoid morphology yet lacking rearranged antigen-specific receptors. ILC include cytotoxic NK cells and diverse helper ILC subsets (ILC1, ILC2, and ILC3) that mirror cytotoxic CD8$^+$ T lymphocytes and Th1/2/17 helper CD4 T lymphocyte subsets, respectively (reviewed in references 28 and 29). While NK cells rely on γc signals delivered through IL-2 and IL-15 for their development and maturation, helper ILC require IL-7 signals for differentiation and survival. As such, *Il2rg*$^{-/-}$ mice have a deficiency in mouse NK cells (as indicated above) but also lack all helper ILC subsets. ILC play diverse roles in immune defense, but one subset of ILC3, called lymphoid tissue inducer cells, is active during the fetal period and promotes the formation of secondary lymphoid tissues (SLT), such as peripheral lymph nodes (LN) and Peyer's patches (30). As such, all HIS mouse models based on *Il2rg* deficiency (*BRGS, NSG, NOG,* and *NRG*) fail to generate SLT. The absence of SLT in *BRGS/NSG/NOG/NRG* HIS mice likely impacts immune performance in these models, since SLT are known to orchestrate and promote effective T and B cell responses.

Very recently, a solution to the SLT deficiency in *Il2rg*-based HIS mouse models was reported (31). Thymic stroma-derived lymphopoietin (TSLP) is an IL-7-like protein that binds the IL-7 receptor but does not require γc for its function (32, 33). TSLP supplementation was able to rescue lymphoid tissue inducer cell function in *Il2rg*$^{-/-}$ mice and restored LN development in *BRGS*-based HIS mice (31). This novel BRGS-TSLP (BRGST) HIS mouse model should find many applications aimed at dissecting the role of LN in human immune and infection-related pathologies.

Human Cytokine and Growth Factor Replacement Mice

Despite high and sustainable human hematopoietic cell engraftment in *BRG/NSG/NOG/NRG*-based HIS mice, the overall composition of human immune subsets remains biased, with prominent T and B lymphocyte development. In contrast, innate lymphocytes (NK cells and ILC), myeloid lineages (neutrophils, eosinophils, and basophils), and monocytes/macrophages are underrepresented in most HIS models (reviewed in references 1–4). Part of the reason for this unbalanced hematopoiesis relates to the fact that several mouse cytokines (including macrophage colony-stimulating factor [M-CSF], granulocyte-macrophage CSF [GM-CSF], IL-3, thrombopoietin, IL-15, and to a lesser extent IL-7) trigger only partially or fail to trigger their corresponding receptors on human hematopoietic target cells. Several studies have reported that injection of human recombinant cytokines, hydrodynamic injection of plasmids expressing human cytokines, or "replacement" of coding exons for mouse cytokines with human counterparts can alleviate this issue and result in enhanced production of human innate lymphocytes (IL-2 and IL-15), dendritic cells (DC) (Flt3L, GM-CSF, and IL-4), and/or macrophages (M-CSF, GM-CSF, and IL-3) (34–39) (Fig. 2).

Combinations of several human cytokines can have dramatic additive effects, leading to almost complete humanization of the mouse bone marrow. For example, *MITRG* and *MISTRG* mice, in which human M-CSF-, IL-3-, GM-CSF-, and thrombopoietin-coding exons are inserted as knock-in alleles on the *BRG* background, have

multilineage human myeloid and monocyte/macrophage development, and strong innate immune responses can be elicited (40). The boost in human myelopoiesis, however, comes at a price, as the expressed human cytokines do not stimulate mouse hematopoietic precursors, resulting in defects in mouse hematopoietic progenitors and phagocytic cells. Subsequent reconstitution of human HSC in these mice shows an increase in human monocytes and macrophages but a decrease in mouse life span due to anemia caused by enhanced phagocytosis of mouse red blood cells (RBC) by human macrophages (40).

APPROACHES TO GENERATE HIS MICE

Mouse models have added considerably to our understanding of pathogenesis and have contributed to the development of numerous prophylactic and therapeutic medications for these devastating diseases. It is generally accepted that animal models (mice as well as other species) will continue to advance our knowledge in this area. Still, the human and mouse immune systems began to diverge roughly 65 million years ago, and since then, significant differences in the structure and function of immune receptors, soluble factors, and signaling pathways have occurred during evolution (reviewed in reference 41). Certain pathogens exhibit unique tropism for humans but not for mice, while many pathogens dis-

Boosting Immune Subsets in Humanized Mice

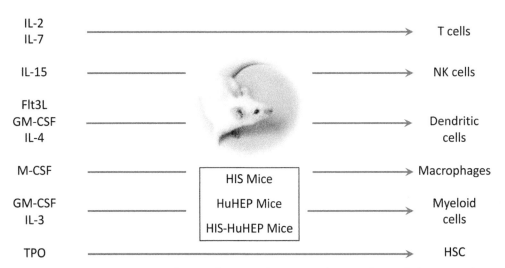

Figure 2 Boosting immune subsets in humanized mice. Cytokines and growth factor supplementation (left) in HIS mice can promote the expansion, differentiation, and function of selected hematopoietic lineages (right). TPO, thrombopoietin.

play distinctly different disease progression and severity in human and mouse models. Such differences can limit the value of mice as preclinical models for certain human infectious diseases. Humanized mice can bypass some of these limitations, and in this regard, accurate modeling of human-specific pathogenesis *in vivo* has been a driving force in the development of improved HIS mouse models. Several humanization strategies for creating HIS mice are available and are described in detail below. As immune responses to infections result from key encounters with specific cell types within the hematopoietic system (antigen-presenting cells, T cell subsets, etc.), putting in place the appropriate HIS mouse model should be carefully considered.

Creating HIS Mice Following Engraftment of Human CD34+ HSC

In order to recapitulate the entire developmental range of human hematopoietic elements in HIS mice, transfer of human CD34+ HSC is required. The sources of human CD34+ HSC may include fetal liver, cord blood, and adult bone marrow-derived cells. These multipotent, self-renewing progenitors are commonly injected into sublethally irradiated *BRG/NSG/NOG/NRG* recipients (newborn or adult mice) via intracardiac or intrahepatic injection. After a period of 8 to 14 weeks, human hematopoietic cells can be detected in tissues and in the circulation. Both adult and newborn mice allow persistent multilineage human hematopoietic engraftment (lasting up to 1 year), but use of newborn pups as hosts is preferred, as T cell development in pups appears to be more robust than that in adults.

The main advantage of the HSC-derived HIS mouse model is its simplicity; only a single injection of CD34+ HSC into an appropriately conditioned (irradiated) host is required. Since the human T cells develop in the context of the mouse thymus, they are "educated" (tolerant) to mouse tissues but remain reactive to foreign antigens. Still, some deficiencies in human immune responses are apparent in HSC-derived HIS mice. While both B and T cells develop, the dynamics are different, with B cells arising after 6 weeks, while T cells require around 12 weeks to emerge from the thymus. As such, T/B cooperation is suboptimal. In this type of HIS model, T cells are selected on the mouse major histocompatibility complex in the thymus, which may explain the delayed T-cell-developmental kinetics. Along these lines, *BRGS/NSG/NOG* strains that express human *HLA-A2*, *DR2*, and *DR4* transgenes have been developed and show improved generation of CD4+ and CD8+ T cells, more rapid T cell emergence, and higher levels of antigen-specific T cell responses (42, 43; Di Santo, manuscript in preparation).

As detailed below, CD34+ HSC HIS mice have been used to study many different types of infectious agents that cause human disease, including viral (HIV, Epstein-Barr virus, cytomegalovirus, and Dengue virus), bacterial (*Salmonella enterica* serovar Typhi, *Mycobacterium tuberculosis*, *Mycobacterium bovis* bacille Calmette-Guérin [BCG], *Staphylococcus aureus*, and others), and parasitic (*Plasmodium falciparum* and *Leishmania major*) infections (reviewed in references 1–4 and 44) (Fig. 3). For example, HIV infection in HSC-based HIS mice leads to preferential depletion of CD4+ T cells and activation of CD8+ T cells, similar to that found in primo-infected patients (reviewed in references 45–47). HIV-infected HIS mice can be treated with highly active antiretroviral therapy (HAART) to suppress HIV replication with the formation of latent viral reservoirs; interruption of HAART leads to a viral rebound in HIS mice similar to that observed in clinics with HAART-treated HIV patients. These studies show the utility of HIS-based mouse models for understanding HIV pathogenesis and for establishing novel therapeutic approaches for eliminating viral reservoirs (HIV "cure").

Improving the quality and breadth of human innate and adaptive immune responses in HIS mice remains a constant challenge. Despite the abundance of mature B and T cells, HIS mice show poor antibody responses, in part due to lack of SLT, as noted above. B cells in immunized or infected HIS mice fail to demonstrate appreciable levels of somatic hypermutation in their Ig genes, suggesting that germinal center reactions are suboptimal (reviewed in references 2, 4, and 44). Providing additional B cell factors (IL-6, BAFF, CXCL13, etc.) (31, 48, 49) in combination and in the context of an appropriate SLT (31) may allow this issue to be resolved.

Creating HIS Mice following Engraftment of Human Fetal Liver, Fetal Thymus, and CD34+ HSC (BLT Mice)

Mucosal tissues (including the gut, lung, skin, and urinary and reproductive tracts), are portals of entry for pathogens. At these sites, strategically placed sentinel cells (epithelial cells, antigen-presenting cells, and macrophages) are targets of infection and/or capture infected cells to initiate immune responses. Innate and adaptive lymphocytes are abundant in mucosal surfaces and include B cells, T cells, NK cells, and various ILC subsets (28, 29). Some viral infections (HIV-1) rely on active replication within the mucosal immune system and form latent reservoirs in this tissue under HAART. Having the

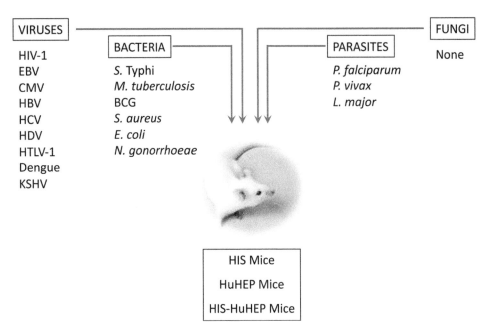

Figure 3 Studying human pathogens in humanized mice. A variety of human pathogens, including viruses, bacteria, and parasites, have been analyzed in HIS mouse models. EBV, Epstein-Barr virus; CMV, cytomegalovirus; HTLV-1, human T cell leukemia virus type 1; KSHV, Kaposi's sarcoma-associated herpesvirus.

capacity to model this aspect of HIV replication in HIS mice may lead to new approaches to target mucosal immunity to a variety of human pathogens.

Mucosal immune system development is essentially absent in HSC-based HIS mice; the reasons for this are not clear but may relate to poor induction of gut-specific homing receptors that guide lymphocytes into these sites (50). In contrast, another technique to generate HIS mice using coengraftment of fetal liver and thymus fragments under kidney capsules of *NOD/SCID* mice followed by CD34$^+$ HSC injection (called BLT mice, for "bone marrow, liver, thymus") results in abundant T cell reconstitution of mucosal tissues (51). The implanted fetal thymus and liver fragment in BLT mice provide autologous thymic epithelium to facilitate HLA-restricted thymocyte development. Moreover, the use of the *NOD/SCID* strain, in which peripheral lymph node and Peyer's patch anlagen exist, allows the reconstitution of SLT (52). As such, BLT mice show strong antigen-specific HLA-restricted T cell responses.

The robust mucosal engraftment of human T cells in BLT mice has allowed several important studies on HIV transmission mechanisms (saliva and breast milk) and for prophylactic prevention strategies (reviewed in references 45–47). Still, the BLT HIS model has several limitations, including the need for access to fetal tissues and special technical and surgical skills to engineer these

mice. Moreover, BLT HIS mice have been reported to have a shorter life span than other HIS models, possibly related to the development of a xenograft-versus-host disease (xeno-GVHD) mediated by human T cells (53). Nevertheless, BLT mice represent an important model for studying T cell immunity against a variety of human pathogens.

Creating HIS Mice Following Engraftment of Human PBL

One of the earliest versions of HIS mice involved transfer of PBL to SCID mice (54). This SCID-PBL HIS model was widely used prior to the advent of *Il2rg*-based immunodeficient hosts and has the advantage that large cohorts of HIS mice can be generated in a very short time frame (weeks). In this model, small numbers of adult PBL (5 to 10 million cells) are injected into *NOD/SCID* recipients; irradiation is not necessary, although it can accelerate the kinetics of humanization. While normal PBL contain several hematopoietic lineages (B cells, T cells, DC, NK cells, neutrophils, etc.), the predominant cell types that expand in this context are mature T cells (both CD4$^+$ and CD8$^+$) (55). Over a period of 2 months, T cell expansion occurs, generating a large population of activated and memory T cells that can be studied in the context of infection or immunization (56). Adoptive transfer of antigen-primed DC into SCID-PBL

HIS mice can also be used to study recall responses to previous vaccines or immunogens (57); these approaches have utility and can be used to monitor pathogen exposure in individuals.

The T cell expansion in this model is driven largely by the sensing of xenodeterminants in the mouse (primarily major histocompatibility complex molecules) by mature human T cells. This process bears some similarity to GVHDs that are T cell mediated and occur in humans following tissue or cell transplantation, and as such, SCID-PBL HIS mice have been used as a model to study some of the immune mechanisms that operate in human GVHD (58). Still, the intensity of xeno-GVHD in this model prevents long-term studies, and the resultant systemic inflammatory reaction makes interpretation of results difficult. Modifications of *BRG/NSG/NOG* mice to eliminate expression of murine class I and class II molecules allows prolonged survival of HIS-PBL mice (58, 59) and may open new avenues of research.

A special type of HIS-PBL mice can be generated to study human erythrocyte biology. Human RBC develop poorly in almost all HIS models due to the inability of mouse erythropoietin to trigger human erythrocytic precursor cells and removal by mouse macrophages (60, 61). In contrast, adoptive transfer of human circulating RBC to macrophage-depleted immunodeficient mice can establish a short-lived pool of human RBC that can then be studied as target for infection by malaria parasites, including *P. falciparum* (62). This RBC transfer approach in HIS mice can be additionally performed in other HIS contexts (CD34$^+$ HSC HIS, BLT HIS, etc.) to create more complex systems for studies involving immunity to malaria parasites.

Creating "Dual" HIS Mice Harboring Additional Nonhematopoietic Tissues

The HIS models described above provide a means to study a multitude of pathogens that directly target human hematopoietic cells. However, several major human diseases result from infection of nonhematopoietic target cells with tissue tropism requirements that are not met by the analogous murine tissue. For example, hepatitis B and C viruses (HBV and HCV) infect human (and some primate) hepatocytes but not mouse hepatocytes (63). In order to create a mouse model for studying human hepatitis virus infection and pathology, genetic engineering of immunodeficient mice was performed to allow humanization of the mouse liver. Several models, including albumin promoter-driven urokinase plasminogen activator (64, 65), albumin-driven thymidine kinase (66), fumarylacetoacetate hydrolase deficiency (*Fah$^{-/-}$*)

(67, 68), and inducible activation of hepatocyte-restricted death-signaling pathways (AFC8) (69), resulted in strong selective pressure against mouse hepatocytes, thereby creating a niche for engraftment of human hepatocytes in mice. By combining these human hepatocyte (HuHEP) mice with existing HIS models, doubly humanized mice bearing both human immune systems and human hepatocytes have been obtained (reviewed in reference 70). HIS-HuHEP mice have been shown to be susceptible to infection by HBV and HCV as well as *P. falciparum* sporozoites, and human immune responses against HBV have been demonstrated that restrict viral replication and spread (70–72). The HIS-HuHEP model is just one example of how multitissue-humanized mice can be generated to address particular aspects of human infections and to provide valuable insights into the role of human immunity in disease progression. As other human tissues can be engrafted in immunodeficient hosts (skin, gut, muscle, fat, etc.), one can envisage ever-more-complex humanized mouse models that can recapitulate the multitissue nature of human disease (following infection but also involving inflammation, autoimmunity, and metabolic stress).

USING HUMAN IMMUNE SYSTEM MICE TO UNDERSTAND THE BIOLOGY OF BACTERIAL INFECTIONS

In this final section, we present some examples of how HIS mouse models can provide an opportunity to study bacterial infections that cause human disease (Fig. 3). Although these studies are somewhat limited in number, they provide evidence for the utility of HIS mice and also suggest avenues for improvements of these models.

Infection of HIS Mice with *S.* Typhi

Typhoid fever is a life-threatening human disease caused by *S.* Typhi. Because of the lack of effective vaccine and the emergence of multidrug-resistant *S.* Typhi strains, this pathogen presents a serious potential threat to global health. The understanding of *S.* Typhi pathogenesis has been impeded by the lack of clinically relevant animal models, as this bacterium exclusively infects humans and does not cause any obvious disease in most laboratory strains of mice. Interestingly, intravenous or intraperitoneal *S.* Typhi infection of CD34$^+$ HSC-engrafted HIS mice showed cardinal clinical features of human typhoid fever, including fever, increased inflammatory cytokines, neurological signs (meningitis), and high mortality (73–75). Increased bacterial burdens in the livers and spleens of HIS mice suggest replication of *S.* Typhi. Importantly, infection of nonhumanized *BRG* and *NSG* host strains showed no disease, demonstrating an obligate role for human hematopoietic cells in this process.

These results show the utility of HIS mice as a novel and valuable tool to investigate the pathological mechanisms of *S.* Typhi infection and to characterize the immune responses of typhoid fever. Still, there appears to be some variability in the severity, kinetics, and clinical symptoms of typhoid fever reported from three independent published studies with HIS mice (73–75). This may reflect differences in the immune reactivity of the different human HSC donors or other experimental variables (such as mouse genetic background and infection routes). Moreover, the natural route of human *S.* Typhi infection is via the digestive tract, whereas studies using HIS mice used intravenous or intraperitoneal routes of infection (76).

Infection of HIS Mice with Mycobacteria

M. tuberculosis infection results in more than 1.4 million deaths per year and is the primary cause of death for HIV-infected patients. Reports of multi-drug-resistant strains of *M. tuberculosis* are on the rise, adding urgency to the need to find new therapeutic approaches to restrain or eliminate persistent *M. tuberculosis* infection. While mouse models of *M. tuberculosis* infection have largely contributed to our understanding of host-pathogen interactions, the inability of *M. tuberculosis*-infected mice to develop latent infections characterized by the formation of organized granulomas (macrophage cores ringed by lymphocytes) has impeded research on this disease (77, 78).

Advances in the development of macrophage and myeloid cell development in HIS mice offered hope that new relevant animal models of *M. tuberculosis* infection might be on the horizon. This appears to be the case, as CD34⁺ HSC-based HIS mice were recently found to form granuloma-type structures in liver and lung after intravenous injection of *M. tuberculosis* or BCG vaccine (79). As was the case for *S.* Typhi infection, granuloma formation was not observed in nonreconstituted *NSG* mice, implying a specific role for human hematopoietic cells in this process.

Latent *M. tuberculosis* infection was not observed in this system, but rather, HIS mice harbored increased numbers of mycobacteria in several organs compared to nonhumanized *NSG* mice; this result was apparently mediated by human CD4⁺ T cells (79). Enhanced macrophage reconstitution in HIS mice following supplementation of human M-CSF resulted in better control of BCG infection (34). Progressive infection was also observed in BLT-based HIS mice after intranasal *M. tuberculosis* infection (80) and in *NSG-HLA-A2* HIS mice after intravenous BCG administration (81). These studies suggest that improved HLA-restricted adaptive T cell responses are not sufficient to contain the active *M. tuberculosis* infection and may even promote infection. Finally, a report of HIV-1–*M. tuberculosis* coinfection using BLT-based HIS mice found that CD4⁺ T cell depletion and CD8⁺ T cell activation following HIV-1 infection exacerbated pulmonary *M. tuberculosis* infection, resulting in more severe lung pathology and increased mycobacterial dissemination (82). The similar findings of enhanced *M. tuberculosis* infection in the context of these two different T cell activation systems in HIS mice suggest a common cellular mechanism that operates to control mycobacterial burden *in vivo*.

Infection of HIS Mice with *Staphylococcus aureus*

S. aureus is a commensal organism with minor representation within human skin and nasopharynx microbiotas that is normally well controlled by the immune system. However, *S. aureus* is also a dangerous pathogen that can cause life-threatening skin infection, pneumonia, peritonitis, endocarditis, and frequently fatal septicemia. A more troubling fact is that the incidence of methicillin-resistant *S. aureus* is increasing, and vaccines targeting this infection have had little preclinical success (83–85).

Several recent studies described *S. aureus* infection in CD34⁺ HSC-based HIS mice (86–88). Comparing to uninfected *NSG* mice or immunocompetent mice, the presence of human immune cells in HIS mice increased the susceptibility to *S. aureus* infection irrespective of the inoculation routes, suggesting that virulence factors of *S. aureus* can appropriately target human cells. Boosting of human myeloid cells in BLT HIS mice using human IL-3 and GM-CSF transgenic hosts enhanced *S. aureus* infection, with a higher bacterial burden in the lung after intranasal infection (86). This increased susceptibility may be explained by the preferential targeting of *S. aureus* to human macrophages via a PVL-C5aR receptor interaction. Hence, these HIS models can be used to better understand human-specific virulent factors that *S. aureus* uses to establish infection and eventually evade immunity.

Using HIS Mice To Study Commensal Microbiota and Their Products

A diverse and resilient microbiota trains the immune system and is thought to play an important role in the prevention of autoimmunity (reviewed in reference 89). Perturbations of microbial communities following antibiotic treatment can have a profound impact on the composition and function of gut immune cells. If these changes occur at critical time windows in human development, long-lasting consequences of these events may eventually occur, leading to alterations in organ (brain) function and increased risk of developing disease (autoimmunity).

In order to study a role for commensal communities in human lymphocyte development, CD34+ HSC-based HIS mice (on the NSG background) were treated with an antibiotic cocktail to reduce the microbiota diversity. Antibiotic treatment lead to increased numbers of effector T cells and development of anti-nuclear autoantibodies (90). Notably, reduced numbers of IL-10-producing macrophage were observed in the guts of antibiotic-treated HIS mice.

Adequate integrity of the intestinal barrier is required to prevent bacterial translocation of commensal microorganisms that can provoke system inflammation. Early in the course of HIV infection, the intestinal barrier is disrupted, in part, by excessive inflammation caused by virus replication in gut T cells and the subsequent immune responses to this infection. On the other hand, dysbiosis caused by shifts in commensal communities may also impact pathogen reservoirs, allowing their activation. These two aspects of mucosal homeostasis have been explored using HIV infection in HIS mice (91, 92).

The study of the impact of intestinal barrier disruption used CD34+ HSC-based HIS mice (on the BRG background) and treatment with dextran sodium sulfate (DSS), which causes lysis of intestinal epithelial cells and promotes bacterial translocation (91). Elevated levels of lipopolysaccharide (LPS) are generated after DSS treatment and are rapidly eliminated by tissue macrophages. However, in HIV-infected HIS mice, macrophage clearance of LPS is compromised, resulting in accentuated T cell activation, which fuels viral replication and T cell loss (91). The inflammation following HIV infection apparently creates a feed-forward loop that comprises mucosal T cell homeostasis at multiple levels.

A study of *Neisseria gonorrhoeae* infection in HIV-infected HIS mice showed the impact of pathogen co-infection at mucosal surfaces (92). CD34+ HSC-based HIS mice (on the NSG background) were infected by HIV-1 Bal, and subsequently, *N. gonorrhoeae* was administered intravaginally. While systemic HIV levels were unchanged in the presence of vaginal *N. gonorrhoeae*, the mucosal shedding of HIV-1 was increased in *N. gonorrhoeae*-infected HIS mice. Although the mechanisms behind this observation remain unclear, this report suggests specific interactions between *N. gonorrhoeae*

and HIV-1 in mucosal sites that can now be dissected using HIS mice.

Using HIS Mice To Study Sepsis

Sepsis is the leading cause of death in critically ill patients and represents a systemic inflammatory response to severe bacterial infection. Sepsis can be modeled experimentally using cecal ligation and puncture (CLP), where leakage of bacterial contents provokes a systemic septic shock syndrome in mice. One report of CLP using CD34+ HSC-based HIS mice demonstrated induced human cytokine responses and lymphocyte apoptosis (93). Severe impairment of human hematopoiesis was observed following CLP-induced sepsis or LPS administration, providing evidence for cross-tissue signaling between the gut and the bone marrow (94). Using BLT-based HIS mice, a small interfering RNA targeting high-mobility group protein 1 in human macrophages and DC reduced the cytokine storm and lymphocyte apoptosis and could rescue HIS mice from CLP-induced mortality (95). Finally, a recent study used HIS mice to model neonatal *Escherichia coli* sepsis and its subsequent immune response (96).

CONCLUDING REMARKS

HIS mice have substantially evolved since their conception almost 6 decades ago and now represent robust models to study human immune development and function. HIS mice can also be used to model a diverse set of human pathologies, especially those caused by pathogenic microorganisms. Advances in gene editing technologies have revolutionized our capacity to modify cellular genomes and provide a means to further refine and optimize HIS mouse models. The ability to multiplex cellular compartments in humanized mice will provide more relevant models that recapitulate the complexity of human tissues. The reliability of HIS mouse models, in terms of quality and reproducibility, suggests that these unique tools can form the basis for preclinical platforms dedicated to drug testing and therapeutic screening.

Citation. Li Y, Di Santo JP. 2019. Modeling infectious diseases in mice with a "humanized" immune system. Microbiol Spectrum 7(2):BAI-0019-2019.

References

1. **Shultz LD, Ishikawa F, Greiner DL.** 2007. Humanized mice in translational biomedical research. *Nat Rev Immunol* 7:118–130.
2. **Shultz LD, Brehm MA, Garcia-Martinez JV, Greiner DL.** 2012. Humanized mice for immune system investigation:

progress, promise and challenges. *Nat Rev Immunol* **12**: 786–798.

3. Ito R, Takahashi T, Katano I, Ito M. 2012. Current advances in humanized mouse models. *Cell Mol Immunol* **9**:208–214.

4. Manz MG. 2007. Human-hemato-lymphoid-system mice: opportunities and challenges. *Immunity* **26**:537–541.

5. Isaacson JHC, Cattanach BM. 1962. Two new 'hairless' mutants—sha and Hfh11. *Mouse News Lett* **27**:31.

6. Schorpp M, Hofmann M, Dear TN, Boehm T. 1997. Characterization of mouse and human nude genes. *Immunogenetics* **46**:509–515.

7. Fogh J, Fogh JM, Orfeo T. 1977. One hundred and twenty-seven cultured human tumor cell lines producing tumors in nude mice. *J Natl Cancer Inst* **59**:221–226.

8. Ganick DJ, Sarnwick RD, Shahidi NT, Manning DD. 1980. Inability of intravenously injected monocellular suspensions of human bone marrow to establish in the nude mouse. *Int Arch Allergy Appl Immunol* **62**:330–333.

9. Bosma GC, Custer RP, Bosma MJ. 1983. A severe combined immunodeficiency mutation in the mouse. *Nature* **301**:527–530.

10. Malynn BA, Blackwell TK, Fulop GM, Rathbun GA, Furley AJ, Ferrier P, Heinke LB, Phillips RA, Yancopoulos GD, Alt FW. 1988. The scid defect affects the final step of the immunoglobulin VDJ recombinase mechanism. *Cell* **54**:453–460.

11. Fulop GM, Phillips RA. 1990. The scid mutation in mice causes a general defect in DNA repair. *Nature* **347**:479–482.

12. Greiner DL, Hesselton RA, Shultz LD. 1998. SCID mouse models of human stem cell engraftment. *Stem Cells* **16**:166–177.

13. Biedermann KA, Sun JR, Giaccia AJ, Tosto LM, Brown JM. 1991. scid mutation in mice confers hypersensitivity to ionizing radiation and a deficiency in DNA double-strand break repair. *Proc Natl Acad Sci USA* **88**:1394–1397.

14. Mombaerts P, Iacomini J, Johnson RS, Herrup K, Tonegawa S, Papaioannou VE. 1992. RAG-1-deficient mice have no mature B and T lymphocytes. *Cell* **68**:869–877.

15. Shinkai Y, et al. 1992. RAG-2-deficient mice lack mature lymphocytes owing to inability to initiate V(D)J rearrangement. *Cell* **68**:855–867.

16. Shultz LD, Lang PA, Christianson SW, Gott B, Lyons B, Umeda S, Leiter E, Hesselton R, Wagar EJ, Leif JH, Kollet O, Lapidot T, Greiner DL. 2000. NOD/LtSz-Rag1null mice: an immunodeficient and radioresistant model for engraftment of human hematolymphoid cells, HIV infection, and adoptive transfer of NOD mouse diabetogenic T cells. *J Immunol* **164**:2496–2507.

17. Shultz LD, et al. 1995. Multiple defects in innate and adaptive immunologic function in NOD/LtSz-scid mice. *J Immunol* **154**:180–191.

18. Takenaka K, Prasolava TK, Wang JC, Mortin-Toth SM, Khalouei S, Gan OI, Dick JE, Danska JS. 2007. Polymorphism in Sirpa modulates engraftment of human hematopoietic stem cells. *Nat Immunol* **8**:1313–1323.

19. Noguchi M, Yi H, Rosenblatt HM, Filipovich AH, Adelstein S, Modi WS, McBride OW, Leonard WJ. 1993. Interleukin-2 receptor gamma chain mutation results in X-linked severe combined immunodeficiency in humans. *Cell* **73**:147–157.

20. Di Santo JP, Müller W, Guy-Grand D, Fischer A, Rajewsky K. 1995. Lymphoid development in mice with a targeted deletion of the interleukin 2 receptor gamma chain. *Proc Natl Acad Sci USA* **92**:377–381.

21. Colucci F, Guy-Grand D, Wilson A, Turner M, Schweighoffer E, Tybulewicz VLJ, Di Santo JP. 2000. A new look at Syk in αβ and γδ T cell development using chimeric mice with a low competitive hematopoietic environment. *J Immunol* **164**:5140–5145.

22. Ito M, Hiramatsu H, Kobayashi K, Suzue K, Kawahata M, Hioki K, Ueyama Y, Koyanagi Y, Sugamura K, Tsuji K, Heike T, Nakahata T. 2002. NOD/SCID/γ_c^{null} mouse: an excellent recipient mouse model for engraftment of human cells. *Blood* **100**:3175–3182.

23. Traggiai E, Chicha L, Mazzucchelli L, Bronz L, Piffaretti JC, Lanzavecchia A, Manz MG. 2004. Development of a human adaptive immune system in cord blood cell-transplanted mice. *Science* **304**:104–107.

24. Ishikawa F, Yasukawa M, Lyons B, Yoshida S, Miyamoto T, Yoshimoto G, Watanabe T, Akashi K, Shultz LD, Harada M. 2005. Development of functional human blood and immune systems in NOD/SCID/IL2 receptor γchain^{null} mice. *Blood* **106**:1565–1573.

25. Legrand N, Huntington ND, Nagasawa M, Bakker AQ, Schotte R, Strick-Marchand H, de Geus SJ, Pouw SM, Böhne M, Voordouw A, Weijer K, Di Santo JP, Spits H. 2011. Functional CD47/signal regulatory protein alpha (SIRPα) interaction is required for optimal human T- and natural killer- (NK) cell homeostasis in vivo. *Proc Natl Acad Sci USA* **108**:13224–13229.

26. Huntington ND, Alves NL, Legrand N, Lim A, Strick-Marchand H, Plet A, Weijer K, Jacques Y, Spits H, Di Santo JP. 2011. Autonomous and extrinsic regulation of thymopoiesis in human immune system (HIS) mice. *Eur J Immunol* **41**:2883–2893.

27. Marodon G, Desjardins D, Mercey L, Baillou C, Parent P, Manuel M, Caux C, Bellier B, Pasqual N, Klatzmann D. 2009. High diversity of the immune repertoire in humanized NOD.SCID.γc$^{-/-}$ mice. *Eur J Immunol* **39**:2136–2145.

28. Spits H, Artis D, Colonna M, Diefenbach A, Di Santo JP, Eberl G, Koyasu S, Locksley RM, McKenzie AN, Mebius RE, Powrie F, Vivier E. 2013. Innate lymphoid cells—a proposal for uniform nomenclature. *Nat Rev Immunol* **13**:145–149.

29. Spits H, Di Santo JP. 2011. The expanding family of innate lymphoid cells: regulators and effectors of immunity and tissue remodeling. *Nat Immunol* **12**:21–27.

30. Eberl G, Marmon S, Sunshine MJ, Rennert PD, Choi Y, Littman DR. 2004. An essential function for the nuclear receptor RORgamma(t) in the generation of fetal lymphoid tissue inducer cells. *Nat Immunol* **5**:64–73.

31. Li Y, Masse-Ranson G, Garcia Z, Bruel T, Kök A, Strick-Marchand H, Jouvion G, Serafini N, Lim AI, Dusseaux M,

Hieu T, Bourgade F, Toubert A, Finke D, Schwartz O, Bousso P, Mouquet H, Di Santo JP. 2018. A human immune system mouse model with robust lymph node development. *Nat Methods* 15:623–630.

32. Verstraete K, van Schie L, Vyncke L, Bloch Y, Tavernier J, Pauwels E, Peelman F, Savvides SN. 2014. Structural basis of the proinflammatory signaling complex mediated by TSLP. *Nat Struct Mol Biol* 21:375–382.

33. Park LS, Martin U, Garka K, Gliniak B, Di Santo JP, Muller W, Largaespada DA, Copeland NG, Jenkins NA, Farr AG, Ziegler SF, Morrissey PJ, Paxton R, Sims JE. 2000. Cloning of the murine thymic stromal lymphopoietin (TSLP) receptor: formation of a functional heteromeric complex requires interleukin 7 receptor. *J Exp Med* 192:659–670.

34. Li Y, Chen Q, Zheng D, Yin L, Chionh YH, Wong LH, Tan SQ, Tan TC, Chan JK, Alonso S, Dedon PC, Lim B, Chen J. 2013. Induction of functional human macrophages from bone marrow promonocytes by M-CSF in humanized mice. *J Immunol* 191:3192–3199.

35. Li Y, Mention JJ, Court N, Masse-Ranson G, Toubert A, Spits H, Legrand N, Corcuff E, Strick-Marchand H, Di Santo JP. 2016. A novel Flt3-deficient HIS mouse model with selective enhancement of human DC development. *Eur J Immunol* 46:1291–1299.

36. Huntington ND, Legrand N, Alves NL, Jaron B, Weijer K, Plet A, Corcuff E, Mortier E, Jacques Y, Spits H, Di Santo JP. 2009. IL-15 trans-presentation promotes human NK cell development and differentiation in vivo. *J Exp Med* 206:25–34.

37. Chen Q, He F, Kwang J, Chan JK, Chen J. 2012. GM-CSF and IL-4 stimulate antibody responses in humanized mice by promoting T, B, and dendritic cell maturation. *J Immunol* 189:5223–5229.

38. Willinger T, Rongvaux A, Takizawa H, Yancopoulos GD, Valenzuela DM, Murphy AJ, Auerbach W, Eynon EE, Stevens S, Manz MG, Flavell RA. 2011. Human IL-3/GM-CSF knock-in mice support human alveolar macrophage development and human immune responses in the lung. *Proc Natl Acad Sci USA* 108:2390–2395.

39. Li Y, Strick-Marchand H, Lim AI, Ren J, Masse-Ranson G, Dan Li, Jouvion G, Rogge L, Lucas S, Bin Li, Di Santo JP. 2017. Regulatory T cells control toxicity in a humanized model of IL-2 therapy. *Nat Commun* 8:1762.

40. Rongvaux A, Willinger T, Martinek J, Strowig T, Gearty SV, Teichmann LL, Saito Y, Marches F, Halene S, Palucka AK, Manz MG, Flavell RA. 2014. Development and function of human innate immune cells in a humanized mouse model. *Nat Biotechnol* 32:364–372.

41. Mestas J, Hughes CC. 2004. Of mice and not men: differences between mouse and human immunology. *J Immunol* 172:2731–2738.

42. Shultz LD, Saito Y, Najima Y, Tanaka S, Ochi T, Tomizawa M, Doi T, Sone A, Suzuki N, Fujiwara H, Yasukawa M, Ishikawa F. 2010. Generation of functional human T-cell subsets with HLA-restricted immune responses in HLA class I expressing NOD/SCID/IL2rγ^{null} humanized mice. *Proc Natl Acad Sci USA* 107:13022–13027.

43. Suzuki M, Takahashi T, Katano I, Ito R, Ito M, Harigae H, Ishii N, Sugamura K. 2012. Induction of human humoral immune responses in a novel HLA-DR-expressing transgenic NOD/Shi-scid/γc^{null} mouse. *Int Immunol* 24:243–252.

44. Walsh NC, Kenney LL, Jangalwe S, Aryee KE, Greiner DL, Brehm MA, Shultz LD. 2017. Humanized mouse models of clinical disease. *Annu Rev Pathol* 12:187–215.

45. Victor Garcia J. 2016. Humanized mice for HIV and AIDS research. *Curr Opin Virol* 19:56–64.

46. Masse-Ranson G, Mouquet H, Di Santo JP. 2018. Humanized mouse models to study pathophysiology and treatment of HIV infection. *Curr Opin HIV AIDS* 13:143–151.

47. Denton PW, García JV. 2011. Humanized mouse models of HIV infection. *AIDS Rev* 13:135–148.

48. Yu H, Borsotti C, Schickel JN, Zhu S, Strowig T, Eynon EE, Frleta D, Gurer C, Murphy AJ, Yancopoulos GD, Meffre E, Manz MG, Flavell RA. 2017. A novel humanized mouse model with significant improvement of class-switched, antigen-specific antibody production. *Blood* 129:959–969.

49. Lang J, Zhang B, Kelly M, Peterson JN, Barbee J, Freed BM, Di Santo JP, Matsuda JL, Torres RM, Pelanda R. 2017. Replacing mouse BAFF with human BAFF does not improve B-cell maturation in hematopoietic humanized mice. *Blood Adv* 1:2729–2741.

50. Cimbro R, Vassena L, Arthos J, Cicala C, Kehrl JH, Park C, Sereti I, Lederman MM, Fauci AS, Lusso P. 2012. IL-7 induces expression and activation of integrin α4β7 promoting naive T-cell homing to the intestinal mucosa. *Blood* 120:2610–2619.

51. Melkus MW, Estes JD, Padgett-Thomas A, Gatlin J, Denton PW, Othieno FA, Wege AK, Haase AT, Garcia JV. 2006. Humanized mice mount specific adaptive and innate immune responses to EBV and TSST-1. *Nat Med* 12:1316–1322.

52. Denton PW, Nochi T, Lim A, Krisko JF, Martinez-Torres F, Choudhary SK, Wahl A, Olesen R, Zou W, Di Santo JP, Margolis DM, Garcia JV. 2012. IL-2 receptor γ-chain molecule is critical for intestinal T-cell reconstitution in humanized mice. *Mucosal Immunol* 5:555–566.

53. Greenblatt MB, Vbranac V, Tivey T, Tsang K, Tager AM, Aliprantis AO. 2012. Graft versus host disease in the bone marrow, liver and thymus humanized mouse model. *PLoS One* 7:e44664 *CORRECTION PLoS One* 8:10.1371/annotation/e413f2a1-5767-4c82-9e27-dd556155f124.

54. Mosier DE, Gulizia RJ, Baird SM, Wilson DB. 1988. Transfer of a functional human immune system to mice with severe combined immunodeficiency. *Nature* 335:256–259.

55. Tary-Lehmann M, Lehmann PV, Schols D, Roncarolo MG, Saxon A. 1994. Anti-SCID mouse reactivity shapes the human CD4+ T cell repertoire in hu-PBL-SCID chimeras. *J Exp Med* 180:1817–1827.

56. Ali N, Flutter B, Sanchez Rodriguez R, Sharif-Paghaleh E, Barber LD, Lombardi G, Nestle FO. 2012. Xenogeneic graft-versus-host-disease in NOD-scid IL-2Rγnull

mice display a T-effector memory phenotype. *PLoS One* 7:e44219.

57. Harui A, Kiertscher SM, Roth MD. 2011. Reconstitution of huPBL-NSG mice with donor-matched dendritic cells enables antigen-specific T-cell activation. *J Neuroimmune Pharmacol* 6:148–157.

58. King MA, Covassin L, Brehm MA, Racki W, Pearson T, Leif J, Laning J, Fodor W, Foreman O, Burzenski L, Chase TH, Gott B, Rossini AA, Bortell R, Shultz LD, Greiner DL. 2009. Human peripheral blood leucocyte non-obese diabetic-severe combined immunodeficiency interleukin-2 receptor gamma chain gene mouse model of xenogeneic graft-*versus*-host-like disease and the role of host major histocompatibility complex. *Clin Exp Immunol* 157: 104–118.

59. Büchner SM, Sliva K, Bonig H, Völker I, Waibler Z, Kirberg J, Schnierle BS. 2013. Delayed onset of graft-*versus*-host disease in immunodeficient human leucocyte antigen-DQ8 transgenic, murine major histocompatibility complex class II-deficient mice repopulated by human peripheral blood mononuclear cells. *Clin Exp Immunol* 173:355–364.

60. Amaladoss A, Chen Q, Liu M, Dummler SK, Dao M, Suresh S, Chen J, Preiser PR. 2015. De novo generated human red blood cells in humanized mice support *Plasmodium falciparum* infection. *PLoS One* 10:e0129825.

61. Hu Z, Van Rooijen N, Yang YG. 2011. Macrophages prevent human red blood cell reconstitution in immunodeficient mice. *Blood* 118:5938–5946.

62. Chen Q, Amaladoss A, Ye W, Liu M, Dummler S, Kong F, Wong LH, Loo HL, Loh E, Tan SQ, Tan TC, Chang KT, Dao M, Suresh S, Preiser PR, Chen J. 2014. Human natural killer cells control *Plasmodium falciparum* infection by eliminating infected red blood cells. *Proc Natl Acad Sci USA* 111:1479–1484.

63. Allweiss L, Dandri M. 2016. Experimental in vitro and in vivo models for the study of human hepatitis B virus infection. *J Hepatol* 64(Suppl):S17–S31.

64. Dandri M, Burda MR, Török E, Pollok JM, Iwanska A, Sommer G, Rogiers X, Rogler CE, Gupta S, Will H, Greten H, Petersen J. 2001. Repopulation of mouse liver with human hepatocytes and in vivo infection with hepatitis B virus. *Hepatology* 33:981–988.

65. Mercer DF, Schiller DE, Elliott JF, Douglas DN, Hao C, Rinfret A, Addison WR, Fischer KP, Churchill TA, Lakey JR, Tyrrell DL, Kneteman NM. 2001. Hepatitis C virus replication in mice with chimeric human livers. *Nat Med* 7:927–933.

66. Hasegawa M, Kawai K, Mitsui T, Taniguchi K, Monnai M, Wakui M, Ito M, Suematsu M, Peltz G, Nakamura M, Suemizu H. 2011. The reconstituted 'humanized liver' in TK-NOG mice is mature and functional. *Biochem Biophys Res Commun* 405:405–410.

67. Azuma H, Paulk N, Ranade A, Dorrell C, Al-Dhalimy M, Ellis E, Strom S, Kay MA, Finegold M, Grompe M. 2007. Robust expansion of human hepatocytes in Fah-/-/Rag2-/-/Il2rg-/- mice. *Nat Biotechnol* 25:903–910.

68. Bissig KD, Le TT, Woods NB, Verma IM. 2007. Repopulation of adult and neonatal mice with human hepatocytes:

a chimeric animal model. *Proc Natl Acad Sci USA* 104: 20507–20511.

69. Washburn ML, Bility MT, Zhang L, Kovalev GI, Buntzman A, Frelinger JA, Barry W, Ploss A, Rice CM, Su L. 2011. A humanized mouse model to study hepatitis C virus infection, immune response, and liver disease. *Gastroenterology* 140: 1334–1344.

70. Kremsdorf D, Strick-Marchand H. 2017. Modeling hepatitis virus infections and treatment strategies in humanized mice. *Curr Opin Virol* 25:119–125.

71. Kaushansky A, Mikolajczak SA, Vignali M, Kappe SH. 2014. Of men in mice: the success and promise of humanized mouse models for human malaria parasite infections. *Cell Microbiol* 16:602–611.

72. Dusseaux M, Masse-Ranson G, Darche S, Ahodantin J, Li Y, Fiquet O, Beaumont E, Moreau P, Riviere L, Neuveut C, Soussan P, Roingeard P, Kremsdorf D, Di Santo JP, Strick-Marchand H. 2017. Viral load affects the immune response to HBV in mice with humanized immune system and liver. *Gastroenterology* 153:1647–1661.e9.

73. Libby SJ, Brehm MA, Greiner DL, Shultz LD, McClelland M, Smith KD, Cookson BT, Karlinsey JE, Kinkel TL, Porwollik S, Canals R, Cummings LA, Fang FC. 2010. Humanized nonobese diabetic-scid *IL2rX^{null}* mice are susceptible to lethal *Salmonella* Typhi infection. *Proc Natl Acad Sci USA* 107:15589–15594.

74. Firoz Mian M, Pek EA, Chenoweth MJ, Ashkar AA. 2011. Humanized mice are susceptible to *Salmonella typhi* infection. *Cell Mol Immunol* 8:83–87.

75. Song J, Willinger T, Rongvaux A, Eynon EE, Stevens S, Manz MG, Flavell RA, Galán JE. 2010. A mouse model for the human pathogen *Salmonella typhi*. *Cell Host Microbe* 8:369–376.

76. Mian MF, Pek EA, Chenoweth MJ, Coombes BK, Ashkar AA. 2011. Humanized mice for *Salmonella typhi* infection: new tools for an old problem. *Virulence* 2:248–252.

77. Hunter RL, Jagannath C, Actor JK. 2007. Pathology of postprimary tuberculosis in humans and mice: contradiction of long-held beliefs. *Tuberculosis (Edinb)* 87: 267–278.

78. Harper J, Skerry C, Davis SL, Tasneen R, Weir M, Kramnik I, Bishai WR, Pomper MG, Nuermberger EL, Jain SK. 2012. Mouse model of necrotic tuberculosis granulomas develops hypoxic lesions. *J Infect Dis* 205: 595–602.

79. Heuts F, Gavier-Widén D, Carow B, Juarez J, Wigzell H, Rottenberg ME. 2013. CD4+ cell-dependent granuloma formation in humanized mice infected with mycobacteria. *Proc Natl Acad Sci USA* 110:6482–6487.

80. Calderon VE, Valbuena G, Goez Y, Judy BM, Huante MB, Sutjita P, Johnston RK, Estes DM, Hunter RL, Actor JK, Cirillo JD, Endsley JJ. 2013. A humanized mouse model of tuberculosis. *PLoS One* 8:e63331.

81. Lee J, Brehm MA, Greiner D, Shultz LD, Kornfeld H. 2013. Engrafted human cells generate adaptive immune responses to *Mycobacterium bovis* BCG infection in humanized mice. *BMC Immunol* 14:53.

82. Nusbaum RJ, Calderon VE, Huante MB, Sutjita P, Vijayakumar S, Lancaster KL, Hunter RL, Actor JK,

Cirillo JD, Aronson J, Gelman BB, Lisinicchia JG, Valbuena G, Endsley JJ. 2016. Pulmonary tuberculosis in humanized mice infected with HIV-1. *Sci Rep* 6:21522.

83. Dantes R, Mu Y, Belflower R, Aragon D, Dumyati G, Harrison LH, Lessa FC, Lynfield R, Nadle J, Petit S, Ray SM, Schaffner W, Townes J, Fridkin S, Emerging Infections Program–Active Bacterial Core Surveillance MRSA Surveillance Investigators. 2013. National burden of invasive methicillin-resistant *Staphylococcus aureus* infections, United States, 2011. *JAMA Intern Med* 173:1970–1978.

84. Klevens RM, Morrison MA, Nadle J, Petit S, Gershman K, Ray S, Harrison LH, Lynfield R, Dumyati G, Townes JM, Craig AS, Zell ER, Fosheim GE, McDougal LK, Carey RB, Fridkin SK, Active Bacterial Core surveillance (ABCs) MRSA Investigators. 2007. Invasive methicillin-resistant *Staphylococcus aureus* infections in the United States. *JAMA* 298:1763–1771.

85. Schaumburg F, Köck R, Mellmann A, Richter L, Hasenberg F, Kriegeskorte A, Friedrich AW, Gatermann S, Peters G, von Eiff C, Becker K, study group. 2012. Population dynamics among methicillin-resistant *Staphylococcus aureus* isolates in Germany during a 6-year period. *J Clin Microbiol* 50:3186–3192.

86. Prince A, Wang H, Kitur K, Parker D. 2017. Humanized mice exhibit increased susceptibility to *Staphylococcus aureus* pneumonia. *J Infect Dis* 215:1386–1395.

87. Knop J, Hanses F, Leist T, Archin NM, Buchholz S, Gläsner J, Gessner A, Wege AK. 2015. *Staphylococcus aureus* infection in humanized mice: a new model to study pathogenicity associated with human immune response. *J Infect Dis* 212:435–444.

88. Tseng CW, Biancotti JC, Berg BL, Gate D, Kolar SL, Müller S, Rodriguez MD, Rezai-Zadeh K, Fan X, Beenhouwer DO, Town T, Liu GY. 2015. Increased susceptibility of humanized NSG mice to Panton-Valentine leukocidin and *Staphylococcus aureus* skin infection. *PLoS Pathog* 11: e1005292.

89. Belkaid Y, Hand TW. 2014. Role of the microbiota in immunity and inflammation. *Cell* 157:121–141.

90. Gülden E, Vudattu NK, Deng S, Preston-Hurlburt P, Mamula M, Reed JC, Mohandas S, Herold BC, Torres R, Vieira SM, Lim B, Herazo-Maya JD, Kriegel M, Goodman AL, Cotsapas C, Herold KC. 2017. Microbiota control immune regulation in humanized mice. *JCI Insight* 2:e91709.

91. Hofer U, Schlaepfer E, Baenziger S, Nischang M, Regenass S, Schwendener R, Kempf W, Nadal D, Speck RF. 2010. Inadequate clearance of translocated bacterial products in HIV-infected humanized mice. *PLoS Pathog* 6:e1000867.

92. Xu SX, Leontyev D, Kaul R, Gray-Owen SD. 2018. *Neisseria gonorrhoeae* co-infection exacerbates vaginal HIV shedding without affecting systemic viral loads in human CD34+ engrafted mice. *PLoS One* 13: e0191672.

93. Unsinger J, McDonough JS, Shultz LD, Ferguson TA, Hotchkiss RS. 2009. Sepsis-induced human lymphocyte apoptosis and cytokine production in "humanized" mice. *J Leukoc Biol* 86:219–227.

94. Skirecki T, Kawiak J, Machaj E, Pojda Z, Wasilewska D, Czubak J, Hoser G. 2015. Early severe impairment of hematopoietic stem and progenitor cells from the bone marrow caused by CLP sepsis and endotoxemia in a humanized mice model. *Stem Cell Res Ther* 6:142.

95. Ye C, Choi JG, Abraham S, Wu H, Diaz D, Terreros D, Shankar P, Manjunath N. 2012. Human macrophage and dendritic cell-specific silencing of high-mobility group protein B1 ameliorates sepsis in a humanized mouse model. *Proc Natl Acad Sci USA* 109:21052–21057.

96. Schlieckau F, Schulz D, Fill Malfertheiner S, Entleutner K, Seelbach-Goebel B, Ernst W. 2018. A novel model to study neonatal *Escherichia coli* sepsis and the effect of treatment on the human immune system using humanized mice. *Am J Reprod Immunol* 80:e12859.

Bacteria and Intracellularity
Edited by Pascale Cossart, Craig R. Roy, and Philippe Sansonetti
© 2019 American Society for Microbiology, Washington, DC
doi:10.1128/microbiolspec.BAI-0007-2019

A Cinematic View of Tissue Microbiology in the Live Infected Host

22

Agneta Richter-Dahlfors[1] and Keira Melican[1]

With each big scientific advancement, plaudits are quickly heaped on the scientists producing these great results as well as recognizing those that came before. Emerging technologies and technological advancements, often crucial to these ground-breaking discoveries, are often overlooked as merely being tools. Each big step forward in our understanding of host-pathogen interaction has been enabled in some way by advancements in technology. These advancements have allowed scientists to look at their problems in a new light, given us more detailed read-outs, or pushed us further toward the clinical environment. Microscopy is a clear example of these types of advancements. The development of the first primitive microscope in the 1670s allowed Antoine van Leeuwenhoek to describe the "animalcules" he saw, which were, in fact, bacteria being visualized for the first time using light-based microscopy (1, 2).

The theory that infectious diseases were caused by these animalcules was spearheaded by the discoveries of Louis Pasteur and Robert Koch (3). For many years, scientists focused on understanding the infectious agent, the microbe. This work resulted in huge advances in understanding the genetics, metabolism, and lifestyles of infectious microbes (3), but nothing exists in isolation, and that is particularly true for microbiologists. Interaction with complementary research fields such as cell biology and immunology has led to the expansion of our knowledge, tools, and understanding of infectious disease. The term "cellular microbiology" was introduced in a *Science* paper in 1996, describing this new field emerging at the interface of cell biology and microbiology (4). Cell biologists could use numerous microbiological tools, such as bacterial toxins, to disrupt and understand cellular pathways. Microbiology likewise benefited from understanding the effect bacterial pro-

teins, toxins, and signaling mechanisms exerted on mammalian cells (4). Later, in 2006, an editorial, "Infection Biology," was published in *Nature* with the tag-line "Immunology and microbiology come together to fight disease" (5). This editorial noted that infection had for too long been studied from two separate angles, where microbiologists studied the pathogen while immunologists studied the host immune response (5). When a bacterial pathogen infects its host, it triggers a cascade of responses, which involve complex intracellular and intraorgan signaling networks. Infection biology aims to understand these complex cascades and to find ways to manipulate them to help prevent the development of disease.

The infected host, commonly the human body, is very complex. A multitude of cell types are organized into tissue structures, which form organs that are interconnected by physiological systems, including the vascular, lymphatic, central nervous, and immune systems (Fig. 1). This complexity is impossible to mimic on the lab bench in *in vitro* systems. *In vivo* experimentation, within the living organism, has thus become a critical aspect of infection biology. The terminology of many scientific papers can, however, be complicated. The scientific definition of "*in vivo*" is not fixed and can vary depending on the context. In bacteriology, "*in vivo*" may refer to ribosomal translation within the bacterial cell (6). The infection of cell cultures has also been termed "*in vivo*." In infection biology "*in vivo*" generally refers to studies performed using animal models, but even these show a level of ambiguity. Sacrificial *in vivo* experiments involve analysis of the infection in dead tissue at the experimental endpoint. So while the experimental infection may be carried out *in vivo*, the analysis is often not (7–10). Explanted organs

[1]Swedish Medical Nanoscience Centre, Department of Neuroscience, Karolinska Institutet, SE-17177, Stockholm, Sweden.

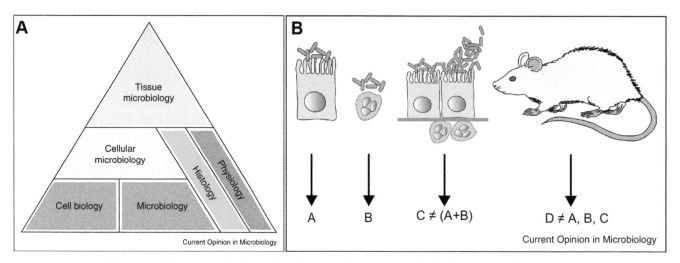

Figure 1 Tissue microbiology. (**A**) Schematic illustration of the development of the research areas leading to the emerging field of tissue microbiology. The base of the pyramid focuses on *in vitro* studies of the bacterial pathogens and cellular biology on the individual host cell types, while cellular microbiology examines the interaction between the two. Tissue microbiology joins cellular microbiology with the physiological and histological aspects. (**B**) Schematic indicating the difficulty of translating *in vitro* cell culture studies *in vivo*. Experimentation *in vivo* includes many variables that are not included *in vitro*. Although essentially correct information is obtained within a given context, reductionistic models do not necessarily represent the complete picture. (Modified from reference 58.)

and tissues, while having the tertiary structures of the tissues, lack the systemic influences of the vascular, immune, and hormonal systems, with often limited usable time spans (11). The use of explants is increasingly described using the term "*ex vivo*," or "outside the living." Each of these descriptions is correct in its context, and it is notable that the definition of "*in vivo*" is evolving, and a driving factor in this evolution is the availability of emerging technologies. In this chapter, we describe the technological advances that have helped drive the push from cellular to tissue microbiology and outline key publications showing this.

INTRAVITAL MICROSCOPY AS A KEY MEDIATOR OF TISSUE MICROBIOLOGY

Over the past decades, imaging technology has developed at an extremely rapid pace. Just before the turn of the millennium, confocal microscopy was relatively new to the scene and was allowing for three-dimensional imaging of infection in tissue. The first example of this was the conclusive demonstration of intracellular *Salmonella* in liver macrophages of infected mice (9). This work demonstrated how the optimization of infection models and three-dimensional imaging could begin to translate *in vitro* knowledge into the *in vivo* setting. We were able to understand how bacteria

interacted with the tissue in three dimensions. "Snapshot" microscopy has continued to develop, and more recently the introduction of "super-resolution" microscopy and single-molecule localization methods have delivered new knowledge of the role of the actin cytoskeleton in this process of *Salmonella* internalization (12).

In 2009, in an invited review in *Current Opinion in Microbiology*, we proposed the term "tissue microbiology." We sought to describe the context of work we developed allowing for the study of bacterial infection within the living tissue with single-cell resolution and spatial/temporal control (13). The key shift with tissue microbiology, as opposed to what had come before, was the ability to watch or image the infection process in real time *in vivo*. The major facilitator of this development was technological. To tell the story from our perspective, in 2004 we joined forces with a leading nephrology group that was developing intravital imaging technology that allowed for real-time imaging within the live kidney. Bruce A. Molitoris and his team at the University of Indiana pioneered the use of multiphoton microscopy to study the dynamics and physiology of the kidney. Their work led to ground-breaking advances in understanding how glomerular filtration, cellular uptake, and ischemia functioned *in vivo* (14–16). Combining our knowledge of infection biology with their expertise and techniques, we were able to facilitate a new level of understanding of how renal tissue responds to bacterial infection. We could follow how a bacterial infection progresses over time, with a particular focus on the first 8 h. We could see how the bacteria multiplied and filled the renal tubules and could follow the tissue response, including the infiltration of immune cells (Fig. 2A and B) (17–19). This gave

us a completely new insight into how the infection occurred *in vivo*. We were, of course, not alone in this advancement. With the expansion of intravital microscopy and an understanding of the importance of the *in vivo* microenvironment, numerous microbiology groups have taken up the technique. Beautiful imagery has been published which shows how different bacteria interact with their target organs *in vivo*. Some

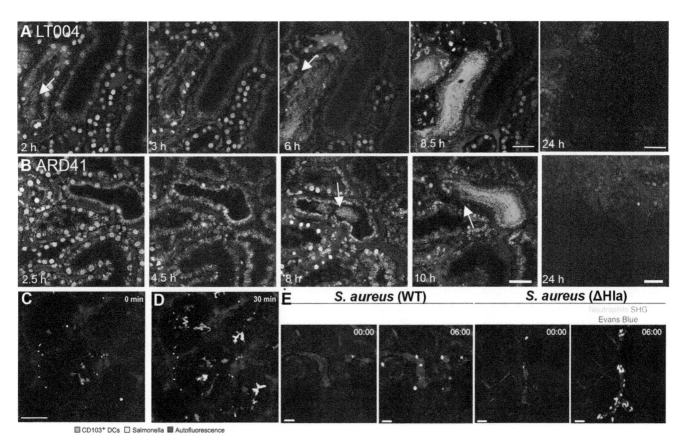

Figure 2 Multiphoton imaging of bacterial infections. (**A, B**) Uropathogenic *E. coli* infection in the kidney. (**A**) Wild-type LT004 bacteria (green, arrow) (*n* = 12) can be seen colonizing the infected tubule (blue outline) within 2 h. As bacteria multiplied, shutdown of the peritubular capillaries was observed by a loss of the red plasma marker within surrounding capillaries (arrow, 6 h). At 24 h bacteria were cleared, leaving behind a scar in the tissue. (**B**) The uropathogenic *E. coli* strain ARD41, which lacks PapG-mediated attachment, showed compromised colonization kinetics with few bacteria visible before 8 h (arrow). At 10 h, bacteria colonized the tubule lumen, and signs of vascular dysfunction appeared (arrow) (*n* = 12). At 24 h the bacteria were cleared, similar to the wild-type infection (panel A). Scale bars: 7 to 10 h = 30 μm, 24 h = 50 μm. (Adapted from reference 19.) (**C, D**) Two-photon microscopy of the epithelial layer in several adjacent villi exposed to *Salmonella*. (**C**) Some intraepithelial YFP^{int} CD103^{+} dendritic cells were already visible at time 0, but within 30 min (**D**) they were joined by several other dendritic cells that had migrated up into the epithelium (scale bar represents 50 μm). (Reprinted from reference 20 with permission from Elsevier.) (**E**) Intravital multiphoton microscopy showing adhesion and extravasation of adoptively transferred *Lyz2*$^{gfp/+}$ neutrophils in ear dermis infected with wild-type or ΔHla *S. aureus*. 00:00, min:s. SHG, second harmonic generation. Scale bars, 30 μm. (Adapted by permission from reference 21. Full figure reused with permission from reference 59.)

examples, which will be discussed in further detail below, include *Salmonella enterica* serovar Typhimurium (Fig. 2C and D) (20), *Staphylococcus aureus* (Fig. 2E) (21), and *Bacillus anthracis* (22).

THE INFECTIOUS MICROENVIRONMENT *IN VIVO*

A key to the development of tissue microbiology has been an appreciation of the complexity of the infectious environment *in vivo*. With the advancement of imaging technology, we have been able to observe how microenvironmental factors such as fluid flow, pH, oxygen tension, and even temperature can affect infection outcome. It became apparent that the conditions in the infectious niche *in vivo* rapidly change over the course of an infection. It is now of great interest to understand how these changing conditions may influence both the pathogen lifestyles and the host's ability to respond. When we used multiphoton microscopy to follow the infection, we could see that vascular flow surrounding a tubular infection was shut down within hours of bacterial introduction (18) (see Video S1). This response, which would have been impossible to observe without intravital microscopy, appears to be a cell-signaling-mediated response that was shown to protect the animal from sepsis (18, 23). These results led us down the unexpected pathway of investigating tissue oxygen tension and renal ischemia as players in infectious pathogenesis. To do this, we again had to borrow techniques from other fields, primarily nephrology, in which renal ischemia had been well studied in ischemia/reperfusion injury (24, 25). Using a microelectrode setup, borrowed from specialists in the field of kidney hypoxia, we were able to measure the tissue oxygen tension in the infected tubule directly and show the rapid decrease in oxygen over the first hours of infection (18).

The roles of tissue oxygen tension and hypoxia are becoming increasingly recognized as influential factors in infection outcome (26). This influence is both from how the host cells may respond to the hypoxic stress and how the bacterial pathogen can adapt its expression of virulence factors and metabolism to an anaerobic environment. Finding ways to measure and monitor these dynamic microenvironmental factors can, however, be more of a challenge. Jennewein et al. used an innovative *in vivo* imaging approach, combining sensor films that allowed for transserosal quantification of cecal tissue oxygen levels and luminescence two-dimensional O_2 imaging on exposed mouse cecum (27). They showed that during *Salmonella* infection, the tissue oxygen in the gut dropped and that this hypoxia allowed

for enhanced replication of *Salmonella* in macrophages. In another study, Marteyn et al. constructed bacterial reporters, based on the expression of luciferase or green fluorescent protein under varying oxygen levels *in vivo*, which they used to show how *Shigella flexneri* can modulate its type III secretion system in response to oxygen concentrations and to show that subtle changes in gut oxygenation may mediate this variation (28). Osteomyelitis infection occurs within the intrinsically hypoxic conditions in the bone. Wilde et al. used a fiber optics-based sensing technique to demonstrate that infection with *S. aureus* reduced the oxygen availability in skeletal tissue even further (29). *S. aureus* was shown to adapt to this lower environmental oxygenation, modifying its quorum sensing and toxin production (29). From the host perspective, hypoxia also affects the regulation of the immune response, such as neutrophil viability and function (30). Hypoxia is believed to affect almost every aspect of macrophage and neutrophil function, including morphology, migration, chemotaxis, adherence to endothelial cells, bacterial killing, differentiation/polarization, and protumorigenic activity (31). This work combined, which demonstrates numerous technical approaches to similar research questions, serves as a demonstration of the importance of the infectious microenvironment to infection outcome. It shows how the infectious niche changes over time and how this needs to be taken into account when trying to understand the roles and functions of multiple virulence factors and immune responses. Beyond oxygenation, the role of changing pH *in vivo* as well as the interaction of infection and the nervous system are all ongoing aspects of development for tissue microbiology.

PHYSIOLOGICALLY RELEVANT INFECTION MODELS FOR TISSUE MICROBIOLOGY

A recurrent theme in tissue microbiology is overcoming experimental constraints to present the most physiologically and clinically relevant model of infection. Pathogens often have very specific infectious niches, and researchers have had to find innovative solutions to allow observation of these pathogens in each niche. In our work, we adapted a number of innovations from Molitoris' group that allowed us to follow infection *in vivo* with unparalleled spatial and temporal control. These innovations included surgery to expose and stabilize the kidney tissue, multicolor imaging, and the use of autofluorescence as a tissue marker. Micropuncture delivery, a rather old technique in nephrology (32), was used to infuse bacteria into a single tubule, allowing us to dictate the time and numbers of bacteria as precisely as in a cell culture experiment, a rarity in *in vivo* models.

Surface-oriented niches such as skin may appear to be more straightforward targets for *in vivo* imaging, but many aspects must be considered. Abtin et al. utilized the mouse ear to study neutrophil migration toward *Staphylococcus* infection in the skin, with the mouse ear being suitable for imaging due to its accessibility and stability. They reported an unexpected role for perivascular macrophages in mediating the translocation of neutrophils toward *Staphylococcus* infection and demonstrated how bacteria could influence this translocation via toxin production (21). Internal organs can prove more challenging, but innovative surgery and stabilization techniques have allowed for imaging of many organs. The liver is of great interest in infection research, and a number of prominent papers have emerged using intravital spinning-disk confocal microscopy to follow the fate of *S. aureus* in the liver. This work has shown the rapid dynamics with which intravascular bacteria are taken up by the liver Kupffer cells, where they form an intracellular reservoir (33). Through a similar setup, the release of neutrophil extracellular traps in liver vasculature following *Staphylococcus* injection was shown (34).

Other organs can prove more of a challenge due to inherent movement issues, such as the gut and the lungs. The gut, a hotbed of interest from the perspective of both invasive gut pathogens and the ever-expanding field of gut microbiota, presents a number of challenges, from its location deep within the body, its continuous peristaltic movement, and its thick, highly autofluorescent mucus. Some groups have found ways to work around a number of these issues. In one study looking at how CD103+ dendritic cells sample bacterial antigens at the gut lumen, an exposed, stabilized setup was used, representing a mid-step between an explant model and noninvasive *in vivo* imaging (20). An informative review of intravital imaging in the gut was recently published reviewing many of the difficulties associated with gut imaging and demonstrating methods with which to overcome this (35).

The breathing motion of the lung is an obvious limitation when it comes to steady intravital imaging, but methods have been developed to minimize such disruptions. One approach is the use of postprocessing tissue motion correction algorithms which produce relatively clear images of living lung tissue (22). This strategy was applied to demonstrate the long-lasting interaction between alveolar macrophages and dendritic cells in response to infection by spores of *B. anthracis*

(22). Another approach has been to optimize stabilization through the use of vacuum stabilization (36, 37).

HUMANIZED MODELS: THE NEXT STEP IN TRANSLATIONAL RESEARCH

A further step in tissue microbiology is the move to humanized infection models. Immunologists have been working for years to develop humanized immune system mice by engrafting human immune cell populations into immunocompromised mice. These mice have been used to study the interaction of human immune cells with a number of human-specific pathogens, such as Epstein-Barr, dengue, and HIV, as well as bacteria including *Mycobacterium tuberculosis* and *S. enterica* serovar Typhi (38, 39). These models take into account the species specificity for some bacterial pathogens, thus allowing studies of human-specific pathogens. *Neisseria meningitidis*, the causative agent of meningococcal septicemia and meningitis, is one example of a pathogen that specifically interacts with human endothelial cells. While huge amounts of work have been performed to understand this interaction *in vitro* (40–42), how this functions *in vivo* was not known. Recently, we were involved in developing a humanized model to address this. By grafting human dermal microvessels in the form of a skin graft onto SCID.bg mice and using spinning-disk confocal intravital imaging, we showed the specificity and speed of *N. meningitidis* adhesion to human dermal microvessels (see Video S2). This adhesion, shown to be type IV pili dependent, led to a rapid human inflammatory response and eventually to the breakdown of the small vessels and local purpura development (43, 44). This work demonstrated how humanized mice can be used as the next step in optimizing our models to more accurately reflect the clinical situation. Obligate human pathogens, such as *N. meningitidis*, are an obvious target, but we foresee that the responses of other bacteria to the distinctly human microenvironment will be further elucidated over the coming years.

TECHNOLOGICAL ADVANCEMENT TO MEET DEVELOPING NEEDS

As intravital imaging has expanded through the field of infection biology, new questions have arisen, and in some cases, it has become apparent that no tools are currently available to address these needs. This leaves us again at the forefront of technological development and needing to seek out new methodologies and approaches to address our questions. In this final section, we will outline two of these issues that have arisen in our lab and how we have sought to address them.

Novel Imaging Probes for Bacterial Lifestyles

When we first began studying bacterial infection in living tissue, we were amazed at the amount of detail, structure, and dynamics that we could now see live. As our experiments progressed and as our research questions became more specific, we started to notice a lack of precise tools. One observation we had made was that uropathogenic *Eschericha coli* bacteria rapidly adhered to the epithelial surface and withstood the shear stress of urine flow when colonizing the renal tubule. When we removed the bacteria's ability to express the type 1 fimbriae, the bacteria were unable to colonize the central parts of the tubule lumen (19). We hypothesized that uropathogenic *E. coli* must adopt a biofilm lifestyle within the kidney tubules to withstand the sheer stress. But then arose the question, how do we confirm biofilm *in vivo*? All biofilm detection techniques at that time were based on nonspecific dyes that were toxic to the animals. We thus needed to look further afield for an answer. Knowing that *E. coli* produces the amyloid protein curli and the polysaccharide cellulose as major constituents of the extracellular matrix, we chose to target these defining elements of the biofilm lifestyle. We therefore approached Peter Nilsson, a chemist from Linköping University, who develops nanoscale probes for the detection of misfolded proteins in diseases such as Alzheimer's disease. The nanoscale optoelectronic probes, termed Optotracers, have a flexible structure, meaning that the conformation of the molecule alters depending on the binding target. Because the conformation is linked to the opto-electronic features of the molecule, binding can be monitored by fluorescent signals emitted at specific wavelengths (45, 46). Starting from the notion that curli fibers have an amyloid structure (47), we began testing whether any Optotracer molecule could be used to detect bacterial biofilm. We recently demonstrated that Optotracer molecules can be used to specifically identify and even differentiate the bacterial expression of curli as well as cellulose (Fig. 3) (48). We showed that the nontoxic Optotracer can be incorporated into live models and are now in the process of optimizing their use for intravital live imaging of biofilm formed *in vivo*. Optotracers represent a new generation of "smart molecules" which can be designed toward their target and display an ON-OFF-like switching of the target-dependent optical signature, allowing for kinetic studies and multitarget differentiation. This work demonstrated how emerging technolo-

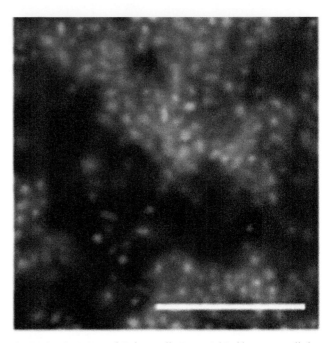

Figure 3 Staining of *Salmonella* (green) biofilm extracellular matrix by luminescent conjugated oligothiophene (LCO) optotracing (red). Scale bar = 10 µm. (Adapted with permission from reference 48.)

gies from outside fields can be applied to infection biology to address unmet needs and tools.

The specificity of innovative probes such as the Optotracers and the increasing sensitivity of imaging information are facilitating another new development toward high-throughput big-data type analysis. As computing power increases exponentially, we are finding new ways of processing and analyzing large volumes of data. In our work, we expanded on the ability of the Optotracers to generate huge amounts of data from each specific spectrum and to specifically identify bacterial cellulose as a diagnostic biomarker for biofilm infections in the urinary tract (49). A workflow was developed in which the Optotracer-generated spectral information from 190 patient urine samples was analyzed by principal component analysis and k-means clustering to identify bacterial cellulose (49). These types of computerized analysis have also been applied to imaging data where artificial intelligence-based screening is being used to identify specific pathologies in tissue slices (50, 51). Such information processing will be increasingly important as we move toward more automated data handling and machine learning-based algorithms. These types of developments hold huge promise for the high-throughput handling of infection biology research and diagnostic data. For a more in-depth review of the applicability of emerging technology, including organic bioelectronics and nano-medicine to infection biology, we have written a number of reviews on the topic in recent years (52–54).

Systemic Response to a Local Infection

Beyond the local infection, a huge advantage of the tissue microbiology models is the ability to study the systemic, holistic response to these small, early-stage infections. In our kidney infection model, we use microinjection to introduce bacteria into 1 of the approximately 30,000 to 35,000 nephrons per kidney. We can use intravital microscopy to follow this infection in real time and have reported the changes that occur locally within the first 8 h. But what happens systemically? How can we study these more global responses? In our lab, a first step to address this was to look at comparative tissue transcriptomics, enabled by the spatial and temporal control of the microinjection approach that allowed us to specifically dissect the local tissue infection site at given time points. We identified rapid inter-organ communication between the kidney and spleen within the first 8 h of infection, mediated by interferon-γ (55). While these data started to give us more of an idea of the global events, the experiments had to be performed at set time points of infection and could not be studied continuously in the animal.

A long-term aim is to be able to quantitatively monitor the earliest indications of the systemic response to local infection in real time. This apparent pipe dream would be a step toward earlier detection of clinical infection in patients as well as being hugely useful in research to monitor the molecular mechanisms of early-phase bacterial infection in animal models. The first step to achieving this required another new approach, and we embraced advances in the field of organic bioelectronics and polymer chemistry. Working together with biomaterial scientists, we developed a biomimetic interface to sense the activation dynamics of the acute-phase reactant C-reactive protein (CRP) (56). Polymer chemistry techniques were used to create a cell-membrane mimetic surface representing a 0.8-nm thick structural analog to a eukaryotic cell membrane. This device was used as a sensor for the activation of CRP by detecting an increase in surface plasmon resonance upon interaction of CRP with the surface. We showed that CRP binding occurred at specific pH and calcium concentrations. We then were able to manipulate the conditions of the surface by combining it with our previously published organic electronic ion pump, which can specifically deliver calcium ions without fluid flow (57). This demonstrated that these types of devices could sense the activation of CRP dependent on minute

changes in the local microenvironment, typical of changes which occur in a localized infection. These types of devices can be used to map the changes in microenvironment and how these changes may affect the action of specific signaling molecules such as CRP. This work is a first step toward the development of real-time sensors for infection that could be applied in combination with our intravital imaging in the future. This work showed that many seemingly challenging experiments can be addressed by using emerging technology.

CONCLUSIONS

The application of emerging technologies is often critical to the advancement of science. As we find new and better ways to address our scientific questions, our knowledge expands. Tissue microbiology is an outgrowth of many generations of work in microbial-host interaction. This outgrowth has relied heavily on novel technologies, including intravital imaging. As outlined here, just one technique is rarely sufficient, and with each step forward we encounter many new challenges. The forefront of addressing these challenges is an exciting and invigorating place to work. The incorporation of emerging technologies from numerous scientific fields is helping bridge these gaps in knowledge and tools. Working at this multidisciplinary interface is challenging for all involved and teaches us new ways to communicate and encourages a wider understanding of biology in general. Understanding how both the host and the pathogen respond and adapt to the infectious microenvironment is a key element in tissue microbiology. The tissue, however, presents numerous dynamic challenges. The tools to address these challenges often exist; we might just have to look outside our own labs to find them.

Video S1 Normal tissue morphology and blood flow in a rat kidney imaged by multiphoton microscopy. Fluorescent 500-kDa dextran labels blood flow (red), cell nuclei are labeled with Hoechst stain (blue), and proximal tubules are identified by dull green autofluorescence. Animation of a series of images collected every second on the same focal plane during a 40-s time period. (From reference 17.) (http://www.asmscience.org/files/BAI-0007-SuppMov1.mov)

Video S2 Intravital microscopy showing a human vessel in the base of a human skin graft on a SCID.bg mouse labeled with UEA lectin (red) and perfused by the mouse circulation. Blood plasma is labeled with a 150-kDa fluorescein isothiocyanate-dextran (green) introduced intravenously. Moving black silhouettes within the plasma are blood cells. (From reference 43.) (http://www.asmscience.org/files/BAI-0007-SuppMov2.mov)

Citation. Richter-Dahlfors A, Melican K. 2019. A cinematic view of tissue microbiology in the live infected host. Microbiol Spectrum 7(3):BAI-0007-2019.

References

1. Hazelwood KL, Olenych SG, Griffin JD, Cathcart JA, Davidson MW. 2007. Entering the portal: understanding the digital image recorded through a microscope, p 3–43. *In* Shorte SL, Frischknecht F (ed), *Imaging Cellular and Molecular Biological Functions*. Springer, Heidelberg, Germany.

2. Ruestow EG. 1996. *The Microscope in the Dutch Republic*. Cambridge University Press, New York, NY.

3. Mims C, Dockrell HM, Goering RV, Roitt I, Wakelin D, Zuckerman M. 2004. *Medical Microbiology*, 3rd ed. Elsevier Mosby, London, United Kingdom.

4. Cossart P, Boquet P, Normark S, Rappuoli R. 1996. Cellular microbiology emerging. *Science* **271**:315–316.

5. Anonymous. 2006. Infection biology. *Nature* **441**:255–256.

6. Richter Dahlfors AA, Kurland CG. 1990. Novel mutants of elongation factor G. *J Mol Biol* **215**:549–557.

7. Deng W, Puente JL, Gruenheid S, Li Y, Vallance BA, Vázquez A, Barba J, Ibarra JA, O'Donnell P, Metalnikov P, Ashman K, Lee S, Goode D, Pawson T, Finlay BB. 2004. Dissecting virulence: systematic and functional analyses of a pathogenicity island. *Proc Natl Acad Sci U S A* **101**:3597–3602.

8. Lecuit M, Vandormael-Pournin S, Lefort J, Huerre M, Gounon P, Dupuy C, Babinet C, Cossart P. 2001. A transgenic model for listeriosis: role of internalin in crossing the intestinal barrier. *Science* **292**:1722–1725.

9. Richter-Dahlfors A, Buchan AM, Finlay BB. 1997. Murine salmonellosis studied by confocal microscopy: *Salmonella typhimurium* resides intracellularly inside macrophages and exerts a cytotoxic effect on phagocytes *in vivo*. *J Exp Med* **186**:569–580.

10. Tam VC, Serruto D, Dziejman M, Brieher W, Mekalanos JJ. 2007. A type III secretion system in *Vibrio cholerae* translocates a formin/spire hybrid-like actin nucleator to promote intestinal colonization. *Cell Host Microbe* **1**:95–107.

11. Chieppa M, Rescigno M, Huang AY, Germain RN. 2006. Dynamic imaging of dendritic cell extension into the small bowel lumen in response to epithelial cell TLR engagement. *J Exp Med* **203**:2841–2852.

12. Han JJ, Kunde YA, Hong-Geller E, Werner JH. 2014. Actin restructuring during *Salmonella typhimurium* infection investigated by confocal and super-resolution microscopy. *J Biomed Opt* **19**:016011.

13. Melican K, Richter-Dahlfors A. 2009. Real-time live imaging to study bacterial infections *in vivo*. *Curr Opin Microbiol* **12**:31–36.

14. Molitoris BA, Sandoval RM. 2009. Techniques to study nephron function: microscopy and imaging. *Pflugers Arch* **458**:203–209.

15. Dunn KW, Sandoval RM, Molitoris BA. 2003. Intravital imaging of the kidney using multiparameter multiphoton microscopy. *Nephron Exp Nephrol* **94**:e7–e11.

16. Molitoris BA, Sandoval RM. 2005. Intravital multiphoton microscopy of dynamic renal processes. *Am J Physiol Renal Physiol* **288**:F1084–F1089.

17. Månsson LE, Melican K, Boekel J, Sandoval RM, Hautefort I, Tanner GA, Molitoris BA, Richter-Dahlfors A. 2007. Real-time studies of the progression of bacterial infections and immediate tissue responses in live animals. *Cell Microbiol* **9**:413–424.

18. Melican K, Boekel J, Månsson LE, Sandoval RM, Tanner GA, Källskog O, Palm F, Molitoris BA, Richter-Dahlfors A. 2008. Bacterial infection-mediated mucosal signalling induces local renal ischaemia as a defence against sepsis. *Cell Microbiol* **10**:1987–1998.

19. Melican K, Sandoval RM, Kader A, Josefsson L, Tanner GA, Molitoris BA, Richter-Dahlfors A. 2011. Uropathogenic *Escherichia coli* P and type 1 fimbriae act in synergy in a living host to facilitate renal colonization leading to nephron obstruction. *PLoS Pathog* **7**:e1001298.

20. Farache J, Koren I, Milo I, Gurevich I, Kim KW, Zigmond E, Furtado GC, Lira SA, Shakhar G. 2013. Luminal bacteria recruit CD103+ dendritic cells into the intestinal epithelium to sample bacterial antigens for presentation. *Immunity* **38**:581–595.

21. Abtin A, Jain R, Mitchell AJ, Roediger B, Brzoska AJ, Tikoo S, Cheng Q, Ng LG, Cavanagh LL, von Andrian UH, Hickey MJ, Firth N, Weninger W. 2014. Perivascular macrophages mediate neutrophil recruitment during bacterial skin infection. *Nat Immunol* **15**:45–53.

22. Fiole D, Deman P, Trescos Y, Mayol JF, Mathieu J, Vial JC, Douady J, Tournier JN. 2014. Two-photon intravital imaging of lungs during anthrax infection reveals long-lasting macrophage-dendritic cell contacts. *Infect Immun* **82**:864–872.

23. Schulz A, Chuquimia OD, Antypas H, Steiner SE, Sandoval RM, Tanner GA, Molitoris BA, Richter-Dahlfors A, Melican K. 2018. Protective vascular coagulation in response to bacterial infection of the kidney is regulated by bacterial lipid A and host CD147. *Pathog Dis* **76**.

24. Sutton TA, Mang HE, Campos SB, Sandoval RM, Yoder MC, Molitoris BA. 2003. Injury of the renal microvascular endothelium alters barrier function after ischemia. *Am J Physiol Renal Physiol* **285**:F191–F198.

25. Molitoris BA, Sutton TA. 2004. Endothelial injury and dysfunction: role in the extension phase of acute renal failure. *Kidney Int* **66**:496–499.

26. Schaffer K, Taylor CT. 2015. The impact of hypoxia on bacterial infection. *FEBS J* **282**:2260–2266.

27. Jennewein J, Matuszak J, Walter S, Felmy B, Gendera K, Schatz V, Nowottny M, Liebsch G, Hensel M, Hardt WD, Gerlach RG, Jantsch J. 2015. Low-oxygen tensions found in *Salmonella*-infected gut tissue boost *Salmonella* replication in macrophages by impairing antimicrobial activity and augmenting *Salmonella* virulence. *Cell Microbiol* **17**:1833–1847.

28. Marteyn B, West NP, Browning DF, Cole JA, Shaw JG, Palm F, Mounier J, Prévost MC, Sansonetti P, Tang CM. 2010. Modulation of *Shigella* virulence in response to available oxygen *in vivo*. *Nature* **465**:355–358.

29. Wilde AD, Snyder DJ, Putnam NE, Valentino MD, Hammer ND, Lonergan ZR, Hinger SA, Aysanoa EE, Blanchard C, Dunman PM, Wasserman GA, Chen J, Shopsin B, Gilmore MS, Skaar EP, Cassat JE. 2015. Bacterial hypoxic responses revealed as critical determinants of the host-pathogen outcome by TnSeq analysis of *Staphylococcus aureus* invasive infection. *PLoS Pathog* **11**:e1005341.

30. Monceaux V, Chiche-Lapierre C, Chaput C, Witko-Sarsat V, Prevost MC, Taylor CT, Ungeheuer MN, Sansonetti PJ, Marteyn BS. 2016. Anoxia and glucose supplementation preserve neutrophil viability and function. *Blood* **128**:993–1002.

31. Egners A, Erdem M, Cramer T. 2016. The response of macrophages and neutrophils to hypoxia in the context of cancer and other inflammatory diseases. *Mediators Inflamm* **2016**:2053646.

32. Roch-Ramel F, Peters G. 1979. Micropuncture techniques as a tool in renal pharmacology. *Annu Rev Pharmacol Toxicol* **19**:323–345.

33. Surewaard BG, Deniset JF, Zemp FJ, Amrein M, Otto M, Conly J, Omri A, Yates RM, Kubes P. 2016. Identification and treatment of the *Staphylococcus aureus* reservoir *in vivo*. *J Exp Med* **213**:1141–1151. (Erratum, 213:3087.)

34. Kolaczkowska E, Jenne CN, Surewaard BG, Thanabalasuriar A, Lee WY, Sanz MJ, Mowen K, Opdenakker G, Kubes P. 2015. Molecular mechanisms of NET formation and degradation revealed by intravital imaging in the liver vasculature. *Nat Commun* **6**:6673.

35. Kolesnikov M, Farache J, Shakhar G. 2015. Intravital two-photon imaging of the gastrointestinal tract. *J Immunol Methods* **421**:73–80.

36. Rodriguez-Tirado C, Kitamura T, Kato Y, Pollard JW, Condeelis JS, Entenberg D. 2016. Long-term high-resolution intravital microscopy in the lung with a vacuum stabilized imaging window. *J Vis Exp* (116):e54603.

37. Looney MR, Thornton EE, Sen D, Lamm WJ, Glenny RW, Krummel MF. 2011. Stabilized imaging of immune surveillance in the mouse lung. *Nat Methods* **8**:91–96.

38. Leung C, Chijioke O, Gujer C, Chatterjee B, Antsiferova O, Landtwing V, McHugh D, Raykova A, Münz C. 2013. Infectious diseases in humanized mice. *Eur J Immunol* **43**:2246–2254.

39. Rämer PC, Chijioke O, Meixlsperger S, Leung CS, Münz C. 2011. Mice with human immune system components as *in vivo* models for infections with human pathogens. *Immunol Cell Biol* **89**:408–416.

40. Soyer M, Charles-Orszag A, Lagache T, Machata S, Imhaus AF, Dumont A, Millien C, Olivo-Marin JC, Duménil G. 2014. Early sequence of events triggered by the interaction of *Neisseria meningitidis* with endothelial cells. *Cell Microbiol* **16**:878–895.

41. Chamot-Rooke J, Mikaty G, Malosse C, Soyer M, Dumont A, Gault J, Imhaus AF, Martin P, Trellet M, Clary G, Chafey P, Camoin L, Nilges M, Nassif X, Duménil G. 2011. Posttranslational modification of pili upon cell contact triggers *N. meningitidis* dissemination. *Science* **331**:778–782.

42. Mairey E, Genovesio A, Donnadieu E, Bernard C, Jaubert F, Pinard E, Seylaz J, Olivo-Marin JC, Nassif X, Duménil G. 2006. Cerebral microcirculation shear stress levels determine *Neisseria meningitidis* attachment sites along the blood-brain barrier. *J Exp Med* **203**:1939–1950.

43. Melican K, Michea Veloso P, Martin T, Bruneval P, Duménil G. 2013. Adhesion of *Neisseria meningitidis* to dermal vessels leads to local vascular damage and purpura in a humanized mouse model. *PLoS Pathog* **9**:e1003139.

44. Melican K, Duménil G. 2013. A humanized model of microvascular infection. *Future Microbiol* **8**:567–569.

45. Sjöqvist J, Maria J, Simon RA, Linares M, Norman P, Nilsson KPR, Lindgren M. 2014. Toward a molecular understanding of the detection of amyloid proteins with flexible conjugated oligothiophenes. *J Phys Chem A* **118**:9820–9827.

46. Klingstedt T, Aslund A, Simon RA, Johansson LB, Mason JJ, Nyström S, Hammarström P, Nilsson KP. 2011. Synthesis of a library of oligothiophenes and their utilization as fluorescent ligands for spectral assignment of protein aggregates. *Org Biomol Chem* **9**:8356–8370.

47. Smith DR, Price JE, Burby PE, Blanco LP, Chamberlain J, Chapman MR. 2017. The production of curli amyloid fibers is deeply integrated into the biology of *Escherichia coli*. *Biomolecules* **7**:E75.

48. Choong FX, Bäck M, Fahlén S, Johansson LB, Melican K, Rhen M, Nilsson KPR, Richter-Dahlfors A. 2016. Real-time optotracing of curli and cellulose in live *Salmonella* biofilms using luminescent oligothiophenes. *NPJ Biofilms Microbiomes* **2**:16024.

49. Antypas H, Choong FX, Libberton B, Brauner A, Richter-Dahlfors A. 2018. Rapid diagnostic assay for detection of cellulose in urine as biomarker for biofilm-related urinary tract infections. *NPJ Biofilms Microbiomes* **4**:26.

50. Komura D, Ishikawa S. 2018. Machine learning methods for histopathological image analysis. *Comput Struct Biotechnol J* **16**:34–42.

51. Melendez J, van Ginneken B, Maduskar P, Philipsen RH, Ayles H, Sanchez CI. 2016. On combining multiple-instance learning and active learning for computer-aided detection of tuberculosis. *IEEE Trans Med Imaging* **35**:1013–1024.

52. Löffler S, Melican K, Nilsson KPR, Richter-Dahlfors A. 2017. Organic bioelectronics in medicine. *J Intern Med* **282**:24–36.

53. Löffler S, Libberton B, Richter-Dahlfors A. 2015. Organic bioelectronic tools for biomedical applications. *Electronics (Basel)* **4**:879–908.

54. Löffler S, Libberton B, Richter-Dahlfors A. 2015. Organic bioelectronics in infection. *J Mater Chem B Mater Biol Med* **3**:4979–4992.

55. Boekel J, Källskog O, Rydén-Aulin M, Rhen M, Richter-Dahlfors A. 2011. Comparative tissue transcriptomics reveal prompt inter-organ communication in response to local bacterial kidney infection. *BMC Genomics* **12**:123.

56. Goda T, Kjall P, Ishihara K, Richter-Dahlfors A, Miyahara Y. 2014. Biomimetic interfaces reveal activa-

tion dynamics of C-reactive protein in local microenvironments. *Adv Healthc Mater* **3:**1733–1738.

57. **Isaksson J, Kjäll P, Nilsson D, Robinson ND, Berggren M, Richter-Dahlfors A.** 2007. Electronic control of Ca2+ signalling in neuronal cells using an organic electronic ion pump. *Nat Mater* **6:**673–679.

58. **Richter-Dahlfors A, Rhen M, Udekwu K.** 2012. Tissue microbiology provides a coherent picture of infection. *Curr Opin Microbiol* **15:**15–22.

59. **Stolp B, Melican K.** 2016. Microbial pathogenesis revealed by intravital microscopy: pros, cons and cautions. *FEBS Lett* **590:**2014–2026.

Bacteria and Intracellularity
Edited by Pascale Cossart, Craig R. Roy, and Philippe Sansonetti
© 2019 American Society for Microbiology, Washington, DC
doi:10.1128/microbiolspec.BAI-0017-2019

Cellular Imaging of Intracellular Bacterial Pathogens

23

Virginie Stévenin[1] and Jost Enninga[1]

INTRODUCTION

Cellular imaging encompasses a large variety of methods that can be considered to be among the most powerful tools for investigating the molecular and cellular details of host-pathogen interactions, particularly when microbes display an intracellular lifestyle. This field has been expanding rapidly during the last 20 years and will likely gain further relevance as it continues to develop. Optical, fluorescence-based approaches are especially popular among infection biologists. In addition, we are witnessing a renaissance of electron microscopy (EM) due to numerous novel ultrastructural approaches changing the perception of EM from that of a confirmatory approach to that of a tool that drives new biological questions.

The explosion of optical, imaging-based studies is based on the following. First, a new generation of microscopes has been brought to the market during the last 2 decades. These microscopes are more easily accessible to biologists, the hardware—especially light sources and detectors—has been dramatically improved, and microscopes are now typically fully automated. Second, molecular and cell biologists have developed a huge catalogue of genetically encoded probes, which started in 1994 with the application of green fluorescent protein (GFP) for cellular imaging (1). Simultaneously, chemists have worked with cell biologists to synthesize a plethora of low-molecular-weight, fluorescent probes or sensors to investigate specific cellular and functional features. Third, computer-assisted analysis of imaging data has moved cellular imaging away from a descriptive and qualitative discipline towards the realm of quantitative studies. Unbiased algorithms are able to extract "high-content" information from the obtained images. These developments are enhanced by open-source and user-friendly software, such as FIJI (http://fiji.sc/Fiji), Cell Pro-

filer (http://www.cellprofiler.org), and ICY (http://icy.bioimageanalysis.org). In addition, analytical pipelines based on artificial intelligence, including deep learning and neural networks, have recently emerged, underlining the interdisciplinary character of this research field.

Cellular imaging for infection research is highly complex, often requiring expertise not only in biology but also in physics (particularly optics), engineering, mathematics, computer science, and chemistry. Therefore, delivering exhaustive information on cellular imaging in a short article on the interaction between pathogens and their hosts is elusive. Here, we provide a short description of some important principles of optical imaging, including methods that breach the diffraction limit of light. In addition, we address some developments commonly considered crucial for the study of host-pathogen interactions, such as labeling, "functionalized" probes, and optogenetic assays. Then we describe screening approaches focusing on the statistical methods used to quantify image-based screening data. Finally, we highlight methods that combine optical imaging with ultrastructural approaches, in particular the game-changing character of large-volume EM methods.

MICROSCOPY AND FLUORESCENCE

Microscopy Principles: Diffraction Limit, Contrast, and Fluorescence

While most microbes are visible by optical microscopy, viruses and some very small bacteria require ultrastructural imaging. Therefore, using imaging techniques to study the interaction of microbes with their host cells is common sense. In doing so, the scholar Antonie Van Leeuwenhoek succeed in discovering the first microbes, or "animalcules," in the late 17th century. Since then,

[1]Institut Pasteur, BCI, Paris 75015, France.

microscopy techniques have continued to be developed, pushing the boundary of what biologists can see. The human eye can distinguish objects down to 100 micrometers, and microscopy is required for anything smaller (Fig. 1). There are numerous excellent textbooks on the fundamental principles of optics and its use in imaging; we recommend *Principles of Fluorescence Spectroscopy* by J. R. Lakowicz for its comprehensive character (2).

Light can be characterized either as a wave or as particles. Its wave characteristics are fully described by the Maxwell equations. It is visible in the range from purple (about 400 nm) to red (800 nm). The wave character of visible light determines the resolution limit of an optical microscope; it is about 250 nm in the x and y directions and about 450 to 700 nm in the z direction. This was formulated by Ernst Abbe in 1870 with the famous equation $d = \lambda/2NA$ (where d is the resolution limit, λ is the wavelength, and NA is the numerical aperture of the objective). As many biological samples do not provide sufficient contrast to be visualized in a light microscope, researchers have developed different contrasting methods throughout the last 100 years. Contrast can be enhanced by using simple bright light illumination, for example, through the phase-contrast procedure (developed by Frits Zernicke in the 1930s), by differential interference contrast (also called Nomarski contrast), or by dark-field contrasting. These techniques do not provide molecular specificity for the imaged objects; therefore, other methods—mainly based on fluorescence—have been established to provide labeling specificity (see "Fluorescent Probes" below for specific examples).

Fluorescence is a widely present phenomenon of light-matter interactions. It describes how molecules interact with light through a defined sequence of light absorption and emission at specific wavelengths at defined energy states. This phenomenon is commonly depicted in a Jablonski diagram (Fig. 2). The light absorption leads to the excitation of the electron cloud of a given molecule to an active state (also called S_1) from its ground state (S_0). The energy from the excited state is emitted within the range of a couple of nanoseconds. Before, energy is lost through collisions or vibrations or crossing to other energy states. The difference between the excitation and emission energy becomes "visible" through the Stokes shift, which is defined as the difference between the excitation peak wavelength and the emission peak wavelength. Fluorescence imaging has become one of the most widely employed techniques in cell biology and infection biology due to its specificity (biomolecules of interest can be labeled) and its sensitivity (single fluorescent molecules can be detected).

Superresolution Microscopy

Objects that are closer to each other than the resolution limit cannot be distinguished as separated. Superresolution techniques break the diffraction limit by temporally or spatially modulating the excitation, or activation, light or by specific postprocessing of the obtained imaging data, exploiting the blinking properties of fluorophores and their point spread functions (3).

Stimulated emission depletion (STED) is a technique that increases the resolution by shaping the excitation light and optically modifying the diffraction limit to reduce its effective diameter. This is achieved by overlaying two excitation beams, one with a doughnut shape and another that is superimposed. The doughnut shape can be modified to enable precise illumination in the subdiffraction range. The two-dimensional resolution

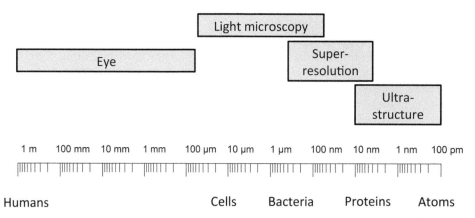

Figure 1 Wavelengths, objects, and their recognition. The sizes of different objects and the tools that can be used for their visualization are shown.

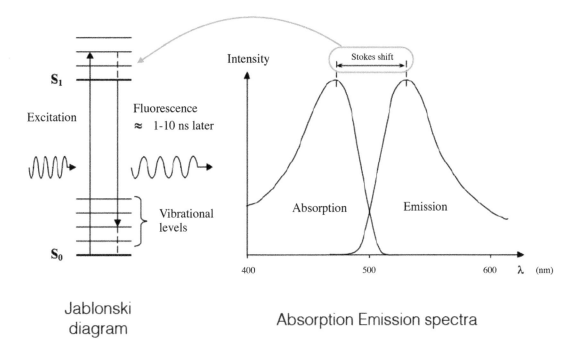

Figure 2 The Jablonski diagram explains the basic principles of fluorescence. Molecules are excited by incoming light to reach a higher energy level (S_1). After vibrational loss of energy (among other losses), the molecule falls back to its low energy level (S_0), emitting fluorescent light. An excitation-and-emission spectrum for a hypothetical fluorophore that could be similar to GFP is shown on the right. Image courtesy of Gael Moneron (Institut Pasteur).

for STED is between 30 and 70 nm, with no increase in axial resolution.

Photo-activated localization microscopy (PALM) and stochastic optical reconstruction microscopy (STORM) techniques are based on single-molecule blinking. They overcome the diffraction limit by using light to turn on only a sparse subset of the fluorescent molecules of interest. Using a mathematical postprocessing step, they estimate the centroids of the localized points to create a reconstructed superresolution image. The difference between PALM and STORM lies in the nature of the fluorescent labels, which are either photoswitchable organic dyes such as Alexa Fluor 647 or Cy5 for STORM or photoswitchable fluorescent proteins for PALM. Currently, these techniques allow localization of the position of the molecule of interest with a precision of 20 nm.

Finally, structured illumination microscopy (SIM) illuminates the entire field with striped patterns of light (4). These excitation patterns mix with the spatial pattern of the sample, and they produce interference patterns, called moiré fringes. To reconstruct a superresolution image, multiple images are taken with different pattern orientations, the information from the frequency space outside the observable region is collected, and the illu-

mination pattern is removed by postprocessing. SIM provides a resolution of about 100 nm in the *x-y* direction and 400 nm axially (5).

Despite a significant improvement of the spatial resolution, standard superresolution techniques provide a lower temporal resolution, and they are further limited because of photobleaching and the phototoxicity, as they require longer time and light exposure to acquire the sample. In addition, most superresolution techniques require special sample preparations, which can be limiting for many experiments.

FLUORESCENT PROBES

The steady development of novel fluorescent probes for the labeling of specific molecular and cellular structures has been a driving force to make fluorescence microscopy a workhorse for cell biologists and infection biologists (6). Fluorescent probes are typically designed to localize low numbers of labeled biomolecules down to individual molecules inside fixed or living cells. While the majority of published studies have employed protein labeling, it is also possible to label all kinds of biomolecules, including nucleic acids, lipids, and sugars. Labeling is achieved through a specific affinity between a small fluorophore and the molecule of interest, such as fluorescently labeled phalloidin intercalating into F-actin structures (Fig. 3).

Additionally, genetically encoded fluorophores allow the expression of fluorescent protein chimeras of molecules of interest or genetically fluorescent sensors (see "Genetically Encoded Probes for Cellular Compartments" below). Numerous engineered GFPs and their derivatives are available, and they span the entire visible spectrum of light. Among them are molecules like mCherry (7), plant-derived fluorescent proteins, such as miniSOG or iLov (8), and others, such as dsRed (6). The physical properties of these fluorophores are highly variable and need to be taken into account by the experimentalist. For example, subtleties of the spectra, bleaching properties, and quantum yield need to be assessed. Also, in some cases, the fluorescent proteins impede the function of the tagged proteins; hence, alternative approaches have been developed to overcome issues arising through the bulkiness of GFP derivatives.

Genetically Encoded Probes for Cellular Compartments

Tagging of host factors is particularly useful for the study of intracellular pathogen trafficking. Within cells, many pathogens can remain within a membrane-enclosed vacuole and avoid fusion with lysosomes to create a unique replicative niche. Alternatively, others escape from this niche, rupturing their vacuole to access the host cytosol for subsequent spread (9). Vacuolar maturation is characterized by the interplay of diverse bacterial effectors and host factors that modulate the lipid and protein composition of the vacuolar membrane. During these processes, small GTPases such as Rabs, ARFs, and Rhos are key regulators of host vesicular trafficking and cytoskeleton dynamics. Tracking their localization by fluorescence microscopy has provided a large amount of information on the host pathways subverted by each pathogen during invasion.

These trafficking events are commonly studied using time-lapse optical microscopy with cells transformed or transfected with DNA coding for fluorescently tagged proteins (Fig. 4). Many pathogens induce membrane ruffles at their entry site or macropinocytic cup formation that can be observed using fluorescently tagged actin or Rac1. Macropinosomes can be followed using Rab5, SNX1/5, or EEA1. Maturing endosomes are monitored with Rab7 as classical probes for late endocytic compartments and with LAMP1 for their endolysosomal identity. The phosphatidylinositol phosphates (PIPs) are lipids that provide a specific identity to each

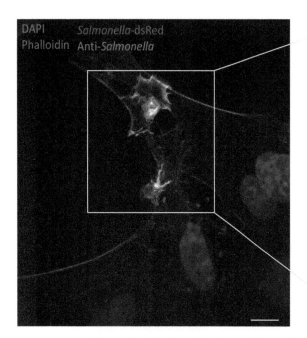
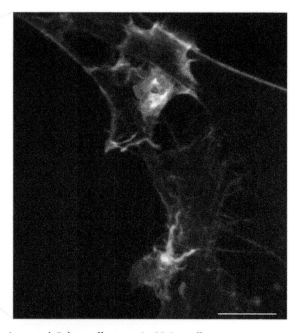

Figure 3 Fixed confocal acquisition of ruffle formations and *Salmonella* entry in HeLa cells. All salmonellae expressed a fluorescent plasmid (in red). *Salmonella* lipopolysaccharide is immunolabeled before cell permeabilization (in green). The host actin cytoskeleton and nuclei are stained with phalloidin (in grey) and DAPI (4′,6-diamidino-2-phenylindole; in blue). Bars, 10 μm.

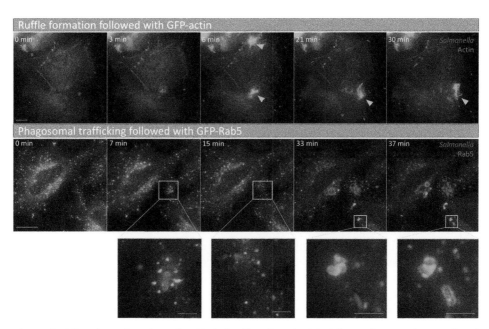

Figure 4 Time-lapse imaging of epithelial cells infected with *Salmonella* using bacterial and host genetically encoded probes. HeLa cells were transfected with GFP-actin (top) or GFP-Rab5 (bottom) to follow the ruffle formation and the phagosomal trafficking upon infection with dsRed-expressing *Salmonella* (yellow arrowheads indicate ruffles). White bars, 10 μm; yellow bars, 2 μm.

endosomal compartment. For example, PI(4,5)P2 can be used to investigate early membrane ruffling, while PI (3,4,5)P3 localizes at the macropinocytic cup, and PI(3)P is enriched on early endosomes after scission from the plasma membrane. Fluorescent biosensors are used to detect the PIPs, such as the lipid-binding PX domain of p40phox or the tandem dimer of the FYVE domain of EEA1 (2xFYVE), which are most frequently used to detect PI(3)P (10, 11). However, considering that pathogens subvert the host in multiple ways to establish unique intracellular pathogen niches, the pathogen-containing endosomal compartment behaves differently from physiological compartments. Therefore, these trafficking markers may behave in unexpected ways in infected cells compared to noninfected cells. Clarity can be obtained only through in-depth studies of the involved trafficking molecules.

Fluorescent reporters have also been developed to differentiate between vacuole-bound and cytosolic bacteria. For example, galectin-3 is a host lectin that can be used as a dynamic marker for vacuolar escape simply by expressing a fluorescently tagged version of the protein within the host cell. As long as the vacuolar integrity is maintained, the galectin-3 fluorescent signal is uniformly distributed within the entire host cell. Upon vacuolar rupture, the signal accumulates in the vicinity of the damaged membrane of bacterium-containing vac-

uoles, forming a readily visible galectin-3 "ghost." This has revealed that *Shigella* escapes into the cytoplasm about 10 minutes after bacterial entry (12, 13). In addition, the galectin-3 marker and other galectins have been successfully used to follow vacuolar rupture in the context of various bacterial pathogens (e.g., *Listeria*, *Salmonella*, *Legionella*, etc.) (13–15).

Functionalized Probes

Molecular switches, such as small GTPases or kinases, regulate the host cytoskeletal and trafficking organization. Upon infection, these proteins are commonly targeted by pathogens to reorganize the host environment. They exist in an active form and an inactive form. To differentiate between these conditions and to delineate the molecular switches, functional fluorescent probes have been developed to measure their activity status through fluorescence energy transfer (FRET). A large catalogue of such probes is now available, and a few of them have been used for bacterial entry. For example, it was shown via ratiometric FRET image analysis that Rac1 is activated at the site of *Yersinia* entry in typically nonphagocytic cells using the interaction of the FRET pair Rac1-CFP with a yellow fluorescent protein fusion of a domain of its downstream adaptor, PAK1 (16). In the case of *Listeria* entry, the same principle was used to monitor Rac1 activation and the implication of small signaling lipids of the inositol-phosphatidyl family (17). Furthermore, FRET sensors were used to investigate vinculin activation during the early entry steps of *Shigella* (18). There are two hurdles that prevent the broad usage of the FRET probes. One issue is that most of them display a limited functionality; for example, it is not clear whether the probes localize in a manner identical to that of the endogenous proteins. Secondly, FRET measurements are often done through relatively slow ratiometric procedures. This can be improved via fluorescence lifetime imaging for measurements in real time, which are important to trace the highly dynamic events during the rapid entry of different pathogens.

We have developed functionalized probes to track vacuolar rupture under both fixed-cell and living-cell conditions in a robust way. This method is based on a cephalosporin-derived FRET probe, CCF4-AM, that can be cleaved by beta-lactamase. Using this assay in real time, we revealed the rapid escape of *Shigella* from the vacuole within less than 10 minutes after cellular entry, which was in line with the results obtained with fluorescently labeled galectins (12). This technique has been successfully adapted for other pathogens, including *Mycobacterium tuberculosis*, *Francisella*, and *Listeria* (19–21). It is highly versatile for high-throughput screening, as described in more detail below. Another fluorescence imaging approach relies on the use of fluorescent dextran, a fluid-phase marker for endocytic compartments that accumulates within the *Salmonella*-containing vacuole. By preloading cells with Alexa488-dextran overnight and challenging them with mCherry-expressing *Salmonella*, the integrity of the *Salmonella*-containing vacuole can be surveyed by time-lapse imaging assessing the colocalization of mCherry-*Salmonella* with Alexa488-dextran a few hours postinfection. This method has been used to demonstrate that the *Salmonella* pathogenicity island 2 type III secretion system is required for bacterial replication within the vacuole but not for cytosolic replication (22). This technique can differentiate between vacuolar and cytosolic bacteria, but unlike the galectin-3 and FRET probe methods, it does not yield precise quantitative information on the timing of vacuolar rupture.

Optogenetics

Optogenetics is a relatively new technique to modulate the localization or the activity status of biomolecules in a spatially and temporally defined way (23). Used in conjunction with regulatory proteins, this technique makes it possible to turn them on and off simply by shining light on the observed specimen.

Notably, optogenetics can be used to induce ruffling and macropinosome formation within chosen regions of a given cell. The pathway associated with receptor tyrosine kinase-induced macropinocytosis can be activated downstream of the receptor tyrosine kinase using optogenetics on modified small GTPases. Fujii and colleagues characterized the activation and deactivation of the small GTPase Rac1 using microscopic photomanipulation (24). Expression of the genetically encoded photoactivatable-Rac1 (PA-Rac1) in RAW264 macrophages enables the local and reversible control of macropinocytosis using blue laser irradiation. The irradiated region of macrophages under the persistent activation of PA-Rac1 displays PI(4,5)P2 accumulation, actin enrichment, membrane ruffling, and unclosed macropinosomes. Deactivation of PA-Rac1 by ceasing irradiation is needed to stop membrane ruffling and lead to the acquisition of maturation markers such as PI(3)P and Rab21 by the preformed macropinosomes. Thus, using an optogenetic technique shows that the targeted activation of Rac1 is sufficient to induce ruffles and macropinosomes. Through this approach, pathogens could be forced to be internalized at specific sites within challenged host cells.

IMAGING-BASED SCREENING

Loss-of-function screens have been instrumental in uncovering numerous features of the host-pathogen cross talk. Loss of function means a targeted depletion or reduction of expression of a specific gene. The most widely used approach still uses RNA interference (RNAi) as a suitable tool for gene function knockdown. The reason for this is the accessibility and the ease of use of small interfering RNA (siRNA) libraries against host genes. siRNA gene knockdowns can be combined with recent advances in imaging technologies (see above), including automated microscopy and image processing software that have been milestones in the development of large-scale screening approaches. Over the past 15 years, image-based RNAi screening has emerged as a powerful technique to unravel the molecular mechanism of intricate cellular processes such as cell division, membrane trafficking, and host-pathogen interactions (25, 26).

RNAi is a conserved posttranscriptional gene silencing process mediated by double-stranded RNAs (dsRNAs). In brief, the double-stranded RNAs are cleaved by the endoribonuclease Dicer, resulting in short fragments, typically of 21 to 23 nucleotides, referred to as siRNAs. These siRNAs are then incorporated into the RNA-induced silencing complex, where one strand of the siRNA, the antisense strand, serves as a guide to specifically recognize and pair with the complementary target mRNA, resulting in mRNA cleavage. siRNA can be chemically synthesized and delivered into the cells, commonly by liposome-based transfection or electroporation. Libraries of siRNAs targeting the entire genome or only subsets of genes involved in specific processes (e.g., membrane trafficking and apoptosis) or family members (kinases and molecular motors) are commercially available for medium- to high-throughput screening applications.

More recently, loss-of-function screens have also been performed via alternative gene-targeting approaches. CRISPR (clustered regularly interspaced short palindromic repeat)-Cas-based gene targeting in particular has become very popular. Through this method, genes can be targeted via small guide RNAs against specific host genes. The targeted genes are deactivated by the Cas9 nuclease, which forms a complex with the guide RNA. Despite the increased usage of CRISPR-based screening methods, they are still less well characterized than siRNA-based approaches, and obtained hits require a careful follow-up characterization with regard to their specificity.

Undoubtedly, image-based loss-of-function screening can yield valuable insight; however, its success requires careful assay design and data analysis. Practically speaking, the experimental pipeline of a screening assay can be divided into the following steps: (i) experimental planning, (ii) assay development and validation, (iii) primary screening, (iv) screen analysis and confirmation, and (v) hit characterization (25, 26). The initial step consists of clearly defining the biological question and appropriate design of the screening assay, including exercising particular care in choosing the model and the knockdown/knockout library (i.e., using a genome-wide library versus a selected subset). One of the most challenging steps (and usually the most time-consuming) is assay development

and validation. Often, this step is underestimated by the experimentalists. Each individual experimental parameter (e.g., the knockdown or knockout procedures, fluorescence biosensor/stain, imaging setup, etc.) needs to be established and optimized, yielding a sensitive, robust, and reproducible assay. In particular, microscopy-based screening requires the development of an automated image analysis algorithm for reliable qualitative and/or quantitative measurements of large data sets.

The reliability of the assay (or quality control) is assessed using statistical tests such as the Z factor (or Z') and the strictly standardized mean difference, which measure the magnitude of the difference between negative and positive controls, ensuring that the selection of effective positive and negative controls is maximal and that the assay can identify hits with a wide range of phenotypic effects (Fig. 5A) (27, 28). Once the assay is statistically validated, the actual screen is usually conducted in plate duplicates, typically taking a few days to weeks depending on the throughput.

Post-primary-screening analysis relies on a number of statistical methods for data normalization and hit selection (Fig. 5B). Data normalization is required to compare and combine data from different plates by removing systematic errors from the raw data. Widely used methods for data normalization are the z score and its variant the robust z score, which basically determine the number of standard deviations from the mean and the median, respectively, for the control population. Because the robust z score is based on the median, it is insensitive to outliers and thus more suitable for knockdown screens. Typically, hit identification relies on a standard deviation threshold, which commonly follow the empirical rule of ±3 standard deviations,

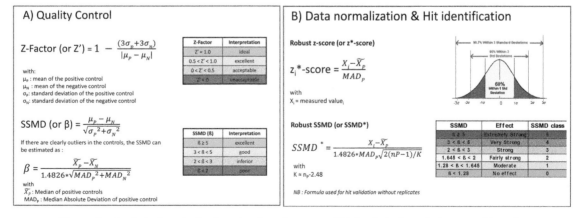

Figure 5 Statistical tools for imaging-based screens. (A) Statistical analysis tests of knockdown screens to assess quality control. (B) Statistical analysis tests for data normalization and hit identification from the screens. Mathematical formulas and interpretation are shown. Adapted from references 27 and 28.

that is directly linked to the *P* value in normally distributed data (i.e., Gaussian distribution).

Alternatively, a more sophisticated method for data normalization and hit identification is the robust strictly standardized mean difference, which has been shown to better measure the effect sizes across experiments. It is noteworthy that this statistical technique grants control of both the false-positive and false-negative rates and provides a valuable classification of the hit effects based on a rigorous probability interpretation (28) (Fig. 5B). Ultimately, the statistical analysis provides a list of target gene candidates that will be further validated and characterized.

Hit characterization usually involves a multidisciplinary approach combining cell biology (e.g., live-cell imaging), bioinformatics (e.g., protein network analysis), and/or biochemistry (e.g., a pull-down assay). Altogether, although they are challenging, image-based loss-of-function screening approaches open exciting avenues for the study of host-pathogen cross talk at the cellular level.

CORRELATIVE LIGHT AND EM OF LARGE VOLUMES

Many of the molecular players and general mechanisms that have roles during host-pathogen cross talk have been identified and characterized in some detail at the level of optical diffraction-limited microscopy. The above-described multidimensional fluorescence microscopy approaches have been instrumental in this, providing dynamic insights into host and pathogen factors during infection, as well as functional information through the development of a multitude of cellular reporters. Nevertheless, how these pathogen and host factors function in the three-dimensional cellular environment at sub-diffraction resolution cannot be resolved by optical approaches. One way to tackle this issue has been the development of superresolution microscopy (see above). Most superresolution approaches rely on fluorescence and can provide increasingly high-resolution information (down to about 10 nm by PALM, STORM, or STED). However, with these methods, one visualizes only the labeled elements, not the complete cellular environment.

This global cellular environment can be imaged at molecular resolution by EM. Nevertheless, EM-based approaches are limited in their ability to fully describe complicated three-dimensional cellular interfaces between the pathogen and host, due to an important and often overlooked factor—their limits of acquisition volume. Only in the past 10 years have we seen the emergence of new EM techniques which have been developed

to not be constrained by these limits. One of these techniques is focused ion beam scanning EM (FIB/SEM), in which large-volume tomograms are acquired (29). Briefly, the principle of large-volume FIB/SEM is that an embedded biological sample is exposed to a focused ion beam capable of removing a thin layer of material (5 to 10 nm thick) in a highly precise manner termed "milling." Between sample millings, a scanning electron beam is used to image the newly exposed surface. By repeating this process hundreds or even thousands of times, a large sample volume can be acquired with up to 5-nm resolution in all axes. Data sets produced by FIB/SEM can be thoroughly examined from any orientation and subjected to detailed quantitative analysis. This allows the high-resolution three-dimensional visualization of intracellular pathogens and their hosts within a large sample volume, providing an unprecedented level of structural detail.

In recent years, FIB/SEM has been combined increasingly frequently with three-dimensional fluorescence microscopy using correlative light EM (CLEM) to address biological questions. CLEM enables the study of a single site of interest using two approaches, each offering unique advantages. Labs routinely employing fluorescence microscopy for the study of pathogens often have a wide arsenal of fluorescent labels (for example, GFP-labeled proteins and organelle-specific stains) that provide precise biological information about the localization of pathogens, proteins, organelles, and compartments. By initially examining samples with fluorescence microcopy, transient or rare biological events as well as specific regions of interest within a pathogen or host cell can be identified. By using a finder grid or another reference system during light microscopy acquisition, samples can be processed for FIB/SEM so that the region of interest that was initially identified can be located again precisely and acquired as part of a large volume.

In CLEM-FIB/SEM, a biological sample is initially imaged by light microscopy (typically three-dimensional confocal or epifluorescence microscopy plus deconvolution) followed by FIB/SEM acquisition at the same location (Fig. 6). Transient or rare biological events can be pinpointed by fluorescent labels prior to FIB/SEM acquisition, allowing imaging of precise stages of pathogen invasion not easily accessible by classic EM investigation. Furthermore, the fluorescent signals can later be correlated to details within the large ultrastructural volume, providing molecular labeling of the observed structures. Therefore, the defining feature of FIB/SEM is its ability to provide access to intricate structural detail placed within a much broader cellular context. Generally, fluorescently labeled pathogens (viruses, bacteria, or parasites) repre-

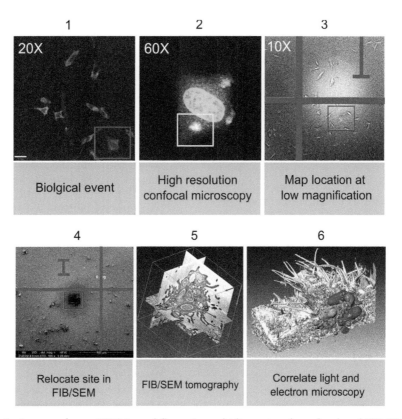

Figure 6 Large-volume CLEM workflow via multidimensional confocal and FIB/SEM imaging. Biological samples are prepared on gridded glass-bottom slides for time-lapse imaging (1), and events are tracked dynamically at high resolution (2). After site identification under the light microscope (3), locations are retrieved in the electron microscope (4), and three-dimensional volumes are obtained by milling and scanning of the prepared specimen (5). Afterwards, both image data sets are correlated and segmented (6). A typical data set spans 10 μm by 10 μm by 10 μm. Invading *Shigella* organisms are depicted, the forming entry foci are segmented (gold), and macropinosomes (orange) in the vicinity of the entering bacteria (blue) are identified. Images were taken by Allon Weiner (Institut Pasteur).

sent objects that can be readily exploited as alignment fiducials for CLEM. The FIB/SEM experimental workflow is relatively fast and simple compared to other advanced EM approaches, allowing quick turnaround times between biological experiments and structural insights. Thanks to this, CLEM-FIB/SEM constitutes a major investigative tool to facilitate ongoing research in a lab.

Correlative FIB/SEM offers several important features: CLEM allows rare or transient biological events to be subjected to ultrastructural investigation. Acquisition of large cellular volumes significantly increases the chance that the event imaged by light microscopy will be fully contained within the ultrastructural volume and therefore unambiguously identified at high resolution. The three-dimensional information obtained by fluorescence microscopy (e.g., confocal) can be directly correlated with the FIB/SEM data, labeling pathogens, compartments, and organelles of interest. As the acquisition volume of

FIB/SEM is much larger than that of conventional tomography, significantly more fluorescent signal can be correlated with ultrastructural data, enhancing the information content. CLEM-FIB/SEM can also be performed in conjunction with even larger-volume micro-computed tomography studies or even *in vivo* imaging (30).

THE NEXT CHALLENGES

"The sky is the limit" describes the feeling that one has in contemplating the ever-increasing number of imaging techniques for the investigation of infection at the cellular level. In this overview, we focus on techniques that we consider will be of key relevance in the coming years. A number of issues need to be tackled in a systematic way.

First, we need to bridge dimensions in imaging. Despite improved CLEM procedures, it is still challenging to obtain molecular resolution in the cellular context. This could be overcome through the consequent implementation of superresolution imaging in the CLEM pipelines. Alternatively, single-molecule methods need to become more accessible. This requires probe development and more sensitive detectors. Another issue is the integration of cellular imaging with tissue imaging that could be achieved either by developing multiphoton imaging or by using more accessible tissue models, for example, organoids.

A second challenge is the need for precise quantification. Cellular reporters need to be fine-tuned to depict the precise process that one wants to study. Also, consequent development of analytical pipelines, including algorithms that use neuronal networks for the analysis of subtle phenotypes, should become routine.

Finally, as imaging is based mainly on probes, one needs to take into account that they interfere with biological processes. In particular, the overexpression of fluorescently tagged proteins often interferes with the processes the protein of interest is involved in. This can be tackled through the labeling of the endogenous proteins using approaches as CRISPR-Cas. Another approach is the consequent development of organic probes with minimal interference, for example, coupling click chemistry with fluorescence imaging.

The consequent integration of the different microscopy-related fields will keep cellular imaging at the forefront of the understanding of the cellular processes taking place during infection.

Citation. Stévenin V, Enninga J. 2019. Cellular imaging of intracellular bacterial pathogens. Microbiol Spectrum 7(2):BAI-0017-2019.

References

1. Chalfie M, Tu Y, Euskirchen G, Ward WW, Prasher DC. 1994. Green fluorescent protein as a marker for gene expression. *Science* **263:**802–805.

2. Lakowicz JR. 2006. *Principles of Fluorescence Spectroscopy*, 3rd ed. Springer Press, New York, NY.

3. Galbraith CG, Galbraith JA. 2011. Super-resolution microscopy at a glance. *J Cell Sci* **124:**1607–1611.

4. Gustafsson MG. 2000. Surpassing the lateral resolution limit by a factor of two using structured illumination microscopy. *J Microsc* **198:**82–87.

5. Schermelleh L, Carlton PM, Haase S, Shao L, Winoto L, Kner P, Burke B, Cardoso MC, Agard DA, Gustafsson MG, Leonhardt H, Sedat JW. 2008. Subdiffraction multicolor imaging of the nuclear periphery with 3D structured illumination microscopy. *Science* **320:**1332–1336.

6. Giepmans BN, Adams SR, Ellisman MH, Tsien RY. 2006. The fluorescent toolbox for assessing protein location and function. *Science* **312:**217–224.

7. Shaner NC, Campbell RE, Steinbach PA, Giepmans BN, Palmer AE, Tsien RY. 2004. Improved monomeric red, orange and yellow fluorescent proteins derived from *Discosoma* sp. red fluorescent protein. *Nat Biotechnol* **22:**1567–1572.

8. Christie JM, Hitomi K, Arvai AS, Hartfield KA, Mettlen M, Pratt AJ, Tainer JA, Getzoff ED. 2012. Structural tuning of the fluorescent protein iLOV for improved photostability. *J Biol Chem* **287:**22295–22304.

9. Fredlund J, Enninga J. 2014. Cytoplasmic access by intracellular bacterial pathogens. *Trends Microbiol* **22:**128–137.

10. Kanai F, Liu H, Field SJ, Akbary H, Matsuo T, Brown GE, Cantley LC, Yaffe MB. 2001. The PX domains of p47phox and p40phox bind to lipid products of PI(3)K. *Nat Cell Biol* **3:**675–678.

11. Lemmon MA. 2008. Membrane recognition by phospholipid-binding domains. *Nat Rev Mol Cell Biol* **9:**99–111.

12. Ray K, Bobard A, Danckaert A, Paz-Haftel I, Clair C, Ehsani S, Tang C, Sansonetti P, Tran Van Nhieu G, Enninga J. 2010. Tracking the dynamic interplay between bacterial and host factors during pathogen-induced vacuole rupture in real time. *Cell Microbiol* **12:**545–556.

13. Paz I, Sachse M, Dupont N, Mounier J, Cederfur C, Enninga J, Leffler H, Poirier F, Prevost MC, Lafont F, Sansonetti P. 2010. Galectin-3, a marker for vacuole lysis by invasive pathogens. *Cell Microbiol* **12:**530–544.

14. Thurston TL, Wandel MP, von Muhlinen N, Foeglein A, Randow F. 2012. Galectin 8 targets damaged vesicles for autophagy to defend cells against bacterial invasion. *Nature* **482:**414–418.

15. Creasey EA, Isberg RR. 2012. The protein SdhA maintains the integrity of the *Legionella*-containing vacuole. *Proc Natl Acad Sci USA* **109:**3481–3486.

16. Wong KW, Isberg RR. 2005. *Yersinia pseudotuberculosis* spatially controls activation and misregulation of host cell Rac1. *PLoS Pathog* **1:**e16.

17. Seveau S, Tham TN, Payrastre B, Hoppe AD, Swanson JA, Cossart P. 2007. A FRET analysis to unravel the role of cholesterol in Rac1 and PI 3-kinase activation in the InlB/Met signalling pathway. *Cell Microbiol* **9:**790–803.

18. Chen H, Cohen DM, Choudhury DM, Kioka N, Craig SW. 2005. Spatial distribution and functional significance of activated vinculin in living cells. *J Cell Biol* **169:**459–470.

19. Juruj C, Lelogeais V, Pierini R, Perret M, Py BF, Jamilloux Y, Broz P, Ader F, Faure M, Henry T. 2013. Caspase-1 activity affects AIM2 speck formation/stability through a negative feedback loop. *Front Cell Infect Microbiol* **3:**14.

20. Simeone R, Bobard A, Lippmann J, Bitter W, Majlessi L, Brosch R, Enninga J. 2012. Phagosomal rupture by *Mycobacterium tuberculosis* results in toxicity and host cell death. *PLoS Pathog* **8:**e1002507.

21. Quereda JJ, Pizarro-Cerdá J, Balestrino D, Bobard A, Danckaert A, Aulner N, Shorte S, Enninga J, Cossart P. 2016. A dual microscopy-based assay to assess *Listeria monocytogenes* cellular entry and vacuolar escape. *Appl Environ Microbiol* **82:**211–217.

22. Malik-Kale P, Winfree S, Steele-Mortimer O. 2012. The bimodal lifestyle of intracellular *Salmonella* in epithelial

cells: replication in the cytosol obscures defects in vacuolar replication. *PLoS One* **7**:e38732.

23. van Bergeijk P, Hoogenraad CC, Kapitein LC. 2016. Right time, right place: probing the functions of organelle positioning. *Trends Cell Biol* **26**:121–134.

24. Fujii M, Kawai K, Egami Y, Araki N. 2013. Dissecting the roles of Rac1 activation and deactivation in macropinocytosis using microscopic photo-manipulation. *Sci Rep* **3**:2385.

25. Conrad C, Gerlich DW. 2010. Automated microscopy for high-content RNAi screening. *J Cell Biol* **188**:453–461.

26. Mohr S, Bakal C, Perrimon N. 2010. Genomic screening with RNAi: results and challenges. *Annu Rev Biochem* **79**:37–64.

27. Zhang XD. 2011. Illustration of SSMD, z score, SSMD*, z* score, and t statistic for hit selection in RNAi high-throughput screens. *J Biomol Screen* **16**:775–785.

28. Zhang XD. 2007. A new method with flexible and balanced control of false negatives and false positives for hit selection in RNA interference high-throughput screening assays. *J Biomol Screen* **12**:645–655.

29. Narayan K, Subramaniam S. 2015. Focused ion beams in biology. *Nat Methods* **12**:1021–1031.

30. Karreman MA, Mercier L, Schieber NL, Solecki G, Allio G, Winkler F, Ruthensteiner B, Goetz JG, Schwab Y. 2016. Fast and precise targeting of single tumor cells in vivo by multimodal correlative microscopy. *J Cell Sci* **129**:444–456.

Bacteria and Intracellularity
Edited by Pascale Cossart, Craig R. Roy, and Philippe Sansonetti
© 2019 American Society for Microbiology, Washington, DC
doi:10.1128/microbiolspec.BAI-0021-2019

Using a Systems Biology Approach To Study Host-Pathogen Interactions

24

Amy Yeung,[1] Christine Hale,[1] Simon Clare,[1] Sophie Palmer,[2]
Josefin Bartholdson Scott,[2] Stephen Baker,[2,3] and Gordon Dougan[2]

INTRODUCTION

Investigations into the mechanisms that influence interactions between microbes and their hosts have exploded over the past ~50 years. These approaches have led to a significantly greater understanding of how pathogens infect their hosts. Data from these experiments can influence therapeutic interventions and aid public health-mediated disease control on local and global scales. Progress in this field has been significant, driven by breakthroughs in several other areas, including molecular biology, biochemistry, immunology, cell biology, and genomics. Each of these independent areas has been underpinned by parallel breakthroughs in laboratory techniques alongside advances in the supporting computational biology (bioinformatics). Progress is ongoing in all of these fields and is continuing apace. Such progress is particularly important as a response to new infection-related threats, such as antimicrobial resistance and the emergence and/or discovery of new pathogens, which challenge our ability to maintain the disease control *status quo* (1–3).

One of the key early steps in developing the field of investigating host-pathogen interactions was the application of genetics to study enteric bacteria, including enterotoxigenic *Escherichia coli* by Herbert Williams Smith, in the 1960s and 1970s (4, 5). This development was followed by the application of gene cloning and the creation of the new field of cellular microbiology, leading to the definition of virulence-associated genes and host susceptibility factors (6–8). Much of the early work was driven by reductionist approaches involving targeted genetic manipulation of the pathogen and the host, which yielded an enormous data resource that came to

define the field. With the creation of next-generation nucleic acid sequencing and developments in mammalian genetics, stem cell biology, and mass spectrometry, new opportunities for genome-wide approaches have emerged that can be applied at scale and in the field. The ability to define how microbial communities influence human health has also emerged as a key technology (9). Combining these approaches will likely be an important route for infection-related research over the next decade. Here, we discuss some of these approaches with a focus on the use of genomics to drive investigations in bacterial pathogenesis.

IMPACT OF WHOLE REFERENCE GENOMES FOR PATHOGENS AND HOSTS

Up until the turn of the millennium, working on pathogen and human genetics was akin to assembling a jigsaw puzzle without an impression of the completed picture. We knew some of the genes within the genome of particular organisms, but we did not have a blueprint of all of the genes in their correct context. This situation changed dramatically with the publication of the first "complete" reference genomes of key organisms. The first finished pathogen genome sequence was that of *Haemophilus influenzae* Rd, which was produced using a shotgun sequencing approach and computer-assisted assembly (10). This work defined the model for a reference genome at the DNA sequence level, and human intervention allowed us to annotate candidate genes and intergenic regions in the full single chromosome. This genome was followed soon after by reference genomes of many classical bacterial pathogens that have shaped the history of

[1]Wellcome Sanger Institute, Wellcome Genome Campus, Hinxton, Cambridge CB10 1SA, United Kingdom; [2]Department of Medicine, University of Cambridge, Addenbrooke's Hospital, Cambridge CB2 0QQ, United Kingdom; [3]Oxford University Clinical Research Unit, The Hospital for Tropical Diseases, Ho Chi Minh City, Vietnam.

humankind. These included *Mycobacterium tuberculosis* (11), *Salmonella enterica* serovar Typhi (12), *Vibrio cholerae* (13), and *Bordetella pertussis* (14). These "brute force" efforts provided us with genetic blueprints for designing genome-wide probes and performing experiments on genes that were not previously known to exist. These new data sets also set the boundaries for whole-genome-based experimental investigations. Several developments quickly followed, including (i) targeted mutagenesis of novel genes or genomic signatures, (ii) genome-wide mutagenesis screens (e.g., Tn-Seq or TraDIS), and (iii) the design of genome-wide probes, including microarray and transcriptome sequencing (RNA-seq) approaches (15–17). All of these technical approaches were paralleled by developments in both bioinformatics and database management. These developments continue apace.

From the perspective of studies involving the host, the publication of the first reference human genomes represented a similarly significant landmark (18, 19). Obviously, this reference was not entirely "complete," in that significant gaps still remained in regions such as those with repetitive sequences, as it was in reality a composite of sequences from multiple humans. Nevertheless, this work stimulated new genome-wide approaches and larger initiatives such as the Case Control Consortium by The Wellcome Trust (https://www.wtccc.org.uk), which heralded a new era in human genetics (20). The generation of reference genomes for non-human organisms used in host-pathogen studies, including the mouse (21) and zebrafish (22), followed, as did reference genomes for various eukaryotic pathogens, including *Plasmodium falciparum* (23) and *Schistosoma mansoni* (24). As was seen with the reference bacterial genomes, these developments in eukaryotic organisms stimulated more ambitious genome-wide experiments, which commonly involved consortia working beyond the limits of individual laboratories. One such example was the Knock Out Mouse Project (KOMP; https://www.komp.org/), which aimed to use recombineering to generate mutations in all the genes in the mouse genome (25). This work resulted in the generation of thousands of novel mutant and transgenic mice that could be exploited for host-pathogen screens (26). Comparable mutant libraries were constructed in zebrafish and eventually in human cell lines. All of these projects provided the impetus as the screening engine to identify novel host-pathogen interaction mechanisms.

Impact of Next-Generation Sequencing Technologies

Shortly after the publication of the multiple reference genomes for microbial pathogens, the commercialization of next-generation nucleic acid sequencing technologies provided a new era in genomic sciences (Fig. 1). Within a comparatively short time, the cost of next-generation sequencing dropped and the efficiency dramatically increased, opening up the possibilities of these technologies across multiple applications and making them more accessible to the broader research community. These technologies meant that literally hundreds of nearly whole genomes could be generated and compared to the original reference sequences, providing an opportunity for comparative genomics and for the definition of phylogenetic structure within pathogens (27–29). The early application of Solexa sequencing (now known as Illumina; www.illumina.com) was used to generate short sequence reads that could be compared to references or assembled into draft genomes. The development of sequencing based on longer reads, such as that available from Pacific Biosciences, facilitated the comparatively cheap and efficient generation of complete draft genomes across populations of bacteria (www.pacb.com; nanoporetech.com).

The rapid generation of multiple genomes provided a platform for studying newly evolving monophyletic lineages within particular species or subtypes. These included the H58 multidrug resistance-associated clade of *S.* Typhi that has become globally dominant (30) and *E. coli* ST131 (31). Such subtypes also became readily accessible to functional genomic analysis. The generation of phylogenetic information within bacterial species and lineages allowed, for the first time, sequence-based identification of evolutionary signatures and the identification and genetic delineation of emerging successful clades. This facilitated improved hypothesis-driven experiments where such genetic signatures could be engineered into laboratory or reference isolates for investigation or evaluation. An excellent example is the identification of mutations influencing serum resistance and potentially the invasiveness of ST313 *S. enterica* serovar Typhimurium in sub-Saharan Africa (32, 33).

Additionally, genome-wide association studies (GWAS) became possible in bacteria (34, 35). The whole-genome-based phylogenetic analysis of pathogens also opened up the possibility of mapping isolates onto geographical space (phylogeographical analysis). This step forward permitted us to map the spread of pathogens in real time between people and within a specific geographical reference frame over time (https://www.sanger.ac.uk/science/tools/microreact). Phylogeographical analysis can be used to track the spread of pathogens across the world or even within particular health care facilities, identifying outbreaks and successful pathogenic clades of bacteria (29, 36). This technology is likely to find favor in the testing of vaccines in the field, in identifying variants

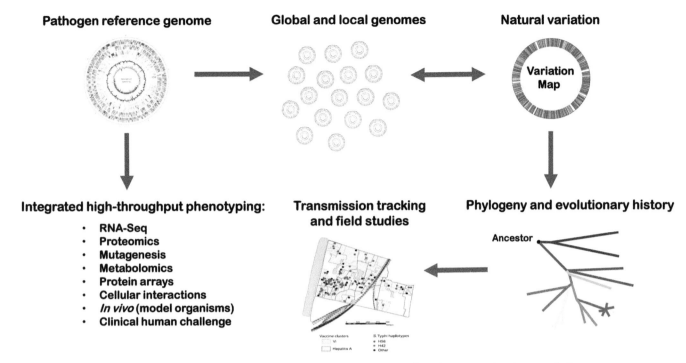

Figure 1 Potential pathways to the functional analysis and exploitation of pathogen whole-genome sequence information. A reference genome (complete and annotated) provides a blueprint for further analysis. The sequencing of populations of related bacteria can be exploited to map sequence variation back onto the reference, providing a map of natural genetic variation on the population. This variation can then be built into phylogeny, providing the evolutionary background of the population. The data can then be collectively used to drive experimental analysis (functional genomics and phenotyping).

that escape vaccine control, or in the monitoring of antimicrobial-resistant variants.

Genome-Wide Screens in Pathogens

As soon as reference bacterial genomes became available, researchers became interested in the concept of genome-wide screens for virulence-associated traits. Some of the initial approaches relied on generating libraries of knock-out mutations representative of all known bacterial genes within a species. This was a labor-intensive approach but was undertaken for several different bacterial species, with different degrees of success, such as *M. tuberculosis* (http://grantome.com/grant/NIH/R24-AI134650-01) and *S.* Typhimurium (37). Libraries of knockouts can be screened for pathogenic traits on a whole-genome, subgenome, or individual-gene basis. Of course, some genes are essential for life or survival in particular environments and therefore cannot be readily inactivated without using specific genetic manipulation.

An alternative genome-wide approach to targeted mutagenesis is using randomly generated transposons, or similar mobile elements, to create libraries that target all genes in the genome. Transposon libraries are generated

within a reference bacterial isolate for which a full genome is available. The resulting library is composed of thousands and potentially millions of individual transposon mutants being pooled for screening. Several research groups independently generated the approach where such libraries are sequenced using primers located on the termini of the transposon that sequence outward and into the adjacent host genome. These sequences can be mapped onto the reference genome, providing both the insertion site and the adjacent sequence for mapping. Terms such as "Tn-Seq" and "TraDIS" have been used to describe these approaches (38–40). Here, the reads obtained from the pools before or after a particular selection are compared to identify genes that are comparatively enriched (positive selection) or depleted (negative selection). Such selections can include antimicrobial exposure, bacteriophage infection, or growth in a particular cellular or *in vivo* system. This approach is similar to methods such as sequence-tagged mutagenesis that were used prior to the generation of reference genome sequences (41). Genome sequencing has become so efficient that it is now possible to identify spontaneous mutations that are selected within a limited phylogenetic lineage, e.g., within an individual host infected with a clonal bacterial population pool or by artificially driving *in vitro* selection (42–44). Such mutations, which are often single nucleotide polymorphisms (SNPs), can be then introduced into reference isolates for validation, which permits the linkage between genotype and phenotype.

A further approach is using RNA-seq or proteome-based approaches to define the transcriptome and proteome generated while the bacteria are cultured under different growth conditions. Here, the transcriptome of the reference bacteria growing at different temperatures can identify RNA populations that are regulated differentially in response to temperature, for example. Such an approach has been used in a pigeon-adapted *S.* Typhimurium strain to identify the role of body temperature in controlling immunogenicity via flagellum regulation (45). A similar approach has been used to identify small noncoding RNA in *S.* Typhimurium influencing the survival of the pathogen inside eukaryotic cells (46). The advent of ultrasensitive mass spectrometry approaches has permitted genome-wide analysis of bacteria, facilitating the identification of posttranscriptional events that influence pathogenesis (47). RNA-seq and proteomics are highly valuable annotation tools in themselves, facilitating the identification of the regulatory and linked operon structure of the transcriptome and proteome, respectively (48). Here, the pool of expressed RNA and proteins can differ greatly under different conditions, thus influencing adaptation and pathogenesis.

Genome-Wide Screens in the Host

Genome-wide association studies

The availability of a draft human genome stimulated interest in identifying host genes and loci that influenced susceptibility to infection and disease outcome. GWAS in humans have been used with some success to identify genes associated with particular traits or diseases (20). GWAS rely on the genotyping of populations of diseased and control humans to identify genetic links through statistical association. As technology has improved, the ability to genotype through SNP arrays or by direct sequencing, both performed in a cost-effective manner, has facilitated the use of a larger number of human DNA samples in the analysis. Many GWAS studies have targeted noncommunicable diseases, such as diabetes, although many noncommunicable diseases, such as inflammatory bowel diseases, have a microbial component, which may be influenced by changes in the microbiota (49). In such diseases, various genes have been identified that fall within immune networks that overlap with other susceptibilities, e.g., leprosy (50). GWAS have the power

to link genetic signatures to infections, but other, more targeted experiments are required to provide supporting evidence of function. The work of applying GWAS-type approaches more broadly in the area of infection has, to some extent, been limited by our inability to effectively diagnose many specific agents of infection. For example, syndromes such as sepsis are caused by multiple pathogens, which can lead to a complicated analysis (51). Some interesting associations have been identified through GWAS, for example, the potential involvement of STAT4 in invasive salmonellosis (52). However, the availability of extremely large genotyped populations, such as those in the United Kingdom in the biobanking programs, has the potential to transform the field, as individuals can be monitored and recalled over time (https://bioresource.nihr.ac.uk).

Cells

Linking genotype to phenotype in humans by association has its challenges. An alternative approach is to screen human cells for cell-associated phenotypes or perform screens within whole model organisms, including mice, flies, or worms. Early screens in human cells exploited libraries of human cell lines that had been assembled to broadly represent human genetic diversity. Such collections included the HapMap lymphoblastoid collection of B cell lines that were assembled to represent major histocompatibility complex diversity in humans as a support to the human genome sequencing program. When this approach was linked with *S.* Typhimurium cell invasion assays, a loss-of-function allele of the gene *CARD8* was associated with increased cell death (53–56). CARD8 is an inhibitor of the proinflammatory protease caspase-1, and the presence of such mutations in human populations indicates a role for this gene in modulating responses to enteric bacterial pathogens. In a related study, a methionine salvage pathway was also linked to this caspase-1-associated response (54). A common SNP associated with reduced expression of apoptotic protease activating factor 1 (APAF1)-interacting protein was associated with increased caspase-1-mediated cell death in response to *Salmonella* infection. Another cellular assay linked a polymorphism on chromosome 18 to decreased pyroptosis and increased the expression of TUBB6 (tubulin β6, class V) (55). Overexpression of TUBB6 can completely disrupt the microtubule network, and cells from individuals with higher levels of TUBB6 expression have lower microtubule stability and a reduced pyroptotic response.

RNA interference (RNAi) technology was revolutionary and quickly became a popular technology for the disruption of expression from any gene of interest, especially in mammalian systems that were previously refractory to genetic manipulations. RNAi enables the study of biological functions of mammalian genes through sequence-specific targeting of mRNA (57). The combination of scalable reagents, efficient cellular delivery, and potent gene knockdown enables genome-wide loss-of function screens to be performed, leading to a wealth of information on gene function involved in diverse processes, including signal transduction, cancer biology, and cellular responses to infection (58–60). The main challenges of RNAi experiments involved incomplete silencing of the target mRNA and the nonspecific knockdown of non-target-related genes (60).

Recent technological advancements in genome editing provided an alternative method of mammalian genetic manipulation using a clustered regularly interspaced short palindromic repeats (CRISPR)-Cas9 system to target DNA directly, leading to complete gene knockout (61). In addition to the ability of CRISPR-Cas9 to target protein-coding sequences, this approach can also target regulatory elements, including promoters, enhancers, and elements transcribing microRNAs and long noncoding RNAs. With improved sensitivity, specificity, and efficiency, CRISPR-Cas9 is now the principal genome engineering system for large-scale loss-of-function and gain-of-function screens. This powerful genetic tool has accelerated the mechanistic discovery of various biological processes, including resistance to chemotherapy drugs, resistance to toxins, cell viability, and host-pathogen interactions (62–64).

Model organisms

Genome-wide screens using live animals pose a significant challenge, particularly if the model animals are vertebrates or even mammals. Screens involving *Caenorhabditis elegans* and *Drosophila melanogaster* have been performed using various subgenomic assays, but these are not reviewed here. The availability of thousands of murine ES cell heterozygous mutant lines through KOMP has facilitated the generation of large numbers of mice for intensive phenotyping, including exposure to immune stimuli and pathogen challenge. Mutant mice are generated on a C57BL/6N background with an *ityS* susceptibility genotype. Efforts in the key genome centers generating live mice from the KOMP resource were eventually combined into the International Mouse Phenotyping Consortium (IMPC; www.mousephenotype.org). In the IMPC, small groups of mice were bred for intensive phenotyping, which included embryonic viability, body morphology, bone structure, behavior, and vision (26). Therefore, each knockout mouse line is intensively phenotyped throughout the early stages of life.

Specialized groups were formed to provide more detailed phenotyping, including the Infection and Immunity Immunophenotyping Consortium (3i; http://www.immunophenotype.org). This group collected hundreds of data points on each mutant mouse line that better defined the immunophenotype in greater detail. Part of the screen utilized pathogen challenge of each mouse line. Over the course of the 3i program and additionally within The Wellcome Trust Sanger Institute, ~1,500 different mutant mouse lines (http://www.mousephenotype.org/) have been challenged at different times with *S.* Typhimurium, *Citrobacter rodentium*, influenza virus, and *Trichuris muris*. These lines have also been widely distributed to other research groups, who have performed their own investigations into host-pathogen interactions.

Many of the genes identified in the mouse pathogen screen belonged to classes already known to be involved in influencing disease outcome, but some of the identified genes were novel. A good example of this is the largely uncharacterized gene BC017643/Eros, where mutant mice are highly susceptible to *Salmonella* (and *Listeria*) challenge. A detailed investigation of the mechanisms driving susceptibility demonstrated that this gene played a critical role in the oxidative burst in neutrophils and macrophages and is likely involved in stabilizing the NADPH oxidase complex (65). More recently, mutations in this gene have been shown to have a similar phenotype in humans, showing the value of this murine screen for identifying candidate human infection susceptibility genes.

Human Challenge Studies

An interesting area where systems biology could have an impact is that of controlled human infection models (CHIMs) with pathogens and vaccines. Collecting data from real human disease in a controlled way is the ultimate approach for studies of host-pathogen interactions, as no cellular or model organism challenge can ever replicate the entire infection process. However, each of these systems can yield valuable data, particularly for comparative analysis that can be validated in CHIMs. As technologies have become more sensitive and can be used with smaller sample volumes, they offer the potential for high-quality clinical investigations. Such analysis made directly from samples can combine DNA and RNA sequencing, enzyme-linked immunosorbent assays, protein assays, proteomics, metabolomics, and fluorescence-activated cell sorting. Samples can be taken from multiple body sites, although blood is the most common fluid for analysis. This systems approach has already been applied to human vaccination studies, where a licensed or experimental vaccine can be administered in a controlled manner and the evolving immune response can be tracked over time (66, 67). Here, technologies measuring B and T cell population changes over time, linked to antibody and cytokine assays, have proved invaluable. Work with live vaccines can give some indication of how the cascade of pathogenesis unfolds during a real infection, particularly at earlier time points.

When patients present in the clinic with a natural infection, it is generally impossible to identify exactly when the pathogen was acquired, what the infecting dose was, or whether the patients were pretreated in any way (e.g., with antimicrobials). CHIMs provide an opportunity to provide some novel insights into these processes through the choice of a particular challenge organism, dose, route of challenge, and time of challenge. Indeed, there are a surprising number of CHIMs that have been approved or are currently active. An excellent example is the typhoid CHIM, which has been running at the University of Oxford for several years (68, 69). Here, volunteers have been challenged with *S.* Typhi or *S.* Paratyphi A with or without prior vaccination. *S.* Typhi and *S.* Paratyphi A are both human-adapted pathogens; consequently, experiments in model organisms have limited utility. A detailed program of sample interrogation has been established in this CHIM; this approach covers many of the modern technologies described here and has provided several novel insights into human typhoid. A detailed transcriptomic analysis identified a previously unrecognized early (12 to 24 h) signature in all pathogen-challenged individuals, which was irrespective of whether they developed symptomatic disease (70). This signature may be driven by a limited number of organisms transiting through the intestinal mucosa. This transcriptional signature was further validated using blood cytokine assays. Other transcriptomic work identified tryptophan metabolism as a key signature of acute typhoid, and this was further validated using complementary murine and macrophage work. A comparison between *S.* Typhi and *S.* Paratyphi A infections has started to define the mechanisms underpinning these two clinically overlapping but microbiologically distinct forms of typhoid. Typhoid toxin has been identified as a key target of the human T cell response, and experiments have been performed in humans using *S.* Typhi mutated to lack the gene(s) encoding this toxin (71). Perhaps of more significance, the typhoid CHIM was used to demonstrate the efficacy of typhoid Vi conjugate vaccines, and these data have been used to influence prequalification of the vaccine, which greatly expands its potential range of use (72). Similar work has been undertaken with other bacterial and parasitic diseases, including malaria and pneumococcal infections (73, 74).

The Potential of Stem Cell Systems

Over the past decade, our ability to manipulate human cells and return them to pluripotent stem cell states has improved substantially. Stem cell lines can be grown directly from tissues such as the intestine, or alternatively, cells from blood or skin can be reprogrammed to stem cell-like states; such cells are known as induced pluripotent stem (IPS) cells (75). Once in the hands of researchers, such stem cells can be analyzed or differentiated into a range of different human cell types using specialized protocols. These protocols, which allow differentiation into cells such as macrophages or organoids representative of the intestine and other tissues, are now in common use (76, 77). Theoretically, such systems can yield large numbers of cells with representative human genomes, potentially from individuals harboring common or rare disease-associated alleles. Additionally, IPS cells are amenable to genetic manipulation, including the use of CRISPR-based approaches, which greatly increase their potential scientific value.

The transcriptional signature of IPS cell-derived macrophages suggests that they are immature in comparison to circulating human equivalent macrophages but have many of the features of naturally differentiated primary cells (78, 79). IPS macrophages derived from different individuals can be infected with *S.* Typhimurium or other pathogens and studied to map transcriptional signatures, including expression quantitative trait loci (80). Alternatively, IPS cells differentiated into intestinal organoids can also be infected using direct pathogen exposure or by microinjection of the bacteria directly into the lumens of individual organoids (81–84). Such intestinal organoids harbor multiple cell types, including enterocytes, enteroendocrine cells, Paneth-like cells, and goblet cells (81). These organoids are also responsive to treatment with cytokines, such as interleukin 22, which greatly enhances their potential for studying pathogen interactions. It will be interesting to see how this field develops in the coming years.

Clinical Samples

Many of the techniques covered in this review have been developed to yield genomic data using a small sample volume. The current direction is to bring these genomic technologies closer to the bedside and validate them for screening clinical samples in real time. Here, there is the potential to analyze pathogens, microbiotas, and host responses directly in the same sample using rapid methods, including real-time PCR, mass spectrometry, and simple bioassays, such as antibody detection (Fig. 2). One of the early developments in this regard is the use of TaqMan

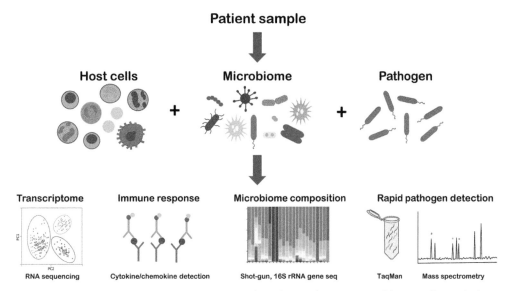

Figure 2 How genomics can empower a clinical sample. It is possible to collect whole-genome or targeted genetic data directly from a clinical sample. This can provide information on the pathogen (TaqMan arrays can cover ~200 pathogens and provide data in hours) or for metagenomics. Metagenomics and 16S analysis can provide data on the microbiota. RNA-seq and other approaches can provide data on the host.

or similar rapid PCR assays that utilize chips comprising targets covering a hundred or more pathogens (www.thermofisher.com/taqman-assay). These assays encompass bacteria, viruses, and fungi as well as potential antimicrobial resistance determinants and can provide data within a few hours. There is the potential to modify these assays to include signatures of the microbiota associated with dysbiotic pathologies involving specific inflammatory markers. Other options include the use of isothermal PCR assays based on dipstick technologies in the field. Again, we anticipate great progress in these areas in coming years.

CONCLUSIONS

The application of genomics and other "-omics" approaches has changed the dynamics of how we can study host-pathogen interactions. The new technologies have become more cost-effective and more sensitive; the trend is to apply these approaches using CHIMs to establish relevant models or in the clinic for improved patient management. Stem cell biology is also starting to open opportunities for a more personalized approach to these studies. Other areas that are likely to have impact include the use of single-cell technologies, initially likely through RNA analysis but potentially through protein analysis in the form of assays including time-of-flight cytometry (85). Other pathogen-specific assays include

matrix-assisted laser desorption ionization–time-of-flight mass spectrometry for rapid bacterial identification (86). Thus, we anticipate that rapid diagnostics will be one of the early translational benefits of this technology.

Acknowledgments. This publication is based on research funded by The Wellcome Trust (098051) and the NIHR Biomedical Research Centres in Cambridge (in particular the NIHR Cambridge BRC AMR Theme) (IS-BRC-1215-20014).

Citation. Yeung A, Hale C, Clare S, Palmer S, Scott JB, Baker S, Dougan G. 2019. Using a systems biology approach to study hostpathogen interactions. Microbiol Spectrum 7(2): BAI-0021-2019.

References

1. Falkow S. 2004. Molecular Koch's postulates applied to bacterial pathogenicity—a personal recollection 15 years later. *Nat Rev Microbiol* **2**:67–72.

2. Baker S, Thomson N, Weill FX, Holt KE. 2018. Genomic insights into the emergence and spread of antimicrobial-resistant bacterial pathogens. *Science* **360**:733–738.

3. Review on Antimicrobial Resistance. 2016. Tackling drug-resistant infections globally: final report and recommendations. Review on Antimicrobial Resitance, London, United Kingdom. https://amr-review.org/sites/default/files/160525_Final%20paper_with%20cover.pdf

4. Smith HW, Halls S. 1967. The transmissible nature of the genetic factor in *Escherichia coli* that controls haemolysin production. *J Gen Microbiol* **47**:153–161.

5. Smith HW, Linggood MA. 1971. Observations on the pathogenic properties of the K88, Hly and Ent plasmids

of *Escherichia coli* with particular reference to porcine diarrhoea. *J Med Microbiol* 4:467–485.

6. Cossart P, Boquet P, Normark S, Rappuoli R. 1996. Cellular microbiology emerging. *Science* 271:315–316.

7. Ko DC, Urban TJ. 2013. Understanding human variation in infectious disease susceptibility through clinical and cellular GWAS. *PLoS Pathog* 9:e1003424.

8. Chapman SJ, Hill AV. 2012. Human genetic susceptibility to infectious disease. *Nat Rev Genet* 13:175–188.

9. Gill SR, Pop M, Deboy RT, Eckburg PB, Turnbaugh PJ, Samuel BS, Gordon JI, Relman DA, Fraser-Liggett CM, Nelson KE. 2006. Metagenomic analysis of the human distal gut microbiome. *Science* 312:1355–1359.

10. Fleischmann RD, Adams MD, White O, Clayton RA, Kirkness EF, Kerlavage AR, Bult CJ, Tomb J, Dougherty BA, Merrick JM, McKenney K, Sutton G, Fitzhugh W, Fields C, Gocyne JD, Scott J, Shirley R, Liu L, Glodek A, Kelley JM, Weidman JF, Phillips CA, Spriggs T, Hedblom E, Cotton MD, Utterback TR, Hanna MC, Nguyen DT, Saudek DM, Brandon RC, Fine LD, Fritchman JL, Fuhrmann JL, Geoghagen NSM, Gnehm CL, McDonald LA, Small KV, Fraser CM, Smith HO, Venter JC. 1995. Whole-genome random sequencing and assembly of *Haemophilus influenzae* Rd. *Science* 269:496–512.

11. Cole ST, Brosch R, Parkhill J, Garnier T, Churcher C, Harris D, Gordon SV, Eiglmeier K, Gas S, Barry CE III, Tekaia F, Badcock K, Basham D, Brown D, Chillingworth T, Connor R, Davies R, Devlin K, Feltwell T, Gentles S, Hamlin N, Holroyd S, Hornsby T, Jagels K, Krogh A, McLean J, Moule S, Murphy L, Oliver K, Osborne J, Quail MA, Rajandream MA, Rogers J, Rutter S, Seeger K, Skelton J, Squares R, Squares S, Sulston JE, Taylor K, Whitehead S, Barrell BG. 1998. Deciphering the biology of *Mycobacterium tuberculosis* from the complete genome sequence. *Nature* 393:537–544.

12. Parkhill J, Dougan G, James KD, Thomson NR, Pickard D, Wain J, Churcher C, Mungall KL, Bentley SD, Holden MT, Sebaihia M, Baker S, Basham D, Brooks K, Chillingworth T, Connerton P, Cronin A, Davis P, Davies RM, Dowd L, White N, Farrar J, Feltwell T, Hamlin N, Haque A, Hien TT, Holroyd S, Jagels K, Krogh A, Larsen TS, Leather S, Moule S, O'Gaora P, Parry C, Quail M, Rutherford K, Simmonds M, Skelton J, Stevens K, Whitehead S, Barrell BG. 2001. Complete genome sequence of a multiple drug resistant *Salmonella enterica* serovar Typhi CT18. *Nature* 413:848–852.

13. Heidelberg JF, Eisen JA, Nelson WC, Clayton RA, Gwinn ML, Dodson RJ, Haft DH, Hickey EK, Peterson JD, Umayam L, Gill SR, Nelson KE, Read TD, Tettelin H, Richardson D, Ermolaeva MD, Vamathevan J, Bass S, Qin H, Dragoi I, Sellers P, McDonald L, Utterback T, Fleishmann RD, Nierman WC, White O, Salzberg SL, Smith HO, Colwell RR, Mekalanos JJ, Venter JC, Fraser CM. 2000. DNA sequence of both chromosomes of the cholera pathogen *Vibrio cholerae*. *Nature* 406:477–483.

14. Parkhill J, et al. 2003. Comparative analysis of the genome sequences of *Bordetella pertussis*, *Bordetella parapertussis* and *Bordetella bronchiseptica*. *Nat Genet* 35:32–40.

15. Leonard EE II, Takata T, Blaser MJ, Falkow S, Tompkins LS, Gaynor EC. 2003. Use of an open-reading frame-specific *Campylobacter jejuni* DNA microarray as a new genotyping tool for studying epidemiologically related isolates. *J Infect Dis* 187:691–694.

16. van Opijnen T, Bodi KL, Camilli A. 2009. Tn-seq: high-throughput parallel sequencing for fitness and genetic interaction studies in microorganisms. *Nat Methods* 6:767–772.

17. Perkins TT, Davies MR, Klemm EJ, Rowley G, Wileman T, James K, Keane T, Maskell D, Hinton JC, Dougan G, Kingsley RA. 2012. ChI-seq and transcriptome analysis of the OmpR regulon of *Salmonella enterica* serovars Typhi and Typhimurium reveals accessory genes implicated in host colonization. *Mol Microbiol* 5:e1000569.

18. International Human Genome Sequencing consortium. 2001. Initial sequencing and analysis of the human genome. *Nature* 409:860–921.

19. Venter JC, et al. 2001. The sequence of the human genome. *Science* 291:1304–1351.

20. Huang H, et al. 2017. Fine-mapping inflammatory bowel disease loci to single-variant resolution. *Nature* 547:173–178.

21. Adams DJ, Doran AG, Lilue J, Keane TM. 2015. The Mouse Genomes Project: a repository of inbred laboratory mouse strain genomes. *Mamm Genome* 26:403–412.

22. Howe K, et al. 2013. The zebrafish reference genome sequence and its relationship to the human genome. *Nature* 496:498–503. *CORRIGENDUM Nature* 505:248.

23. Gardner MJ, et al. 2002. Genome sequence of the human malaria parasite *Plasmodium falciparum*. *Nature* 419:498–511.

24. Berriman M, et al. 2009. The genome of the blood fluke *Schistosoma mansoni*. *Nature* 460:352–358.

25. Bradley A, et al. 2012. The mammalian gene function resource: the International Knockout Mouse Consortium. *Mamm Genome* 23:580–586.

26. White JK, et al. 2013. Genome-wide Generation and Systematic Phenotyping of Knockout Mice Reveals New Roles for Many Genes. *Cell* 154:452–464.

27. Holt KE, Parkhill J, Mazzoni CJ, Roumagnac P, Weill FX, Goodhead I, Rance R, Baker S, Maskell DJ, Wain J, Dolecek C, Achtman M, Dougan G. 2008. High-throughput sequencing provides insights into genome variation and evolution in *Salmonella* Typhi. *Nat Genet* 40:987–993.

28. Chan CX, Ragan MA. 2013. Next-generation phylogenomics. *Biol Direct* 8:3–4.

29. Klemm E, Dougan G. 2016. Advances in understanding bacterial pathogenesis gained from whole-genome sequencing and phylogenetics. *Cell Host Microbe* 19:599–610.

30. Wong VK, et al. 2015. Phylogeographical analysis of the dominant multidrug-resistant H58 clade of *Salmonella* Typhi identifies inter- and intracontinental transmission events. *Nat Genet* 47:632–639.

31. Nicolas-Chanoine MH, Bertrand X, Madec JY. 2014. *Escherichia coli* ST131, an intriguing clonal group. *Clin Microbiol Rev* 27:543–574.

32. Okoro CK, Kingsley RA, Connor TR, Harris SR, Parry CM, Al-Mashhadani MN, Kariuki S, Msefula CL, Gordon MA, de Pinna E, Wain J, Heyderman RS, Obaro S, Alonso PL, Mandomando I, Maclennan CA, Tapia MD, Levine MM, Tennant SM, Parkhill J, Dougan G. 2012. Intracontinental spread of human invasive *Salmonella* Typhimurium pathovariants in sub-Saharan Africa. *Nat Genet* 44:1215–1221.

33. Hammarlöf DL, Kröger C, Owen SV, Canals R, Lacharme-Lora L, Wenner N, Schager AE, Wells TJ, Henderson IR, Wigley P, Hokamp K, Feasey NA, Gordon MA, Hinton JCD. 2018. Role of a single noncoding nucleotide in the evolution of an epidemic African clade of *Salmonella*. *Proc Natl Acad Sci USA* 13:115–119.

34. Chewapreecha C, Marttinen P, Croucher NJ, Salter SJ, Harris SR, Mather AE, Hanage WP, Goldblatt D, Nosten FH, Turner C, Turner P, Bentley SD, Parkhill J. 2014. Comprehensive identification of single nucleotide polymorphisms associated with beta-lactam resistance within pneumococcal mosaic genes. *PLoS Genet* 10:e1004547.

35. Sheppard SK, Didelot X, Meric G, Torralbo A, Jolley KA, Kelly DJ, Bentley SD, Maiden MCJ, Parkhill J, Falush D. 2013. Genome-wide association study identifies vitamin B5 biosynthesis as a host specificity factor in *Campylobacter*. *Proc Natl Acad Sci USA* 110:11923–11927.

36. Alam MT, Petit RA III, Crispell EK, Thornton TA, Conneely KN, Jiang Y, Satola SW, Read TD. 2014. Dissecting vancomycin-intermediate resistance in *Staphylococcus aureus* using genome-wide association. *Genome Biol Evol* 6:1174–1185.

37. Porwollik S, Santiviago CA, Cheng P, Long F, Desai P, Fredlund J, Srikumar S, Silva CA, Chu W, Chen X, Canals R, Reynolds MM, Bogomolnaya L, Shields C, Cui P, Guo J, Zheng Y, Endicott-Yazdani T, Yang HJ, Maple A, Ragoza Y, Blondel CJ, Valenzuela C, Andrews-Polymenis H, McClelland M. 2014. Defined single-gene and multi-gene deletion mutant collections in *Salmonella enterica* sv Typhimurium. *PLoS One* 9:e99820.

38. Langridge GC, Phan M-D, Turner D, Perkins T, Parts L, Haase J, Charles I, Maskell DM, Peters S, Dougan G, Wain J, Parkhill J, Turner KA. 2009. Simultaneous assay of every *Salmonella* Typhi gene using one million transposon mutants. *Genome Res* 19:2308–2316.

39. Troy EB, Lin T, Gao L, Lazinski DW, Lundt M, Camilli A, Norris SJ, Hu LT. 2016. Global Tn-seq analysis of carbohydrate utilization and vertebrate infectivity of *Borrelia burgdorferi*. *Mol Microbiol* 101:1003–1023.

40. Pickard D, Kingsley RA, Hale C, Turner K, Sivaraman K, Wetter M, Langridge G, Dougan G. 2013. A genomewide mutagenesis screen identifies multiple genes contributing to Vi capsular expression in *Salmonella enterica* serovar Typhi. *J Bacteriol* 195:1320–1326.

41. Hensel M, Shea JE, Gleeson C, Jones MD, Dalton E, Holden DW. 1995. Simultaneous identification of bacterial virulence genes by negative selection. *Science* 269:400–403.

42. Klemm EJ, Gkrania-Klotsas E, Hadfield J, Forbester JL, Harris SR, Hale C, Heath JN, Wileman T, Clare S, Kane L, Goulding D, Otto TD, Kay S, Doffinger R, Cooke FJ, Carmichael A, Lever AM, Parkhill J, MacLennan CA,

Kumararatne D, Dougan G, Kingsley RA. 2016. Emergence of host-adapted *Salmonella* Enteritidis through rapid evolution in an immunocompromised host. *Nat Microbiol* 1:15023.

43. Didelot X, Walker AS, Peto TE, Crook DW, Wilson DJ. 2016. Within-host evolution of bacterial pathogens. *Nat Rev Microbiol* 14:150–162.

44. Lieberman TD, Michel JB, Aingaran M, Potter-Bynoe G, Roux D, Davis MR, Skurnik D, Leiby N, LiPuma JJ, Goldberg JB, McAdam AJ, Priebe GP, Kishony R. 2011. Parallel bacterial evolution within multiple patients identifies candidate pathogenicity genes. *Nat Genet* 43:1275–1280.

45. Kingsley RA, Kay S, Connor T, Barquist L, Sait L, Holt KE, Sivaraman K, Wileman T, Goulding D, Clare S, Hale C, Seshasayee A, Harris S, Thomson NR, Gardner P, Rabsch W, Wigley P, Humphrey T, Parkhill J, Dougan G. 2013. Genome and transcriptome adaptation accompanying emergence of the definitive type 2 host-restricted *Salmonella enterica* serovar Typhimurium pathovar. *mBio* 4:e00565-13.

46. Westermann AJ, Förstner KU, Amman F, Barquist L, Chao Y, Schulte LN, Müller L, Reinhardt R, Stadler PF, Vogel J. 2016. Dual RNA-seq unveils noncoding RNA functions in host-pathogen interactions. *Nature* 529:496–501.

47. Florio W, Tavanti A, Barnini S, Ghelardi E, Lupetti A. 2018. Recent advances and ongoing challenges in the diagnosis of microbial infections by MALDI-TOF mass spectrometry. *Front Microbiol* 9:1097–1099.

48. Toledo-Arana A, Dussurget O, Nikitas G, Sesto N, Guet-Revillet H, Balestrino D, Loh E, Gripenland J, Tiensuu T, Vaitkevicius K, Barthelemy M, Vergassola M, Nahori MA, Soubigou G, Régnault B, Coppée JY, Lecuit M, Johansson J, Cossart P. 2009. The *Listeria* transcriptional landscape from saprophytism to virulence. *Nature* 459:950–956.

49. Walker AW, Sanderson JD, Churcher C, Parkes GC, Hudspith BN, Rayment N, Brostoff J, Parkhill J, Dougan G, Petrovska L. 2011. High-throughput clone library analysis of the mucosa-associated microbiota reveals dysbiosis and differences between inflamed and non-inflamed regions of the intestine in inflammatory bowel disease. *BMC Microbiol* 11:7–10.

50. Liu H, Irwanto A, Tian H, Fu X, Yu Y, Yu G, Low H, Chu T, Li Y, Shi B, Chen M, Sun Y, Yuan C, Lu N, You J, Bao F, Li J, Liu J, Liu H, Liu D, Yu X, Zhang L, Yang Q, Wang N, Niu G, Ma S, Zhou Y, Wang C, Chen S, Zhang X, Liu J, Zhang F. 2012. Identification of IL18RAP/IL18R1 and IL12β as leprosy risk genes demonstrates shared pathogenesis between inflammation and infectious diseases. *Am J Hum Genet* 91:935–941.

51. Goh C, Knight JC. 2017. Enhanced understanding of the host-pathogen interaction in sepsis: new opportunities for omic approaches. *Lancet Respir Med* 5:212–223.

52. Gilchrist JJ, Rautanen A, Fairfax BP, Mills TC, Naranbhai V, Trochet H, Pirinen M, Muthumbi E, Mwarumba S, Njuguna P, Mturi N, Msefula CL, Gondwe EN, MacLennan JM, Chapman SJ, Molyneux ME, Knight JC, Spencer CCA, Williams TN, MacLennan CA, Scott JAG, Hill AVS. 2018. Risk of nontyphoidal *Salmonella* bacte-

raemia in African children is modified by STAT4. *Nat Commun* 9:1014–1019.

53. Ko DC, Shukla KP, Fong C, Wasnick M, Brittnacher MJ, Wurfel MM, Holden TD, O'Keefe GE, Van Yserloo B, Akey JM, Miller SI. 2009. A genome-wide in vitro bacterial-infection screen reveals human variation in the host response associated with inflammatory disease. *Am J Hum Genet* 85:214–227.

54. Miller SI, Chaudhary AA. 2016. Cellular GWAS approach to define human variation in cellular pathways important to inflammation. *Pathogens* 26:5.

55. Ko DC, Gamazon ER, Shukla KP, Pfuetzner RA, Whittington D, Holden TD, Brittnacher MJ, Fong C, Radey M, Ogohara C, Stark AL, Akey JM, Dolan ME, Wurfel MM, Miller SI. 2012. Functional genetic screen of human diversity reveals that a methionine salvage enzyme regulates inflammatory cell death. *Proc Natl Acad Sci USA* 109:E2343–E2352.

56. Salinas RE, Ogohara C, Thomas MI, Shukla KP, Miller SI, Ko DC. 2014. A cellular genome-wide association study reveals human variation in microtubule stability and a role in inflammatory cell death. *Mol Biol Cell* 25:76–86.

57. Fire A, Xu S, Montgomery MK, Kostas SA, Driver SE, Mello CC. 1998. Potent and specific genetic interference by double-stranded RNA in *Caenorhabditis elegans*. *Nature* 391:806–811.

58. Warner N, Burberry A, Franchi L, Kim YG, McDonald C, Sartor MA, Núñez G. 2013. A genome-wide siRNA screen reveals positive and negative regulators of the NOD2 and NF-κB signalling pathways. *Sci Signal* 6:rs3.

59. Kühbacher A, Emmenlauer M, Rämo P, Kafai N, Dehio C, Cossart P, Pizarro-Cerdá J. 2015. Genome-wide siRNA screen identifies complementary signaling pathways involved in *Listeria* infection and reveals different actin nucleation mechanisms during *Listeria* cell invasion and actin comet tail formation. *mBio* 6:e00598-15.

60. Sasaki K, Kurahara H, Young ED, Natsugoe S, Ijichi A, Iwakuma T, Welch DR. 2017. Genome-wide in vivo RNAi screen identifies ITIH5 as a metastasis suppressor in pancreatic cancer. *Clin Exp Metastasis* 34:229–239.

61. Sun J, Katz S, Dutta B, Wang Z, Fraser IDC. 2017. Genome-wide siRNA screen of genes regulating the LPS-induced THF-α response in human macrophages. *Sci Data* 4:170007.

62. Schultz N, Marenstein DR, De Angelis DA, Wang WQ, Nelander S, Jacobsen A, Marks DS, Massagué J, Sander C. 2011. Off-target effects dominate a large-scale RNAi screen for modulators of the TGF-β pathway and reveal microRNA regulation of TGFBR2. *Silence* 2:3.

63. Mali P, Yang L, Esvelt KM, Aach J, Guell M, DiCarlo JE, Norville JE, Church GM. 2013. RNA-guided human genome engineering via Cas9. *Science* 339:823–826.

64. Koike-Yusa H, Li Y, Tan EP, Velasco-Herrera MDC, Yusa K. 2014. Genome-wide recessive genetic screening in mammalian cells with a lentivirus CRISPR-guide RNA library. *Nat Biotechnol* 32:267–273.

65. Thomas DC, et al. 2017. Eros is a novel transmembrane protein that controls the phagocyte respiratory burst and is essential for innate immunity. *J Exp Med* 214:1111–1128.

66. Akondy RS, Fitch M, Edupuganti S, Yang S, Kissick HT, Li KW, Youngblood BA, Abdelsamed HA, McGuire DJ, Cohen KW, Alexe G, Nagar S, McCausland MM, Gupta S, Tata P, Haining WN, McElrath MJ, Zhang D, Hu B, Greenleaf WJ, Goronzy JJ, Mulligan MJ, Hellerstein M, Ahmed R. 2017. Origin and differentiation of human memory CD8 T cells after vaccination. *Nature* 552:362–367.

67. Kazmin D, Nakaya HI, Lee EK, Johnson MJ, van der Most R, van den Berg RA, Ballou WR, Jongert E, Wille-Reece U, Ockenhouse C, Aderem A, Zak DE, Sadoff J, Hendriks J, Wrammert J, Ahmed R, Pulendran B. 2017. Systems analysis of protective immune responses to RTS,S malaria vaccination in humans. *Proc Natl Acad Sci USA* 114:2425–2430.

68. Waddington CS, Darton TC, Jones C, Haworth K, Peters A, John T, Thompson BA, Kerridge SA, Kingsley RA, Zhou L, Holt KE, Yu LM, Lockhart S, Farrar JJ, Sztein MB, Dougan G, Angus B, Levine MM, Pollard AJ. 2014. An outpatient, ambulant design, controlled human infection model using escalating doses of *Salmonella* Typhi challenge delivered in sodium bicarbonate solution. *Clin Infect Dis* 58:1230–1240.

69. Dobinson HC, Gibani MM, Jones C, Thomaides-Brears HB, Voysey M, Darton TC, Waddington CS, Campbell D, Milligan I, Zhou L, Shrestha S, Kerridge SA, Peters A, Stevens Z, Podda A, Martin LB, D'Alessio F, Thanh DP, Basnyat B, Baker S, Angus B, Levine MM, Blohmke CJ, Pollard AJ. 2017. Evaluation of the clinical and microbiological response to *Salmonella* Paratyphi A infection in the first paratyphoid human challenge model. *Clin Infect Dis* 64:1066–1073.

70. Blohmke CJ, et al. 2016. Interferon-driven alterations of the host's amino acid metabolism in the pathogenesis of typhoid fever. *J Exp Med* 213:1061–1077.

71. Napolitani G, et al. 2018. Clonal analysis of Salmonella-specific effector T cells reveals serovar-specific and cross-reactive T cell responses. *Nat Immunol* 19:742–754.

72. Jin C, Gibani MM, Moore M, Juel HB, Jones E, Meiring J, Harris V, Gardner J, Nebykova A, Kerridge SA, Hill J, Thomaides-Brears H, Blohmke CJ, Yu LM, Angus B, Pollard AJ. 2017. Efficacy and immunogenicity of a Vi-tetanus toxoid conjugate vaccine in the prevention of typhoid fever using a controlled human infection model of *Salmonella* Typhi: a randomised controlled, phase 2b trial. *Lancet* 390:2472–2480.

73. Murugan R, Buchauer L, Triller G, Kreschel C, Costa G, Pidelaserra Martí G, Imkeller K, Busse CE, Chakravarty S, Sim BKL, Hoffman SL, Levashina EA, Kremsner PG, Mordmüller B, Höfer T, Wardemann H. 2018. Clonal selection drives protective memory B cell responses in controlled human malaria infection. *Sci Immunol* 16:eaap8029.

74. Collins AM, Wright AD, Mitsi E, Gritzfeld JF, Hancock CA, Pennington SH, Wang D, Morton B, Ferreira DM, Gordon SB. 2015. First human challenge testing of a pneumococcal vaccine. Double-blind randomized controlled trial. *Am J Respir Crit Care Med* 192:853–858.

75. Takahashi K, Tanabe K, Ohnuki M, Narita M, Ichisaka T, Tomoda K, Yamanaka S. 2007. Induction of pluripo-

tent stem cells from adult human fibroblasts by defined factors. *Cell* **131**:861–872.

76. Hale C, Yeung A, Goulding D, Pickard D, Alasoo K, Powrie F, Dougan G, Mukhopadhyay S. 2015. Induced pluripotent stem cell derived macrophages as a cellular system to study *Salmonella* and other pathogens. *PLoS One* **10**:e0124307.

77. Heo I, Dutta D, Schaefer DA, Iakobachvili N, Artegiani B, Sachs N, Boonekamp KE, Bowden G, Hendrickx APA, Willems RJL, Peters PJ, Riggs MW, O'Connor R, Clevers H. 2018. Modelling *Cryptosporidium* infection in human small intestinal and lung organoids. *Nat Microbiol* **3**:814–823.

78. Alasoo K, Martinez FO, Hale C, Gordon S, Powrie F, Dougan G, Mukhopadhyay S, Gaffney DJ. 2015. Transcriptional profiling of macrophages derived from monocytes and iPS cells identifies a conserved response to LPS and novel alternative transcription. *Sci Rep* **5**:12524.

79. Alasoo K, Rodrigues J, Mukhopadhyay S, Knights AJ, Mann AL, Kundu K, Hale C, Dougan G, Gaffney DJ, HIPSCI Consortium. 2018. Shared genetic effects on chromatin and gene expression indicate a role for enhancer priming in immune response. *Nat Genet* **50**:424–431.

80. Yeung ATY, Hale C, Lee AH, Gill EE, Bushell W, Parry-Smith D, Goulding D, Pickard D, Roumeliotis T, Choudhary J, Thomson N, Skarnes WC, Dougan G, Hancock REW. 2017. Exploiting induced pluripotent stem cell-derived macrophages to unravel host factors influencing *Chlamydia trachomatis* pathogenesis. *Nat Commun* **8**:15013–15019.

81. Forbester JL, Goulding D, Vallier L, Hannan N, Hale C, Pickard D, Mukhopadhyay S, Dougan G. 2015. The interaction of *Salmonella enterica* serovar Typhimurium with intestinal organoids derived from human induced pluripotent stem cells. *Infect Immun* **83**:2926–2934.

82. Karve SS, Pradhan S, Ward DV, Weiss AA. 2017. Intestinal organoids model human responses to infection by commensal and Shiga toxin producing *Escherichia coli*. *PLoS One* **12**:e0178966.

83. Nigro G, Hanson M, Fevre C, Lecuit M, Sansonetti PJ. 2016. Intestinal organoids as a novel tool to study microbes-epithelium interactions. *Methods Mol Biol* [Epub ahead of print].

84. Leslie JL, Huang S, Opp JS, Nagy MS, Kobayashi M, Young VB, Spence JR. 2015. Persistence and toxin production by *Clostridium difficile* within human intestinal organoids result in disruption of eithpelial paracellular barrier function. *Infect Immun* **83**:138–145.

85. Berger CN, Crepin VF, Roumeliotis TI, Wright JC, Carson D, Pevsner-Fischer M, Furniss RCD, Dougan G, Dori-Bachash M, Yu L, Clements A, Collins JW, Elinav E, Larrouy-Maumus GJ, Choudhary JS, Frankel G. 2017. *Citrobacter rodentium* subverts ATP flux and cholesterol homeostasis in intestinal epithelial cells in vivo. *Cell Metab* **26**:738–752.E6.

86. Oviaño M, Bou G. 2018. Matrix-assisted laser desorption ionization-time of flight mass spectrometry for the rapid detection of antimicrobial resistance mechanism and beyond. *Clin Microbiol Rev* **32**:e00037-18.

Index